ONE HUNDRED BOOKS FAMOUS IN MEDICINE

Conceived, organized, and with an introduction by

HASKELL F. NORMAN, M.D.

Catalogue edited by Hope Mayo

Based on an exhibition held at

THE GROLIER CLUB

20 September – 23 November 1994

ONE HUNDRED BOOKS FAMOUS IN MEDICINE

THE GROLIER CLUB
NEW YORK · 1995

ISBN 0-910672-12-1

Dedicated as an expression of esteem for members of the Grolier Club
who inspired this exhibition:

Le Roy Crummer
MEMBER 1919–1933

Harvey Cushing
MEMBER 1925–1936

Bern Dibner
MEMBER 1957–1979

John F. Fulton
MEMBER 1939–1943

Robert B. Honeyman, Jr.
MEMBER 1958–1970

Harrison D. Horblit
MEMBER 1947–1988

Warren R. Howell
MEMBER 1954–1984

Josiah K. Lilly, Jr.
MEMBER 1928–1966

Sir William Osler
MEMBER 1902–1919

CONTENTS

INTRODUCTION

THE 1958 GROLIER CLUB exhibition, One Hundred Books Famous in Science, curated by Harrison D. Horblit (Grolier Club Member 1947–1988) did much to stimulate the collecting of rare books in the history of science. Inclusion of a "book" in this exhibition (and later in the 1964 catalogue) gave the item an official sanction, and was no doubt responsible for the increased prices and demand for items which previously had been more or less neglected. Even those who might have publicly frowned upon the use of lists as a guide for collecting wanted to include Horblit's "high spots" in their libraries. For example, the Houghton Library catalogue of selected acquisitions for 1942–1967 indicated that the Harvard Library "already possessed 106 of the titles he [Horblit] described—an agreeable paradox explained by the fact that, counting alternates, the Horblit list actually contains 130 books."[1]

Josiah K. Lilly, Jr. (Grolier Club Member 1928–1966), whom David A. Randall (Grolier Club Member 1944–1975) described as "the *beau idéal* of the perfect collector" decided after World War II to collect, among others, classic books in the history of medicine and science from the beginnings to the present time. Lilly, who liked to collect from lists such as the Grolier "One Hundreds" of American and English Literature, A. E. Newton's "One Hundred Good Novels," and Asa Don Dickinson's *One Thousand Best Books*, did not know of anything comparable at the time in medicine and science, and therefore set out to create his own list. He asked W. R. LeFanu, librarian of the Royal College of Surgeons, to compile "Two Hundred Key Books in the History of Medicine and Surgery," and Professor I. Bernard Cohen, then managing editor of *Isis*, to do the same for science. David A. Randall, the eminent book dealer and later Lilly librarian, wrote that Lilly's interest in lists was not because he lacked imagination but rather that he used them as springboards from which to begin his collection.[2] Neither the LeFanu nor the Cohen list was ever published. W. R. LeFanu advised me that plans were made in the early seventies to publish the medical list with descriptions and bibliography, but this project was later limited to books in the Lilly Library and published in 1976 as *Notable Medical Books*.[3]

Lists and exhibitions such as these limit their total entries to round numbers—ten, twenty, one hundred, two hundred, or one thousand—in part because these figures seem to possess magical qualities. Bern Dibner (Grolier Club Member 1957–1979), referring in the preface of his *Heralds of Science* to his choice of two hundred, said, "This magic is of no more importance than a landing in a long staircase. It is a stopping point at which one can pause, catch one's breath, and look around."[4] We, like Harrison Horblit, have followed the Grolier Club tradition of one hundred. We understand that there has been some criticism of Horblit for not limiting himself to precisely that number, since occasionally he added, in subordination to some entries, other books which served to introduce, amplify, or complete the meaning of the specific item; however, I doubt that any serious bibliophile was offended by this deviation. As I recall, I welcomed these additions, and eventually several of these books found their way into my library.

My decision to propose an exhibition of One Hundred Books Famous in Medicine was based partly on the Grolier Club's tradition of such exhibitions. The first Grolier One Hundred exhibition was One Hundred Books Famous in English Literature in 1903, followed by One Hundred Illustrated Books in 1921, One Hundred Books Influential in American Literature in 1946, and the above-mentioned One Hundred Books Famous in Science in 1958.[5]

Another reason I proposed this exhibition and its catalogue was that, like J. K. Lilly, I value such lists as guides. I recall that in 1960 I asked Dr. Ernst Weil, then the leading antiquarian bookseller in medicine and science, to list for me the ten most important books in medicine. Weil was not constrained by the number ten and sent me a list of sixteen instead. The authors he named were Auenbrugger (1761), Avicenna (1473), Celsus (1478), Fleming (1929), Fracastoro (1530), Fuchs (1542), Galen (1490), Harvey (1628), Jenner (1798), Ketham (1491), Koch (1881, 1884), Pander (1817), Pasteur (1857), Servetus (1790), Virchow (1858), and Wolff (1759). Of these he checked off nine, I suppose in an effort to comply with my request, leaving me presumably to guess which one might be the tenth. Auenbrugger, Avicenna, Celsus, Galen, and Harvey were listed as very rare. For Ketham, Weil listed the 1491, 1493, and 1495 editions, with the notation that the 1491 edition was hopelessly rare. Jenner and Koch were simply checked. For the Servetus, he noted that there was no point in thinking of the 1553 edition, since there were only two and a half copies in existence. As I look back on his list now, I am amazed that he did not include Vesalius. Perhaps it was to be the tenth item.

Horblit dealt with the question, "What is a book?" by ignoring it. To him an article was as acceptable an exhibition entry as a "book." He was not restricted by the modern technical definition of a book issued by UNESCO: "a non-periodical printed publication of at least 49 pages, excluding covers."[6] In this respect, we have followed Horblit's example. But we differ from his preference for the original journal number or volume rather than the offprint of the article. Horblit's argument was that it was in the original journal that the articles were first printed and achieved exposure. He felt that "the journal is the thing" and tended to minimize the merit of the offprint. The eminent William A. Jackson (Grolier Club Member 1931–1964) had a different perspective which coincides with ours. Writing in 1956, he stated, "The importance of offprints has yet to be generally recognized, certainly by institutional libraries which normally reject them, if excerpted from serials already on their shelves, and yet to the author they often seem the real first edition. It is in that form that he thinks of his work, for it is his copies of the offprints he presents to his friends. In the collecting of offprints of scientific literature the private collector, as so often happens, has realized their importance far sooner and more clearly than has the librarian."[7] This was written in reference to a copy of the Darwin-Wallace offprint "On the Tendency of Species to Form Varieties," which is inscribed in Darwin's hand on the front wrapper "C. D. and R. W." and on the back wrapper "Wallace & self." "[It] is a true offprint, not an extract, for it has separate pagination and a 'slug' reading 'Reprinted from the Journal of proceedings of the Linnean Society'" on the first page. Jackson felt that this Darwin offprint, because of its rarity and significance, was the most desirable of the Darwin material. The experience of the book trade confirms that the author's own copy of a book or an offprint is usually regarded as the most precious and valued accordingly.

Since the seventeenth century, when the publication of scientific and medical journals began, authors have reported their discoveries in them. This has become progressively more common during the nineteenth and twentieth centuries. Accordingly, a number of our selections are represented either by the journal volume, the single number of the journal, or the offprint of the article. Where we have been able to locate the offprint or the first separate publication, we have, unlike Horblit, favored it. For example, the Dutch microscopist Antoni van Leeuwenhoek first reported his discoveries in letters written in Dutch to the Royal Society of London, which then published the abbreviated English translations in its *Philosophical Transactions.* In Leeuwenhoek's case, we decided to exhibit the separate Dutch publication announcing his discovery of bacteria (1684), in our opinion his single most important letter, rather than the abbreviated English version in the journal volume. Luigi Galvani also published his important paper, "De viribus electricitatis in motu musculari commentarius" (1791) as one of the "Opuscula" in the proceedings of the Bolognese academy, *De Bononiensi Scientiarum et Artium Instituto atque Academia Commentarii.* The two offprints of this article were the earliest offprints in our exhibition.

Before we could begin the actual selection of works for this exhibition, it was necessary to define the particular kind of medical classic we were searching for. We turned to Sir William Osler (Grolier Club Member 1902–1919), who has served as an inspiration and model for bibliophiles interested in science and medicine. In the arrangement of his *Bibliotheca Osleriana,* Sir William differentiated between writers of the first rank whose books were milestones in the evolution of science and medicine (Bibliotheca Prima), and those who made notable contributions that nevertheless were not up to the level of the first group (Bibliotheca Secunda).[8] Commingling the Prima and the Secunda with the traditional Grolier choice of the word "famous" gave us our basic guidelines and also allowed us considerable leeway. A book that is "famous" need not be one that is most important, nor need it announce the author's major discovery or, for that matter, any discovery at all. It is likely that some of our choices will be disputed as insufficiently important. However, much will depend on one's perspective.

In defining the time frame to be covered in our exhibition, it seemed reasonable to adopt one similar to Horblit's, namely, ancient times to the twentieth century. (Horblit began with fifteenth-century editions of the works of several ancient authors, including Aristotle and Galen, and ended with Einstein's *Die Grundlage der allgemeinen Relativitätstheorie* [1916].) When we presented this plan to our colleagues, one of them, a librarian knowledgeable about rare medical and scientific books, argued that we should begin with the work of Semmelweis, who first demonstrated the importance of asepsis in the prevention of puerperal fever. A second colleague objected to our time frame because many of the books we planned to exhibit were already well known from previous exhibitions and catalogues. He suggested that we concentrate on twentieth-century classics, most of which had never been exhibited before. In response to this point we added a few more representatives of twentieth-century medicine, including Hounsfield's first paper on computed tomography (1973).

In order to select the material, I assembled a committee of colleagues whom I knew would be both qualified and interested in the challenge of preparing the list of books. The committee consisted of medical bibliophiles and antiquarian booksellers, all of whom have been building collections or cataloguing rare medical books for at least twenty, and in some instances forty or more, years. I asked each member of the committee to prepare a list of one hundred books and to submit it to me. I also prepared my own. The result, with a few exceptions, was a fairly good consensus on about two-thirds of the titles. Thereafter, a meeting of the participants was arranged to fill in gaps, emphasizing nineteenth- and twentieth-century material. As the curator of the exhibition, I made the final decisions as to which titles and which copies would be exhibited.

After the list was drawn up we concentrated on the catalogue. Participants, consultants, and selected authorities were invited to contribute 300–500 word descriptions of the books that pertained to their fields of interest. The narratives were submitted to me and to Diana H. Hook, who was responsible for the initial editing. The final editing was done by Hope Mayo (Grolier Club Member 1990–), working with the Publications Committee of the Grolier Club.

In keeping with our bibliophilic aspirations, we tried to locate and borrow from private collectors and medical or other libraries the most interesting copy of each book, judging by standards such as author's copy, dedication copy, presentation copy, important provenance, binding, condition, and rarity. Because this was to be a Grolier Club exhibition, we wanted to have an example of the books bound for Jean Grolier, the famous sixteenth-century French bibliophile. From Gabriel Austin's catalogue, we discovered that Grolier had once owned a copy of the Latin *editio princeps* of Hippocrates' *Opera* (1525), but that it had been lost at the time of the Commune in 1871.[9] The Grolier copy of Aristotle's *De animalibus* (1476) is in the Herzog August Bibliothek, Wolfenbüttel. The

Grolier Celsus, which Sir William Osler had stated was the best copy he had seen, is according to Gabriel Austin not the first edition of 1478, but the fourth edition of 1497.[10] We soon discovered that it was not practical for us to borrow from European libraries or collectors. Fortunately, the Pierpont Morgan Library owns Jean Grolier's copy of Volume II of Aristotle's *Opera* in Greek.

Nearly all the American libraries we contacted were cooperative, and we were pleased with what we were able to assemble. Nevertheless, finding suitable books was not always without difficulty. We wanted to borrow the Huntington Library's copy of Dioscorides' *De materia medica* (1478), which had belonged to the fifteenth-century physician Nicolaus Pol, and its drawing for the title page of Vesalius's *De humani corporis fabrica* (1543), but regrettably, this library is bound by its charter not to lend. We were most successful where we had access to catalogues of special exhibitions, as at the Lilly Library,[11] the College of Physicians of Philadelphia,[12] and Yale University,[13] or catalogues of special collections, such as the Osler Library at McGill University,[14] the Harvey Cushing Library at Yale,[15] the Reynolds Collection at the University of Alabama,[16] and the Benjamin Collection at UCLA.[17] We also relied on the occasional journal article, e.g., John Fulton on Boerhaave.[18] For incunabula we used Goff.[19] Thereafter, we were fortunate to have contact with librarians who had an intimate knowledge of their books.[20] We also obtained some assistance from the publication of our lists in *The Watermark*, the newsletter of the Archivists and Librarians in the History of the Health Sciences.

In older libraries, several of the books we wanted had been acquired years before, primarily for their content, and were bound in library bindings that made them less desirable for our exhibition. We made an effort to stress condition to the degree that it was possible, but in some instances we gave provenance priority over condition. Few libraries, either public or private, had an abundance of special copies. With the exception of the few journal volumes, all of our books are rare, several extremely rare, many of legendary rarity, and a few unique at least in their state. The random ownership of special copies by institutional libraries suggested that possession of special copies was almost accidental. We were surprised and very pleased to locate books from the libraries of two significant fifteenth-century physicians, Hartmann Schedel, the author of the *Nuremberg Chronicle*, and Nicolaus Pol, physician to the Holy Roman Emperor Maximilian I.

As an example of the sort of challenges and problems we encountered, I mention the *Liber ad Almansorem*, the most renowned work of the great tenth-century Arab clinician and encyclopedist, Rhazes. Of this work, the ninth book, *Liber nonus Almansoris*, which deals with pathology and therapeutics, is the most famous. It was first published in part in Gianmatteo Ferrari's *Practica cum textu noni ad Almansorem* (1472), copies of which are housed at the National Library of Medicine and the Pierpont Morgan Library. However, we preferred the complete text of this book, which was published separately in 1476.

Copies of this are found in the Dibner Collection at the Smithsonian, at the British Library (willed to them by Sir William Osler, who thought he possessed the only copy of this edition), and at an Italian library. When we were unable to borrow any of these copies, we settled on the first edition of the complete *Liber ad Almansorem* (1481).

Selections from the fifteenth and sixteenth centuries provided us with an opportunity to study the coloring of woodcuts. From the most famous herbal of the sixteenth century, Leonhart Fuchs's *De historia stirpium commentarii* (1542), we learned that professionally colored copies—which had characteristics distinguishing them from less professional ones—could be purchased from the publishers at the time of printing. We asked a number of specialists, including Bernadette Callery, Professor W. Stearn, and Dr. Frederick Meyer, to assist us in our quest for the correct Fuchs, and finally located two in the United States: one at the National Agricultural Library, Beltsville, Md., and the other at the Holden Arboretum, Cleveland, Ohio. A similar effort was made to locate a correct colored copy of Georg Bartisch's *Augendienst* (1583), a woodcut book that gave ophthalmology its name. While we were aware of three special copies in Europe, to our knowledge there was only one in the United States, at the Trent Collection at Duke University. Our conclusion from comparing the various editions is that the coloring of the botanical specimens in Fuchs enhanced its educational value by providing a closer approximation to nature, but that the coloring of woodcuts in Ketham, Gersdorff, Paracelsus, Vesalius, Paré, and Bartisch was mainly decorative and presumably for patrons or other wealthy individuals.

One of the surprises of the seventeenth century was Marcello Malpighi's *De pulmonibus observationes anatomicae* (1661). Malpighi used the microscope to discover the structure of the lungs and observe the capillaries. His observations confirmed Harvey's description of the circulation of the blood as a hydraulic system. Malpighi wrote the mathematician Giovanni Alfonso Borelli about his observations, and his letters were subsequently published as a small book. Until recently it was thought that the only copy of this in the United States was at the National Library of Medicine. We were therefore intrigued to discover others at Yale University and in the Crerar Collection at the University of Chicago.

Seventeenth-century books with special provenances are very rare in American libraries or private collections. However, we were able to borrow one of the more interesting ones, Descartes' *De homine* (1662), about which W. W. Francis, the first Osler librarian, relates this story:

> This 1662 copy, in old stiff vellum, and with Sir Charles Sherrington's name, 1888, on the title-page, was come by honestly, no doubt, though it is not always safe to lend precious old books to an ardent collector, no matter how honest. When I was cataloguing the library, Sherrington picked this book off the shelf and brought it to me with a twinkle in his eye and told me he had lent it to W. O. in 1914. While waiting in the library about 1916 he found it and saw that W. O. had written on the fly-leaf that Sherrington had given it to him in 1914, so, not having the heart to disillusion him, he quietly wrote

above Osler's inscription his own Latin one acquiescing in the expropriation. It is a rare book and Sherrington had never succeeded in getting another copy. I wanted to restore it to him but he would not accept it, even for his life-time. It bears three book-plates, in two different forms, of a James Scott, M.D., so Sherrington, whose middle name is Scott, may have inherited it. It was apparently acquired in Paris in 1820 for the equivalent of £2.6.0. Sherrington, in the B.M.J. of 9 July 1949, tells of a similar incident in connection with the Macer Floridus herbal, no. 5100.[21] One would be inclined to think that this couldn't happen twice, but the dates of the inscription in no. 5100 bear out his statement, so it is not a question of his 92-year-old memory against my youthful septuagenarian one.[22]

In addition to this copy of Descartes, works by Osler and Sherrington were also included in our exhibition.

We were particularly pleased to exhibit John Morgan's copy of Giovanni Morgagni's great classic of pathology, *De sedibus, et causis morborum* (1761), from the library of the College of Physicians of Philadelphia. After receiving his medical degree from Edinburgh University in 1763, the young American physician John Morgan, then twenty-six years old, went on a grand tour of Europe. While there, he visited the elder Morgagni, age eighty-one, and presented him with a copy of his thesis. In return Morgan received this copy of Morgagni's work, with presentation inscriptions in Latin as a tribute from Morgagni to his American namesake.

It is known that Charles Darwin broke up his manuscript of *On the Origin of Species* (1859) and that some of the pages were actually used as scratch paper by his children. It is rare to find more than a single page in a collection. Accordingly, the earliest possible version of the complete text is the proof copy which Robert B. Honeyman, Jr., presented to Lehigh University Library. It is the complete final page proofs with corrections in Darwin's hand, and was part of our exhibition.

Wilhelm Roentgen sent offprints of his ten-page article announcing the discovery of X-rays, *Eine neue Art von Strahlen* (1895), along with original X-ray photographs, to a number of prominent scientists. Many of these were inscribed to their recipients, for example the one sent to his friend Hippel, on which Roentgen wrote: "Sent to you to indicate what the truth is and what the damn papers dreamed up."[23] Our exhibition included copies of Roentgen's first and second papers with presentation inscriptions in English, borrowed from the Osler Library at McGill University, along with original X-ray photographs of Roentgen's wife's hand and of the barrel of his gun, which we borrowed from the Francis A. Countway Library of Medicine in Boston.

As science became increasingly technical, and publication became more rapid, bibliographical complexities made it more difficult to determine precisely where certain discoveries were first published. Certain specialists assisted us in the selection process. For example, Professor Arthur Silverstein informed us that our choice of Karl Landsteiner's paper "Zur Kenntniss der antifermentativen, lytischen und agglutinierenden Wirkungen des Blutserums und der Lymphe" (1900) as a "first" was wrong:

> I assume that it was included as the first observation on the existence of human blood groups, for which he received the Nobel Prize . . . [but in the 1900 paper] Landsteiner merely reports briefly in a footnote the observation that normal blood sera may agglutinate the erythrocytes of other normal humans. He does not discuss the implications of this, nor does he present the data. It is only in a subsequent paper (*Wien. klin. Wochenschr.* 14, 1132–34) that Landsteiner presents the data, suggests the existence of different blood groups, and points to the implications of this for blood transfusion and for forensics analysis.

We of course accepted his correction.

Similarly, Dr. W. Bruce Fye informed us that our choice of Willem Einthoven's "Die galvanometrische Registrirung des menschlichen Elektrokardiogramms, zugleich eine Beurtheilung der Anwendung des Capillar-Elektrometers in der Physiologie" (1903) was not the first publication on the electrocardiogram. Instead, he proposed and we accepted Einthoven's "Galvanometrische registratie van het menschelijk electrocardiogram" (1902), a contribution to a Dutch *Festschrift* that preceded the more widely known German paper by a year.

Deciding on a work that would best represent modern nutrition was not easy. Nicolai Lunin (1853–1937) began the era of modern research on vitamins with his paper "Ueber die Bedeutung der anorganischen Salze für die Ernährung des Thiers" (1881), in which he demonstrated that animals could not live on a synthetic milk diet because it lacked an accessory component necessary for growth. In 1896 Christiaan Eijkman (1858–1930) produced beriberi in fowls by feeding them a diet of polished rice, which led to the understanding that beriberi in humans resulted from a dietary deficiency. In "The Importance of Individual Amino-Acids in Metabolism" (1906), Sir Frederick Gowland Hopkins (1861–1947) predicted the importance of accessory food factors, and his pioneering work led eventually to the discovery of vitamins. However, we decided to follow the example of W. R. LeFanu, who composed J. K. Lilly's list, in choosing *Die Vitamine* (1914) by Casimir Funk (1884–1967). We consulted with Mr. LeFanu about his choice and received the following reply:

> I first thought of using Hopkins as the representative of discovery of the vitamins. He was, I consider, the chief surveyor of the subject of dietary deficiencies. The others whom you mention—Lunin and Eijkman (and two or three more)—did most important work, but on special aspects.
>
> Two reasons led me to choose Funk—he invented the word vitamin(e), and his research and publication in five countries (and four language-areas) made the knowledge

> of the necessity of vitamins, in preventing illnesses of dietary deficiency origin, widespread among the educated public as well as to research scientists. . . .
>
> Funk's book, published in Germany when he was thirty, elaborated his previous reports. He called it "a first attempt, incorporating besides facts the personal observations of the author, new questions, ideas and plans of work . . . much fragmentary, much hypothetical, but a first step in a new direction for physiology and pathology. A superstructure loosely built on firm and sure foundations." He dealt in turn with several diseases which he first showed to be due to nutritional deficiencies, and described nutritional defects in infants and deficiency diseases in cattle. He discussed the chemistry of growth and the role of the vitamins in growth and metabolism. Funk's book opened the way for vast advances in preventive and therapeutic medicine.

The papers of Frederick Banting, discoverer of insulin, have continued to puzzle us. In the collections of both J. K. Lilly and Harvey Cushing, we located his first publications of 1922. In both collections Banting had autographed for presentation his paper, "*The Internal Secretion of the Pancreas*, by F. G. Banting and C. H. Best (Read before the Academy of Medicine, February 7th, 1922)." However, the paper with the same title published in the February 1922 issue of the *Journal of Laboratory and Clinical Medicine* is usually described as his first paper. In neither collection was this paper inscribed. After considerable deliberation, we were able to locate and speak with Michael Bliss, author of *The Discovery of Insulin* (1982), and *Banting: A Biography* (1984; revised edition, 1992). Mr. Bliss confirmed from his knowledge of the Banting archives that the first paper was in fact that which appeared in the journal. The paper which Banting inscribed had been privately printed later by the Academy. Why Banting inscribed the one and not the other is a question that still remains unanswered.

ISSUED AS THEY ARE in small numbers of twenty-five or fifty, offprints of important discoveries are the rare medical books of today. Several years ago the late Warren R. Howell of John Howell Books offered for sale the offprint of Sir Alexander Fleming's paper, published in the *British Journal of Experimental Pathology* (1929), announcing his discovery of penicillin. Almost simultaneously, similar offprints were offered by other prominent booksellers. Since these offprints were presumed to be very rare, the group of copies on the market created excitement in the small circle of booksellers and collectors interested in such things. It was not long, however, before Howell and others discovered that what had been presumed to be the original offprint was in fact a later reprinting which Fleming, faced with numerous reprint requests for a paper originally published years earlier, had commissioned in 1944 for private distribution. Two hundred fifty copies were made of this "reprint," which corresponded to the extremely rare original offprint, except that the text was reset, the pagination was changed to pp. 1–12, and there was a reprint statement at the head of page 1.

We had a parallel experience with the paper on DNA by James D. Watson and Francis H. C. Crick, "A Structure for Deoxyribose Nucleic Acid" (1953). In our effort to obtain authors' copies for our exhibition, we contacted Dr. Watson, one of the co-authors, and asked if he would be willing to lend us his signed copy of the offprint, which he agreed to do. We also learned of another copy, signed by Watson, Crick, Maurice Wilkins, and Ray Gosling, and thought we would like to exhibit it as well. When we received photographs of both, we were surprised to discover that they differed: the offprint from Watson consisted of a single leaf printed in double columns on both sides and contained Watson and Crick's paper only, whereas the other offprint consisted of fourteen pages printed in single columns and contained three papers under the over-all heading "Molecular Structure of Nucleic Acids"—a reflection of the similar arrangement in the journal *Nature*, where the articles had originally been published. The three papers were Watson and Crick's "A Structure for Deoxyribose Nucleic Acid" (three pages); "Molecular Structure of Deoxypentose Nucleic Acids" by M.H.F. Wilkins, A. R. Stokes, and H. R. Wilson (six pages); and "Molecular Configuration in Sodium Thymonucleate" by Rosalind D. Franklin and R. G. Gosling (five pages). We compared both versions of the offprint with the original in the journal and found that neither was an exact replica of the journal article, although interestingly enough, the two offprints appear to have been printed from the same setting of type. Although we were unable initially to contact Dr. Watson directly, we had a number of conversations about the offprint with members of his staff. At one point, we were advised that the single-sheet offprint was the first to have appeared. Because some forty years have elapsed since the initial publication, it is understandable that scientists who have been preoccupied with much more important matters may have difficulty remembering what for them is a relatively minor point. Nonetheless, this has made it difficult for us to clarify the matter of priority. The persons with whom we communicated at the journal *Nature* dismissed our inquiry with the statement that scientists are free to have additional reprints made. Our effort to locate the original printer seemed to indicate that he was no longer in business. We did contact Francis Crick and Maurice Wilkins and found that neither recalled the single-paper offprint but did remember the three-paper one. In another effort to clarify, if possible, the issue of priority, we wrote to James D. Watson asking him if he would help resolve the matter. We very much appreciated his letter dated 22 September 1993:

> My memory of the reprint orders for our original DNA paper is vague. My best guess now is that the three-paper reprint came second, being given in the fall of 1953 by the National Foundation for Infantile Paralysis which had sponsored me during my second year at Cambridge. Given the awkward personality situations then existing, I doubt that Francis Crick and I would have asked in the spring of '53 that all three papers be bound together. Favoring this view is the fact that the one-page reprint exactly reflects the size of the *Nature* page.

With this letter, we thought that we had concluded our investigation of the priority of the Watson and Crick offprint more or less satisfactorily.

This, however, was not to be the case. By chance, I came upon a copy of Francis Crick's book, *What Mad Pursuit*, in which I found the statement that "mainly due to Max Delbruck, copies of the three initial papers were distributed to all those attending the 1953 Cold Spring Harbor symposium, and Watson's talk on DNA was added to the program."[24] It seemed reasonable to write to Dr. Crick to ascertain the date of the symposium and to inquire whether it was the three-paper offprint that had been circulated at that time. Dr. Crick responded to my letter by telephone. He was able to date the symposium to 5-11 June 1953, but could not verify what was distributed then because he had not attended the symposium. Since Max Delbruck was no longer alive, Dr. Crick referred me back to Dr. Watson. During this conversation, I asked Dr. Crick if he had seen the single-paper offprint, and he replied that he thought he had. I then wrote to the archives department of the California Institute of Technology, where Delbruck had worked, to see if there was any information in their files about this matter. They did have copies of correspondence between Watson and Delbruck which indicated that the copies of the three DNA papers that had been distributed at the symposium were mimeographed copies. Neither the single-leaf nor the three-paper offprint was in Delbruck's file. At this point I was still inclined to consider the single-paper offprint as the first issue.

We had earlier involved in the investigation one of our London contributors, Nigel Phillips, a bookseller who had sold two autographed copies of the three-paper offprint, signed by Watson, Crick, and others, for a San Francisco bibliophile. Both Phillips and his client were adamant that the three-paper offprint was the first issue. On 28 October 1993 I received a letter from Phillips advising me that he had contacted all the living British authors of the three DNA papers—Wilkins, Stokes, Wilson, and Gosling—and that not one of them was aware of the single-leaf offprint. We ourselves had contacted Dr. Peter Pauling, son of Dr. Linus Pauling, who had been on the scene, and who had sold the proof copy of the three-paper offprint which he had obtained from Francis Crick; Dr. Peter Pauling was also of the opinion that the three-paper offprint was the original. On 22 November 1993 we received another letter from Phillips with the following enclosures, which we now reprint. The first is a letter dated 1 November 1993 from Sir Aaron Klug, recipient of the Nobel Prize for Chemistry in 1982 and director of the Laboratory of Molecular Biology, Medical Research Council, Cambridge. (Watson and Crick did their DNA research at the Cavendish Laboratory, Cambridge University.) The relevant part of Sir Aaron's letter reads as follows:

> . . . The copy of Francis Crick's Ph.D. thesis, which he gave me in about 1957, has a pocket at the back containing a reprint of the April 1953 *Nature* papers. This is in the one-column format and has the Watson & Crick paper bound together with the two papers from King's. I therefore do not believe that there was an "original" reprint in

which the Watson & Crick paper was published alone in the full-page format. In those days *Nature* did not use that format.

To check this I asked Max Perutz what he remembered, and I enclose a copy of my query and his reply. He confirms that the reprint received by the MRC Unit in 1953 was not in the full-page format, and showed me the bound collected papers of the Unit for that year. The reprint is of the one-column format and contains all three papers. I hope this settles this matter to the satisfaction of the Museum Curator.

I confirm, as I told you on the 'phone, that I raised the matter with Jim Watson when I saw him in Chicago at the 50th anniversary meeting in October. He seemed quite unsure about the history and did not press the view that the one-page "reprint" given out at Cold Spring Harbor earlier this year was the true original.

It seems to me that at some point somebody made a copy of the Watson & Crick paper alone from the actual pages of *Nature* and this is now being presented as the original. In view of the above I do not think there is any evidence for this.

Next we quote from the undated letter that Sir Aaron Klug sent to Max F. Perutz (Nobel Laureate in Chemistry in 1962), at King's College, University of London, where Wilkins and the others had worked:

> Max, Could you possibly help settle a dispute that has arisen (among archivists) about the reprint(s) of the Watson-Crick and two King's papers in *Nature* April 1953? Most people (including myself) have a reprint of all three papers bound together in the old style one-column format—with the overall title Molecular Structure of Nucleic Acids. Recently Cold Spring Harbor have produced what they say is the original reprint of the W-C paper, namely one printed on its own (without the King's papers) and in full-page format. This, of course, was not the style of *Nature* reprints in those days. Francis says he can't remember (although the copy in his Ph.D. thesis was of the one-column, three-paper format). Jim is now unsure. Do you remember? Or indeed do you have a copy of the "original" reprint? I attach copies.

Perutz's reply, also undated, stated:

> The reprints received in 1953 were not in the full-paper format as shown by the original bound into the collected papers of the M.R.C. unit.

On 23 November 1993 I received Dr. Watson's second letter, which reads as follows:

> After your letter of 19 October arrived, I saw Francis Crick at a meeting in Houston. He feels very strongly that the three-paper reprint was in fact the first one, and that the two-page reprint was printed afterward for the National Foundation. He is probably correct, but to be certain you should check directly with the editors of *Nature.*

As Dr. Watson suggested, we contacted the editors of *Nature* again. The reply we received, in a letter dated 13 January 1994, was that they did not know the answer. The editor who responded guessed that both reprints were done at the same time. In the interim, a letter from Dr. Linus Pauling (winner of the Nobel Prize in Chemistry in 1952 and the Peace Prize in 1962), to whom I had also written, disclosed his thought that he had received a copy of the single-paper version, but that he was unable to locate it at that time. He did not remember having received a copy of the three-paper offprint.

The details of these efforts have been added as a cautionary note. They explain the great difficulty that we have had with the bibliography of this relatively recent landmark paper, both authors of which are still alive. Thanks to the cooperation of the many distinguished scientists who gave time and thought to the matter, it is now our tentative conclusion that the three-paper offprint is the first issue. However, I doubt that any serious bibliophile would turn away from a signed copy of the single-paper offprint, which appears to be the rarer of the two.[25]

SINCE THE ANCIENTS, the "book" has served as an instrument of education for the physician, as well as a means of communication between physicians and scientists. With the development of medical and scientific societies in the seventeenth and eighteenth centuries, journal publication became more frequent, a trend that is now almost exclusive in the twentieth century. In this exhibition we have attempted to highlight this panorama of medical progress as documented in print, from the Greeks to the second half of the twentieth century. Had we accepted the suggestion of our colleague who proposed we begin with Semmelweis (1861), we would have exhibited a few books, several bound volumes of journals, occasional single numbers of journals, and offprints (preferably signed). This tendency would have been even more pronounced had we limited ourselves to the twentieth century, as another colleague advised. The few single numbers of journals and the offprints we were able to assemble came from the authors, private collections, and the librarians who had the foresight to collect them or were the beneficiaries of private collections.

As I conclude this introduction I have been informed that various medical journals are beginning to be published in electronic form, such as CD-ROM, in addition to traditional printed form. Media for the recording and distribution of information have changed more in the past ten years than in the previous five hundred since Gutenberg's invention of movable type. Exactly what form a future exhibition of twenty-first century classics of medicine might take is hard to imagine at this time, considering the increasingly rapid rate of change in this area. Yet I venture to say that however communication technology evolves, there will always be repositories of information and collectors of classic achievements in science and medicine.

HASKELL F. NORMAN, M.D.

1. *The Houghton Library 1942–1967: A Selection of Books and Manuscripts in Harvard Collections* (Cambridge, Mass., 1967), p. 161.
2. David A. Randall, *Dukedom Large Enough* (New York, 1969), pp. 339–54; *Medicine: An Exhibition of Books Relating to Medicine and Surgery from the Collection Formed by J. K. Lilly* (Bloomington, 1966), pp. 3–9.
3. Personal communication from W. R. LeFanu to Haskell F. Norman; *Notable Medical Books from the Lilly Library, Indiana University*, prepared by W. R. LeFanu (Indianapolis, 1976).
4. Bern Dibner, *Heralds of Science*, 2d ed. (Washington, D.C., 1980), p. 5.
5. The catalogues or exhibition handlists were published as: *One Hundred Books Famous in English Literature* (New York, 1902); *Bibliographical Notes on One Hundred Books Famous in English Literature* (New York, 1903); *One Hundred Illustrated Books, 1472–1896* (New York, 1921); *One Hundred Influential American Books Printed before 1900* (New York, 1947); *One Hundred Books Famous in Science* (New York, 1964).
6. Quoted in Daniel J. Boorstin, *The Discoverers* (New York, 1983), p. 524.
7. William A. Jackson, *The Houghton Library Report of Accessions for the Year 1955–56* (Cambridge, Mass., 1956), pp. 46–47.
8. *Bibliotheca Osleriana: A Catalogue of Books Illustrating the History of Medicine and Science* (Oxford, 1929; reprinted , Montreal & London, 1969).
9. Gabriel Austin, *The Library of Jean Grolier: A Preliminary Catalogue* (New York, 1971).
10. Ibid.
11. *Medicine* (Bloomington, 1966); and *Notable Medical Books* (Indianapolis, 1976).
12. *Legacies of Genius: A Celebration of Philadelphia Libraries*, edited by Edwin Wolf 2nd (Philadelphia, 1988); Thomas A. Horrocks, "A Selection of Treasures from the Historical Collections of the Library of the College of Physicians of Philadelphia," *Transactions and Studies of the College of Physicians of Philadelphia*, series 5, 9, no. 1 (1987): 3–24.
13. *Exhibitions in Yale University on the Occasion of the Sesquicentennial Celebration of the School of Medicine* (New Haven, 1960).
14. *Bibliotheca Osleriana* (Oxford, 1929).
15. *The Harvey Cushing Collection of Books and Manuscripts* (New York, 1943).
16. *Rare Books and Collections of the Reynolds Historical Library: A Bibliography* (Birmingham, Ala., 1968).
17. *Catalogue of the Medical History Collection Presented to UCLA by Dr. and Mrs. John A. Benjamin in Honor of Bennet M. Allen and Boris Krichesky* (Los Angeles, 1964).
18. John F. Fulton, "The Influence of Boerhaave's *Institutiones Medicae* on Modern Physiology," *Nederl. tijdschrift voor geneeskunde* 82, no. 40 (1 October 1928): 4860–66.
19. Frederick R. Goff, *Incunabula in American Libraries: A Third Census of Fifteenth-Century Books Recorded in North American Collections* (Millwood, N.Y., 1973).
20. Michael T. Ryan (Grolier Club Member 1988–), formerly Director of Special Collections at Stanford University and now in a similar capacity at the University of Pennsylvania, was an early supporter and made a number of inquiries on our behalf.
21. *Bibliotheca Osleriana*, no. 5100, quotes the following note: "Given to me by my colleague Sherrington. [W.O.]."
22. We are indebted to the Osler Library, McGill University, for permission to reprint this quotation.
23. Bern Dibner, *The New Rays of Professor Röntgen* (Norwalk, Conn., 1963), p. 19. This copy is now in the Smithsonian.
24. Francis Crick, *What Mad Pursuit* (New York, 1988), p. 76.
25. Subsequently we learned from the English bookseller William Patrick Watson, who in 1994 offered for sale a copy of the three-paper offprint signed by all six living authors, that in 1985 Zeitlin and VerBrugge (catalogue 281, no. 391) offered for sale Max Delbruck's copy. This was also the three-paper offprint. It was unsigned and unbound, with Max Delbruck's stamps and notations. Watson also made an additional comment:

> Only a very small number of copies of the offprint were printed (in contrast with highly specialised journals, where offprints were produced in fairly large quantities as authors' main means of disseminating their writings among colleagues, *Nature* had a very wide circulation and the call for offprints was consequently restricted). The format is smaller, the journal being printed in double columns, whereas the

offprint is in a single column. *Nature* was set in Monotopye, and an electrotype plate was made from the standing type; the journal was printed from the plate and not directly from the type. The offprint, however, was printed from the standing type, reset only so far as the diagram of the double-helix is here printed at the head of page two, whereas in the journal it was embedded in the text [William Patrick Watson, *Catalogue No. 5: Science, Medicine and Natural History* (1994), no. 145].

On inquiry, Mr. Watson informed us that his source for this printing information was Nicolas Barker, who in the 1950s was production manager of Macmillans, who were the publishers of *Nature* at the time.

EDITOR'S PREFACE

THIS CATALOGUE seeks not only to chronicle the importance in medical history of the one hundred, and more, "books" selected by Haskell F. Norman for exhibition at the Grolier Club. It also aims to give a complete bibliographical account of the first publication of these works, both as a contribution to the further study of the scientific, intellectual, and social importance of the discoveries announced in them, and as an illustration of the history of printing and publishing in the field of medicine.

Each entry in the catalogue consists of two parts: a heading, which gives title and publication information and bibliographical descriptions for each work included in the entry, and an essay that discusses the medical and historical significance and bibliographical history of the works described. Characteristics of the copies exhibited are recorded in a separate section. The catalogue essays were commissioned by Dr. Norman and are signed by their contributors, and Dr. Norman also provided special notes concerning the provenance of some of the copies exhibited; these sections were edited for uniformity of presentation and bibliographical content. The editor is responsible for the formulation of title and publication information, the bibliographical descriptions, and the physical details of copy description and provenance evidence. These are based on information provided by the lenders to the exhibition, on Diana H. Hook's knowledge of copies in the Haskell F. Norman Library of Science and Medicine, and on the editor's examination of the exhibition copies and copies at the New York Academy of Medicine, the College of Physicians of Philadelphia, the National Library of Medicine, the Harvey Cushing/John Hay Whitney Medical Library at Yale University, the Augustus C. Long Health Sciences Library at Columbia University, and the Adelaide Nutting Historical Nursing Collection at the Teachers College of Columbia University.

The editions featured in the exhibition were those selected by Dr. Norman, as explained in his Introduction. For the most part, these were the first editions of the works in question, including both the first Latin and the first Greek editions of ancient Greek authors (cat. nos. 1, 2, 3, and 5). However, in the case of two works first printed in the fifteenth century (cat. nos. 7 and 8), copies of the first editions were not available in North America, and later editions were shown. For the three works first published in fascicles (cat. nos. 51, 55, and 86), the organizers of the exhibition were unable to locate full sets of parts, and so exhibited bound copies of composite volumes containing the complete text. In the case of medical discoveries first published in journals, as has been increasingly the case in the nineteenth and twentieth centuries, Dr. Norman preferred to identify and exhibit offprints rather than journal numbers or bound volumes (see his discussion of this point in the Introduction). And when a work was published simultaneously in Britain and in the United States (cat. nos. 66, 68, 71, 76, 82, and 90), or simultaneously in two journals (cat. nos. 78 and 91A), the exhibition included only one version. All of these selections have been fully described in the bibliographical sections and among the copies exhibited.

In addition, so that the catalogue may serve as a complete record of the first appearances in print of the works it features, the bibliographical sections include descriptions of all the initial manifestations of each work. Where a later version was exhibited, the first is also described. For works whose first publication was in parts, the differences between the fascicles and the combined volumes are described insofar as they could be determined. For articles published in journals, both the journal number (or volume) and the offprint are described, and an effort made to characterize the typographical relationship between the two. And for works published simultaneously in England and America, both publications are described and their textual and bibliographical relationship identified.

Identifying these multiple manifestations, describing them, and characterizing their relationships involved the investigation of various kinds of bibliographical evidence and provided illustrations of many kinds of bibliographical relationships. The process of reviewing the early printings of the works of Rhazes (cat. no. 6), as described by Dr. Norman in the Introduction, illustrated the problem of identifying and choosing among versions of a text. The preparation of the catalogue entry for the works of Avicenna (cat. no. 7) required consideration of recent arguments for dating the early editions of this author on the basis of paper and type evidence as well as textual relationships. Examination of the works published in fascicles showed how the relation between the parts and composite volumes may vary from work to work and copy to copy: in the case of Baillie (cat. no. 51), the complete volumes appear to be bound from the parts, with the first fascicle reprinted; in the case of Willan (cat. no. 55), the first two fascicles were reset with slightly different collation and content, so that complete copies may include either the originals or what are in fact the second editions of the first two parts; for Ramón y Cajal (cat. no. 86), the only copy I have seen was bound from the parts, as indicated by the wrappers bound in at the end and by slight differences in the paper from part to part.

The bibliographical and historical complexities resulting from simultaneous publication in Britain and the United States are well-known to students of nineteenth-century literature. On the evidence of the present catalogue, the same questions can be seen to apply also to medical and scientific works. The bibliographical and textual relationships of the American and English publications, their relative timing, and the absolute dates of their appearance in each country, all potentially affected the reception of the ideas announced in each work as well as subsequent understanding of each publication's influence. A work published in one country might be pirated—released in one or more unauthorized versions—in the other, as was the case with Florence Nightingale's *Notes on Nursing* (1860; cat. no. 71), which was published in London and republished independently from new settings of type in both New York and Boston. The later appearance might be a corrected resetting, as was the Philadelphia edition of Gray's *Anatomy* (1859, based on the 1858

London edition; cat. no. 68); this was presumably an authorized edition, since the American publisher was able to import a set of blocks for printing the illustrations. In some instances when the text was reset, the direction of transmission and the source of the resetting have yet to be determined: Sims (cat. no. 66) was an American but was living in London when *Clinical Notes on Uterine Surgery* (1866) was published in both London and New York. In other circumstances, one publisher might sell the book in printed sheets to his counterpart on the other continent, as was the case with Osler (*The Principles and Practice of Medicine*, 1892; cat. no. 82), whose British issue was furnished with a cancel title leaf, and with Sherrington (*The Integrative Action of the Nervous System*, 1906; cat. no. 90), where the first quire was apparently reset to provide an integral title leaf with the imprint of the London publisher. In the case of Ferrier (*The Functions of the Brain*, 1876; cat. no. 76), copies with the London imprint, generally considered to be first, are identical in setting with those bearing the New York imprint, but there is no evidence in the form of cancel leaves or printers' colophons to indicate the nature of the bibliographical relationship between the two. For these authors and works, this catalogue describes both the English and the American first appearances, even if further research will be required to clarify their exact chronological and textual relationships. In general, the criteria for including both were the existence of British and American first appearances apparently identical in setting, or representing two settings of the same text, and published within a year of each other.

The question of offprints is particularly important in dealing with medical and scientific publications. Dr. Norman, in the Introduction, comments on this subject from the bibliophilic point of view and explains the collector's preference for offprints—of which he has assembled an impressive collection—while also taking note of Horblit's choice of the journal as embodying the intended original appearance of an article. To the bibliographer both journal and offprint are of interest, and one of the objectives of the bibliographical sections of this catalogue is to elucidate the relationships that exist between the two. An offprint may be defined as a pamphlet printed from a portion of the typesetting prepared for a journal number. To judge from the terminology employed by the offprints catalogued in this volume, medical and scientific journals refer to "reprints" rather than "offprints"; bibliographically, however, it is preferable to use the term "offprint" to refer to those copies that represent substantially the same setting of type as the journal and to avoid the term "reprint," which can have other meanings. To assume that the type was set for the purpose of producing the journal volume or number and that the offprints were printed from that type does not exclude nuances of chronological or typographical relationship. Chronologically, depending on the distribution system used by the journal, the offprints of an article may actually be available for the author to distribute before the journal volume has been released. Typographically, the journal may have been printed from plates while the offprint was printed from the original typesetting (as in the case of cat. no.

99; see also the Introduction), or copies of individual articles may be reproduced by offset, possibly at a later period. All of these, however, represent the same setting of type, whatever the historical circumstances surrounding their production and distribution.

Separate distribution of the text of journal articles may also take forms other than the offprint; these may be mentioned parenthetically here. Articles in journals or the "offprints" of them are sometimes "reprinted" from type reset for the purpose, as happened with works by Henry Jacob Bigelow (cat. no. 64A) and Alexander Fleming (cat. no. 96), but bibliographically these are new editions. Contributions to journals may also be circulated in the form of "preprints." No examples of this form are included in the present catalogue, but those with which I am familiar have consisted of copies of the typescript of an article or copies of the proofs, distributed privately by the author before the publication of the journal.

Even though journal article and offprint were printed from the same setting of type, other aspects of their bibliographical relationship may vary. In the journal, the placement and layout of the article are determined by the over-all composition and layout of the journal. The offprint, in its simplest form bibliographically, consists of an overrun of the type pages as set for the journal, or a separate printing of them, sometimes with a statement of reprinting added to the first or last page. In offprints of this type, the pages correspond to the appropriate section of the journal in layout, pagination, and imposition; the offprint may be folded and gathered in sections corresponding to those of the journal, or its folds may have been removed so that it takes the form of separate leaves that may or may not be fastened at the spine. Frequently, however, offprints were produced by reimposing the type pages or columns from the journal, sometimes with different page breaks, in order to form an independent pamphlet that often differs from the article in collation, pagination, layout, or size. Many, though not all, offprints are provided with wrappers, which may give a title and imprint for the individual offprint or may be generic wrappers intended to be used on all offprints from a given journal. A few offprints have separate title pages printed for the purpose.

In an effort to clarify these relationships, this catalogue includes bibliographical descriptions both of the journal number or journal volume in which an article appeared and also of any offprints. Descriptions of the offprints have been given in every case where I was aware of the existence of one and was able to gain access to a copy of it; in addition, in the two instances of resetting already referred to, the catalogue includes descriptions of the "reprints" of the "offprints," so as to make clear the distinction between the original publication and the later appearance of a reset text. Both the journal number or volume and the offprint are fully described according to the same principles applied to the bibliographical description of books. (Only in four instances, cat. nos. 97, 98A, 98B, and 100, was I unable to find a copy of the journal number which retained its original folds or other evidence of its original form of binding, so that the collation had to be omitted.) In addition to the usual elements of description, the location of the article within the journal volume is given in terms both of collation and of pagination, in order to facilitate comparison with the bibliographical composition of the offprint. Any differences in the layout of the offprint are characterized with brief notes, such as "Reimposed, with different page breaks," "Reimposed in single-column pages," or "Partially reset, to accommodate the different placement of the figure." Except for the offprints described in cat. no. 99, which I have collated completely against one another in every possible combination, I have judged identity of setting by the rough-and-ready criteria of comparing line lengths, collating line-endings, and spot-checking texts; these tests, of course, do not necessarily suffice for detecting all resettings, some of which may remain to be discovered, and evaluated, by future bibliographers. Although it is hoped that these observations on the subject of offprints will contribute to the systematic analysis of this class of publication, many questions, both bibliographical and historical, remain concerning these ephemeral items. In the present catalogue, such complexities are well exemplified in Dr. Norman's discussion of the offprints of Watson and Crick's article on DNA (see cat. no. 99 and the Introduction).

THE EDITORIAL PRINCIPLES that inform the bibliographical sections of this catalogue are here summarized for the convenience of the reader:

Title and Publication Information. For fifteenth-century books the titles and imprints are taken from standard reference works, such as Goff, or have been supplied by the editor, as in the case of the title for the first Greek edition Aristotle's works (cat. no. 2B). For later books, journal articles, and offprints the title transcriptions reproduce the orthography of the items being described, but capitalize according to the rules of the language in question. In the case of a few sixteenth-century books (e.g., cat. nos. 13, 16, etc.) abbreviations have been expanded. Imprints for books give the city in English, followed by the publisher's statement as found on the title page or in the colophon, and the date in arabic numerals. Journal citations are given in standard form, in order to facilitate reference to the original and to later scholarship. For offprints, the title is taken from the title page, when there is one, or from the wrapper (designated "[wrapper title]"), or from the head of the first page of the text (designated "[head title]"). The statement of reprinting is transcribed from the same sources, but an imprint is given only when one appears on the title page or the wrapper. Except in these cases, no place, publisher, or printer is given for journals or offprints; it can be assumed that this information is the same for journals and their offprints. Book titles, names of journals, and the titles of offprints (as separate publications) are italicized; titles of articles in journals are printed in roman type.

The order of the catalogue entries, roughly chronological, was determined by Dr. Norman, as was the choice of the principal work in each entry. The author or authors of the principal work form the heading for each entry; the authors of subordinate works are given within the entries, immediately preceding the titles of the additional works. Subordinate works or editions within an entry are distinguished by the letters B and C. An alphabetical index of all the authors whose works are featured in the catalogue will be found at the end of the book.

Bibliographical Descriptions. The same principles have been applied to books, offprints, and journal numbers (or volumes, when there was no evidence that the volume was published in separate numbers), and to publications of both the hand-press and the machine-press periods. The bibliographical descriptions attempt to describe ideal copies, although it is possible that there are variants that have escaped the editor's attention. The topics covered are, as applicable:

Format: Given for all books for which it is possible to determine from the watermarks and/or chain lines of the paper how the sheet was folded.

Collation: Given for all books, offprints, and journal numbers, including those of the machine-press period. The formula represents the structure of the gatherings as bound into the book, journal, or offprint, and it uses the symbols employed by the printer. Unsigned publications were collated wherever possible, and the collations given by assigning bracketed numbers. (See above for a reference to four cases in which I was unable to locate copies of journal numbers suitable for collation.) Details of signing within quires, and the erroneous signing of individual leaves, are not reported. Repeated sequences of signing are given without the addition of preliminary superscripts to distinguish them, and within sequences each alphabet is recorded separately. In the case of some fifteenth- and sixteenth-century books (see, e.g., cat. nos. 4, 21), where discrete sequences of signing correspond to separate texts or tables, some copies may be bound with the parts in an order other than the one represented here.

Leaf count: This corresponds to the total represented by the collation.

Foliation or pagination: Reported in the terms used in the publication. The principal sequences are given in arabic or roman numerals, including erroneous disjunctures that affect the numbering of major sections within sequences (see, e.g., cat. nos. 1, 17), but minor errors in numbering are not noted. Where the last printed number of a sequence is in error, the printed number is reported, and a correction is given in brackets. Unnumbered sequences for which no numbers can be inferred are represented by a total in brackets. Unnumbered pages at the beginning of a sequence, for which numbers can be inferred, are represented by italicized numbers, but unnumbered leaves or pages after the last printed number of a sequence are given as a total in brackets. This system has several advantages: it is not necessary to infer numbers with respect to a final printed number that may be erroneous; the use of unbracketed roman type to report the first and last printed numbers of a sequence facilitates comparison with the publication; and ending each sequence with the last printed number permits easier comparison with descriptions based on library cataloguing rules, which give the extent of the item in these terms.

Illustrations: This section includes a collation of the illustrations using the terms, if any, employed in the publication. It distinguishes inserted plates from illustrations printed with the text, identifies the technique or techniques, notes the use of printed color (hand-coloring is described as a feature of individual copies), and identifies the artists when illustrations are signed or the artists are named in the publication. Other aspects of the illustrations or questions of attribution may be discussed in the essays.

Bindings: Publishers' bindings, including printed wrappers and printed boards, are noted here, since they are part of the item as published. No effort has been made to describe the details of cloth grain or labeling, and it is possible that not all color variants have been identified. Detailed descriptions of the particular publishers' bindings exhibited and of other bindings will be found with the copy descriptions.

References: These include standard works of medical bibliography, other standard bibliographical works, and bibliographies of the works of the authors featured in the catalogue.

Copies Exhibited. These listings include the following information, as applicable, for each copy exhibited: catalogue number; abbreviated author, title, and imprint; binding description; leaf size; additional copy description; provenance; comments; references; and lender. In instances where more than one copy was exhibited, the descriptive information is repeated for each. Where the catalogue gives a bibliographical description of more than one edition or other published version of a work, the copy description identifies the item exhibited as well as describing it. The following principles lie behind the selection and organization of this information as it relates to the individual copies:

Author, title, and imprint: Derived from the information in the main catalogue entry.

Binding: Descriptions briefly characterize the covering material and its style of decoration, without as a rule noting details of labeling. Binding supports are assumed to be pasteboards; wooden boards, wrappers, and other forms of binding are described explicitly. Printed wrappers, printed boards, and publisher's cloth are identified and described as they are found on the copy exhibited. Bindings are dated and localized to the extent possible from general or specific evidence, and binders are identified where possible, either by comparison with repertories of binders' tools for early bindings, or from binders' stamps or tickets for later bindings.

Leaf size: The figures given represent the vertical and horizontal measurements of an average leaf of paper in the copy in question.

Additional copy description: This includes comments on illumination or rubrication, hand-coloring, annotations, etc.

Provenance: Successive owners are listed, often with identifying phrases, and with reference to the evidence for their ownership; where possible, inscriptions are quoted and translated; the presence of illegible and deleted ownership marks is noted.

Comments: Remarks supplied by Dr. Norman regarding the special characteristics of certain books.

References: Given in a few instances where the copy in question or its binding has been recorded or described in a published reference work.

Lender: Briefly identified. A list of lenders to the exhibition is also given elsewhere in the catalogue.

HOPE MAYO

ACKNOWLEDGMENTS

MANY PEOPLE gave of their time and energy to this project, and we would like to thank them here. Apart from the contributors of book lists, descriptions, and books, who are noted elsewhere, we are indebted to the following people: Gabriel Austin; Michael Bliss, University of Toronto; Inci A. Bowman, Blocker History of Medicine Collections, Moody Medical Library, University of Texas Medical Branch at Galveston; Clare Bunce, Cold Spring Harbor Laboratory Archives; William R. Cagle and Joel Silver, Lilly Library, Indiana University; Bernadette G. Callery, New York Botanical Garden; Elizabeth Carroll-Horrocks and Roy Goodman, American Philosophical Society; Susan Case, Clendening History of Medicine Library, University of Kansas Medical Center; Helen Challacombe, Wangensteen Historical Library, University of Minnesota; Francis Crick, Salk Institute; Geoffrey Davenport, Royal College of Physicians; Katherine E. Donahue, Louise Darling Biomedical Library, University of California at Los Angeles; Leonard J. Eddy, Kornhauser Health Sciences Library, University of Louisville; Richard Eimas, Hardin Library, University of Iowa; Norman Fiering, John Carter Brown Library, Brown University, H. George Fletcher, Pierpont Morgan Library; Allen Fusone, National Agricultural Library; Ferenc Gyorgyey and Grethe Shepherd, Harvey Cushing/John Hay Whitney Medical Library, Yale University; Thomas A. Horrocks, College of Physicians of Philadelphia; Sir Godfrey Newbold Hounsfield; Barbara S. Irwin, George F. Smith Library of the Health Sciences, University of Medicine & Dentistry of New Jersey; Glen P. Jenkins, Rare Book Library, Historical Division, Cleveland Medical Library Association; Stanley H. Johnston, Jr., Holden Arboretum; Alan Jutzi, Huntington Library; Diane E. Kaplan, Manuscripts and Archives, Yale University Library; W. R. LeFanu; Eric v.d. Luft, Health Science Center, State University of New York, Syracuse; M. G. McGuinn, Reynolds Historical Library, University of Alabama, Birmingham; Helen Meranda, Alfred Taubman Medical Library, University of Michigan; Philip A. Metzger and Marie C. Boltz, Linderman Library, Lehigh University; Edward T. Morman, Institute of Medicine, Johns Hopkins University; P. G. Naiditch, Department of Special Collections, University of California at Los Angeles; Linda Ordogh, June Schachter, and Faith Wallace, Osler Library of the History of Medicine, McGill University; Leslie Overstreet and Ellen Wells, Special Collections, Smithsonian Institution; Ann Pasquale Haddad, New York Academy of Medicine; Suzanne Porter, History of Medicine Collections, Duke University Medical Center Library; Margaret Rogers, History of Science Collections, Cornell University Library; Bernard Rosenthal; Henri Schiller; Robert A. Schindler, M.D.; Alice Schreyer and Bill Pugh, Joseph Regenstein Library, University of Chicago; Lilli Sentz, Robert L. Brown History of Medicine Collection, State University of New York at Buffalo; Eugene R. Sheridan, The Papers of Thomas Jefferson, Princeton

University Library; Professor W. T. Stearn; Roger E. Stoddard and Dennis Marnon, Houghton Library, Harvard University; Larry E. Sullivan and Peter VanWingen, Rare Book and Special Collections Division, Library of Congress; Charlotte Tancin, Hunt Botanical Library, Carnegie Mellon University; Marvin J. Taylor and Susan Jacobson, Augustus C. Long Health Sciences Library, Columbia University; Philip Teigen and Margaret Kaiser, National Library of Medicine; Thomas Tottie, Uppsala University; James D. Watson, Cold Spring Harbor Laboratory; Richard J. Wolfe, Francis A. Countway Library of Medicine; Helen Yam, McGoogan Library of Medicine, University of Nebraska Medical Center; David Zeidberg, Special Collections, University of California at Los Angeles; and Nancy W. Zinn, Special Collections, University of California, San Francisco.

Special thanks go to the officers and staff of the Grolier Club, in particular the following: Kenneth A. Lohf, President when this project was conceived; William B. Warren, President when it was brought to completion; Martin W. Hutner, Chair of the Exhibitions Committee; William Reese, Chair of the Publications Committee when the project was begun; James O'Halloran, Chair of the Publications Committee when it was completed; Martin Antonetti, Librarian; and Kimball Higgs, Eric Holzenberg, and Nancy Houghton, who saw to the practical details of arranging the loans and installing the exhibition.

William H. Helfand deserves special thanks for his invaluable support and endless favors. He assisted in the coordination of our efforts with several Eastern libraries and served as a liaison with the staff of the Grolier Club and the Publications Committee.

My secretary, Pamela Castaldi, also deserves special thanks. For several years she handled our huge correspondence and dealt with the innumerable revisions which continued up to the last day.

Finally, I am especially indebted to Diana H. Hook of Jeremy Norman & Co., Inc., whose efforts in the assembly and preliminary editing of the catalogue were essential to its successful completion.

Without the support of the officers and staff of the Grolier Club and these last three people, the exhibition would not have taken place.

HASKELL F. NORMAN, M.D.

The editor would like to thank the following individuals and institutions for their contributions to the final preparation of the catalogue. I am indebted to Haskell F. Norman for the opportunity to participate in the project and to Diana H. Hook for her substantial contributions to the organization of the catalogue and its initial editing. At the Grolier Club, William B. Warren, President, Helmut N. Friedlaender, Vice President, James O'Halloran, Chair of the Publications Committee, Martin Antonetti, Librarian, and

William H. Helfand provided invaluable support. Paul Needham and G. Thomas Tanselle gave welcome advice on questions of descriptive and historical bibliography; the latter was especially generous with his time and expertise, and the form and content of the bibliographical descriptions result in large part from policies worked out in consultation with him. John Parascandola and Charles E. Rosenberg read the text as historians of medicine. Ursula Bauermeister, Nina Musinsky, Diane Shaw, Joel Silver, Victor Skretkowicz and David Vander Meulen answered specific questions. Mary Kiffer and Kathy Talalay assisted with the general editing, and Spring Harvey prepared the text for computer typesetting. The design and layout of the printed catalogue are the work of Jerry Kelly.

In the course of preparing the bibliographical descriptions and editing the catalogue text, I had occasion to consult rare and reference books at the New York Academy of Medicine; the Harvey Cushing/John Hay Whitney Medical Library, Historical Library, Yale University; the College of Physicians of Philadelphia; the National Library of Medicine; the Augustus C. Long Health Sciences Library, Columbia University; and the Adelaide Nutting Historical Nursing Collection, Department of Special Collections, Milbank Library, Teachers College, Columbia University. I wish to thank the librarians of these institutions, and especially Ann Pasquale Haddad, Lois Fischer Black, and Shaw Kinsley of the New York Academy of Medicine, for their cooperation.

HOPE MAYO

CONTRIBUTORS TO THE CATALOGUE

DANIEL M. ALBERT, M.D.
Frederick Allison Davis Professor and Chairman, Department of Ophthalmology
University of Wisconsin-Madison

SUSAN ALON
Washington University, St. Louis

HAROLD ATTWOOD, M.D., F.R.C.P.A.
Professor Emeritus of Pathology and Curator of Medical History Unit
University of Melbourne, Australia

THOMAS D. BROCK, PH.D.
Professor Emeritus
University of Wisconsin-Madison

JOHN THORNE CRISSEY, M.D.
Professor of Clinical Medicine
University of Southern California School of Medicine

EUGENE S. FLAMM, M.D.
Philadelphia, Pennsylvania

W. BRUCE FYE, M.D.
Marshfield, Wisconsin

RICHARD L. GOLDEN, M.D.
State University of New York at Stony Brook

RICHARD D. GURNEY
London, England

ANN PASQUALE HADDAD, M.L.S.
The New York Academy of Medicine

WILLIAM H. HELFAND
New York, New York

THOMAS A. HORROCKS
Director of the Francis C. Wood Institute for the History of Medicine and Director of the Library for Historical Services
The College of Physicians of Philadelphia

PAUL A. KLIGFIELD, M.D.
Professor of Medicine
Cornell University Medical College

LAWRENCE D. LONGO, M.D.
Loma Linda University

ARTHUR E. LYONS, M.D.
San Francisco, California

FREDERICK G. MEYER
U.S. National Arboretum (Retired)

GEORGE MORA, M.D.
Narragansett, Rhode Island

RODNEY B. NELSON III, M.D.
Geneva, Illinois

HASKELL F. NORMAN, M.D.
Ross, California

JEREMY M. NORMAN
San Francisco, California

DENNIS G. PAPPAS, M.D.
Birmingham, Alabama

NIGEL PHILLIPS
London, England

IRWIN J. PINCUS, M.D.
Beverly Hills, California

PAUL POTTER, M.D.
London, Ontario, Canada

MICHAEL T. RYAN
Director of Special Collections
University of Pennsylvania Libraries

ROBERT A. SCHINDLER, M.D.
Professor and Chair of the Department of Otolaryngology, Head and Neck Surgery
University of California, San Francisco

ARTHUR M. SILVERSTEIN, PH.D.
Johns Hopkins University

GARFIELD TOURNEY, M.D., LITT.D.
Professor Emeritus of Psychiatry and Human Behavior
University of Mississippi School of Medicine
Honorary Physician, University Hospital

ABBREVIATIONS

ABRAMS

Paul Needham. *The George Abrams Collection.* Sotheby's London, 16 November 1989.

ADAMS

H. C. Adams. *Catalogue of Books Printed on the Continent of Europe, 1501–1600, in Cambridge Libraries.* 2 vols. Cambridge, 1967.

AHMANSON-MURPHY

A Catalogue of the Ahmanson-Murphy Aldine Collection at UCLA. Compiled by Nicolas Barker, et al. Los Angeles, 1989– .

AUSTIN

Gabriel Austin. *The Library of Jean Grolier: A Preliminary Catalogue.* New York, 1971.

BAL

Bibliography of American Literature. Compiled by Jacob Blanck; edited and completed by Michael Winship. 9 vols. New Haven, 1955–91.

BENJAMIN

Catalogue of the Medical History Collection Presented to UCLA by Dr. and Mrs. John A. Benjamin in Honor of Bennet M. Allen and Boris Krichesky. Los Angeles, 1964.

BISHOP

P. James Bishop. "A Bibliography of Auenbrugger's 'Inventum novum' (1761)," *Tubercle* 42 (1961): 75–90.

BISHOP & GOLDIE

W. J. Bishop and Sue Goldie. *A Bio-Bibliography of Florence Nightingale.* London, 1962.

BLAKE

John B. Blake. *A Short Title Catalogue of Eighteenth Century Printed Books in the National Library of Medicine.* Bethesda, Md., 1979.

BMC

British Museum. *Catalogue of Books Printed in the XVth Century Now in the British Museum.* London, 1908– .

BSB-INK.

Bayerische Staatsbibliothek Inkunabelkatalog. Edited by Elmar Hertrich. Wiesbaden, 1988– .

CHASE

Merrill W. Chase, et al. "The Bibliography of Dr. Karl Landsteiner," *Journal of Immunology, Virus Research and Experimental Chemotherapy* 48 (1944): 5–16; reprinted as "Karl Landsteiner-Bibliographie," in Paul Speiser, *Karl Landsteiner, Entdecker der Blutgruppen: Bibliographie eines Nobelpreisträgers aus der Wiener Medizinischen Schule* (Vienna, 1961), pp. 97–111.

CHOULANT-FRANK

Ludwig Choulant. *History and Bibliography of Anatomic Illustration.* Translated and annotated by Mortimer Frank. New York, 1945.

CIBN

Bibliothèque National. *Catalogue des Incunables.* Edited by Ursula Baurmeister, Annie Charon-Parent, and Dominique Coq. Paris, 1981– .

COLEBROOK

L. Colebrook. "Alexander Fleming," *Biographical Memoirs of Fellows of the Royal Society,* 1956, 2: 117–27.

CRAINZ

Franco Crainz. "The Editions and Translations of Dr. Matthew Baillie's *Morbid Anatomy,*" *Medical History* 16 (1982): 443–52.

CUSHING

Harvey Cushing. *A Bio-Bibliography of Andreas Vesalius.* New York, 1943; reprinted, Hamden, Conn., 1962.

CUSHING SOCIETY

Harvey Cushing Society. *A Bibliography of the Writings of Harvey Cushing: Prepared on the Occasion of His Seventieth Birthday, April 8, 1939.* Springfield, Ill., 1939.

DOBELL

Clifford Dobell. *Antony van Leeuwenhoek and His "Little Animals."* New York, 1932; reprinted, New York, 1960.

DOE

Janet Doe. *A Bibliography of the Works of Ambroise Paré.* Chicago, 1937.

DOHENY

Felix de Marez Oyens and Paul Needham. *The Estelle*

Doheny Collection. Part I: *Fifteenth-Century Books.* Christie's New York, 22 October 1987.

DURLING

Richard J. Durling. *A Catalogue of Sixteenth Century Printed Books in the National Library of Medicine.* Bethesda, Md., 1967.

EFDT

En français dans le texte: dix siècles de lumières par le livre. Paris: Bibliothèque Nationale, 1990.

FISCH

Max H. Fisch. *Nicolaus Pol Doctor 1494.* New York, 1947.

FRATI

Carlo Frati. "Bibliografia Malpighiana: catalogo descrittivo delle opere a stampa di Marcello Malpighi e degli scritti che lo riguardano," *Pizzoli,* 1897: 281–338; reprinted, London, 1960.

FREEMAN

R. B. Freeman. *The Works of Charles Darwin: An Annotated Bibliographical Handlist.* 2d ed. Folkestone, 1977.

FULTON

John F. Fulton. *Two Oxford Physiologists: Richard Lower, 1631–1691; John Mayow, 1643–1679.* Oxford, 1935.

FULTON *Sherrington*

John F. Fulton. "Sir Charles Scott Sherrington, O.M. (1857–1952), *Journal of Neurophysiology* 15 (1952): 166–90; bibliography reprinted in *Selected Writings of Sir Charles Sherrington,* compiled and edited by D. Denny-Brown (Oxford, 1979), pp. 516–29.

FULTON & STANTON

John F. Fulton and Madeline E. Stanton. "A Bibliography of Galvani's Writings on Animal Electricity," in Luigi Galvani, *Commentary on the Effects of Electricity on Muscular Motion,* translated by Margaret Glover Foley (Norwalk, Conn., 1953).

GM

Leslie Morton. *Morton's Medical Bibliography: An Annotated Check-List of Texts Illustrating the History of Medicine (Garrison and Morton).* Edited by Jeremy M. Norman. 5th ed. London, 1991.

GOFF

Frederick R. Goff. *Incunabula in American Libraries: A Third Census.* New York, 1964; reprinted with additions, Millwood, N.Y., 1973. *Supplement.* New York, 1972.

GOLDEN & ROLAND

Richard L. Golden and Charles G. Roland. *Sir William Osler: An Annotated Bibliography with Illustrations.* San Francisco, 1988.

Great Names in Neurology

Great Names in Neurology: Bibliography of Writings by Joseph Babinski, Sir Victor Horsley, Sir Charles Sherrington and Arthur Van Gehuchten. Prepared for the First International Congress of Neurological Sciences, Brussels, Belgium, July 21–28, 1957. Bethesda, Md., 1957.

GRINSTEIN

Alexander Grinstein. *The Index of Psychoanalytic Writings.* 14 vols. New York, 1956–75.

GRMEK

M. D. Grmek. *Catalogue des manuscrits de Claude Bernard avec la bibliographie de ses travaux imprimés et des études sur son oeuvre.* Paris, 1967.

GROLIER *American*

Grolier Club. *One Hundred Influential American Books Printed before 1900.* New York, 1947.

GW

Gesamtkatalog der Wiegendrucke. Leipzig (etc.), 1925– .

Heirs of Hippocrates

Heirs of Hippocrates: The Development of Medicine in a Catalogue of Historic Books in the Hardin Library for the Health Sciences, the University of Iowa. Compiled and edited by Richard Eimas. 3d ed. Iowa City, 1990.

HILL

William Hill. "Richard Bright—A Bio-Bibliography," *Guy's Hospital Gazette* 64 (1950): 454–57, 472–84; reprinted as "Richard Bright: A Bibliography," *Guy's Hospital Reports* 107 (1958): 531–42.

HOBSON

Anthony Hobson. *Humanists and Bookbinders: The Origin and Diffusion of the Humanistic Bookbinding 1459–1559, with a Census of Historiated Plaquette and*

Medallion Bindings of the Renaissance. Cambridge, 1989.

HORBLIT

Harrison D. Horblit. *One Hundred Books Famous in Science.* New York: The Grolier Club, 1964.

HUNT

Jane Quinby and Alan Stevenson. *Catalogue of Botanical Books in the Collection of Rachel McMasters Miller Hunt.* 3 vols. Pittsburgh, 1958–61.

IGI

Indice generale degli incunaboli delle biblioteche d'Italia. Rome, 1943–81.

KEYNES

Geoffrey Keynes. *A Bibliography of the Writings of Dr. William Harvey 1578–1637.* 3d ed., revised by Gweneth Whitteridge and Christine English. Winchester, 1989.

KLEBS

A. C. Klebs. *Incunabula scientifica et medica.* Bruges, 1938.

KRIVATSY

Peter Krivatsy. *A Catalogue of Seventeenth Century Printed Books in the National Library of Medicine.* Bethesda, Md., 1989.

KYRISS

Ernst Kyriss. *Verzierte gotische Einbände im alten deutschen Sprachgebiet.* 4 vols. Stuttgart, 1951–58.

LEFANU

William LeFanu. *A Bibliography of Edward Jenner.* 2d ed. Winchester, 1985.

LEFANU *Lister*

William LeFanu. *A List of the Original Writings of Joseph Lord Lister*, O. M. Edinburgh & London, 1965.

LINDEBOOM

G. A. Lindeboom. *Bibliographia Boerhaaviana: List of Publications Written or Provided by H. Boerhaave or Based Upon His Works and Teaching.* Leiden, 1959.

MALLOIZEL

G. Malloizel. "Bibliographie des travaux scientifiques: Mémoires, lectures et communications aux Académies et Sociétés savantes," in *L'Oeuvre de Claude Bernard* (Paris, 1881).

MAUROIS

André Maurois. "Bibliography," in *The Life of Sir Alexander Fleming, Discoverer of Penicillin,* translated by Gerard Hopkins (New York, 1959), pp. 281–86.

NEEDHAM

Paul Needham. *Twelve Centuries of Bookbindings, 400–1600.* New York, 1979.

NICHOLAS

J. S. Nicholas. "Ross Granville Harrison," *Biographical Memoirs of the National Academy of Sciences of the United States of America* 35 (1961): 132–62.

NIXON

Howard M. Nixon. *Sixteenth-Century Gold-Tooled Bookbindings in the Pierpont Morgan Library.* New York, 1971.

NORMAN

Diana H. Hook and Jeremy M. Norman. *The Haskell F. Norman Library of Science and Medicine.* 2 vols. San Francisco, 1991.

OSLER

Bibliotheca Osleriana: A Catalogue of Books Illustrating the History of Medicine and Science. Oxford, 1929; reprinted, Montreal & London, 1969.

OSLER *Incunabula medica*

William Osler and Victor Scholderer. *Incunabula medica: A Study of the Earliest Printed Medical Books 1467–1480.* Oxford, 1923.

PELLECHET

Marie Pellechet (and Marie-Louise Polain). *Catalogue général des incunables des bibliothèques publiques de France.* Paris, 1897–1909.

PETERS & FULTON

Charlotte H. Peters and John F. Fulton. "William Beaumont's Letter to His New Haven Bookseller, Hezekiah Howe, with a Bibliographical Description of the Editions of Beaumont's Book," *Yale Journal of Biology and Medicine* 6 (1933–34): 9–17.

PMM

Printing and the Mind of Man: A Descriptive Catalogue Illustrating the Impact of Print on the Evolution of Western Civilization during Five Centuries. Compiled and edited by John Carter and Percy H. Muir, et al. London & New York, 1967.

RAVITCH

Mark M. Ravitch, ed. "Curriculum Vitae and Bibliography," in *The Papers of Alfred Blalock* (2 vols., Baltimore, 1966), vol. 2, pp. 1982–92.

RENOUARD

Antoine-Auguste Renouard. *Annales de l'imprimerie des Alde.* 3d ed. Paris, 1834.

SACHS

H. Sachs. "Bibliographie," in *Paul Ehrlich: Eine Darstellung seines wissenschaftlichen Wirkens* (Jena, 1914), pp. 625–57.

SCHWALBE

J. Schwalbe. *Virchow-Bibliographie 1843–1901.* Berlin, 1901.

SKRETKOWICZ

Victor Skretkowicz. "Florence Nightingale's Notes on Nursing: The First Version and Edition," *The Library,* 6th series, 15 (1993): 24–46.

STC

A Short-Title Catalogue of Books Printed in England, Scotland, and Ireland and of English Books Printed Abroad 1475–1640. First compiled by A. W. Polland and G. R. Redgrave. 2d ed., revised and enlarged, begun by W. A. Jackson and F. S. Ferguson, completed by Katharine F. Pantzer. 3 vols. London, 1976–91.

STEVENSON

Lloyd Stevenson. "Bibliography," in *Sir Frederick Banting* (rev. ed., London, 1947), pp. 438–40.

STILLWELL

Margaret B. Stillwell. *The Awakening Interest in Science During the First Century of Printing 1450–1550: An Annotated Checklist of First Editions Viewed from the Angle of Their Subject Content.* New York, 1970.

SUDHOFF

Karl Sudhoff. *Versuch einer Kritik der Echtheit der Paracelsischen Schriften.* 2 vols. Berlin, 1894–99.

VIETS

Henry R. Viets. "Some Editions of Laennec's Work on Mediate Auscultation," *Boston Medical and Surgical Journal* 195 (1926): 213–17.

WALLER

H. Sallander. *Bibliotheca Walleriana: The Books Illustrating the History of Medicine and Science Collected by Dr. Erik Waller.* Stockholm, 1955.

WELLCOME

A Catalogue of Printed Books in the Wellcome Historical Medical Library. London, 1962– .

WING

Short-Title Catalogue of Books Printed in England, Scotland, Ireland, Wales, and British America and also of English Books Printed in Other Countries 1641–1700. Compiled by Donald Wing. 2d ed. 3 vols. New York, 1972–88.

ZANELLI

Renato Zanelli. "Catalogo ragionato delle edizioni morgagnane in ordine cronologico," in *Le onoranze a G. B. Morgagni, Forlì, 24 maggio 1931–IX.* Siena, 1931.

ONE HUNDRED BOOKS
FAMOUS IN MEDICINE

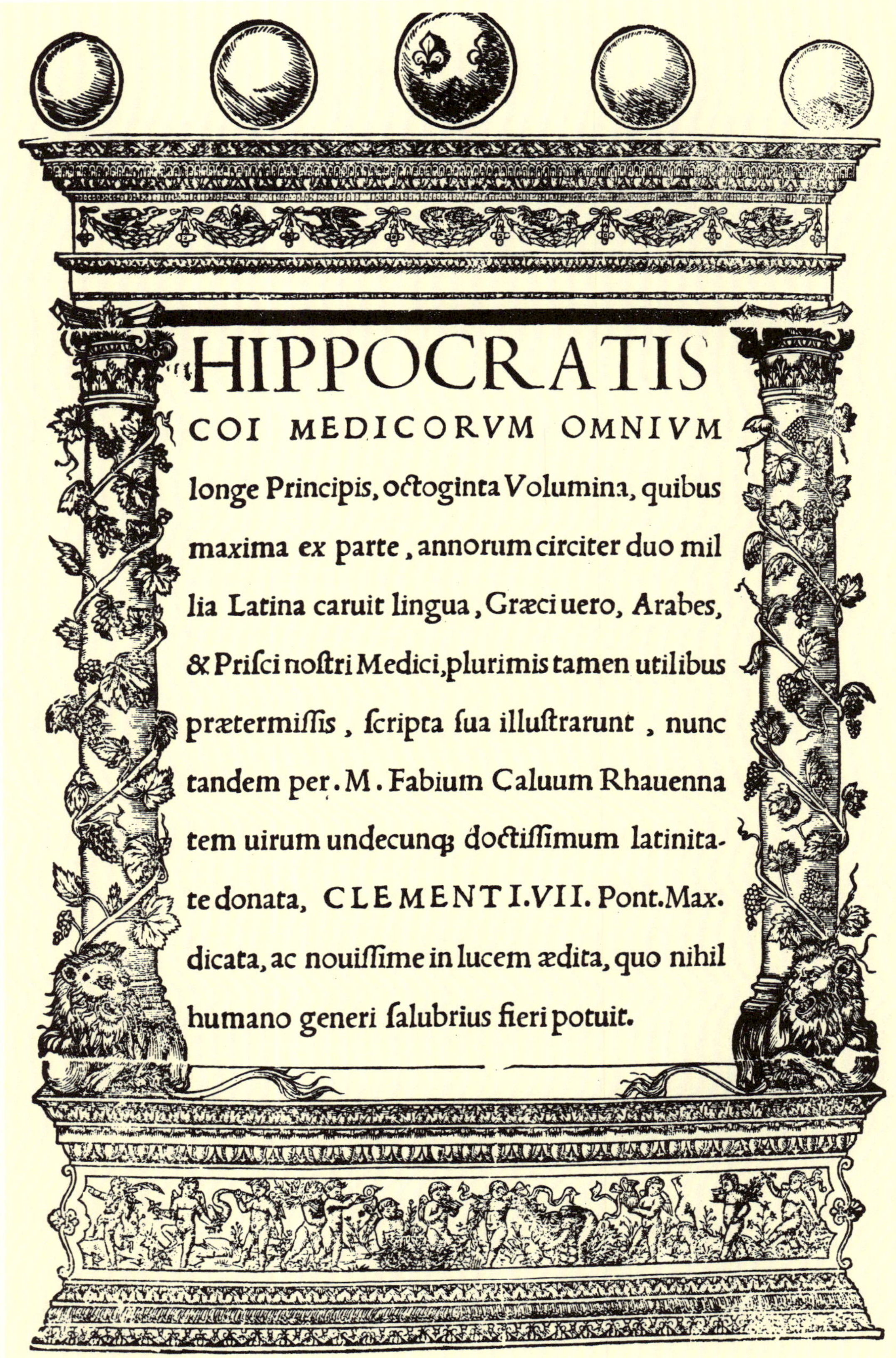
HIPPOCRATIS
COI MEDICORVM OMNIVM
longe Principis, octoginta Volumina, quibus
maxima ex parte, annorum circiter duo mil
lia Latina caruit lingua, Græci uero, Arabes,
& Priſci noſtri Medici, plurimis tamen utilibus
prætermiſſis, ſcripta ſua illuſtrarunt, nunc
tandem per. M. Fabium Caluum Rhauenna
tem uirum undecunq; doctiſſimum latinita-
te donata, CLEMENTI.VII. Pont.Max.
dicata, ac nouiſſime in lucem ædita, quo nihil
humano generi ſalubrius fieri potuit.

Fig. 1. No. 1A. Hippocrates. Title page of the Latin *editio princeps* (1525).

I

HIPPOCRATES

(460 B.C.–ca. 370 B.C.)

A] *Hippocratis Coi medicorum omnium longe principis, octoginta volumina, quibus maxima ex parte, annorum circiter duo millia Latina caruit lingua . . . nunc tandem per M. Fabium Caluum . . . latinitate donata.*

Rome: Ex aedibus Francisci Minitii Calvi, 1525.

2°: π–2π4 A–E6 F4 A–Z6 AA–ZZ6 AAA–OOO6 PPP8. 410 leaves, pp. [84] I–DLXXV DLXXVII–DCCXXXIII [i.e., 732] [4].

Adams H–567. Durling 2320. cf. GM 13. *Heirs of Hippocrates* 10. Norman 1076. Osler 149. PMM 55. Stillwell 406, 657. Waller 4495. Wellcome 3177.

B] Ἅπαντα τὰ τοῦ Ἱπποκράτους. *Omnia opera Hippocratis.*

Venice: In aedibus Aldi, & Andreae Asulani soceri, May 1526.

2°: *6 A–Z8 AA–EE8 FF10. 240 leaves, ff. [6] 1–233 [1].

Adams H–563. Durling 2316. cf. GM 13. Norman 1077. Osler 142. Renouard 1526.1 (p. 102). Stillwell 405, 656. Wellcome 3173.

C] Iusiurandum [Hippocratic Oath]. In: *Articella.*

Venice: Hermannus Liechtenstein, 29 March 1483.

2°: a–d8 e6 f–s8 t–u6 v–z8 A–C8 D6. 216 leaves, ff. *1* 2–150 [4] 151–212.

BSB–Ink. A–786. cf. GM 1757.90. Goff A–1143. GW 2679. Klebs 116.2. Stillwell 414. Wellcome 493.

The texts assigned to Hippocrates are "Hippocratic" in the sense that the manuscript tradition routinely labelled them as such. It is uncertain which of them, if any, are directly connected with the historical physician Hippocrates of Cos, who flourished in the latter half of the fifth century B.C. Through the writings attributed to him Hippocrates is credited with developing the first system of empirical medicine based on clinical experience, and the Hippocratic *Oath* has long been regarded as expressing the fundamental ethical and moral standards of the medical profession.

The Hippocratic corpus, brought together probably in Alexandria from the writings attributed to Hippocrates and his school, has exerted a most profound influence on all

ἍΠΑΝΤΑ ΤᾺ ΤΟΥ͂ ἹΠΠΟΚΡΆΤΟΥΣ.

OMNIA OPERA HIPPOCRATIS.

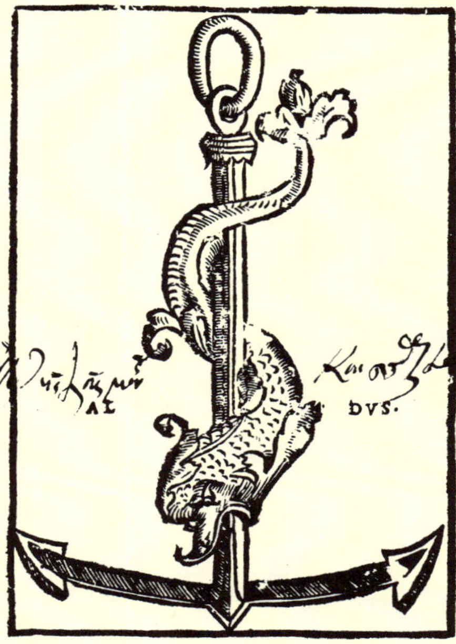

Ne quis alius impune, aut Venetiis, aut uſquam lo-
corum hos Hippocratis libros imprimat, &
Clementis VII. Pont. Max. & Sena-
tus Veneti decreto cau-
tum eſt.

Fig. 2. No. 1B. Hippocrates. Title page of the Greek *editio princeps* (1526).

subsequent Western medical thought. Aristotle quoted from the *Nature of Man*; Diocles of Carystus and Herophilus of Chalcedon each alluded to several treatises; Apollonius of Citium built the discussion in his treatise *On Joints* around the Hippocratic book of the same title; and Erotian in the first century A.D. devoted a dictionary to difficult Hippocratic words; it is in the preface to this work that the first list of Hippocratic titles (about forty) is found. Galen dealt at great length with many of the writings and raised "Hippocrates" to a quasi-divine status as first discoverer of the medical art.

This reputation carried the figure, if not the writings, triumphantly through the Middle Ages. Of the writings, the most popular, judging from the number of Arabic and Latin translations and commentaries, were undoubtedly the *Aphorisms* and *Prognostic*, with *Regimen in Acute Diseases*, *Epidemics*, *Nature of Man*, *Airs, Waters and Places*, and the *Oath* distant followers. There was apparently no attempt, as in the case of Galen (see no. 5), to translate the bulk of the corpus into Arabic in the ninth century, or into Latin in the thirteenth and fourteenth centuries, so that when printing was introduced in the fifteenth century, only this relatively small group of works, with a few later and partly apocryphal additions, found its way into the new medium.

The project of preparing a complete Latin translation of the Hippocratic corpus was undertaken by Marcus Fabius Calvus (ca. 1440–1527) of Ravenna toward the end of the first decade of the sixteenth century. As a first step, he wrote out by hand his own Greek text (Vaticanus graecus 278) based on the collation of at least three authorities: Parisinus graecus 2140 (XIV cent.), Vaticanus graecus 277 (XIV cent.), and Laurentianus graecus 74.1 (XV cent.); this, as he recorded on the last page of his copy, he completed in Rome on 24 July 1512. Translation into Latin was completed on 14 August 1515. Why publication did not follow until ten years later is nowhere explained, but perhaps the dedication of the printed edition to Pope Clement VII (1523–34) indicates belated support from that quarter.

Calvus's stoic character and his paternal relationship with the young Raphael of Urbino, for whom he prepared an Italian translation of the Roman architectural writer Vitruvius in 1514, are portrayed in a letter of 1519 from Celio Calcagnini to Jakob Ziegler.[1]

In spite of ten-year privileges granted by Pope Clement VII and King Francis I of France, Calvus's edition was reprinted the following year in Basel by Andreas Cratander with only a few substitutions: Calvus's translations of *Regimen in Acute Diseases* and *Prognostic* were replaced by those of Wilhelm Cop (1487–ca. 1562), his *Aphorisms* by the version of Niccolò Leoniceno (1428–1524), and his *Nature of Man* by the translation of Andrea Brenta (1460–ca. 1485). Complete reprints of Calvus's translations appeared in Rome in 1549, 1610, and 1619.

The Greek *editio princeps* of the Hippocratic corpus was published in 1526 by the successors of Aldus Manutius. It presented no special difficulties to the Aldine press, since the text was neither exceptional among ancient writings for length, fitting neatly into one fo-

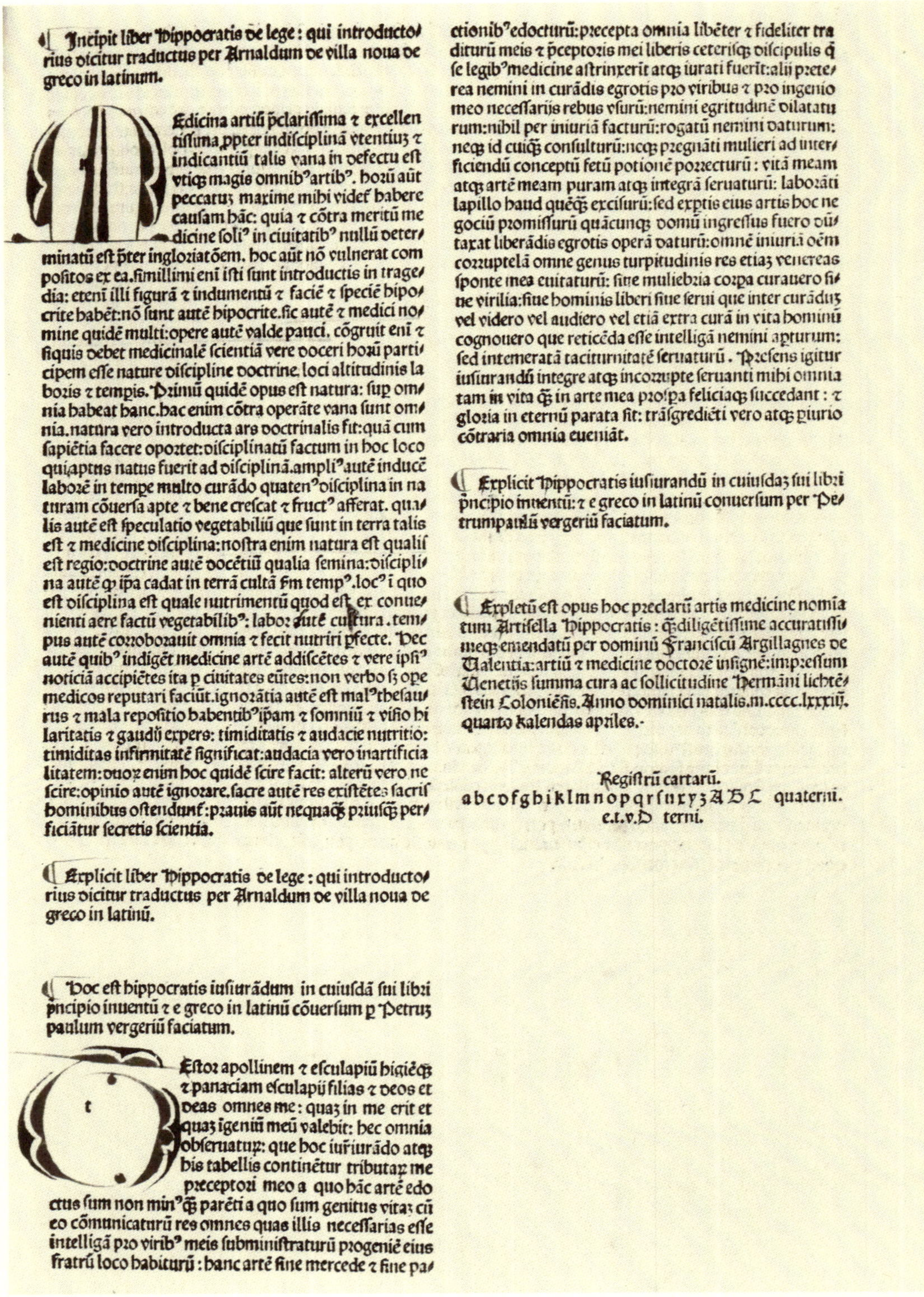

Incipit liber Hippocratis de lege: qui introductorius dicitur traductus per Arnaldum de villa noua de greco in latinum.

Medicina artiū pclarissima ꝛ excellentissima ppter indisciplinā ꝟtentiuꝫ ꝛ indicantiū talis vana in defectu est vtiqꝫ magis omnibꝰ artibꝰ. horū aūt peccatuꝫ maxime mihi videt habere causam hāc: quia ꝛ cōtra meritū medicine soliꝰ in ciuitatibꝰ nullū determinatū est pter inglorātōem. hoc aūt nō vulnerat compositos ex ea. simillimi enī isti sunt introductis in tragedia: etenī illi figurā ꝛ indumentū ꝛ faciē ꝛ speciē hipocrite habēt: nō sunt autē hipocrite. sic autē ꝛ medici nomine quidē multi: opere autē valde pauci. cōgruit enī ꝛ siquis debet medicinalē scientiā vere doceri horū participem esse nature disciplinę doctrine. loci altitudinis laboris ꝛ tempis. Primū quidē opus est natura: sup omnia habeat hanc. hac enim cōtra operāte vana sunt omnia. natura vero introducta ars doctrinalis fit: quā cum sapiētia facere opoztet: disciplinatū factum in hoc loco qui aptus natus fuerit ad disciplinā. ampliꝰ autē inducē laborē in tempe multo curādo quatenꝰ disciplina in naturam cōuersa apte ꝛ bene crescat ꝛ fructꝰ afferat. qualis autē est speculatio vegetabiliū que sunt in terra talis est ꝛ medicine disciplina: nostra enim natura est qualis est regio: doctrine autē docētiū qualia semina: disciplina autē qꝫ ipa cadat in terrā cultā fm tempꝰ. locꝰ i quo est disciplina est quale nutrimentū quod est ex conuenienti aere factū vegetabilibꝰ: labor autē cultura. tempus autē corroborauit omnia ꝛ fecit nutriri pfecte. Hec autē quibꝰ indigēt medicine artē addiscētes ꝛ vere ipsiꝰ noticiā accipiētes ita p ciuitates eūtes: non verbo sꝫ ope medicos reputari faciūt. ignorātia autē est malꝰ thesaurus ꝛ mala repositio habentibꝰ ipam ꝛ somniū ꝛ visio hilaritatis ꝛ gaudij expers: timiditatis ꝛ audacie nutritio: timiditas infirmitatē significat: audacia vero inartificialitatem: duoꝫ enim hoc quidē scire facit: alterū vero nescire: opinio autē ignorare. facre autē res existētes facris hominibus ostendunt: prauis aūt nequaqꝫ priusqꝫ perficiātur secretis scientie.

Explicit liber Hippocratis de lege: qui introductorius dicitur traductus per Arnaldum de villa noua de greco in latinū.

Hoc est hippocratis iusiurādum in cuiusdā sui libri pncipio inuentū ꝛ e greco in latinū cōuersum p Petruꝫ paulum vergeriū faciatum.

Testor apollinem ꝛ esculapiū higiēqꝫ ꝛ panaciam esculapij filias ꝛ deos et deas omnes me: quaꝫ in me erit et quaꝫ igeniū meū valebit: hec omnia obseruatup: que hoc iurirādo atqꝫ his tabellis continētur tributap me preceptori meo a quo hāc artē edoctus sum non minꝰ qꝫ parēti a quo sum genitus vitaꝫ cū eo cōmunicaturū res omnes quas illis necessarias esse intelligā pro viribꝰ meis subministraturū progeniē eius fratrū loco habiturū: hanc artē sine mercede ꝛ sine pactionibꝰ edocturū: precepta omnia libēter ꝛ fideliter traditurū meis ꝛ pceptoris mei liberis ceterisqꝫ discipulis qꝫ se legibꝰ medicine astrinxerit atqꝫ iurati fuerit: alij preterea nemini in curādis egrotis pro viribus ꝛ pro ingenio meo necessarijs rebus vsurū: nemini egritudinē dilataturum: nihil per iniuriā facturū: rogatū nemini daturum: neqꝫ id cuiqꝫ consulturū: neqꝫ pregnāti mulieri ad interficiendū conceptū fetū potionē porrecturū: vitā meam atqꝫ artē meam puram atqꝫ integrā seruaturū: laborāti lapillo haud queqꝫ excisurū: sed exptis eius artis hoc negociū promissurū quācunqꝫ domū ingressus fuero dūtaxat liberādis egrotis operā daturū: omnē iniuriā oēm corruptelā omne genus turpitudinis res etiaꝫ venereas sponte mea euitaturū: siue muliebria corpa curauero siue virilia: siue hominis liberi siue serui que inter curāduꝫ vel videro vel audiero vel etiā extra curā in vita hominū cognouero que reticēda esse intelligā nemini apturum: sed intemeratā taciturnitatē seruaturū. Presens igitur iusiurandū integre atqꝫ incorrupte seruanti mihi omnia tam in vita qꝫ in arte mea prospa feliciaqꝫ succedant: ꝛ gloria in eternū parata sit: trāsgredieti vero atqꝫ piurio cōtraria omnia eueniāt.

Explicit Hippocratis iusiurandū in cuiusdaꝫ sui libri pncipio inuentū: ꝛ e greco in latinū conuersum per Petrumpaulū vergeriū faciatum.

Expletū est opus hoc preclarū artis medicine nomiatum Articella Hippocratis: qꝫ diligētissime accuratissimeqꝫ emendatū per dominū Franciscū Argillagnes de Ualentia: artiū ꝛ medicine doctorē insignē: impressum Venetijs summa cura ac sollicitudine Hermāni lichtestein Colonieñs. Anno dominici natalis. m. cccc. lxxxiij. quarto kalendas apriles.

Registrū cartarū.
abcdfghiklmnopqrsturyꝫ A B C quaterni.
e.t.v.D terni.

Fig. 3. No. 1c. Hippocrates. The first printing of the Hippocratic Oath, in the *Articella* (1483). The text of the Oath ("Iusiurandum") begins at the foot of the left-hand column.

lio volume, nor difficult to assemble, as it was frequently to be found almost complete in one manuscript. The manuscript that served as printer's copy for this edition, Parisinus graecus 2141 (XV cent.), displays between its lines and in its margins the many changes and additions that the editor, Franciscus Asulanus, made in preparation for printing. These corrections derive in the main—there are a few isolated variants from other manuscripts, and even fewer original conjectures—from the tenth-century Marcianus graecus 269. This manuscript was one of the original 468 Greek manuscripts that Cardinal Bessarion (1403–72) collected from all over the Greek world and donated in 1468 to the Venetian Republic in order to preserve the endangered heritage of Antiquity for future generations. Although donated on the condition that there be "free access to all who wish to read and study them," in fact the manuscripts lay largely inaccessible for half a century, until Andrea Navagero, who became librarian in 1515, attempted to recover what had gone astray and order what had lain unsorted. Thus, although Aldus himself evidently never had the use of Bessarion's collection, by the 1520s his successors did have access to this inestimable treasure.

The Aldine Greek edition of Hippocrates marked a significant advance over Calvus's Latin translation. As Franciscus Asulanus pointed out in his notice to the reader, it repaired a considerable number of accidental omissions and one long repetition that Calvus—"whose industry is otherwise worthy of immortal praise"—made because he followed only one manuscript. Moreover, by presenting the original text, it laid the necessary foundation for all further philological and medical study of the corpus.

The Hippocratic *Oath* first appeared in print in a collection of medical works whose roots can be traced back to the School of Salerno, the earliest center of organized medical instruction in medieval Europe, and to the early twelfth century. By that time a core of five theoretical, medical texts in Latin translation had coalesced, which, with various accretions, went on to play a significant role in European medical education well into the sixteenth century. The earliest manuscripts contain these writings: Ḥunayn ibn Isḥāq (808–873), *Questions on Medicine* (= Johannitii *Isagoge*); Hippocrates, *Aphorisms*; Hippocrates, *Prognostic*; Theophilus Protospatharius (VII cent.), *On Urines*; and Philaretus (IX/X cent.), *On Pulses.*

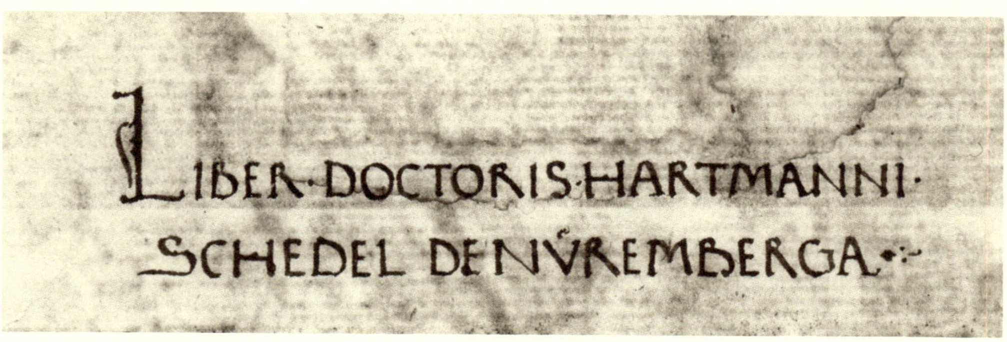

Fig. 4. No. 1C. Hartmann Schedel's mark of ownership in his copy of the *Articella.*

About the middle of the twelfth century Galen's *Medical Art* (=*Ars parva*=*Microtegni*) was added to the collection, and early in the thirteenth century the Hippocratic *Regimen in Acute Diseases.* Manuscripts of the succeeding two and a half centuries contain this canon of seven writings, often supplemented by Latin versions of Greek, Arabic, and contemporary commentaries on them, and by various other medical texts. The first printed edition, which appeared about 1476 in Padua, contained the seven traditional treatises (BSB–Ink. A–785). The second edition, dated 1483, bears the title *Artisella Hippocratis,* derived from the Galenic *Ars parva* and usually standardized to *Articella.* It contains, besides the seven treatises of the earlier edition, a second version of the *Aphorisms* and these additional works: Hippocrates, *Epidemics VI*; Hippocrates, *Nature of the Child*; Gentile da Foligno (d. 1348), *Division of Galenic Books*; and Hippocrates, *Law* and *Oath.*

From the time of this printing of the Hippocratic *Oath* in the Latin translation of Pier Paolo Vergerio (1370–1444), the document became popular, appearing in the four subsequent incunable editions of the *Articella,* as well as in several selected editions of medical and other works, including an undated edition of Perottus's *De generibus metrorum* that was printed before 6 June 1483 (IGI 7430). The *Oath* also appeared in the collected Hippocratic editions beginning with Calvus (1525).

About the origins of the *Oath,* W.H.S. Jones has said with truth:

> . . . its exact relationship to the history of medicine is unknown, and apparently, in our present state of knowledge, unknowable. The student must, at every stage of the inquiry, confess his ignorance. What is the date of the *oath*? Is it mutilated or interpolated? Who took the *oath,* all practitioners or only those belonging to a guild? What binding force had it beyond its moral sanction? Above all, was it ever a reality or merely a "counsel of perfection"? To all these questions the honest inquirer can only say that for certain he knows nothing.[2]

The *Oath* is first mentioned in the first century A.D., in the list of Hippocratic works given in the introduction to Erotian's *Hippocratic Glossary,* and also in a prefatory letter to the *Compositiones* of Scribonius Largus (I cent.). Scribonius, who was physician to the emperor Claudius, integrated the Hippocratic ideals into a Roman framework of *humanitas*:

> Hippocrates, the founder of our profession, passed down the principles of our discipline in an oath, which forbids a physician to give or reveal to a pregnant woman any drug that causes abortion of the fetus; in this way Hippocrates sought to forcefully cultivate humanity in the souls of his students. . . . He holds it to be of great importance that physicians preserve the name and reputation of medicine through pure and holy hearts, and practice according to his principles. For medicine is the art of healing, not of harming.[3]

The *Oath* was also referred to by Soranus of Ephesus (I/II cent.) and maintained a secure place in the Hippocratic corpus through the Middle Ages. It was translated into

Arabic by Ḥunayn, playing a fundamental role in Islamic medical deontology, and appeared several times in Latin translation from the twelfth century onwards. The first edition in English is found in a collection of surgical works entitled *A Most Excellent and Compendious Method of Curing Woundes in the Head, and in Other Parts of the Body . . .* (London, 1588), edited by John Read, and headed by the first English translation of Francesco Arceo's *De recta curandorum vulnerum ratione* (STC 723). It was, however, the inclusion of the *Oath* in the *Articella* and the *Opera omnia* of Hippocrates that secured for it a central place in the European medical consciousness, a role that, once achieved, it has never relinquished.

PP

1. Quoted by E. Littré, ed., *Oeuvres complètes d'Hippocrate* (10 vols., Paris, 1839–61) I, p. 542.
2. *Hippocrates* (Loeb Classical Library, London, 1923) I, p. 291.
3. Scribonius Largus, *Compositiones* (Bibliotheca Teubneriana, Leipzig, 1983), p. 2.

See color plate 1.

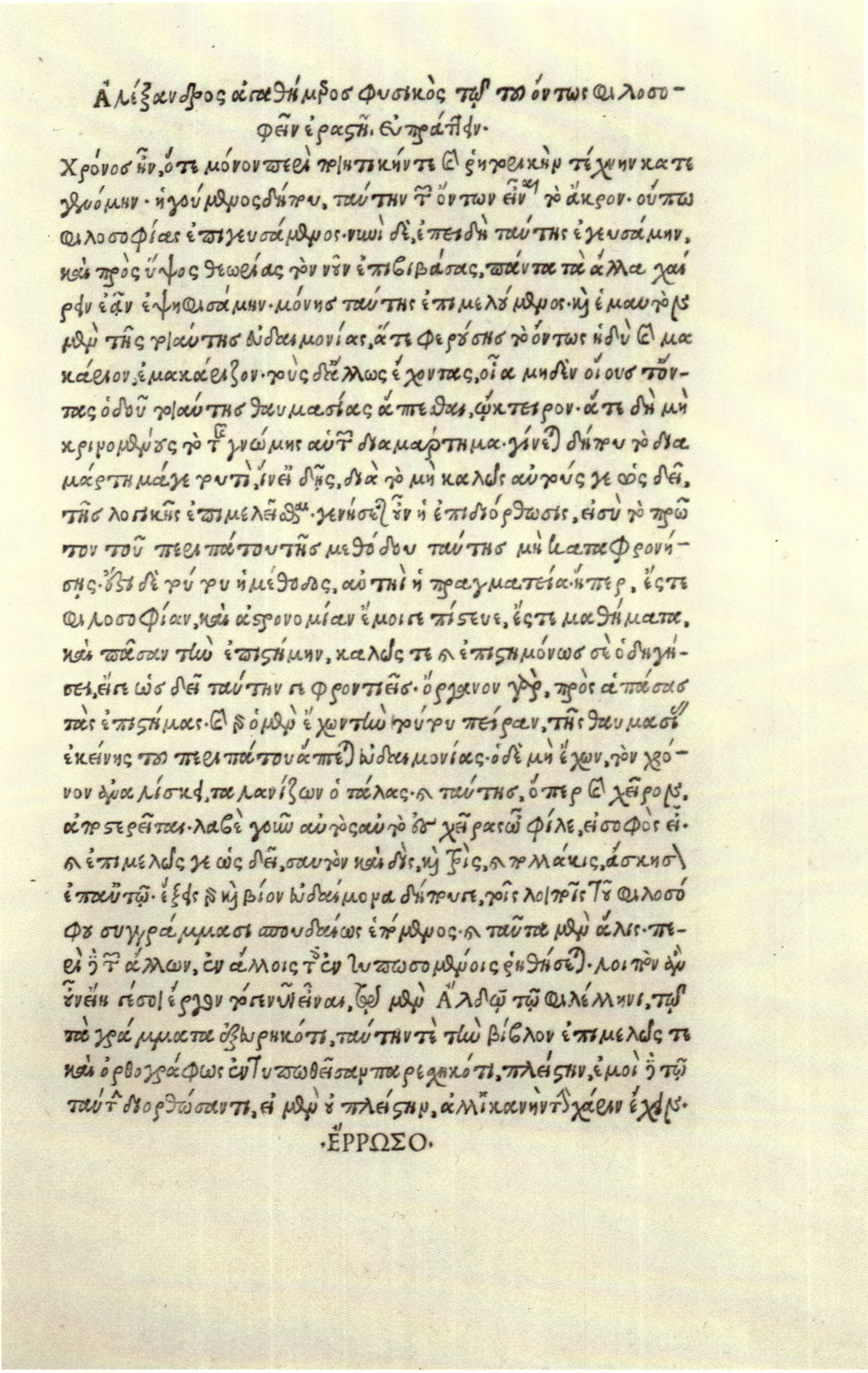
Ἀλέξανδρος ἀγαθήμερος φυσικὸς τῷ τῷ ὄντως φιλοσο-
φεῖν ἐρασθέντι εὖ πράττειν.

Χρόνος ἦν, ὅτε μόνον περὶ ἰατρικήν τε καὶ χειρουργικὴν τέχνην κατε-
γινόμην· ἡγούμενος δήπου, ταύτην τῶν ὄντων εἶναι τὸ ἄκρον· οὔπω
φιλοσοφίας ἐπιγευσάμενος· νυνὶ δὲ, ἐπειδὴ ταύτης ἐγευσάμην,
καὶ πρὸς ὕψος θεωρίας τὸν νοῦν ἐπιβιβάσας, πάντα τὰ ἄλλα χαί-
ρειν ἐᾶν ἐψηφισάμην· μόνης ταύτης ἐπιμελούμενος· καὶ ἐμαυτὸν
μὲν τῆς τοιαύτης εὐδαιμονίας, ἅτε φερούσης τὸ ὄντως ἡδὺ καὶ μα-
κάριον, ἐμακάριζον· τοὺς δὲ ἄλλως ἔχοντας, οἷα μηδὲν οἵους τε ὄν-
τας ὁδοῦ τοιαύτης θαυμασίας ἅπτεσθαι, ᾤκτειρον· ἅτε δὴ μὴ
κρινομένους τὸ τῆς γνώμης αὐτῶν διαμάρτημα· γίνεται δήπου τὸ δια-
μάρτημα γε τουτὶ, ἵν᾽ εἰδῇς, διὰ τὸ μὴ καλῶς αὐτούς γε ὡς δεῖ,
τῆς λογικῆς ἐπιμελεῖσθαι· γενήσεται γοῦν ἡ ἐπιδιόρθωσις, εἰ σὺ τὸ πρῶ-
τον τοῦ περιπάτου τῆς μεθόδου ταύτης μὴ καταφρονή-
σῃς· ἔστι δὲ τοῦ τοῦ ἡ μέθοδος, αὐτὴ ἡ πραγματεία ἥπερ, ἔστι
φιλοσοφίαν, καὶ ἀστρονομίαν ἐμοί γε πίστευε, ἔστι μαθήματα,
καὶ πᾶσαν τὴν ἐπιστήμην, καλῶς τε καὶ ἐπιστημόνως σε ὁδηγή-
σει, εἴ γε ὡς δεῖ ταύτην σε φροντιεῖς· ὄργανον γάρ, πρὸς ἁπάσας
τὰς ἐπιστήμας· καὶ γὰρ ὁ μὲν ἔχων τὴν τούτου πεῖραν, τῆς θαυμασί-
ας ἐκείνης τοῦ περιπάτου ἅπτεται εὐδαιμονίας· ὁ δὲ μὴ ἔχων, τὸν χρό-
νον ἀναλίσκει, ταλανίζων ὁ τάλας· καὶ ταύτης, ὅπερ καὶ χεῖρόν ἐστιν,
ἀποστερεῖται· λαβὲ γοῦν αὐτὸς αὐτὸ εἰς χεῖρας ὦ φίλε, εἰ σοφὸς εἶ·
καὶ ἐπιμελῶς γε ὡς δεῖ, σαυτὸν καὶ δὶς, καὶ τρίς, καὶ πολλάκις, ἄσκησον
ἐν τούτῳ· ἐξῆς δὲ καὶ βίον εὐδαίμονα δήπου γε, τοῖς λοιποῖς τοῦ φιλοσό-
φου συγγράμμασι σπουδαίως ἑπόμενος· καὶ ταῦτα μὲν ἅλις· περὶ
δὲ τῶν ἄλλων, ἐν ἄλλοις τοῖς ἐντυπωσομένοις ἐκτεθήσεται· λοιπὸν ἂν
εἴη σοι ἔργον τὸ συνιέναι, τῷ μὲν Ἄλδῳ τῷ φιλέλληνι, τῷ
τὰ γράμματα ἐξευρηκότι, ταύτην τε τὴν βίβλον ἐπιμελῶς τε
καὶ ὀρθογράφως ἐντυπωθεῖσαν παρεσχηκότι, πλείστην, ἐμοὶ δὲ τῷ
ταύτην διορθώσαντι, εἰ μὲν οὐ πλείστην, ἀλλ᾽ ἱκανήν τινα χάριν ἔχειν.

·ἜΡΡΩΣΟ·

Fig. 5. No. 2B. Aristotle. Opening page of Volume I (1495) of the *Opera omnia*, showing Aldus Manutius's first Greek type.

2

ARISTOTLE
(384–322 B.C.)

A] *De animalibus.*

Venice: Johannes de Colonia and Johannes Manthen, 1476.

2°: a–b^{10} c–d^{8} e–k$^{10/8}$ l–t^{10} u^{8} x^{10} aa–dd^{10} ee^{8} ff^{6}. 252 leaves.

BMC V, 232. Goff A–973. GW 2350. Klebs 85.1. Norman 69. Osler 239. Osler *Incunabula medica* 106. Stillwell 573. Waller 16. Wellcome 425.

B] *Opera* [Greek].

Venice: Aldus Manutius Romanus, 1 November 1495, February 1497, January [Greek colophon: 29 January] 1497, 1 June 1497, June 1498.

[Vol. I] 2°: A–C^{8} Δ^{8} E–K^{8} L–N^{6} a–c^{8} d–e^{6} f–i^{8} κ^{8} l–q^{8} r–s^{6}. 234 leaves.

[Vol. II] 2°: *^{8} ※^{8} +^{8}@^{8} aα–oξ^{8} pπ–rς^{8} sσ–zψ^{8} &ω^{8} A–B^{8} CΓ^{6} DΔ–HΘ^{8} I^{8} K^{6}. 300 leaves, ff. [32] 1–268.

[Vol. III] 2°: aaαα–iiιι^{10} κκ^{10} llλλ–zzψψ^{10} &&ωω^{10} AA–ΠΠ^{10} χPP^{2}(–χPP$_{2}$) PP–ΦΦ^{10} XX^{8}※^{8}. 467 leaves, ff. 1–400 [1] 401–457 [1] [8].

[Vol. IV] 2°: [+]^{2} aaaααα–iiiιιι^{8} κκκ^{8} lllλλλ–zzzψψψ^{8} &&&ωωω^{8} AAA–BBB^{8} CCCΓΓΓ^{8} DDDΔΔΔ^{10}; AAAaaa–MMMmmm^{8} NNNnnn–ΞΞΞooo^{10} α′a–δ′d^{8} ε′e^{10} a′α–b′β^{6} AAAααα–OOOξξξ^{8} PPPooo^{10}. 520 leaves, ff. 1 [1] 1–226; 1–116, 1–42, 1–12, 1–121 [1].

[Vol. V] 2°: αααα–ιιιι^{10} κκκκ^{4} λλλλ–φφφφ^{10} χχχχ^{6} ψψψψ^{12} ωωωω^{10} AAAA–BBBB^{10} ΓΓΓΓ^{6} ΔΔΔΔ–IIII^{10} KKKK^{12}. 330 leaves, ff. *1* 2–209 [1] [12] 210–316 [1].

BMC V, 553, 556, 555, 556, 558. Doheny, lot 105. cf. GM 17. Goff A–959. GW 2334. Klebs 83.1. Norman 70. Osler 229. PMM 38. Stillwell 570. Wellcome 414.

Aristotle, pupil of Plato and tutor of Alexander the Great, made substantial contributions not only to the disciplines of logic and philosophy but also to the body of scientific knowledge and theory that became part of the heritage of classical Antiquity to Western culture. Aristotle's works formed the basis of philosophical and scientific instruction in European universities from the thirteenth century to the seventeenth, and the character of modern scientific thought still reflects features of his method: the conviction that only individual substances are real, that observation is the foundation of knowledge, that classification of phenomena is the key to clear thought about the nature of things, that knowledge is advanced by generalizing from particulars and by formulating and testing hypotheses based on what is observed.

Aristotle took considerable interest in natural history and medicine, and his treatises on zoology make up a quarter of his extant works. Although his knowledge of human anatomy and physiology was weak, he left several works of descriptive zoology that embody information based on observation, and sometimes on dissection, of both familiar and exotic animals. When three of these texts were published in Latin in 1476, this was the first collection of treatises on biology to be printed.

Included in the eighteen books of *De animalibus* are Latin translations of Aristotle's main zoological works: *Historia animalium* (Inquiry into animals), Books 1–9; *De partibus animalium* (Parts of animals), Books 1–4; and *De generatione animalium* (Generation of animals), Books 1–5. The Greek manuscript on which the translator Theodorus Gaza (ca. 1400–75) based his translations lacked *Historia animalium*, Book 10, now thought to be spurious. Gaza also changed the order of *Historia animalium*'s later books on the basis of a remark Aristotle made in *Historia animalium*, Book 5, to the effect that his account of reproduction in man would come last. This account, Book 9 of the manuscripts, belonged, according to Gaza, after the account of reproduction in animals (Books 5 and 6), not at the end of the whole work after Book 8, where he supposed Aristotle's heirs had mistakenly placed it; thus he moved the book from ninth to seventh position, with the result that Books 7 and 8 of the manuscripts became Books 8 and 9 in the printed edition. This rearrangement was accepted by the editor of the 1497 Aldine Greek *Opera*, and in fact by all subsequent editors.

Historia animalium is an immense collection of biological data—anatomical, physiological, behavioral—on over five hundred species of animals. Aristotle's interest lay in identifying and classifying groups of animals and in explaining their functioning as a part of nature, and it was the data reported in *Historia animalium* that provided the basis for his philosophical analyses of relationships between structure, function, and purpose. In *De partibus animalium* he explored these "links of causation" in the various groups of animals. In *De generatione animalium* he dealt with the principles of animal generation, including organs and secretions, gave a detailed account of generation in the different groups of animals, answered various questions connected with generation, and finally gave an explanation of development after birth and of the differences between individuals of the same species. Joseph Needham, in his history of embryology, called *De generatione animalium* "the first great compendium of embryology ever written."[1]

The keen interest in Aristotle in fifteenth-century Italy, particularly in connection with the Platonic-Aristotelian debate, stimulated a new round of translations, directly from the Greek, to replace earlier medieval Latin versions by such translators as Michael Scotus (died ca. 1235) and William of Moerbeke (ca. 1215–ca. 1286). In 1450 Pope Nicholas V (1447–55) called a number of scholars, including several Greek exiles, to Rome to carry out Aristotelian translations. Many of these translations appeared in print in the later decades of the century: a Latin version of the *Rhetoric* (Paris, ca. 1476–77; CIBN A–535), translated by George Trapezuntius (1395–1472); and Latin translations by John Argyropoulos (1393/94–1487) of the *Nicomachean Ethics* (Florence, ca. 1480; Goff A–981), the *Physics* (Rome, 1481; BMC IV, 130), and *On the Soul* (Venice, ca. 1500; Goff A–972). Theodorus Gaza's translation of *De animalibus*, here discussed, was commissioned by Pope Nicholas V and completed no later than 1458, but before it was printed in 1476 it was rededicated to Pope Sixtus IV (1471–84)—the illuminated presentation manuscript, written in 1473–74, survives as Vaticanus latinus 2094.[2] Gaza also produced translations of Theophrastus's *Enquiry into Plants* and *Causes of Plants*, completed in 1451 and published in Treviso in 1483 (Goff T–155).[3]

Besides working as a translator, Theodorus Gaza taught literature and philosophy, wrote an influential Greek grammar book, translated Cicero's *De amicitia* and *De senectute* into Greek, and collaborated with the printers then developing a method of printing Greek quotations in such Latin works as Aulus Gellius's *Noctes Atticae* (Rome, 1469). Aldus Manutius called Gaza *facile princeps* among the classical scholars of his age. He recommended the comparative study of his own Greek text and Gaza's "wonderfully successful" Latin version of *De animalibus* as a way of learning Greek, and he twice reprinted Gaza's translation (1504, 1513).

The importance attributed to the works of Aristotle by the learned world of the fifteenth century is attested by the frequency with which these texts and commentaries on them were printed. Besides innumerable editions of individual or selected works, eight Latin *Opera*, some accompanied by Latin versions of the Arabic commentaries, appeared between 1472/74 (Padua; Klebs 82.1) and 1497 (Cologne; Klebs 82.8), five of them in Venice (1482, 1483, 1489, 1495/96, and 1496; Klebs 82.2–82.7). The Greek *editio princeps*, in five folio volumes, was brought out by Aldus in the same city. It was among the earliest Greek texts to be printed, appearing before the first editions of Plato (1513), the dramatists (1498 etc.), the astronomers (1499), the historians (1502), the mathematicians (Euclid 1533; Archimedes 1544), and the medical writers (Dioscorides 1499, see no. 3B; Galen 1525, see no. 5B; Hippocrates 1526, see no. 1B). Complementing these editions were three folio volumes of Greek commentaries on the works of Aristotle and related texts, all printed in Venice at the turn of the century: Simplicius on the *Categories* in 1499 (Goff S–535), Ammonius on Porphyrius's *Introduction* in 1500 (Goff A–565), and Ammonius on *De interpretatione* in 1503. The first two were printed by Zacharias Callierges for Nicholas Blastus and the last by Aldus himself.

Aldus Manutius (ca. 1452–1515) was born at Bassiano in the region of Sermoneta, about forty miles southeast of Rome—hence his frequent references to himself as "Romanus." When he made the decision to become a printer, about 1488, he already had a long and respectable career as a scholar and teacher behind him. By the time he printed his first book in 1494, Aldus had worked for five years developing a method of printing Greek, a problem greatly complicated by the several diacritical marks (accents, breathings, iota subscripts) that have to be set above or below certain vowels. In preparing his edition of Aristotle, he relied on manuscripts located or copied by contemporary Greek scholars in Italy. For the biological works at least three manuscripts were consulted: Ambrosianus graecus I 56 sup., Vaticanus graecus 267, and Parisinus suppl. graecus 212. Ironically, the superior thirteenth-century Marcianus graecus 208, which was among the manuscripts Cardinal Bessarion had donated to the Venetian Republic in 1468, was not available to Aldus.[4] Book 10 of the *Historia animalium* became known to him only after Volume III, which includes the zoological works, had been printed; it was therefore added at the end of this volume.

The first volume of Aristotle's works, containing the *Organon,* or logical tracts, appeared on 1 November 1495. Three further volumes appeared in January, February, and June 1497, and the final volume in June 1498. Together these five Greek folios contain all the works of Aristotle and Theophrastus then known, together with ancient biographies and other miscellaneous treatises such as Porphyrius's *Introduction,* pseudo-Galen's *History of Philosophy,* and Alexander of Aphrodisias's *Problems.* With the addition of the *Poetics* and the *Rhetorica,* published by Aldus in the *Rhetores graeci* of 1508, this edition determined the text of Aristotle until the nineteenth century.

PP

1. Joseph Needham, *A History of Embryology,* 2d ed., revised (New York, 1959), p. 39.

2. Nancy G. Siraisi, "Life Sciences and Medicine in the Renaissance World," in *Rome Reborn: The Vatican Library and Renaissance Culture,* ed. Anthony Grafton (Washington, D.C., 1993), pp. 176–77.

3. Theophrastus (ca. 371 B.C.–ca. 287 B.C.), Aristotle's associate and successor, who also inherited his library, was the author of several treatises on botany that correspond to Aristotle's works on zoology. These were transmitted with the Aristotelian corpus and were printed in Greek in the Aldine edition of Aristotle.

4. A detailed account of how Aldus went about collecting and collating manuscripts for his edition of Aristotle is given in Martin Sicherl, *Handschriftliche Vorlagen der* Editio princeps *des Aristoteles* (Mainz, 1976).

See color plates II and III.

3

DIOSCORIDES
(fl. A.D. 50–70)

A] *De materia medica.*

Colle: Johannes de Medemblick, July 1478.

2°: a^{10} b–c^{8} d^{4} e^{8} f–g^{6} h^{8} A–B^{6} C–F^{8} $[G]^{2}$. 104 leaves.

BMC VII, 1078. Goff D–261. cf. GM 1786. GW 8436. Klebs 342.1. Osler *Incunabula medica* 161. PMM 20. Stillwell 354, 618.

B] Περὶ ὕλης ἰατρικῆς.

Venice: Aldus Manutius, Romanus, July 1499.

2°: $*^{6}$ α–o^{8} π^{10} A–Δ^{8} E^{6} α^{10}. 184 leaves. Quire α^{10}, scholia on Nicander, is not present in all copies.

BMC V, 560. Goff D–260. cf. GM 1786. GW 8435. Klebs 343.1. Osler 334. Renouard 1499.4 (p. 21). Wellcome 1776.

The most important classical guide to pharmacy and medical botany was Dioscorides' *De materia medica*, composed between A.D. 50 and 70. It contained over eight hundred entries, more than any preceding compilation. Dioscorides' descriptions covered more than 600 plants and plant ingredients, 90 minerals, and 35 animal products, including most of the *materia medica* previously described by Hippocrates. A large number of these substances can be found in modern guides to pharmacognosy, and many still find use in medicine today, including opium, aloes, asafoetida, squill, aconite, ginger, and castor oil. However, nomenclature has changed, and many of the descriptions in *De materia medica* resist identification with present-day botanical species.

Dioscorides, who may have been a physician with the Roman army, studied plants and other sources of medicines in travels around the eastern Mediterranean. His descriptions of *materia medica* included details on synonyms, habitat, botanical description, properties or actions, medical usage, side effects, and dosage; methods of harvesting, production, and storage; and veterinary, magical, and other non-medical uses. Methods of adulteration, where applicable, were described, and the means of detecting adulteration, including such procedures as drug solubility variations, specific gravity measurements, and differences in the way products burned, were discussed. Dioscorides identified natural families of plants long before Linnaeus's practical classification system of the eighteenth century; thus his work also has significance in the history of biology and taxonomy.

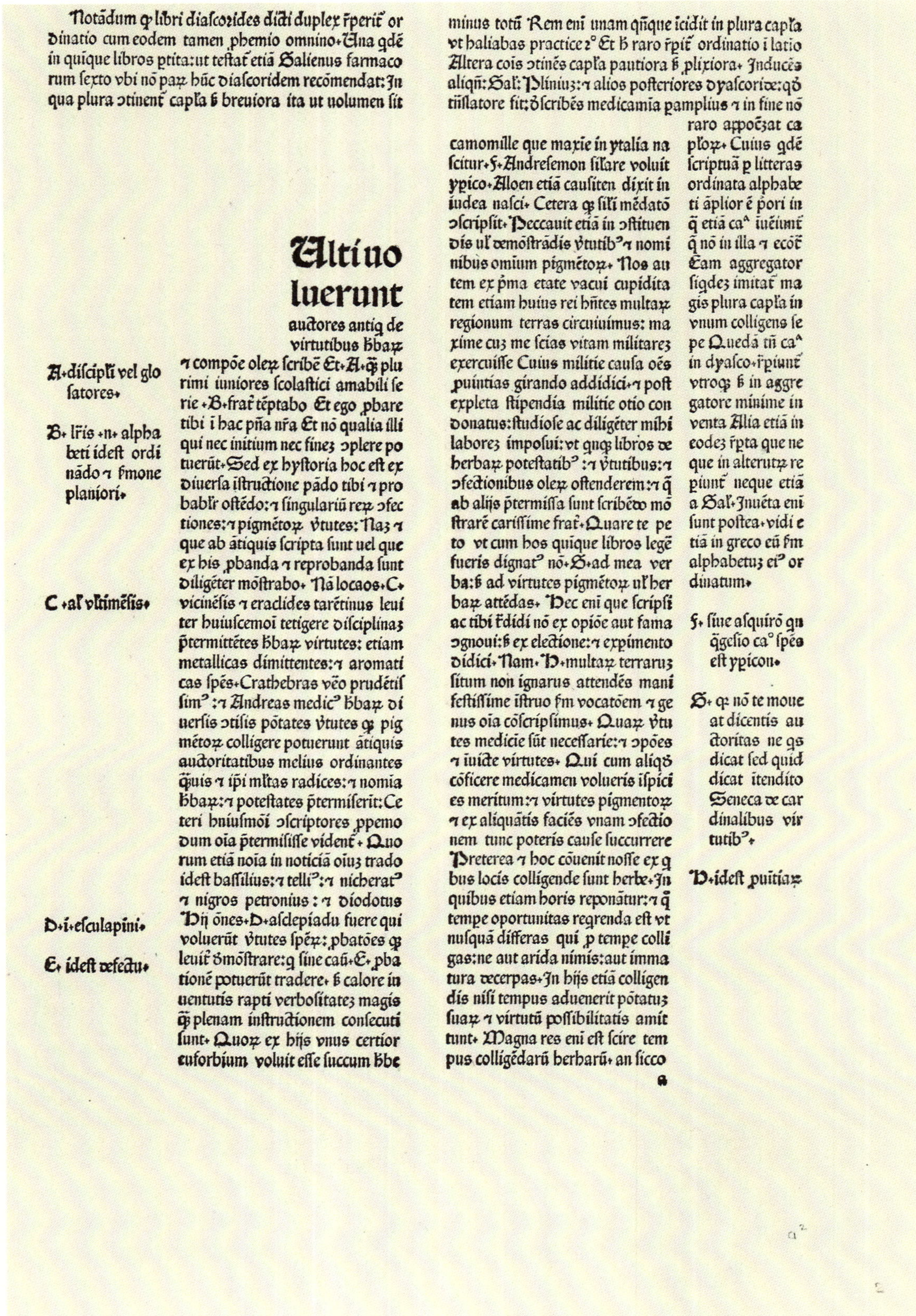

Notãdum q libri diascorides dicti duplex reperit' or dinatio cum eodem tamen phemio omnino. Una qdē in quinque libros ptita: ut testat' etiā Galienus farmaco rum sexto vbi nō paz hūc diascoridem recōmendat: In qua plura ɔtinent' capl'a s breuiora ita ut uolumen sit minus totū Rem eni unam qnque icidit in plura capl'a vt haliabas practice 2° Et h raro rpit' ordinatio i latio Altera cois ɔtinēs capl'a pautiora s plixiora. Inducēs aliqn: Gal: Pliniuz: ⁊ alios posteriores dyascoride: qd tnslatore fit: d scribēs medicamia pamplius ⁊ in fine nō raro appōzat ca

Ultiuo luerunt

auctores antiq de virtutibus hbaz ⁊ compōe olez scribē Et. A. q plu rimi iuniores scolastici amabili se rie. B. frat' tēptabo Et ego pbare tibi i hac pña nra Et nō qualia illi qui nec initium nec finez ɔplere po tuerūt. Sed ex hystoria hoc est ex diuersa istructione pādo tibi ⁊ pro babl'r ostēdo: ⁊ singulariū rez ɔfec tiones: ⁊ pigmētoz vtutes: Naz ⁊ que ab ātiquis scripta sunt uel que ex his pbanda ⁊ reprobanda sunt diligēter mōstrabo. Nā locaos. C. vicinēsis ⁊ eraclides tarētinus leui ter huiuscemoi tetigere disciplinaz ptermittētes hbaz virtutes: etiam metallicas dimittentes: ⁊ aromati cas spēs. Crathebras vēo prudētis sim⁹: ⁊ Andreas medic⁹ hbaz di uersis ɔtisis pōtates vtutes q pig mētoz colligere potuerunt ātiquis auctoritatibus melius ordinantes q̄uis ⁊ ipi mltas radices: ⁊ nomia hbaz: ⁊ potestates ptermiserit: Ce teri huiusmōi ɔscriptores ppemo dum oia ptermisisse vident'. Quo rum etiā noia in noticiā oiuz trado idest bassilius: ⁊ telli⁹: ⁊ nicherat⁹ ⁊ nigros petronius: ⁊ diodotus Hij ōnes. D. asclepiadu fuere qui voluerūt vtutes spēz: pbatōes q leuit' dmōstrare: q sine cau. E. pba tionē potuerūt tradere. s calore in uentutis rapti verbositatez magis q plenam instructionem consecuti sunt. Quoz ex hijs vnus certior euforbium voluit esse succum hbe camomille que maxie in ytalia na scitur. F. Andresemon silare voluit ypico. Aloen etiā causiten dixit in iudea nasci. Cetera q sili mēdatō ɔscripsit. Peccauit etiā in ɔstituen dis ul' demōstrādis vtutib⁹ ⁊ nomi nibus omium pigmētoz. Nos au tem ex pma etate vacui cupidita tem etiam huius rei hñtes multaz regionum terras circuiuimus: ma xime cuz me scias vitam militarez exercuisse Cuius militie causa oēs puintias girando addidici. ⁊ post expleta stipendia militie otio con donatus: studiose ac diligēter mihi laborez imposui: vt qnq libros de herbaz potestatib⁹: ⁊ vtutibus: ⁊ ɔfectionibus olez ostenderem: ⁊ q ab alijs ptermissa sunt scribēdo mō strarē carissime frat'. Quare te pe to vt cum hos quique libros legē fueris dignat⁹ nō. G. ad mea ver ba: s ad virtutes pigmētoz ul' her baz attēdas. Hec eni que scripsi ac tibi rdidi nō ex opiōe aut fama ɔgnoui: s ex electione: ⁊ expimento didici. Nam. H. multaz terraruz situm non ignarus attendēs mani festissime istruo sm vocatōem ⁊ ge nus oia cōscripsimus. Quaz vtu tes medicie sūt necessarie: ⁊ ɔpōes ⁊ iuicē virtutes. Qui cum aliqd cōficere medicamen volueris ispici es meritum: ⁊ virtutes pigmentoz ⁊ ex aliquātis faciēs vnam ɔfectio nem tunc poteris cause succurrere Preterea ⁊ hoc cōuenit nosse ex q bus locis colligende sunt herbe. In quibus etiam horis reponātur: ⁊ q tempe oportunitas regrenda est vt nusquā differas qui p tempe colli gas: ne aut arida nimis: aut imma tura decerpas. In hijs etiā colligen dis nisi tempus aduenerit pōtatuz suaz ⁊ virtutū possibilitatis amit tunt. Magna res eni est scire tem pus colligēdarū herbarū an sicco

a

A. discipli vel glo satores.

B. lris .n. alpha beti idest ordi nādo ⁊ smone planiori.

C. al' vltimēsis.

D. i. esculapini.

E. idest defectu.

raro appōzat ca ploz. Cuius qdē scriptuā p litteras ordinata alphabe ti āplior ē pori in q etiā ca^a iueniut' q nō in illa ⁊ ecōt' Eam aggregator siqdez imitat' ma gis plura capl'a in vnum colligens se pe Quedā tū ca^a in dyasco. rpiunt' vtroq s in aggre gatore minime in venta Alia etiā in eodez rpta que ne que in alterutz re piunt' neque etiā a Gal. Inuēta eni sunt postea. vidi e tiā in greco eū sm alphabetuz ei⁹ or dinatum.

F. siue asquirō qn qgesio ca° spēs est ypicon.

G. q nō te moue at dicentis au ctoritas ne qs dicat sed quid dicat itendito Seneca de car dinalibus vir tutib⁹.

H. idest puitiaz

Fig. 6. No. 3A. Dioscorides. First page of the Latin *editio princeps* (1478).

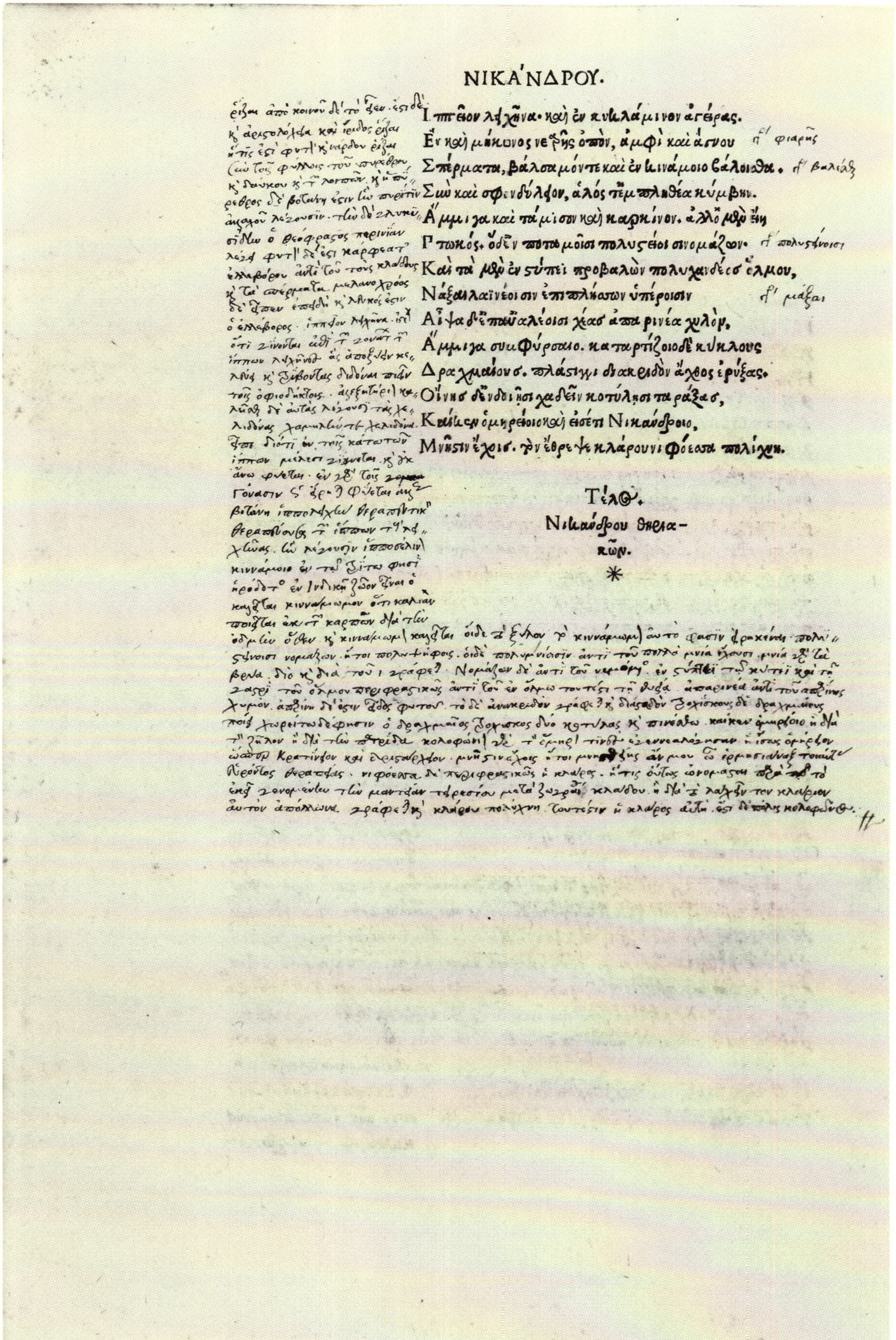

ΝΙΚΑΝΔΡΟΥ.

Ἴππειον λειχῆνα, καὶ ἐν κυκλάμινον ἀγείρας.
Ἐν καὶ μήκωνος νεαρῆς ὀπόν, ἀμφὶ καὶ ἄγνου
Σπέρματα, βάλσαμόν τε καὶ ἐν κινάμοιο βάλοιο.
Σὺν καὶ σφονδύλιον, ἁλὸς πέμπληθέα κύμβην.
Ἄμμιγα καὶ πάμισον καὶ καρκίνον. ἄλλο μὲν ἤ
Πτωκός. ὅδ' ἐν ποταμοῖσι πολυστέοισ' ὀνομάζων.
Καὶ τὰ μὲν ἐν στύπει προβαλὼν πολυχανδέος ὅλμου,
Ναξίαι λαΐνεοισιν ἐπιπλήσσων ὑπέροισιν
Αἶψα δὲ τοῦ παλέοισι χέας ἀπαρινέα χυλόν,
Ἄμμιγα συμφύρσαιο. καταρτίζοιο δὲ κύκλους
Δραχμαίους. πλάσιγγι διακρείδον ἄχθος ἐρύξας.
Οἴνης δ' ἐν δυοῖ ἢ σὺ χαδεῖν κοτύλησι ταράξας,
Καί κεν ὁμηρείοιο καὶ εἰσέτι Νικάνδροιο,
Μνῆστιν ἔχοις. τὸν ἔθρεψε Κλάρου νιφόεσσα πολίχνη.

Τέλος.
Νικάνδρου θηρια-
κῶν.
*

Fig. 7. No. 3B. Dioscorides. Page of the Greek *editio princeps* (1499), which included the work of Nicander, showing early annotations.

The *editiones principes* in Latin and Greek were the only editions of Dioscorides to appear in the fifteenth century. Five editions of the Greek text and six new Latin translations were published in the sixteenth century. By the end of the seventeenth century there existed thirty-six different Latin commentaries in ninety-six separate printings, and more than forty editions in Italian, French, German, Spanish, and other modern vernacular languages. These publications, a number of which were illustrated with woodcuts of herbs and animals, played a significant role in pharmaceutical and botanical studies during and after the Renaissance.

WHH

An illustrated Latin "herbarium" of Dioscorides is mentioned by Cassiodorus in the sixth century, although identification of this work with *De materia medica* is not secure, some scholars arguing that Cassiodorus meant the treatise known as *Ex herbis femininis*, a compilation of late Antiquity that was based on the works of Dioscorides and others. In any case, linguistic evidence strongly suggests that the oldest Latin translation of *De materia medica*, as contained in the ninth-century manuscript Parisinus latinus 12,995, does in fact go back at least to the sixth century, if not further. This translation, which follows the original nonalphabetic order of Dioscorides' work, is generally accurate and quite complete, although it omits some chapters, especially in Book II.

In the eleventh or twelfth century, this Latin translation was partly alphabetized: i.e., it was rearranged by grouping the entries alphabetically according to their *first* letters (within the individual letters items are not arranged alphabetically). In this reworking, a considerable amount of original material was discarded and an even greater amount of new information (approximately a third) was added from Latin, Greek, and Arabic sources. A note in a thirteenth-century Bamberg manuscript ascribes this reworking to Constantine the African (died 1087), which may also indicate a connection with the School of Salerno. Two centuries later, Peter of Abano (ca. 1250–1316) took this alphabetic version as the basis for a complete commentary on the work in the form of glosses to the individual chapters. Peter probably carried out this work while he was lecturer in Padua, after his return from Constantinople in 1303.

It was this medieval Latin text and commentary that were printed for the first time in 1478, by John of Medemblick at Colle di Val d'Elsa, about thirty miles south of Florence. This translation and commentary were reprinted at Lyons in 1512, but they were then definitively superseded by two independent new Latin translations made directly from the Greek and published in 1516 in Venice and Paris, the first by Ermolao Barbaro (1454–95), whose version was accompanied by a commentary entitled *Corollarium*, and the second by Jean Ruel (ca. 1474–1537). Although the manuscript tradition of Dioscorides is known for a number of magnificently illustrated codices with texts in Greek or Arabic, the first printed editions in both Latin and Greek were unillustrated.

The Greek *editio princeps* of Dioscorides' work was printed by Aldus Manutius; included in it were not only *De materia medica*, but also the Greek *editiones principes* of two pharmacological poems, *Theriaca* and *Alexipharmaca*, by Nicander of Colophon (III or II cent. B.C.). Some copies also contain an additional gathering of scholia on Nicander. In his foreword, Aldus directed Dioscorides' work particularly to the attention of students of Pliny (*qui in pliniana lectione versati*), whose *Natural History* was at the time the center of a heated controversy as scientists struggled to reconcile Pliny's account of natural phenomena with what they themselves were observing.

In the preface, dedicated to his friend and colleague Areius of Tarsus, Dioscorides explained the principles his work was to follow. Besides indicating the need to add plants omitted by his predecessors, he insisted on the advantage of fact over theory, of personal observation over reading, and of the new arrangement based on drug properties that he was introducing in preference to simply listing drugs according to the alphabetical order of their names. Following the scheme "one agent, one chapter," the five books of *De materia medica* described medicinal substances derived from the plant, animal, and mineral kingdoms. First dividing the substances into large groups according to their main characteristics or origin (e.g., aromatics, oils, salves, trees, shrubs, animals), Dioscorides then arranged the chapters within each group in a manner perhaps best called "associative." Similarities of botanical form, method of extraction, mode of drug action (e.g., warming, astringent, diuretic), and specific medical application all played varying roles in determining a complex web of associations that gave the final system an apparent order and made it easier to remember.

Dioscorides' work dominated the field of pharmacology from its own time through the Middle Ages; it was translated into both Latin and Arabic at an early date, and served as the source of countless other texts and commentaries. By the time of Photius (IX cent.), two additional texts had been added to the original five books, one on *Poisons and Antidotes*, and one on *Poisonous Animals and the Treatment of Their Wounds*.

In spite of Dioscorides' rejection of alphabetical order in his preface, *De materia medica* is found already in this form in the earliest extant copy, a splendid illustrated manuscript prepared about 512 for Anicia Juliana, daughter of the emperor Flavius Olybrius, and now in the Austrian National Library, in Vienna. In fact, the majority of the Greek manuscripts contain *De materia medica* in the alphabetized form, testifying to the popularity of this arrangement with Byzantine physicians and scholars. Aldus, no doubt taking into account Dioscorides' statement on alphabetic order, chose as the basis of his edition the original nonalphabetic arrangement, as he found it in the fifteenth-century manuscript Parisinus graecus 2183. He also included in his Dioscorides the works mentioned by Photius, the *Poisons and Antidotes*, in one book, and the *Poisonous Animals*, here divided into three books.

PP

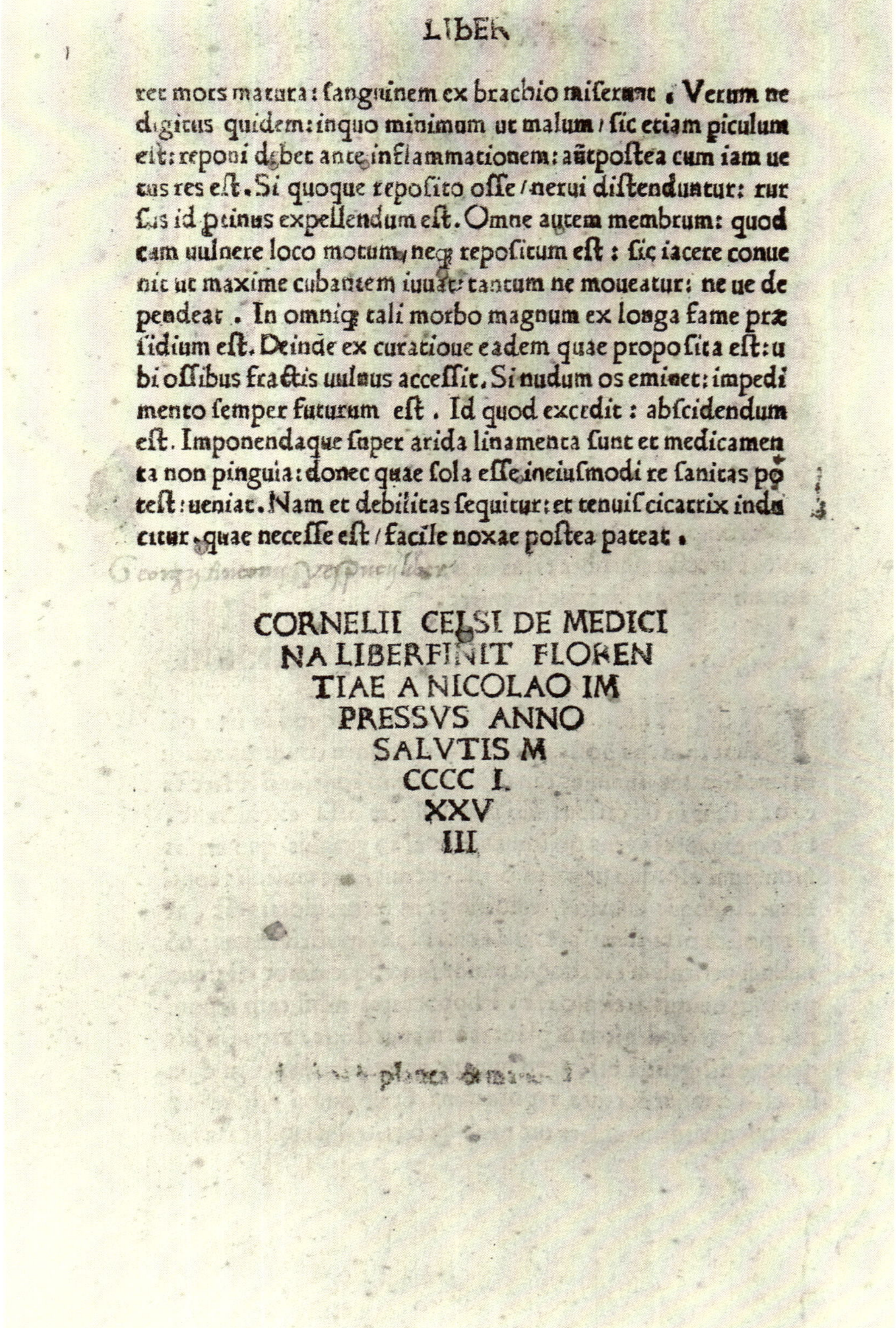

LIBER

ret mors matura: sanguinem ex brachio miserunt. Verum ne
digitus quidem: inquo minimum ut malum / sic etiam piculum
est: reponi debet ante inflammationem: aūtpostea cum iam ue
tus res est. Si quoque reposito osse / nerui distenduntur: rur
sus id pctinus expellendum est. Omne autem membrum: quod
cum uulnere loco motum / neq repositum est: sic iacere conue
nit ut maxime cubantem iuuat: tantum ne moueatur: ne ue de
pendeat. In omniq tali morbo magnum ex longa fame præ
sidium est. Deinde ex curatione eadem quae proposita est: u
bi ossibus fractis uulnus accessit. Si nudum os eminet: impedi
mento semper futurum est. Id quod excedit: abscidendum
est. Imponendaque super arida linamenta sunt et medicamen
ta non pinguia: donec quae sola esse ineiusmodi re sanitas po
test: ueniat. Nam et debilitas sequitur: et tenuis cicatrix indu
citur, quae necesse est / facile noxae postea pateat.

CORNELII CELSI DE MEDICI
NA LIBER FINIT FLOREN
TIAE A NICOLAO IM
PRESSVS ANNO
SALVTIS M
CCCC L
XXV
III

Fig. 8. No. 4. Celsus. The signature of Giorgio Antonio Vespucci is faintly visible beneath the final paragraph, above the colophon.

4

AULUS CORNELIUS CELSUS

(fl. A.D. 25)

De medicina.

Florence: Nicolaus Laurentii, Alamanus, 1478.

2° and 4°: π^6 a^4 b–i^6 l–z^6 $\&^6$ aa–gg^6 hh^4 A^8. 196 leaves.

BMC VI, 627. GM 20. Goff C–364. GW 6456. Klebs 260.1. Norman 424. Osler 286. Osler *Incunabula medica* 147. Stillwell 331, 610. Waller 44. Wellcome 1392.

Aulus Cornelius Celsus's *De medicina* is the oldest Western medical document after the Hippocratic writings and the earliest Western history of medicine. The eight books of *De medicina* formed part of an encyclopedia entitled *Artes*, which also contained sections (now lost) on agriculture, military science, and possibly rhetoric, philosophy, and jurisprudence. *De medicina* begins with a proem, in which Celsus portrays the history of medicine from its mythical beginnings down to his own time and justifies the eclectic position he is to take among contemporary medical sects. This is followed by two books on diet in health, two on diseases treated by diet, two on diseases treated by medicaments, and two on surgery. The text, which gives an account of the whole of medicine and surgery, is based on a thorough and impartial use of Greek material from the last two centuries B.C., carefully worked into a harmonious and effective unity, and expressed in elegant Ciceronian Latin.

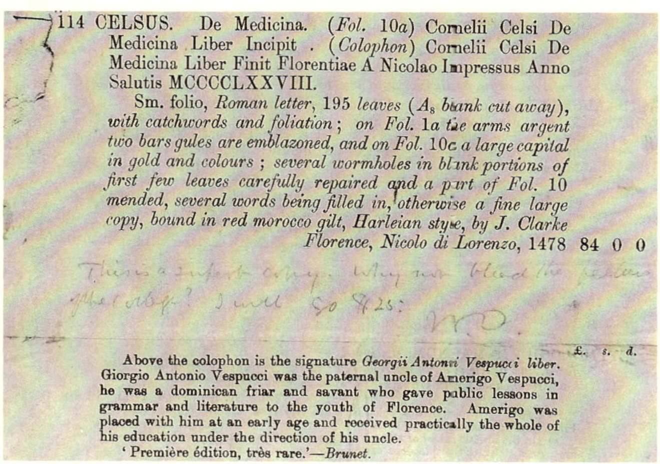

114 CELSUS. De Medicina. (*Fol.* 10*a*) Cornelii Celsi De Medicina Liber Incipit . (*Colophon*) Cornelii Celsi De Medicina Liber Finit Florentiae A Nicolao Impressus Anno Salutis MCCCCLXXVIII.

Sm. folio, *Roman letter*, 195 *leaves* (*A_8 blank cut away*), *with catchwords and foliation*; *on Fol.* 1*a the arms argent two bars gules are emblazoned, and on Fol.* 10*c a large capital in gold and colours*; *several wormholes in blank portions of first few leaves carefully repaired and a part of Fol.* 10 *mended, several words being filled in, otherwise a fine large copy, bound in red morocco gilt, Harleian style, by J. Clarke*

Florence, Nicolo di Lorenzo, 1478 84 0 0

£. s. d.

Above the colophon is the signature *Georgii Antonii Vespucci liber.* Giorgio Antonio Vespucci was the paternal uncle of Amerigo Vespucci, he was a dominican friar and savant who gave public lessons in grammar and literature to the youth of Florence. Amerigo was placed with him at an early age and received practically the whole of his education under the direction of his uncle.

'Première édition, très rare.'—*Brunet*.

Fig. 9. No. 4. Celsus. Dealer's description (circa 1913) of the Vespucci copy. Osler's pencilled note beneath the description reads: "This is a superb copy. Why not bleed the Fellows of the College? I will go $25. W.O."

In the books of *De medicina* that deal with diseases treatable by diet and regimen are found the earliest uses of the terms *insania* and *cardiacus* to refer to insanity and heart disease. The surgical chapters contain the first accounts of the use of ligature, excellent descriptions of lateral lithotomy and herniotomy, and the earliest discussions of what is now called plastic surgery. *De medicina's* interest for historians of ancient medicine is heightened by the fact that only very limited source material has survived from the period between the formation of the Hippocratic corpus (ca. 350 B.C.) and Celsus, so that for reconstructing the development of medicine during these four centuries *De medicina* plays a crucial role. Thus Celsus reports, for example, that Diocles of Carystus invented an instrument called a *cyathiscus* to remove missiles embedded in the flesh, that Herophilus and Erasistratus dissected living prisoners handed over to them by the kings of Egypt, that Asclepiades of Bithynia demanded that practitioners cure their patients "safely, speedily, and pleasantly," and that Themison of Laodicea established the three "methodist" *genera* of diseases: *adstrictum*, *fluens*, and *mixtum*.

In fact, *De medicina* was more than an exhaustive medical compendium for educated Romans that later became a treasure-trove for medical historians: for four centuries it proved to be an eminently useful handbook of medicine for practitioners. Although the text seems to have enjoyed little notice in Antiquity and the Middle Ages, the discovery of a tenth-century manuscript by Guarino of Verona in Bologna in 1426, and of another by Giovanni Lamola the following year in Milan, led to an avid recopying (no fewer than twenty fifteenth-century manuscripts survive), and to the publication by Nicolaus Laurentii Alamanus of the *editio princeps*, edited by Bartolomeo Fonzio (1445–1513) from the manuscript Laurentianus Plut. 73,4 (XV cent.). *De medicina* was printed three more times in the fifteenth century (1481, 1493, and 1497; Goff C–365, C–366, C–367) and at least fifteen times in the sixteenth century. By the middle of the nineteenth century it had been published in a total of over fifty editions, eloquent testimony to its immense and long-standing popularity with medical teachers and students.

PP

See color plates IV *and* V.

5

GALEN

(A.D. 129/130–199/200)

A] *Opera.*

Venice: Philippus Pincius, 27 August 1490.

[Vol. I] 2º: π^{6} aa–bb^{8} ee–zz^{8} ⁊⁊^{4} ꝯꝯ^{10} t–x^{8} y–z^{6}. 224 leaves.

[Vol. II] 2º: a–g^{8} h^{6} iI^{8} kK^{6} lL^{4} llL^{4} mM^{10} i–r^{8} A–I^{8} K^{4} ꝶ^{6}. 248 leaves.

Goff G–37. GW 10481. Horblit 34. Klebs 432.1. PMM 33. Stillwell 375, 642. Wellcome 2509.

B] Γαληνου Α′ [–Ε′]. *Galeni librorum pars prima [–quinta].*

Venice: In aedibus Aldi, et Andreae Asulani soceri, April–August 1525.

[Vol. I] 2º: [*]^{4} Αα–Γγ^{8} a–e^{8} f^{4} g–l^{8} m^{4} n–o^{8} p^{10} q^{4} r–x^{8} y^{10} z^{8} &^{6} A–L^{8} M^{12} N^{8}. 318 leaves, ff. [4] 1–24, 1–180 [i.e., 181] [1], 1–108.

[Vol. II] 2º: **^{4} aa–kk^{8} ll^{6} mm–yy^{8} zz^{10} a–g^{8} h^{6} i–n^{8} o^{4}. 294 leaves, ff. [4] 1–184, 1–160 [i.e. 106].

[Vol. III] 2º: [***]^{4} a–i^{8} k^{12} l–m^{8} n^{6} aaa–bbb^{8} ccc^{10} ddd–ggg^{8} hhh–lll^{6} mmm^{8} nnn–ooo^{6} ppp–ttt^{8} uuu^{4} xxx^{10}. 266 leaves, ff. [4] 1–106, 1–155 [1].

[Vol. IV] 2º: [*]^{4} AAa^{8} BBb^{6} CCc^{4} DDd–PPp^{8} aaaa–cccc^{8} dddd–eeee^{6} ffff–iiii^{8} kkkk^{6} **^{6} 1–6^{8} 7^{6} 8^{4}. 256 leaves, ff. [4] 1–113 [1], 1–74, 1–3 [i.e., 6], 1–55 [i.e., 57] [1].

[Vol. V] 2º: *^{4} Aa^{8} Bb^{10} Cc–Ff^{8} Gg^{6} Hh–Mm^{8} Nn–Oo^{6} Pp–Xx^{8} Yy^{10} Zz^{8} Aaa–Fff^{8} Ggg–Hhh^{12} Iii^{10} Κκκ–Ννν^{8} Οοο–Τττ^{8} Υυυ^{10} ΑΑΑ^{6}. 356 leaves, ff. [4] 1–327 [i.e., 346], 1–6.

Adams G–32. Durling 1748. GM 27. Osler 350. Renouard 1525.3 (p. 101). Stillwell 374, 641. Wellcome 2507.

Galen, who was born at Pergamum, in Asia Minor, studied medicine there and in Smyrna, Corinth, and Alexandria. For several years he served as physician to the gladiators at Pergamum, but he spent most of his career in Rome, where he practiced medicine in influential circles, gave public anatomical lectures and demonstrations, and engaged in disputations on medical subjects. In his numerous writings he sought to reconcile Hippocrates with Plato and presented Hippocrates' teachings as the basis for his own medical thought, including his greatly influential theory of the four humors. In anatomy and physiology his theories were informed by a teleological point of view derived from Aristotle, even as he emphasized the importance of experiment.

The foundation for Galen's position of authority in the medicine of the Middle Ages was laid in late Antiquity in Constantinople and Alexandria. Oribasius of Pergamum (ca. 320–403), a physician and friend of the emperor Julian, first excerpted the works of Galen and then, at the request of the emperor, compiled a seventy-book *Collectiones medicae* that contained extracts from the writings of the more important Greek physicians. In the preface to this monumental work, of which about a third has survived, he emphasized Galen's standing:

> I have left nothing that Galen said aside, since he surpasses all who have written on these subjects; he employs the securest methods and distinctions, following meticulously the principles and opinions of Hippocrates.[1]

In the sixth century, Alexandrine medical scholars established a canon of sixteen Galenic works that formed the center of their activities as teachers and commentators. Thus, when Greek medicine passed to the East in the seventh and eighth centuries, it was explicitly centered about Galen the philosopher-physician and Galen the prophet of Hippocrates. The Syrian Nestorian scholar and translator Ḥunayn ibn Isḥāq knew the titles of 129 Galenic works, of which he himself had translated about ninety from Greek into Syriac and about forty into Arabic. This work of translation was continued by Ḥunayn's followers, so that by the ninth century most of the Galenic corpus was available in Arabic.

With the gradual assimilation of Arabic medical learning in the medieval universities of Western Europe, especially at Bologna and Montpellier, the authority of Galen grew, and there followed an active translation of his works into Latin, either through the Arabic or directly from Greek. It is these medieval translations that were collected and edited by Diomedes Bonardus and printed by Philippus Pincius in Venice in 1490. Of the seventy-eight titles listed in the tables of contents of this two-volume edition, one translation has been identified as the work of Constantine the African (died 1087), four have been assigned to Burgundio of Pisa (ca. 1110–93), five to Gerard of Cremona (ca. 1114–87), one to Mark of Toledo (XII cent.), one to Accursio of Pistoia (1182–1260), one to William of Moerbeke (ca. 1215–ca. 1286), three to Peter of Abano (ca. 1250–1316), and thirty-nine to Nicholas of Reggio (ca. 1280–ca. 1350), leaving twenty-three of the translations unattributed. The collection included a wide range of introductory, theoretical, and clinical works, among them *De interioribus* (=*De locis affectis*), *De sectis*, *Microtegni* (=*Ars medica*), *De iuvamentis membrorum* (=*De usu partium*), *De virtutibus naturalibus* (=*De temperamentis*), *De simplici medicina* (=*De simplicium medicamentorum temperamentis et facultatibus*), *De accidenti et morbo* (=*De morborum differentiis*, etc.), *De regimine sanitatis* (=*De sanitatis tuenda*), *De ingenio sanitatis* (=*Methodus medendi*), and *De febribus* (=*Ad Glauconem de medendi methodo*). Notably absent were *De anatomicis administrationibus*, *De placitis Hippocratis et Platonis*, and the Hippocratic commentaries. Bonardus, a physi-

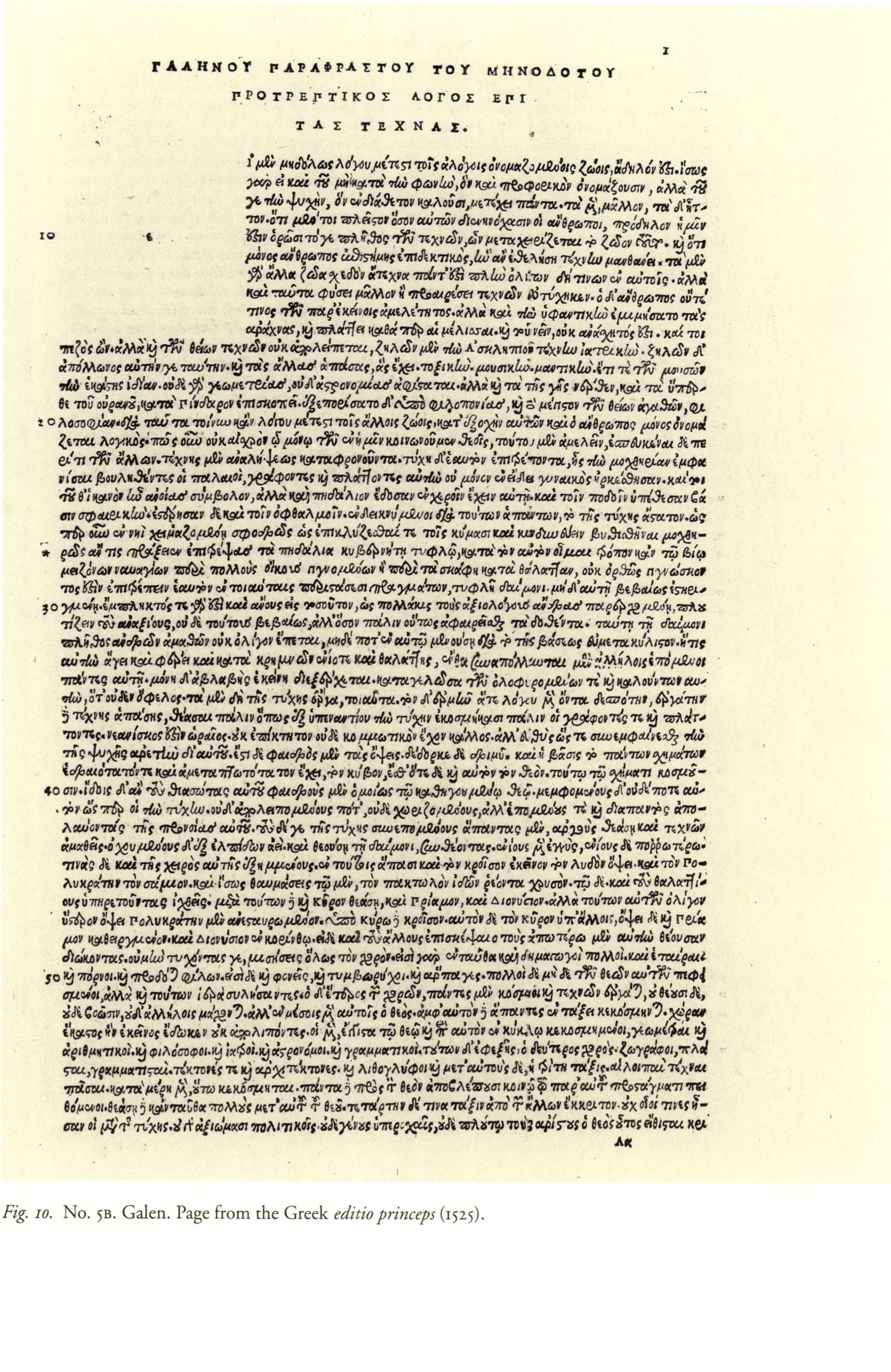

1

ΓΑΛΗΝΟΥ ΠΑΡΑΦΡΑΣΤΟΥ ΤΟΥ ΜΗΝΟΔΟΤΟΥ ΠΡΟΤΡΕΠΤΙΚΟΣ ΛΟΓΟΣ ΕΠΙ ΤΑΣ ΤΕΧΝΑΣ.

Ι μὲν μηδ' ὅλως λόγου μέτεστι τοῖς ἀλόγοις ὀνομαζομένοις ζώοις, ἄδηλόν ἐστι. ἴσως γὰρ εἰ καὶ μὴ τοῦ κατὰ τὴν φωνήν, ὃν καὶ προφορικὸν ὀνομάζουσιν, ἀλλὰ τοῦ γε κατὰ τὴν ψυχήν, ὃν ἐνδιάθετον καλοῦσι, μετέχει πάντα. τὰ μὲν μᾶλλον, τὰ δ' ἧττον. ὅτι μέντοι πλεῖστον ὅσον αὐτῶν διενηνόχασιν οἱ ἄνθρωποι, πρόδηλον ἢ μὴν ἐστὶν ὁρῶσι τό γε πλῆθος τῶν τεχνῶν, ὧν μεταχειρίζεται τὸ ζῶον τοῦτο. καὶ ὅτι μόνος ἄνθρωπος ἐπιστήμης ἐπιδεκτικός, ἣν ἂν ἐθελήσῃ τέχνην μανθάνει. τὰ μὲν γὰρ ἄλλα ζῶα σχεδὸν ἄτεχνα πάντ' ἐστὶ πλὴν ὀλίγων δή τινων ἐν αὐτοῖς. ἀλλὰ καὶ ταῦτα φύσει μᾶλλον ἢ προαιρέσει τεχνῶν ἐπιτύχηκεν. ὁ δ' ἄνθρωπος οὐ τινος τῶν παρ' ἐκείνοις ἀμελέτητος. ἀλλὰ καὶ τὴν ὑφαντικὴν ἐμιμήσατο τὰς ἀράχνας, καὶ πλάττει καθάπερ αἱ μέλισσαι. καὶ νεῖν οὐκ ἀδύνατός ἐστι. καί τοι πεζὸς ὤν. ἀλλὰ καὶ τῶν θείων τεχνῶν οὐκ ἀπολείπεται, ζηλῶν μὲν τὴν Ἀσκληπιοῦ τέχνην ἰατρικήν. ζηλῶν δ' Ἀπόλλωνος αὐτήν γε ταύτην. καὶ τὰς ἄλλας ἁπάσας, ἃς ἔχει. τοξικήν. μουσικήν. μαντικήν. ἔτι τε τῶν μουσῶν τὴν ἑκάστης ἰδίαν. οὐδὲ γὰρ γεωμετρίας, οὐδ' ἀστρονομίας ἀπείρατος. ἀλλὰ καὶ τὰ τῆς γῆς νέρθεν, καὶ τὰ ὕπερθε τοῦ οὐρανοῦ, κατὰ Πίνδαρον ἐπισκοπεῖ. ἐξεπορίσατο δ' ἀπὸ φιλοπονίας, καὶ ὃ μέγιστον τῶν θείων ἀγαθῶν, φιλοσοφίαν. διὰ ταῦτα τοίνυν κἂν λόγου μέτεστι τοῖς ἄλλοις ζώοις, κατ' ἐξοχὴν αὐτῶν καὶ ὁ ἄνθρωπος μόνος ὀνομάζεται λογικός. πῶς οὖν οὐκ αἰσχρὸν ᾧ μόνῳ τῶν ἐν ἡμῖν κοινωνοῦμεν θεοῖς, τούτου μὲν ἀμελεῖν, ἐσπουδακέναι δὲ περί τι τῶν ἄλλων. τέχνης μὲν ἀναλήψεως καταφρονοῦντα, τύχῃ δ' ἑαυτὸν ἐπιτρέποντα, ἧς τὴν μοχθηρίαν ἐμφανίσαι βουληθέντες οἱ παλαιοί, γράφοντές τε καὶ πλάττοντες αὐτήν, οὐ μόνον ἐν εἴδει γυναικὸς ἠρκέσθησαν. καίτοι γε ἱκανὸν ἦν ἀνοίας σύμβολον, ἀλλὰ καὶ πηδάλιον ἔδοσαν ἐν χεροῖν ἔχειν αὐτῇ. καὶ τοῖν ποδοῖν ὑπέθεσαν βάσιν σφαιρικήν. ἐστέρησαν δὲ καὶ τοῖν ὀφθαλμοῖν. ἐνδεικνύμενοι διὰ τούτων ἁπάντων, τὸ τῆς τύχης ἄστατον. ὡς γὰρ οὖν ἐν νηῒ χειμαζομένῃ σφοδρῶς ὡς ἐπικλύζεσθαί τε τοῖς κύμασι καὶ κινδυνεύειν βυθισθῆναι, μοχθηρῶς ἄν τις πράξειεν ἐπιτρέψας τὰ πηδάλια κυβερνήτῃ τυφλῷ, κατὰ τὸν αὐτὸν οἶμαι τρόπον καὶ τῷ βίῳ μειζόνων ναυαγίων περὶ πολλοὺς οἴκους γιγνομένων ἢ περὶ τὰ σκάφη κατὰ θάλατταν, οὐκ ὀρθῶς γιγνώσκοντος ἐστὶν ἐπιτρέπειν ἑαυτὸν ἐν τοιαύταις περιστάσεσι πραγμάτων, τυφλῇ δαίμονι. μὴ δ' αὐτῇ βεβαίως ἱσταμένῃ. ἔμπληκτός τε γάρ ἐστι καὶ ἀνόητος εἰς τοσοῦτον, ὡς πολλάκις τοὺς ἀξιολόγους ἄνδρας παρερχομένη, πλουτίζειν τοὺς ἀναξίους, οὐδὲ τούτους βεβαίως, ἀλλ' ὅσον πάλιν οὕτως ἀφαιρεῖσθαι τὰ δοθέντα. ταύτῃ τῇ δαίμονι πλῆθος ἀνδρῶν ἀμαθῶν οὐκ ὀλίγον ἕπεται, μηδέ ποτ' ἐν αὐτῷ μενούσῃ διὰ τὸ τῆς βάσεως εὐμετακύλιστον. ἥτις αὐτὴν ἄγει καὶ φέρει καὶ κατὰ κρημνῶν ἐνίοτε καὶ θαλάττης, ἔνθα συναπόλλυνται μὲν ἀλλήλοις ἑπόμενοι πάντες αὐτῇ. μόνη δ' ἀβλαβὴς ἐκείνη διεξέρχεται. καταγελῶσα τῶν ὀλοφυρομένων τε καὶ καλούντων αὐτήν, ὅτ' οὐδὲν ὄφελος. τὰ μὲν δὴ τῆς τύχης ἔργα, τοιαῦτα. τὸν δ' Ἑρμῆν ἅτε λόγου μὲν ὄντα δεσπότην, ἐργάτην δὲ τέχνης ἁπάσης, θέασαι πάλιν ὅπως ἐξ ὑπεναντίου τὴν τύχην ἐκοσμήκασι πάλιν οἱ γράφοντές τε καὶ πλάττοντες. νεανίσκος ἐστὶν ὡραῖος. οὐκ ἐπίκτητον οὐδὲ κομμωτικὸν ἔχων κάλλος. ἀλλ' ἀληθὲς ὥστε συνεμφαίνεσθαι τὴν τῆς ψυχῆς ἀρετὴν δι' αὐτοῦ. ἔστι δὲ φαιδρὸς μὲν τὰς ὄψεις. δέδορκε δὲ δριμύ. καὶ ἡ βάσις τὸ πάντων σχημάτων ἑδραιότατόν τε καὶ ἀμεταπτωτότατον ἔχει, τὸν κύβον, ἔσθ' ὅτε δὲ καὶ αὐτὸν τὸν θεόν. τούτῳ τῷ σχήματι κοσμοῦσιν. ἴδοις δ' αὖ τοὺς θιασώτας αὐτοῦ φαιδροὺς μὲν ὁμοίως τῷ καθηγουμένῳ θεῷ. μεμφομένους δ' οὐδέποτε αὐτὸν ὥσπερ οἱ τὴν τύχην. οὐδ' ἀπολειπομένους ποτ', οὐδὲ χωριζομένους, ἀλλ' ἑπομένους τε καὶ διαπαντὸς ἀπολαύοντας τῆς προνοίας αὐτοῦ. τοὺς δέ γε τῆς τύχης συνεπομένους ἅπαντας μέν, ἀργοὺς θεάσῃ καὶ τεχνῶν ἀμαθεῖς. ὀχουμένους δ' ὑπ' ἐλπίδων ἀεί. καὶ θεούσῃ τῇ δαίμονι, συνθέοντας. ἐνίους μὲν ἐγγύς, ἐνίους δὲ πορρωτέρω. τινὰς δὲ καὶ τῆς χειρὸς αὐτῆς ἐξηρτημένους. ἐν τούτοις ἅπασι καὶ τὸν Κροῖσον ἐκεῖνον τὸν Λυδὸν ὄψει. καὶ τὸν Πολυκράτην τὸν Σάμιον. καὶ ἴσως θαυμάσεις τῷ μέν, τὸν Πακτωλὸν ἰδὼν ῥέοντα χρυσόν. τῷ δὲ καὶ τοὺς θαλαττίους ὑπηρετοῦντας ἰχθύας. μετὰ τούτων δὲ καὶ Κῦρον θεάσῃ, καὶ Πρίαμον, καὶ Διονύσιον. ἀλλὰ τούτων αὐτῶν ὀλίγον ὕστερον ὄψει Πολυκράτην μὲν ἀνεσταυρωμένον. ὑπὸ Κύρου δὲ Κροῖσον. αὐτὸν δὲ τὸν Κῦρον ὑπ' ἄλλοις, ὄψει δὲ καὶ Πρίαμον καθειργμένον. καὶ Διονύσιον ἐν Κορίνθῳ. εἰ δὲ καὶ τοὺς ἄλλους ἐπισκέψαιο τοὺς πορρωτέρω μὲν αὐτὴν θέουσαν διώκοντας. οὐ μὴν τυχόντας γε, μισήσεις ὅλως τὸν χορόν. εἰσὶ γὰρ ἐνταῦθα καὶ δημαγωγοὶ πολλοί. καὶ ἑταῖραι καὶ πόρνοι. καὶ προδόται φίλων. εἰσὶ δὲ καὶ φονεῖς, καὶ τυμβωρύχοι. καὶ ἅρπαγες. πολλοὶ δὲ μὴ δὲ τῶν θεῶν αὐτῶν πεφεισμένοι, ἀλλὰ καὶ τούτων ἱεροσυλήσαντες. ὁ δ' ἕτερος τῶν χορῶν, πάντες μὲν κόσμιοί καὶ τεχνῶν ἐργάται, οὐ θέουσι δέ, οὐδὲ βοῶσιν, οὐδ' ἀλλήλοις μάχονται. ἀλλ' ἐν μέσοις μὲν αὐτοῖς ὁ θεός. ἀμφ' αὐτὸν δὲ ἅπαντες ἐν τάξει κεκόσμηνται. χώραν ἕκαστος ἣν ἐκεῖνος ἔδωκεν οὐκ ἀπολιπόντες. οἱ μέν, ἐγγύτατα τῷ θεῷ καὶ περὶ αὐτὸν ἐν κύκλῳ κεκοσμημένοι, γεωμέτραι καὶ ἀριθμητικοί. καὶ φιλόσοφοι. καὶ ἰατροί. καὶ ἀστρονόμοι. καὶ γραμματικοί. τούτων δ' ἐφεξῆς, ὁ δεύτερος χορός. ζωγράφοι, πλάσται, γραμματισταί. τέκτονές τε καὶ ἀρχιτέκτονες. καὶ λιθογλύφοι καὶ μετ' αὐτοὺς δέ, ἡ τρίτη τάξις. αἱ λοιπαὶ τέχναι πᾶσαι. κατὰ μέρη μέν, οὕτω κεκόσμηνται. πάντα δὲ πρὸς τὸν θεὸν ἀποβλέπουσι κοινῷ τῷ παρ' αὐτοῦ προστάγματι πειθόμενοι. θεάσῃ δὲ κἀνταῦθα πολλοὺς μετ' αὐτοῦ τοῦ θεοῦ. τετάρτην δέ τινα τάξιν ἀπὸ τῶν ἄλλων ἔκκειτον. οὐχ οἷοί τινες ἦσαν οἱ μετὰ τῆς τύχης. οὐ τοῖς ἀξιώμασι πολιτικοῖς. οὐδὲ γένους ὑπεροχαῖς, οὐδὲ πλούτῳ τοὺς ἀρίστους ὁ θεὸς οὗτος εἴθισται κρί-

Αα

Fig. 10. No. 5B. Galen. Page from the Greek *editio princeps* (1525).

cian of Brescia, told in his preface of the corrupt state of the manuscripts he had to depend upon and the difficulties he had locating the dispersed volumes of Galen in the "gymnasia" of Italy. He ended with a solemn vow:

> I swear by God, that I have carried out this task not in the hope of wealth, but only through a trust in learning and truth, believing there to be no possession of man that is better or more divine.

Aldus Manutius's intention to print the Greek medical writers was first signaled in the preface to the February 1497 volume of the *Opera* of Aristotle (see no. 2B), addressed to his patron Alberto Pio of Carpi:

> We will also publish the collected works of Hippocrates and Galen, and of the other writers famous in medicine. . . . Truly, if I live long enough, there shall be no shortage of good books in fine literature and the liberal arts for scholars.

When Aldus died on 6 February 1515, this promise was unredeemed. The press passed to his partner and father-in-law, Andreas Asulanus (1451–1528), whose experience in printing dated from 1474, and who had printed Aldus's Latin grammar, *Institutiones grammaticae*, in 1493. Asulanus, with the help of his sons Franciscus and Fredericus, continued Aldus's tradition, bringing out a number of Greek *editiones principes*: Pausanias (1516), Strabo (1516), Aeschylus (1518), Artemidorus (1518), and Lucian (1522). The five folio volumes of Galen, however, represented the largest single body of text the house had ever printed. To meet this challenge, the Pavian professor of medicine Giovanni Battista Oppizzoni (ca. 1485–ca. 1532) was placed in charge of a large group of assistants recruited mainly from northern medical scholars then studying in Italy: John Clement (ca. 1495–1572), Edward Wotton (1492–1555), William Rose (ca. 1490–1525), and Thomas Lupset (1495–1530), all Englishmen and followers of Thomas Linacre (ca. 1460–1524); and the Saxon Georgius Agricola (1495–1555), author of *De re metallica*. The 106 treatises they edited were collected and collated from numerous Greek manuscripts, most of which seem to have been in the area of Venice and Padua at the time. The following have been identified: Marcianus graecus 279 and 281–285; Marcianus graecus App. Cl. V. 4–5 and 8; Vaticanus Reginensis graecus 172–173; and Parisinus graecus 2148 and 2164–2168.

The significance of the first printing of a classical author cannot be overestimated, especially a prolific one like Aristotle or Galen, whose works were not to be found in a single or even very few manuscripts, but whose corpus had to be assembled from as many manuscripts as the printer could find. Such texts, when printed, were made available throughout the scholarly world in a standardized and corrected form, and their influence was often enhanced. In the case of Galen, the numerous editions and translations of his works that were published later in the sixteenth century were based on the Aldine Greek text.[2] At the Aldine press, the Greek *editio princeps* of Galen's works was followed by those of Hippocrates in 1526 (see no. 1B), Paul of Aegina (VII cent.) in 1528, and the first eight books (of sixteen) of the *Medical Compendium* of Aëtius of Amida (VI cent.) in 1534.

PP

Galen's dominance throughout the centuries owed as much to his philosophical views as to his medical expertise. His teleological interpretations of medical and physiological phenomena appealed to Christian, Jewish, and Muslim theologians, who found in his writings a scientific basis for their own theology; likewise, his intense dogmatism and almost dictatorial manner attracted disciples who required an unequivocal master. For these reasons, and because of the enormous range covered by the writings attributed to him, Galen's teachings were central to the curriculum of the medical schools of late Antiquity and the Middle Ages. Although his authority was challenged during the Renaissance, even then his influence was far from eliminated. Many of the greatest medical discoveries of the early modern period built on Galen while also correcting him.

Today Galen is honored as the founder of experimental physiology and as the sole proponent of this discipline in Western medicine until the time of William Harvey some fifteen centuries later. Galen demonstrated the normal presence of blood in the arteries (correcting Erasistratus) and made a number of important neurophysiological observations. He distinguished between motor and sensory nerves, demonstrated that the recurrent laryngeal nerve controls speech, produced various types of paralysis by sectioning the spinal cord at different levels, and observed the effects of lesions of the cerebrum and cerebellum. Galen's anatomy, based almost entirely on the dissection of animals, was erroneous in many respects, but he contributed several significant anatomical observations, including the identification of seven out of the twelve pairs of cranial nerves.

HFN

1. Quoted in Photius, *Bibliotheca*, 217.

2. Nikolaus Mani, "Die griechische *Editio princeps* des Galens (1525), ihre Entstehung und ihre Wirkung," *Gesnerus* 13 (1956): 29–52.

See color plate VI.

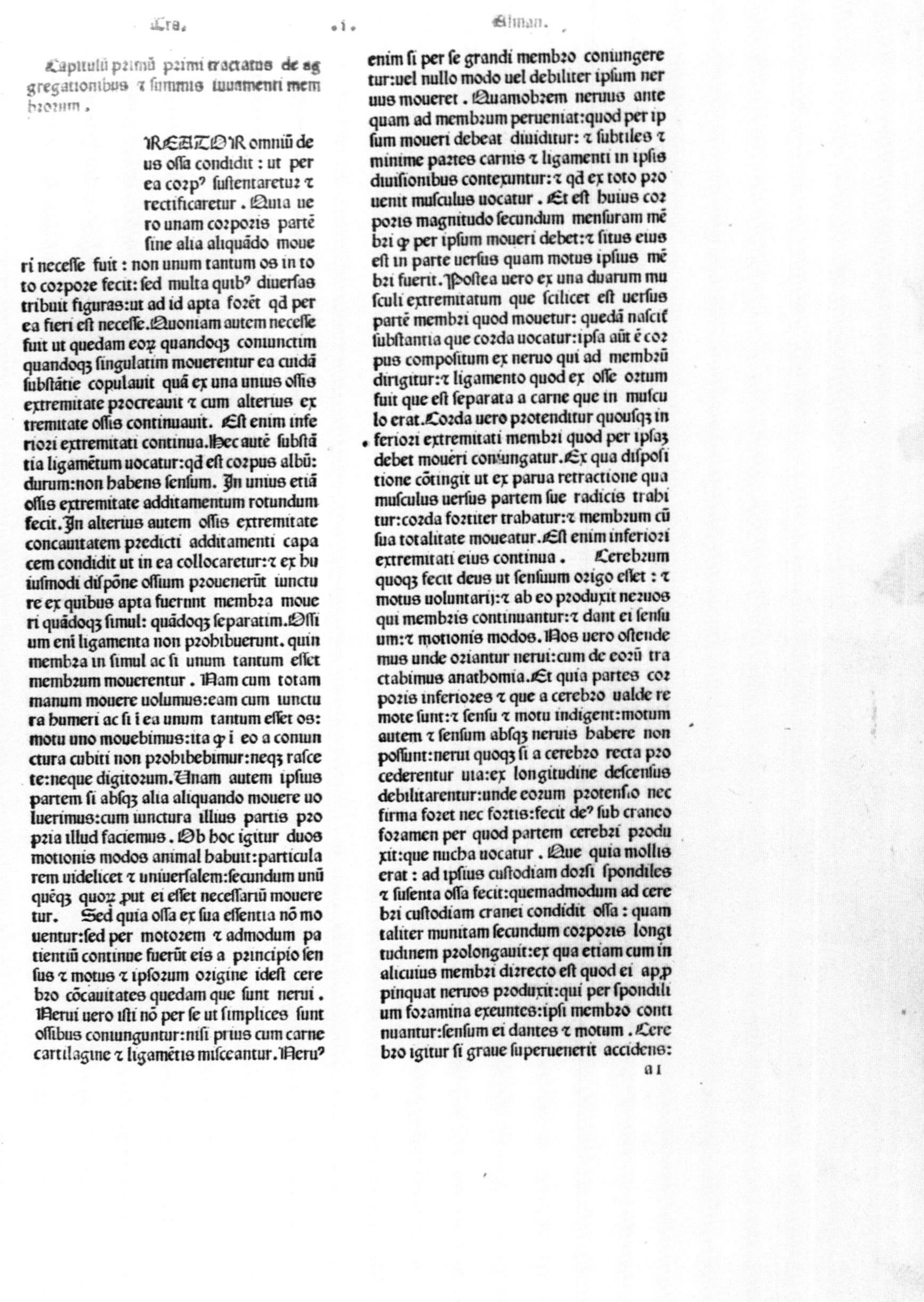

Tra. .i. Alman.

Capitulū primū primi tractatus de aggregationibus & summis iuuamenti membrorum.

CREATOR omniū deus ossa condidit : ut per ea corp⁹ sustentaretur & rectificaretur. Quia uero unam corporis partē sine alia aliquādo moueri necesse fuit : non unum tantum os in toto corpore fecit: sed multa quib⁹ diuersas tribuit figuras:ut ad id apta forēt qd per ea fieri est necesse. Quoniam autem necesse fuit ut quedam eorū quandoqȝ coniunctim quandoqȝ singulatim mouerentur ea cuidā substātie copulauit quā ex una unius ossis extremitate procreauit & cum alterius extremitate ossis continuauit. Est enim inferiori extremitati continua. Hec autē substātia ligamētum uocatur:qd est corpus albū: durum:non habens sensum. In unius etiā ossis extremitate additamentum rotundum fecit. In alterius autem ossis extremitate concauitatem predicti additamenti capacem condidit ut in ea collocaretur:& ex huiusmodi dispōne ossium prouenerūt iuncture ex quibus apta fuerunt membra moueri quādoqȝ simul: quādoqȝ separatim. Ossium enī ligamenta non prohibuerunt, quin membra in simul ac si unum tantum esset membrum mouerentur. Nam cum totam manum mouere uolumus:eam cum iunctura humeri ac si i ea unum tantum esset os: motu uno mouebimus:ita ꝙ i eo a coniunctura cubiti non prohibebimur:neqȝ rascete:neque digitorum. Unam autem ipsius partem si absqȝ alia aliquando mouere uoluerimus:cum iunctura illius partis propria illud faciemus. Ob hoc igitur duos motionis modos animal habuit:particularem uidelicet & uniuersalem:secundum unū quēqȝ quorū ꝓut ei esset necessariū moueretur. Sed quia ossa ex sua essentia nō mouentur:sed per motorem & admodum patientiū continue fuerūt eis a principio sensus & motus & ipsorum origine idest cerebro cōcauitates quedam que sunt nerui. Nerui uero isti nō per se ut simplices sunt ossibus coniunguntur:nisi prius cum carne cartilagine & ligamētis misceantur. Neru⁹ enim si per se grandi membro coniungeretur:uel nullo modo uel debiliter ipsum neruus moueret. Quamobrem neruus antequam ad membrum perueniat:quod per ipsum moueri debeat diuiditur: & subtiles & minime partes carnis & ligamenti in ipsis diuisionibus contexuntur:& qd ex toto prouenit musculus uocatur. Et est huius corporis magnitudo secundum mensuram mēbri ꝙ per ipsum moueri debet:& situs eius est in parte uersus quam motus ipsius mēbri fuerit. Postea uero ex una duarum musculi extremitatum que scilicet est uersus partē membri quod mouetur: quedā nascit substantia que corda uocatur:ipsa aūt ē corpus compositum ex neruo qui ad membrū dirigitur:& ligamento quod ex osse ortum fuit que est separata a carne que in musculo erat. Corda uero protenditur quousqȝ inferiori extremitati membri quod per ipsaȝ debet moueri coniungatur. Ex qua dispositione cōtingit ut ex parua retractione qua musculus uersus partem sue radicis trahitur:corda fortiter trahatur:& membrum cū sua totalitate moueatur. Est enim inferiori extremitati eius continua. Cerebrum quoqȝ fecit deus ut sensuum origo esset : & motus uoluntarij:& ab eo produxit neruos qui membris continuantur:& dant ei sensuum:& motionis modos. Nos uero ostendemus unde oriantur nerui:cum de eorū tractabimus anathomia. Et quia partes corporis inferiores & que a cerebro ualde remote sunt:& sensu & motu indigent:motum autem & sensum absqȝ neruis habere non possunt:nerui quoqȝ si a cerebro recta procederentur uia:ex longitudine descensus debilitarentur:unde eorum protensio nec firma foret nec fortis:fecit de⁹ sub craneo foramen per quod partem cerebri produxit:que nucha uocatur. Que quia mollis erat : ad ipsius custodiam dorsi spondiles & susenta ossa fecit:quemadmodum ad cerebri custodiam cranei condidit ossa : quam taliter munitam secundum corporis longitudinem prolongauit:ex qua etiam cum in alicuius membri directo est quod ei appinquat neruos produxit:qui per spondilium foramina exeuntes:ipsi membro continuantur:sensum ei dantes & motum. Cerebro igitur si graue superuenerit accidens:

a i

Fig. 11. No. 6. Rhazes. Page from the first Latin edition of the *Liber ad Almansorem* (1481).

6

RHAZES [ABŪ BAKR MUḤAMMAD IBN ZAKARIYYĀ AL-RĀZĪ]
(ca. 854–925)

Liber ad Almansorem (with other medical tracts).

Milan: Leonardus Pachel and Uldericus Scinzenzeler, 14 February 1481.

2°: π^6 a–l^8 m^4 n–z^8 $ꝛ^8$ $ꝯ^8$ $ꝶ^6$ $℞^{10}$. 218 leaves.

BMC VI, 749. Goff R–175. Klebs 826.1. Norman 1800. Stillwell 500, 689.

Rhazes, a Persian philosopher and physician, was born near Teheran and during the course of his career directed hospitals in his hometown and in Baghdad. A follower of Galen in his medical thinking, he nevertheless did not hesitate to question traditional authority when it was contradicted by his experience. He also brought a considerable knowledge of chemistry to his clinical studies. His major works include the one known in Latin as *Continens* (Kitāb al-ḥāwī), the *Liber ad Almansorem* or *Liber Almansoris* (Kitāb al-Manṣūrī), and a work on smallpox and measles (Kitāb al-jadarī wal-ḥaṣba). The *Liber ad Almansorem* contains ten books, the first six on physiology, dietetics, and rules of health, the seventh on surgery, the eighth on poisons, the ninth on pathology, and the last on fevers. It was translated into Latin in the twelfth century, and this version was published by Leonardus Pachel and Uldericus Scinzenzeler in Milan in 1481. Excerpts from the ninth book, which was popular as a therapeutic guide, had appeared earlier in Gianmatteo Ferrari's commentary, conventionally entitled *Practica*, printed in Milan before 29 October 1472 (GW 9830). The first separate edition of Book 9 was published in Padua, 8 June 1476 (IGI 8343; BMC VII, 906), and this portion of the work often appeared separately.

Although he was an important clinician, Rhazes' great contribution to medicine was as an encyclopedist. His compilations included extensive information from diverse sources and provided original clinical histories and the results of therapeutic experiments. Rhazes is credited with the earliest written description of smallpox, even though some imprecise statements about the disease had been recorded as early as the sixth century. Fielding Garrison thought Rhazes' description of smallpox so vivid and complete that it could be considered almost modern.[1] Rhazes also furnished the earliest authentic description of measles and made contributions to obstetrics and ophthalmology. He took an interest in pharmaceutical dosage forms, considering both efficacy and palatability, and recommended pills as vehicles of choice for the administration of medicines.

WHH

1. Fielding H. Garrison, *An Introduction to the History of Medicine*, 4th ed. (Philadelphia, 1929), p. 129.

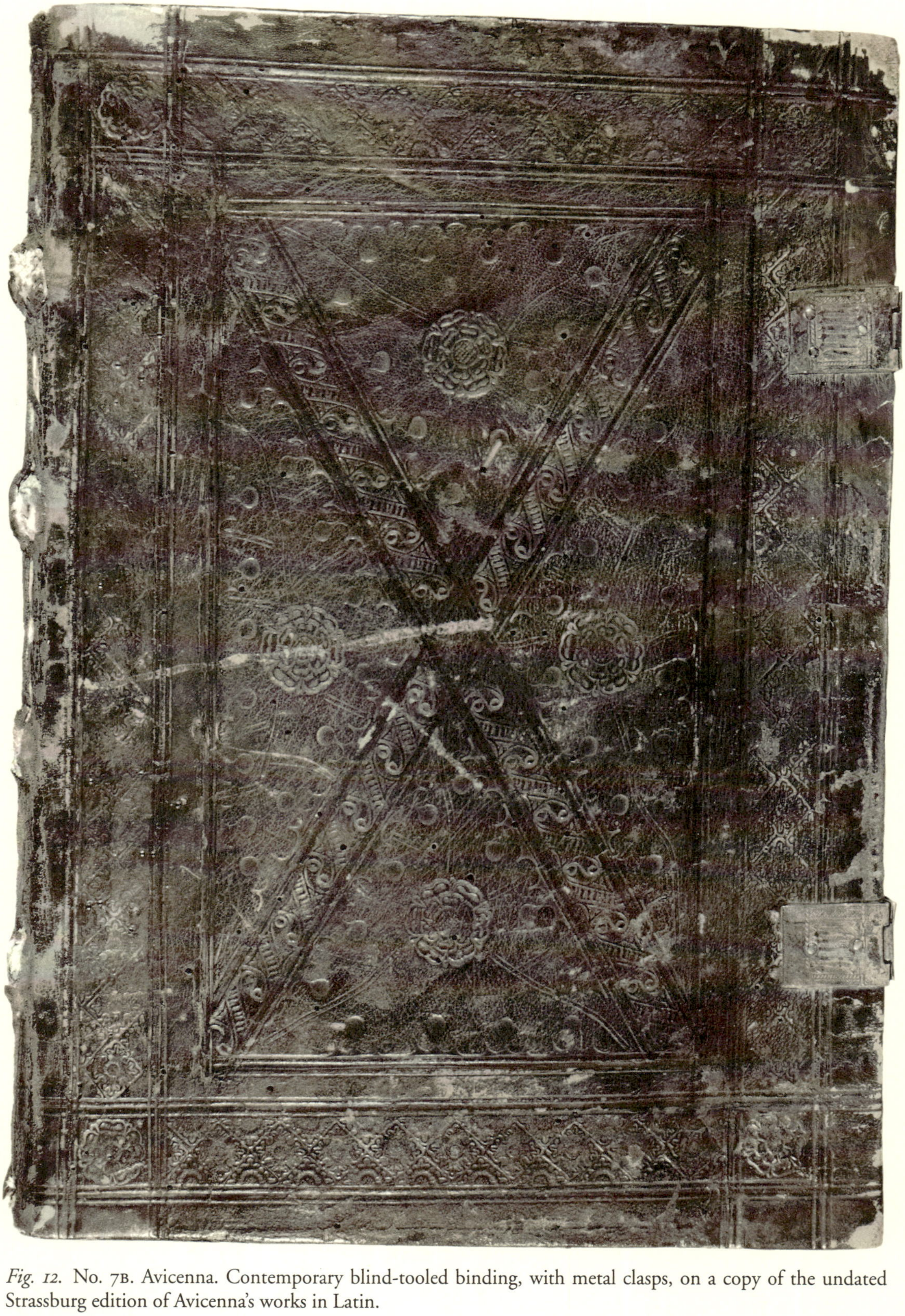

Fig. 12. No. 7B. Avicenna. Contemporary blind-tooled binding, with metal clasps, on a copy of the undated Strassburg edition of Avicenna's works in Latin.

7

AVICENNA [ABŪ 'ALĪ AL-ḤUSAYN IBN 'ABDALLAH IBN-SĪNĀ] (980–1037)

A] *Canon medicinae.*

Milan: Philippus de Lavagnia, 12 February 1473.

2°: [1–7^{10} 8^{8} 9^{10} 10^{4} (10_{1} + 1), 11–17^{10} 18^{8} 19^{6}, 20^{12} 21–25^{10} 26–27^{8} 28–34^{10} 35^{6} 36–42^{10} 43^{8} 44^{4}, 45^{4} 46–57^{10}, 58–61^{10}]. 93 (Book I), 84 (Book II), 236 (Book III), 124 (Book IV), 40 (Book V) [= 577] leaves.

BMC VI, 700. CIBN A–806. GM 43. GW 3115. Klebs 131.2. Osler *Incunabula medica* 35. Stillwell 287, 589.

B] *Canon medicinae.*

[Strassburg: The R-Printer (Adolf Rusch), not before 1475, not after 1477].

2°: [1–7^{10} 8^{8} 9^{10} 10^{4} (10_{1} + 1), 11–17^{10} 18^{8} 19^{6}, 20^{6} 21^{12} 22–26^{10} 27^{8} 28^{6} (28_{1} + 1) 29–35^{10} 36^{6} 37–43^{10} 44^{8}, 45^{4} 46–57^{10}, 58–61^{10}]. 93 (Book I), 84 (Book II), 237 (Book III), 124 (Book IV), 40 (Book V) [= 578] leaves.

BMC I, 65. CIBN A–807. Goff A–1417. GW 3114. Horblit 7. Klebs 131.3. Osler *Incunabula medica* 186. PMM 11.

In his *Canon medicinae*, the Persian physician Ibn-Sīnā, known as Avicenna, tried to consolidate medical knowledge and to reconcile medieval medical concepts with his own observations and those of Hippocrates, Aristotle, Galen, Rhazes, and other early medical writers. His encyclopedic Arabic text, containing about one million words, influenced generations of physicians and pharmacists. Even today Arabic editions remain in print, and in the Islamic world Avicenna continued to be cited as a medical authority into this century.[1] His work was translated into Latin by Gerard of Cremona in the twelfth century, and this version was printed in Milan in 1473. An undated Strassburg edition by the R-Printer, formerly regarded as the *editio princeps*, was reprinted from the Milan edition between 1475 and 1477; this edition may also postdate the one issued at Padua, 28 September–12 December 1476 (Goff A–1418).[2] The Arabic text was first printed in Rome by the Stamperia Medicea in 1593.

Although Avicenna was the prolific author of more than a hundred books on philosophy, theology, metaphysics, law, astronomy, and medicine, it is on his contributions to the last subject that his reputation rests. Physician to the ruling caliphs, he also served as chief physician of the Baghdad hospital. Among his many contributions were the earliest descriptions of the properties and preparation of alcohol and sulfuric acid and recognition of the communicable nature of a number of diseases such as tuberculosis and dysentery. He also perceived the hereditary nature of conditions such as premature baldness and gout. Two of the five books of the *Canon* discuss pharmaceutical matters, the nature of simple drugs, poisons, compound mixtures, and procedures for the gilding and silvering of pills; more than 750 drugs are discussed and there is also a long list of medicinal recipes, including examples from Galen and Dioscorides. Certain critics, including Albrecht von Haller, have faulted the *Canon* for its unwieldy organization, possibly because of its alphabetical arrangement, while others, such as Fielding Garrison, have felt that it set back the progress of surgery by claiming the surgical art to be inferior to medicine and by substituting cautery for the knife.[3] According to the German historian of medicine Max Neuberger, the *Canon* was the "epitome of all precedent development, the final codification of Graeco-Arabic medicine."[4]

WHH

1. In a manuscript note dated 7 August 1915, made in his copy of Martin Winter's *Über Avicennas Opus egregium de anima* (Munich, 1903), William Osler wrote that "Dr. Neligan, physician to the British embassy, Teheran, told me today that he had a consultation on a case of fever with a native physician who quoted Avicenna and said he did not think the case was one of typhoid as it did not correspond with the symptoms laid down in the Canon" (quoted in *Bibliotheca Osleriana*, [Oxford, 1939], p. 44).
2. Arguments for the dating of the Strassburg edition have been kindly supplied by Paul Needham; see his remarks in Doheny, lot 16, and Abrams, lots 22 and 108. See also CIBN A–806 and A–807, and Jean-Luc Kahn, "Mentelin et l'imprimerie à Strasbourg jusqu'en 1475," *Bulletin du bibliophile,* 1990: 345–70.
3. Fielding H. Garrison, *An Introduction to the History of Medicine*, 4th ed. (Philadelphia, 1929), pp. 130–31.
4. Max Neuberger, *Geschichte der Medizin*, vol. 2 (Stuttgart, 1911), p. 181.

See color plate VII.

8

GUY DE CHAULIAC

(ca. 1298–ca. 1368)

A] *Chirurgia* [French].

Lyons: [Nicolaus Philippi and Marcus Reinhart for] Barthélemy Buyer, 28 March 1478.

2°: a^8 b–c^{10} d–t^8 v^6 x–z^8 $ꝛ^8$ A–I^8. 266 leaves. Woodcut figures of surgical instruments in text.

GM 5556. Klebs 491.1. Osler *Incunabula medica* 164. Pellechet 3533. PMM 21. Stillwell 398, 650.

B] *Chirurgia* [Italian].

Venice: Nicolaus Girardengus, de Novis, 2 November 1480.

2°: a^8 b^4 c^8 d^{10} e–f^8 g^{10} h^8 i^{10} k^8 l–n^{10} o^8 p–q^{10} R^{10} S–T^6 r–u^8 x–z^6 A–C^6 D^{10}. 240 leaves.

BMC V, 273. Goff G–562. Klebs 492.1. Osler *Incunabula medica* 194. Waller 69.

The importance of the *Chirurgia* lies not in its description of technical advances but in its systematization of surgery and its recognition of the responsibilities of the surgeon and the needs of his patients, which have not changed in the six hundred years since the work was written. Guy de Chauliac studied medicine in Toulouse, Montpellier, and Bologna, where he was a pupil of Mondino's successor Niccolo Bertruccio. He later served as physician to three successive popes in exile in Avignon. His major work, *Chirurgia*, was completed in 1363, a few years before his death.

The *Chirurgia* is one of the landmarks in the history of surgery. With its 3,300 references to more than one hundred authors, including numerous quotations from Avicenna, Albucasis, Rhazes, Haly Abbas, Hippocrates, and Galen, it represented the most complete compilation of surgical material prepared to that date, and it remained authoritative in Western medicine until the seventeenth century. The book's seven sections cover a broad range of subjects, from cancers to wounds and fractures to dentistry. Its preface (*Capitulum singulare*) contains both a brief history of medicine and Guy's essay on what all surgeons should know about the liberal arts, diet, surgical instruments, and operating methods. Guy himself regarded his book as a compendium of the best medical ideas of his time, stating that only a few things were original with him, yet he often used his own experiences as a basis for criticism of the classical Greek and Arabic medical writings.

Chirurgia exists in many manuscripts copied between 1363 and the late fifteenth century, including versions in Latin, French, English, Italian, Provençal, Dutch, and Hebrew; the existence of so many early translations into the vernacular is an indication of the es-

Nel nome de dio cōmeza lo inuētario o uer colectorio che apartiē ala parte đ la cirogia: cōposto e compido del āno de la incarnation del nostro signore Mccc.lxiii. p lo clarissimo e famoso dōtor maistro. Guidon de gualiaco ciroico i lo clarissio studio de mompolier.

Rubrica.

O A poi che pria hauero reso gratie a dio: elq̄l dona la uita perpetua a le anime: sāita a li corpi: e medega le grā de egritudine: p la gratia laqual lui a dato a ogno carne: p le uirtu che cōseruāo la sāita e che defēdeno da lāgorii e da. A intēdere la r☙ de la medecia e īgenio đ la sāita ali diuini e anemosi ītelligēti. daro opera a comēta e a sumar. In prima adōcha Io comēzādo alguna comētation o uero collectiō de la arte de la cirugia. Rendo gratia a dio uiuo e uero: elquale da a ognuno le ser: sēza elqual nesū pricipio dritamēte se fūda. Adio deuotissia mēte rcorādo e cō tute le forze del mio cuor supplicando che ī questa opera & ī tute le altr māde a mi lo aiuto suo sācto. e de sion me aiute dando felice pricipio e piu felice mezo gouernādo & cōande cōpir quelo che sia utile a fi bon dedugādo. La rasō de questa comētatiō ouer colectiō nō fo per difetō de libri ma piu tosto per unita e perfectiō: certo nō e possibile zascuno hauer tuti li libri e se ancora ciascadūo li hauesse: seria tediō a legerli e seria cosa diuina retignir ogni cosa a mēte. La lection de diuerse cose delectare. la certa zoua e ne lo cōstrution sempre occore meioramēti certe le scientie sono fate per aditamēti. perche nō e possibile un medeīso comenzar e finir. Nui siemo puti nel colo del gigāte: per che posēo ueder zascaduna cosa che uede el gigāte e alguna cosa piu e adōcha ī le cōstrution e assūation unita e perfetion Ma perche come dice plato quele cose lequal se scriueno piu brieuemente de quelo che se cōuien sono diminute e obscur e quele che sono scrite piu lōge fastidisseno li studiāti nō e quasi libro che fuza reprēsiōe. e perzo a mi a solazo de la uechieza e exercitio de la mēte: a oto signori mei medici đ mōpolier e da bologna e da parix e da uignō. specialmēte papali liquali me a cōpagnasti nel seruitio de li romāi pōtifici cō liquali aldēdo lezando e operādo fu nudrido obseruādo la mediocrita con moderada breuita: restrēzero li principali diti de li saui liquali ī diuersi uolumi de libri de cirogia hano tratado per laqual cosa questo libro sera chiamado inuentario o uer coletorio đ cirugia. Ne li o azōto del mio ꝓprio alguna cosa: se nō forsi pochissie leq̄le segōdo el mio pocho īgenio ho reputado utile e se algua cosa īperfecta: dubia. supfiua e obscura sera a la corretiō uostra me sotometo e supplico che a la puocha mia scientia sia perdōado Capitulo sīgular ī lo qual se pmete algune cose cōmune molto necessarie a

ai

Fig. 13. No. 8B. Guy de Chauliac. Page from the first edition in Italian (1480).

teem in which the book was held in the later Middle Ages. Although probably written in Latin, the work was first published in a French translation by Nicolaus Panis, printed in Lyons in 1478. This was followed by editions in Italian (1480), Catalan (1492; Klebs 493.1), and Spanish (1493; Klebs 493.2). The first Latin edition was published in Venice in 1498 (Goff G–558). Following the manuscript tradition, which included depictions of surgical instruments, the first and many later editions of the *Chirurgia* contained woodcut illustrations of such instruments. In the first Italian edition, however, spaces were left for the figures to be supplied.

ESF

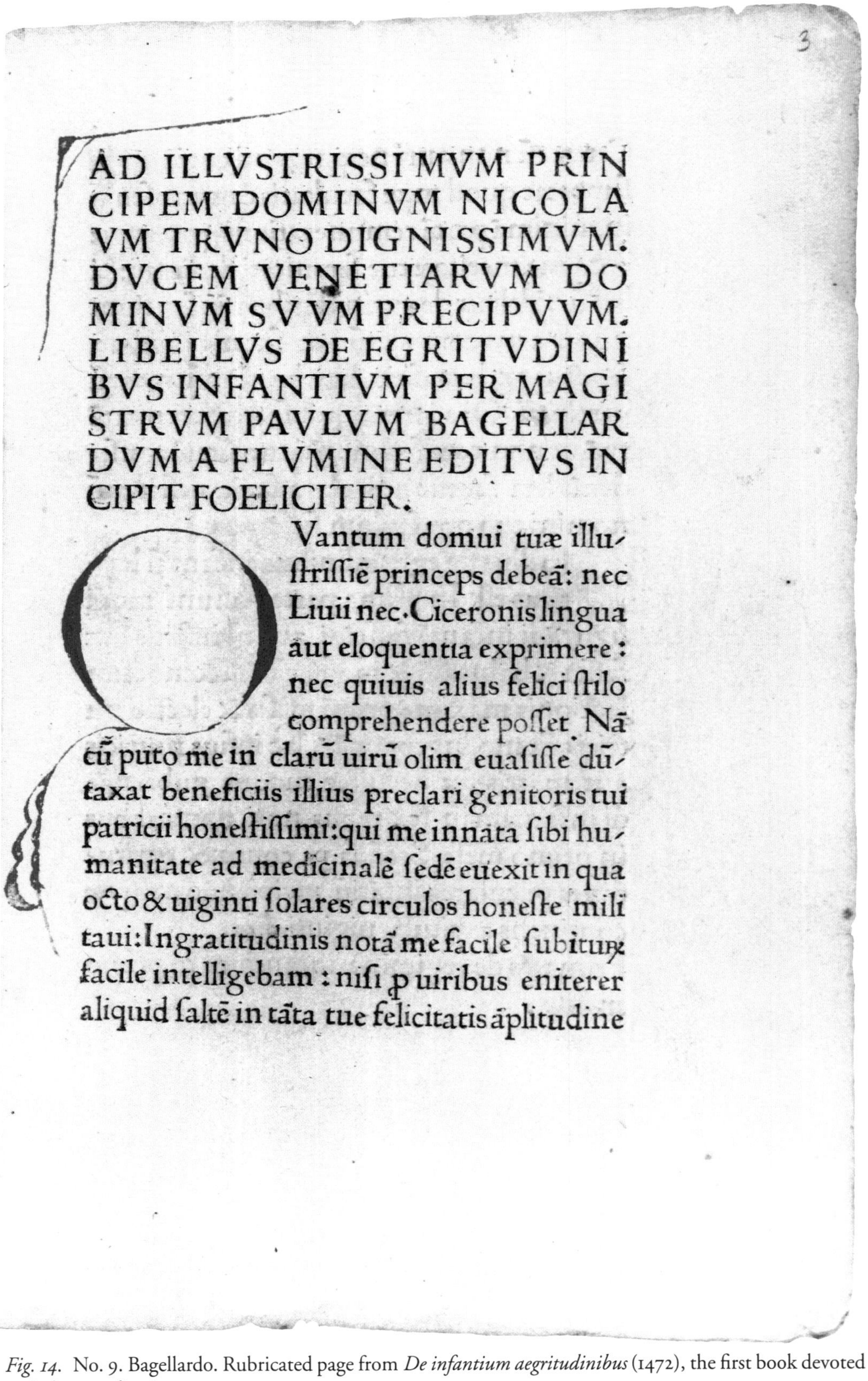
3

AD ILLVSTRISSIMVM PRINCIPEM DOMINVM NICOLAVM TRVNO DIGNISSIMVM. DVCEM VENETIARVM DOMINVM SVVM PRECIPVVM. LIBELLVS DE EGRITVDINIBVS INFANTIVM PER MAGISTRVM PAVLVM BAGELLARDVM A FLVMINE EDITVS INCIPIT FOELICITER.

QVantum domui tuæ illustrissiē princeps debeā: nec Liuii nec. Ciceronis lingua aut eloquentia exprimere: nec quiuis alius felici stilo comprehendere posset. Nā cū puto me in clarū uirū olim euasisse dūtaxat beneficiis illius preclari genitoris tui patricii honestissimi: qui me innata sibi humanitate ad medicinalē sedē euexit in qua octo & uiginti solares circulos honeste militaui: Ingratitudinis notā me facile subiturū facile intelligebam: nisi ꝓ uiribus eniterer aliquid saltē in tāta tue felicitatis āplitudine

Fig. 14. No. 9. Bagellardo. Rubricated page from *De infantium aegritudinibus* (1472), the first book devoted entirely to pediatrics.

9

PAOLO BAGELLARDO
(d. 1492)

De infantium aegritudinibus et remediis.

[Padua]: Bartholomaeus de Valdezoccho and Martinus de Septem Arboribus, 21 April 1472.

4°: [1^2 2–3^{10} 4^8 5^{10}]. 40 leaves.

BMC VII, 904. Goff B–10. GM 6315. GW 3166. Klebs 139.1. Norman 102. Osler 7417. Osler *Incunabula medica* 20. Stillwell 291. Waller 26.

Bagellardo's treatise, the title of which translates as "On the diseases of children and their cure," has three marks of distinction: (1) as the first medical book to make its earliest appearance in print rather than in manuscript form; (2) as one of the first two medical books submitted to the press by a living author; and (3) as the first printed book to deal exclusively with pediatrics. Little is known about the author beyond the fact that he was educated at Padua and practiced medicine there until his death in 1492. In his book he noted that he had been in practice for twenty-eight years at the time of its publication.

Bagellardo's book is a compendium of the pediatric practice of his time. The influence of Rhazes, Avicenna, Hippocrates, and Galen, among others, is acknowledged, but Bagellardo also recorded his own observations, experience, and opinions. The book is divided into two parts: the first deals with infant management during the early months of life, and the second discusses the treatment of different diseases, including diarrhea, constipation, worms, epilepsy, and afflictions of the eyes and ears. The historian of pediatrics John Ruhräh commented favorably on Bagellardo's treatment of wakefulness: "He advises that 'the curing begins with the lighter remedies, since all things which provoke sleep are narcotic and in a certain measure are stupefying.' Sound advice indeed!"[1]

De infantium aegritudinibus et remediis was reprinted in Padua in 1487 (Goff B–11), in Lyons early in the sixteenth century (Waller 599), and again in Lyons in 1538 with an introduction by Petrus Toletus (Durling 433). An Italian translation was published in Brescia in 1486 (Goff B–12). It was reproduced in facsimile by Karl Sudhoff in 1925 and translated into English in the same year.[2]

HFN

1. John Ruhräh, *Pediatric Biographies* (Chicago, 1932), p. 7.
2. Facsimile in Karl Sudhoff, ed., *Erstlinge der pädiatrischen Literatur: Drei Wiegendrucke über Heilung und Pflege des Kindes* (Munich, 1925). Translation in John Ruhräh, *Pediatrics of the Past* (New York, 1925), pp. 28–70.

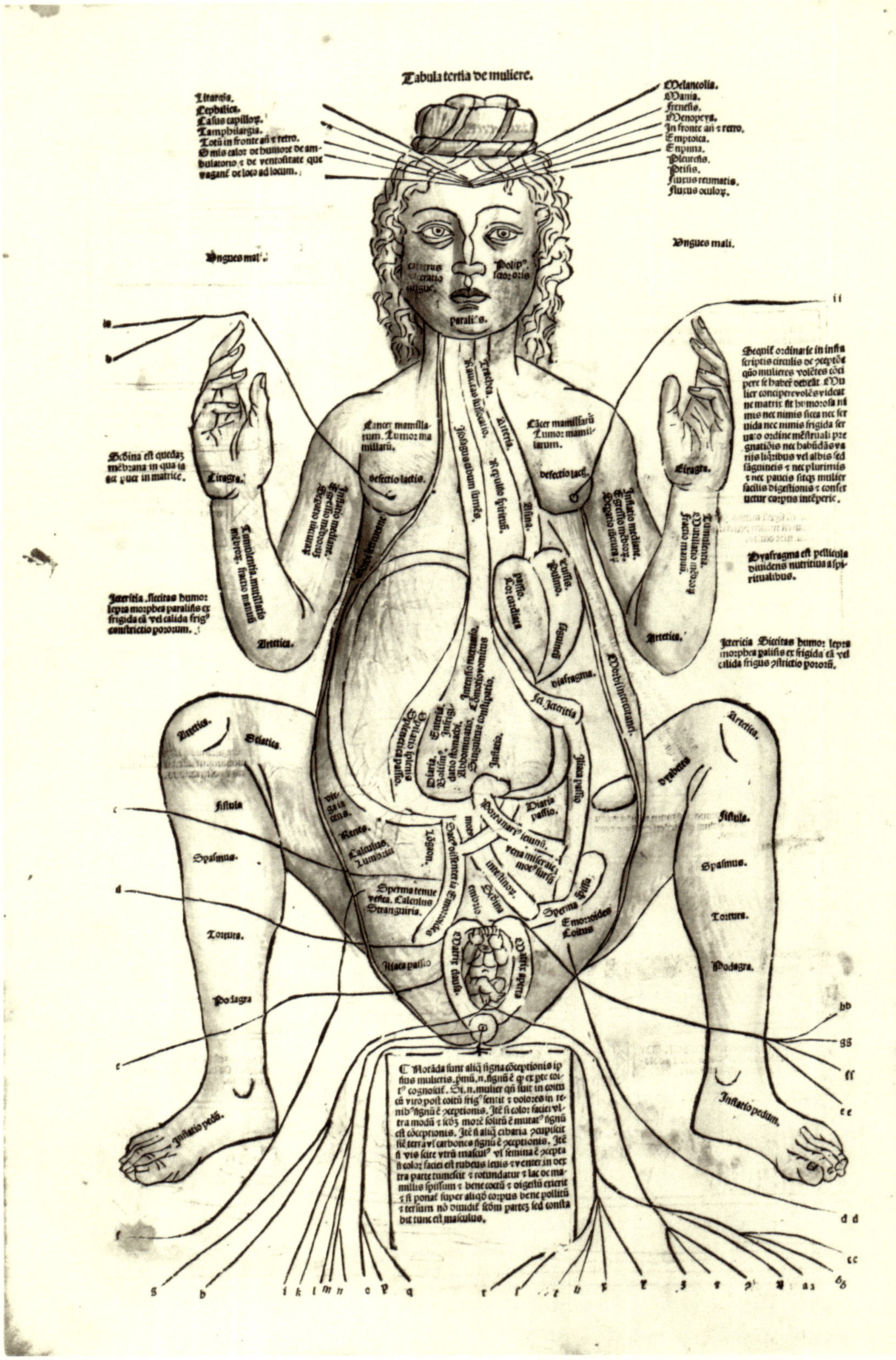

Fig. 15. No. 10A. Johannes de Ketham. Female figure from the first edition (1491), showing the traditional squatting posture and distorted abdomen.

10

JOHANNES DE KETHAM
(fl. 1455–1470)

A] *Fasciculus medicinae.*

Venice: Joannes and Gregorius de Gregoriis, de Forlivio, 26 July 1491.

2°: a–b⁸. 16 leaves. 6 full-page woodcuts in text.

Choulant-Frank, pp. 115–16. GM 363. Goff K–13. Klebs 573.1. Stillwell 436, 667.

B] *Fascicolo di medicina.*

Venice: Joannes and Gregorius de Gregoriis, 5 February 1493/94.

2°: a–h⁶ i⁴. 52 leaves. 10 full-page woodcuts in text.

BMC V, 344. Choulant-Frank, pp. 116–19. GM 363.1. Goff K–17. Klebs 574.1. PMM 36. Waller 86.

This collection of short medical treatises, some dating as far back as the thirteenth century, circulated widely in manuscript before the brothers De Gregoriis of Forlì printed the first edition at their Venetian press in 1491. The "Ketham" to whom the printers attributed the collection was probably Johann von Kircheim, a physician and professor of medicine in Vienna who is supposed to have assembled these practical texts and diagrams for educational purposes: "Ketham" is a plausible corruption of "Kircheim."[1] The first edition was the first printed medical book to contain anatomical illustrations, if one discounts the crude phlebotomy figure that occurs in a Flemish collection of medical texts by Lanfranc of Milan, Guy de Chauliac, and Avicenna (Louvain, 1481; BMC IX, 159), and the woodcut of the three cerebral ventricles printed in the *Philosophia pauperum* of pseudo-Albertus Magnus (Brescia, 1490; Goff A–296). The anatomical illustrations prepared for the first edition of *Fasciculus medicinae* included the following: (1) phlebotomy man; (2) zodiacal man; (3) seated figure of a pregnant woman, showing the internal organs; (4) wound man; and (5) disease man. Another woodcut, with captions printed in red, shows a schematic representation of urine glasses arranged in a circle. All of these illustrations have well-established precedents in the manuscript tradition.

The 1491 Latin edition of the *Fasciculus medicinae* was followed by an Italian translation published in 1493/94 and a Spanish translation printed in 1495 (Goff K–18). The Italian version, by Sebastianus Manilius, made no reference to Ketham, but added to the compilation an Italian translation of the *Anatomia* of Mondino de' Luzzi, a fourteenth-century compendium by a professor of medicine at Bologna that included observations based on the dissection of human cadavers. For the Italian translation of *Fasciculus medicinae*, all the illustrations save that of the "disease man" were redrawn and recut, and four new illustrations were added: (1) a doctor identified as "Petrus de Montagnana" in his study (frontispiece); (2) Petrus, his students, and an attendant with a flask of urine; (3) a doctor's visit to a plague patient; and (4) a lesson in dissection. There has been much speculation about the identity of the artist of these strikingly beautiful woodcuts, but he was certainly close to the school of Bellini. Hind states that "Lesson in dissection," which prefaces Mondino's work, is sometimes found "printed from three colour-blocks in red, green and yellow, in addition to the outline in black," the color probably applied by hand-held blocks rather than the printing press.[2] Others, including Harvey Cushing, have speculated that the coloring in these examples may have been applied using a stencil, citing as evidence the red coloring of the professor's right hand and the prosecutor's left hand, which would have "had to be included in the opening of the stencil."[3] Coloring in the other plates, when it occurs, was added by hand.

It is in the woodcuts prepared for the Italian edition that the transition from medieval to modern anatomical illustration is first evident. In the 1491 edition, the woodcut of the female viscera, like those of the other anatomical figures, was derived from the traditional nonrepresentational squatting figure found in medieval medical manuscripts. However, the illustrations for the Italian edition "included an entirely redesigned figure showing female anatomy. . . . The scholastic figure from 1491 must have irritated the eyes of the artistic Venetians to such a degree that they immediately abandoned it. After this the female figure actually sits in an armchair, so that the traditional position corresponds to a real situation."[4]

ESF

1. Johannes de Ketham, *The Fasciculus Medicinae of Johannes de Ketham Alemanus. Facsimile of the First (Venetian) Edition . . . with introduction by Karl Sudhoff*, trans. and ed. Charles Singer (Milan, 1924), pp. 42–45.

2. Arthur M. Hind, *An Introduction to a History of Woodcut* (New York, 1935), pp. 494–96.

3. Cushing's note in the Yale copy of the 1493/94 Italian edition.

4. Robert Herrlinger, *History of Medical Illustration from Antiquity to A.D. 1600*, trans. Graham Fulton-Smith (London, 1970), p. 66.

See color plates VIII and IX.

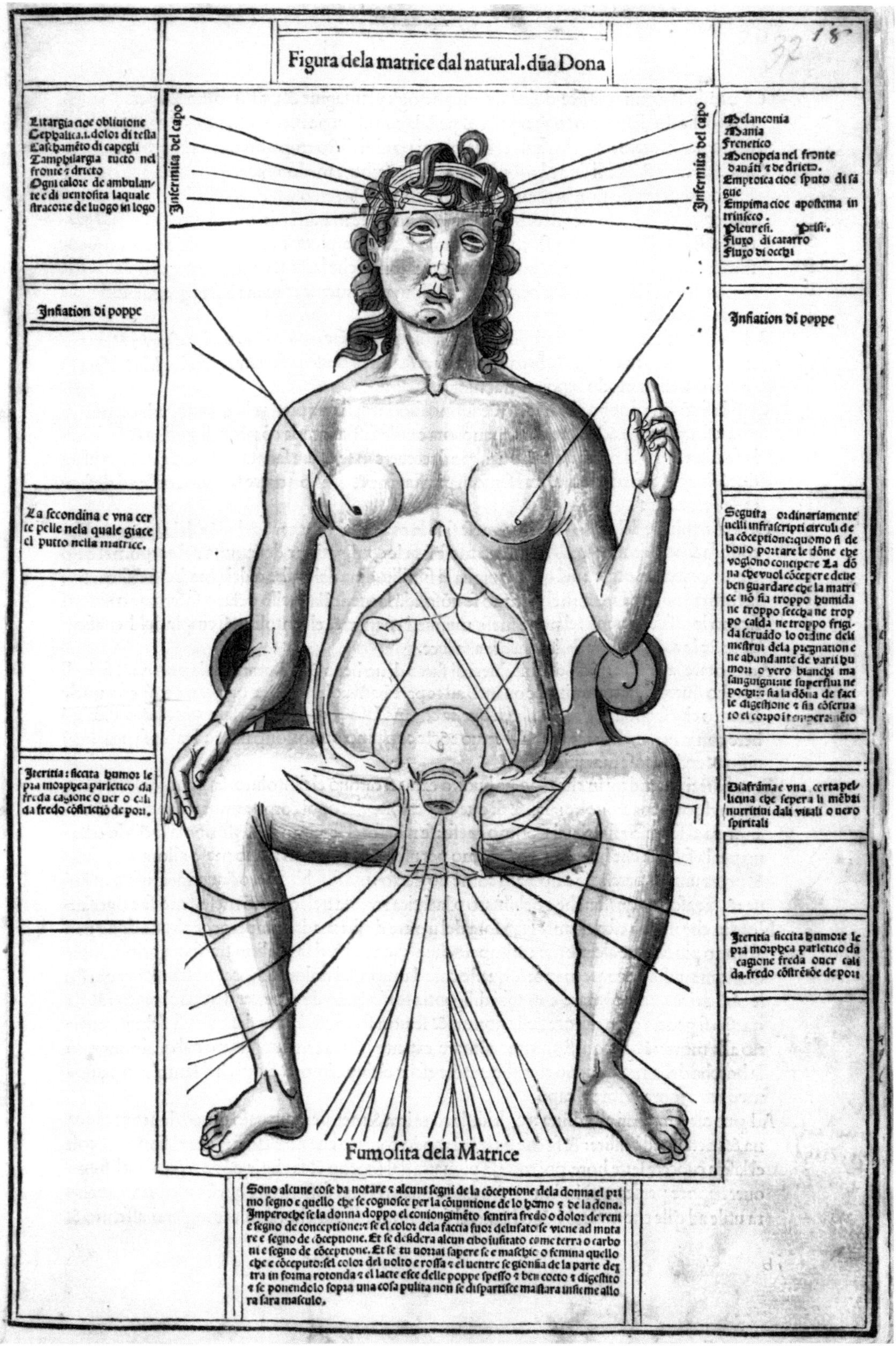

Fig. 16. No. 10B. Johannes de Ketham. Female figure from the 1493 Italian edition, showing a more realistic posture and abdominal configuration.

GABRIELIS ZERBI VERONENSIS
AD INNOCENTIVM. VIII. PON. MAX.
GERENTOCOMIA FELICITER INCI-
PIT. PROLOGVS.

Ntiquo ac paterno oim fere ꝯsẽsu natura ⁊ rõe
ducente ꝯfessuꝫ est imenso numine aliquo cũcta
disponi cuiꝰ nutu sũmoto tueri seipm põt nihil. Hꝫ
numen deus siue quolibeat nomine appellet perfectionis
eius exuberantia oia singulis vt decet impartit ⁊ abundã
tius tribuit etsi sepenumero ineptitudine eius qđ subijcit
nequeãt adipisci. Licꝫ aũt esse ipsum ⁊ viuere diuturnita
tisqꝫ vite ⁊ salutis appetentia sicuti ⁊ ꝑfectões alie a deo
emanãtes rebus nature ꝯstantibus cõicent nulla bonita-
te que illis cõgruit retenta apud eũ in primo reꝝ exordio
homini tñ vni animantiũ oim meliori (nescio an dicam)
eius fato seu tristiori adeo imensam parens natura dedit
viuendi cupidinem ⁊ iocunditatẽ eius vite comites indi-
uiduas vt vitã hãc ꝗuis temporalis sit ac labore plenissi
ma tã senes ꝗ iuuenes cupiãt ⁊ hi qui miseri sunt nolint
interire etiã cũ se miseros esse sentiãt. quo fit vt hoim ple
riqꝫ senescere cupiant ꝗuis senectutem accusent adepti.
Adeo etiã blanda est spirandi ꝑ se cuiqꝫ dulcedo vt nemo
sit tã senex morte etiã in foribus deplorate iam vite exũte
cuilicꝫ interposito metu spes tñ adhuc annue vite non su
persit. Nõ explet aũt cuiuslibet hominis vita quam tan-
topere exoptant periodo equali paucis aut nullis eoꝝ ad
vltimũ humane vite finem naturalem imo vix ad senectu
tis principia ꝑuenientibus desidia nõ modo ⁊ luxuria bo
nos mores (vt aiunt) vitiantibus quibus humana corpa
affligi ꝯsueuerũt verumetiam accidentibus pluribus atqꝫ
offensaculis sibi oppositis intercipiẽtibus prius vitã quo

Fig. 17. No. 11. Zerbi. First page of the first book devoted to geriatrics.

11

GABRIELE ZERBI
(1445–1505)

Gerontocomia.

Rome: Eucharius Silber, 27 November 1489.

4°: [1^6 $2–17^8$ 18^2]. 136 leaves. Quire 18, the "Emendationes errorum," is not found in all copies.

BMC IV, 110. GM 1589.1. Goff Z–26. *Heirs of Hippocrates* 137. Klebs 1057.1. Stillwell 558. Waller 150.

Zerbi is considered the founder of the science of geriatrics, and his *Gerontocomia*, a practical manual of geriatrics, was the earliest monograph on the subject to be printed. In spite of its emphasis on classical sources, it is a most remarkable and innovative piece of work. In his dedication to Pope Innocent VIII (1484–92), Zerbi described his aim thus: "One must labor to protect the old from the torture of their bodies, to ward off death by proper care of their health . . . and to stand guard against those forces which bring on premature death, so that with their health intact, the old people may live out the rest of their lives as peacefully as possible."

The longest section of the work, filling twenty chapters, deals with diet and nutrition, discussing the suitability for the elderly of every type of food and drink then available in Italy. Zerbi also included a chapter on the running of an old peoples' home, which must be one of the earliest accounts of one in medical literature. The details are practical: the assistants or special nurses (*gerontocomes*) should be clean, well-dressed, cheerful, and polite. It should be their task to prepare for the comfort of the inmates, to see that they have suitable clothes and bedclothes, and that they take baths and regular exercise. As well as physical activity, mainly in the form of walking and swimming, Zerbi stressed the importance of the old retaining mental interests and occupations. It is these often small details that make *Gerontocomia* a pioneering work, not only in geriatrics but also in preventive medicine.

Zerbi himself did not enjoy the peaceful old age he advocated for others. At the age of sixty, after achieving some distinction as professor of anatomy at Padua, he was brutally murdered by the sons of a Turkish pasha whom he had failed to cure. His book on old age was long ignored, presumably because of the rarity of the original and only early edition. Its reassessment as a medical classic follows the recent publication of an English translation.[1]

RDG

1. Gabriele Zerbi, *Gerontocomia: On the Care of the Aged* . . . , trans. L. R. Lind (Philadelphia, 1988).

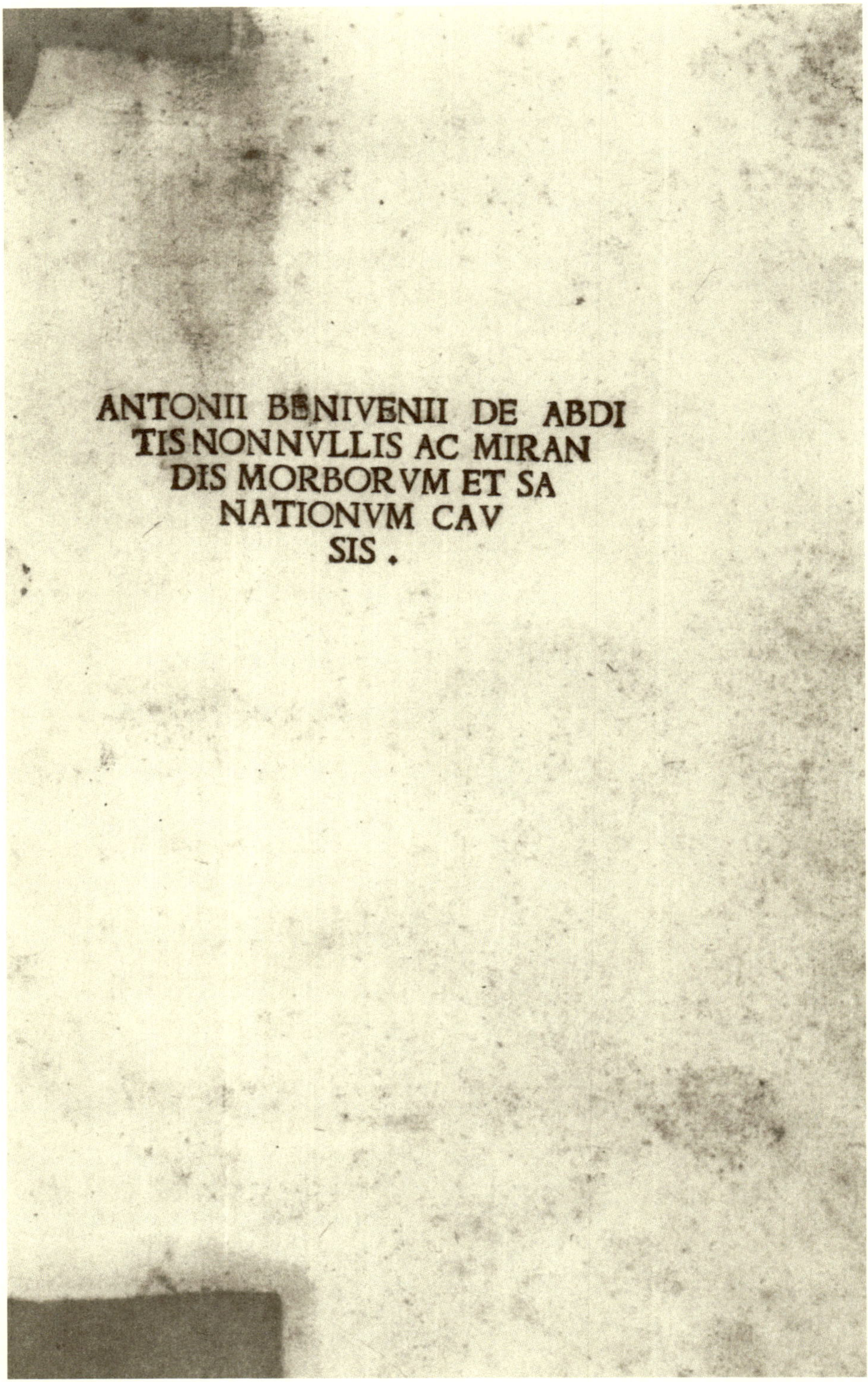
ANTONII BENIVENII DE ABDI
TIS NONNVLLIS AC MIRAN
DIS MORBORVM ET SA
NATIONVM CAV
SIS.

Fig. 18. No. 12. Benivieni. Title page.

12

ANTONIO BENIVIENI
(1443–1502)

De abditis nonnullis ac mirandis morborum et sanationum causis.

Florence: Opera & impensa Philippi Giuntae, 24 September 1507.

4°: a–f^8 g^6. 54 leaves.

Adams B–664. Durling 528. GM 2270. Norman 183. Stillwell 299, 597. Waller 894.

Jean Cruveilhier, the famous French pathologist, called Benivieni the father of pathological anatomy, and the distinguished French historian of surgery J. F. Malgaigne wrote of Benivieni that "he was the first to make experience a necessity and to give his successors the useful example of seeking in the cadaver . . . the 'hidden causes' of diseases."[1]

Antonio Benivieni was a friend and colleague of several of his distinguished contemporaries, including Angelo Poliziano, Marsilio Ficino, Benedetto Varchi, and Lorenzo de' Medici; during his thirty years of medical practice he attended the most important families in Florence. However, his fame today rests on the posthumous *De abditis*, edited by his brother, the poet Girolamo Benivieni, and the physician Giovanni Rosati. The title of the book, which translates as "On the several hidden and strange causes of disease and cure," reflects the author's interest in ascertaining, via postmortem examination, the reasons for death in cases where diagnosis during life had been obscured. It is probable that the title of Benivieni's book was suggested by the phrase *abditae morborum causae* employed by Celsus, as it is known that he possessed in his library a copy of Celsus's *De medicina* (see no. 4).[2] Later editions of *De abditis* were published in Venice (1516), Paris (1528), Basel (1529), Cologne (1581), and Leiden (1585).

In keeping with his time, Benivieni's anatomy and physiology were influenced by Galen; however, he seems to have escaped the restraint on new ideas that was part of the heritage of medieval scholasticism. Benivieni was the first physician known to have requested permission of his patients' relations to perform autopsies to clarify the causes of illness and death, and the records of postmortems that he and his colleagues performed were the first of their kind to be published. His necropsies were limited, however, by the fact that he merely incised the bodies (*incidere*), rather than dissecting the organs out (*decidere*) as Morgagni did over two and a half centuries later (see no. 46).

De abditis was derived from the large number of manuscript records that Benivieni left behind him at his death. The work was originally conceived as a treatise of 300 sections to be published in three series or *centuriae*; however, Benivieni completed only 160 sections, and of these the editors selected 111. The autograph manuscript of *De abditis* was rediscovered by Francesco Puccinotti in 1855, and although it subsequently disappeared again, a transcription survives. This indicates that Benivieni performed twenty autopsies and that he observed gallstones, urinary calculi, scirrhous cancer of the stomach, fibrous tumor of the heart, and peritonitis arising from intestinal perforation. He was one of the first physicians to study syphilis, and he gave an account of this disease at the beginning of the manuscript, describing its superficial manifestations and the transmission of it to the fetus. Benivieni was a competent surgeon, and several important examples of pathology are given in his descriptions of surgical procedures. In fact, *De abditis* is as important for the history of surgery as it is for the history of pathology.

Interest in Benivieni's book revived in 1843 when it was translated into Italian by Carlo Burci, the first ordinary professor of pathological anatomy in Italy.[3] In America it was cited by Esmond Long, professor of pathology at the University of Chicago, in his *History of Pathology* (1928), and Long also wrote a biographical appreciation of Benivieni for the English translation of *De abditis* that he and Charles Singer published in 1954.[4] Long summed up his evaluation of Benivieni's observations as follows: "To be sure, his explanations of what he saw were based entirely on the old humoral pathology, but he took the great step forward of searching out, as well as he could, the organic seat of disease."[5] The medical historian Ralph Major wrote in 1935: "Benivieni's *De abditis* marks the beginning of a new method of thinking in medical science. . . . He was unquestionably a pathfinder in medicine, who blazed a new path which physicians waited for more than two centuries and a half to follow."[6]

HFN

1. J. F. Malgaigne, *Surgery and Ambroise Paré*, ed. and trans. Wallace Hamby (Norman, Okla., 1965), p. 114.

2. Pietro Franceschini, "Benivieni, Antonio," in *Dictionary of Scientific Biography*, vol. 1 (New York, 1970), p. 612.

3. Carlo Burci, *Di alcune ammirabili ed occulte cause di morbi e loro guarigioni. Libro di Antonio Benivieni con un elogio storico intorno alla vita e alle opere dell'autore* (Florence, 1843).

4. Antonio Benivieni, *De abditis nonnullis ac mirandis* . . . , trans. by Charles Singer, with a biographical appreciation by Esmond R. Long (Springfield, Ill., 1954).

5. Esmond R. Long, *A History of Pathology*, 2d ed. (New York, 1965), p. 35.

6. Ralph Major, "Antonio di Pagolo Benivieni," *Bulletin of the History of Medicine* 3 (1935): 749.

See color plate X.

13

EUCHARIUS RÖSSLIN
(d. 1526)

A] *Der swangern Frauwen vnd Hebammen Rosegarten.*

Strassburg: Martinus Flach iunior impressit, 6 March 1513.

4°: A–N4 O6. 58 leaves. Woodcut title border; in text, 4 full-page woodcuts (2 images, each repeated) and 20 smaller woodcuts (including 2 repeats).

Choulant-Frank, pp. 73–74. Durling 3893. Stillwell 507.

B] *Der swangern Frawen vnd Hebammen Roszgarten.*

[Hagenau]: Heinrich Gran (device), [ca. 1515].

4°: A–O4. 56 leaves. Woodcut title border incorporating printer's device; in text, 2 full-page woodcuts and 20 smaller woodcuts (including 2 repeats).

GM 6138. Osler 3818. Waller 8093.

C] *Der swangern Frawen vnd Hebammen Rosegarten.*

[Cologne: Arnt von Aich, ca. 1518].

4°: A–O4. 56 leaves. Woodcut title border, title-page woodcut; in text, 1 full-page woodcut and 20 smaller woodcuts (including 2 repeats).

Durling 3894. Waller 8091.

Rösslin was the first to publish an illustrated obstetrical manual for the use of midwives. With the exception of Ortolff von Bayerland's *Büchlein der schwangeren Frauen*, also called *Frauenbuchlein*, a small volume of thirteen pages published about 1495 (Goff O–113), this work is the first printed book dealing exclusively with the subject of obstetrics as distinct from medicine and surgery. It contains little that is original, but instead relies on the medical authorities of Antiquity and the Middle Ages, including Hippocrates, Galen, Soranus, Rhazes, Avicenna, and Albertus Magnus. Rösslin began with a preface in verse inveighing against contemporary obstetrical practice and against the ignorance, carelessness, and superstition of midwives, who brought about unnecessary deaths of numberless newborn infants. The instructions in Rösslin's work were simple and direct. He described most of the important fetal positions and discussed the use of podalic version in difficult deliveries, positions for delivery, and methods of assisting at delivery. He also included instructions on the care of the child from birth until weaning and described the diseases of infancy.

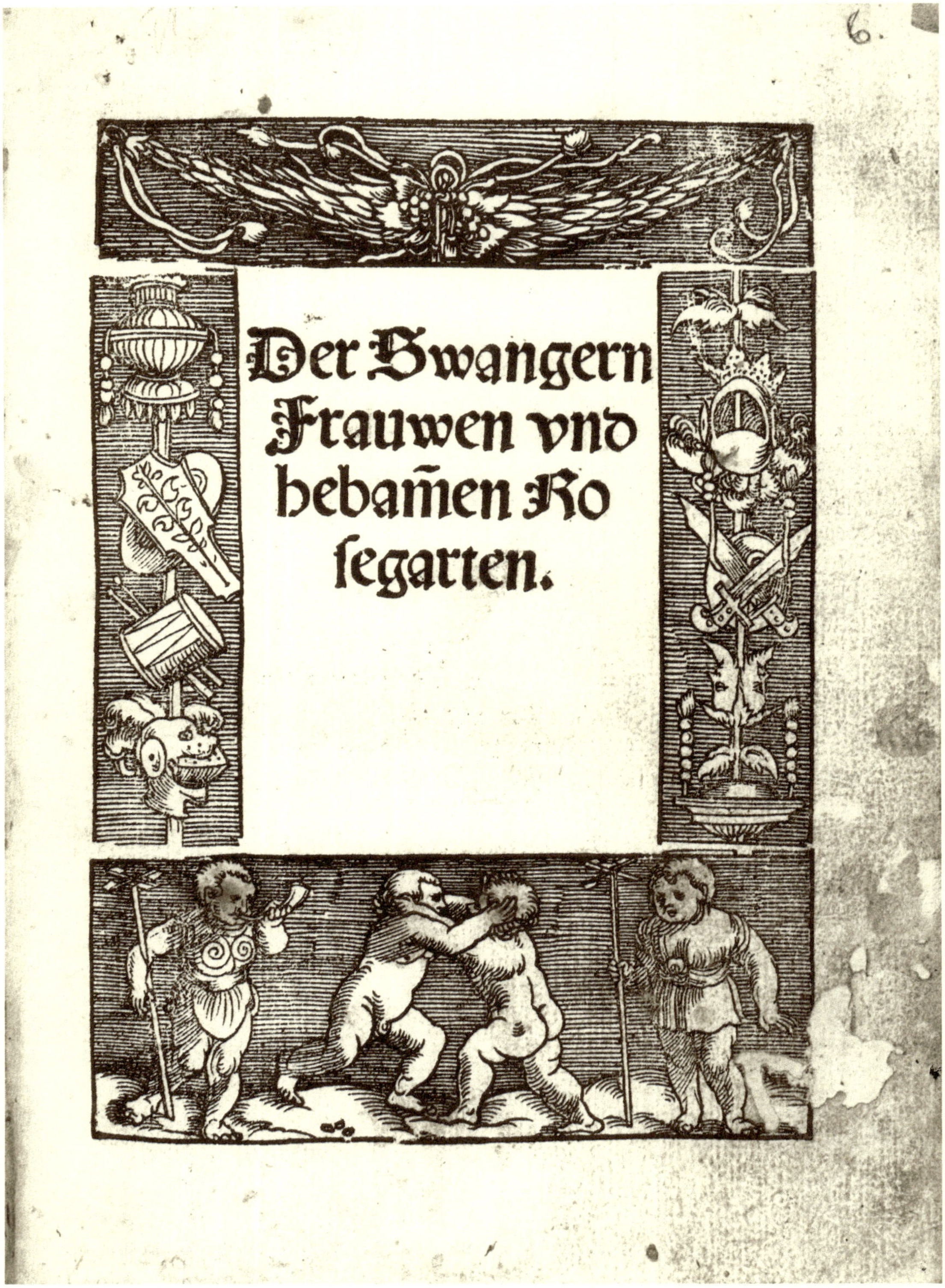

Fig. 19. No. 13A. Rösslin. Title page from the first edition (1513).

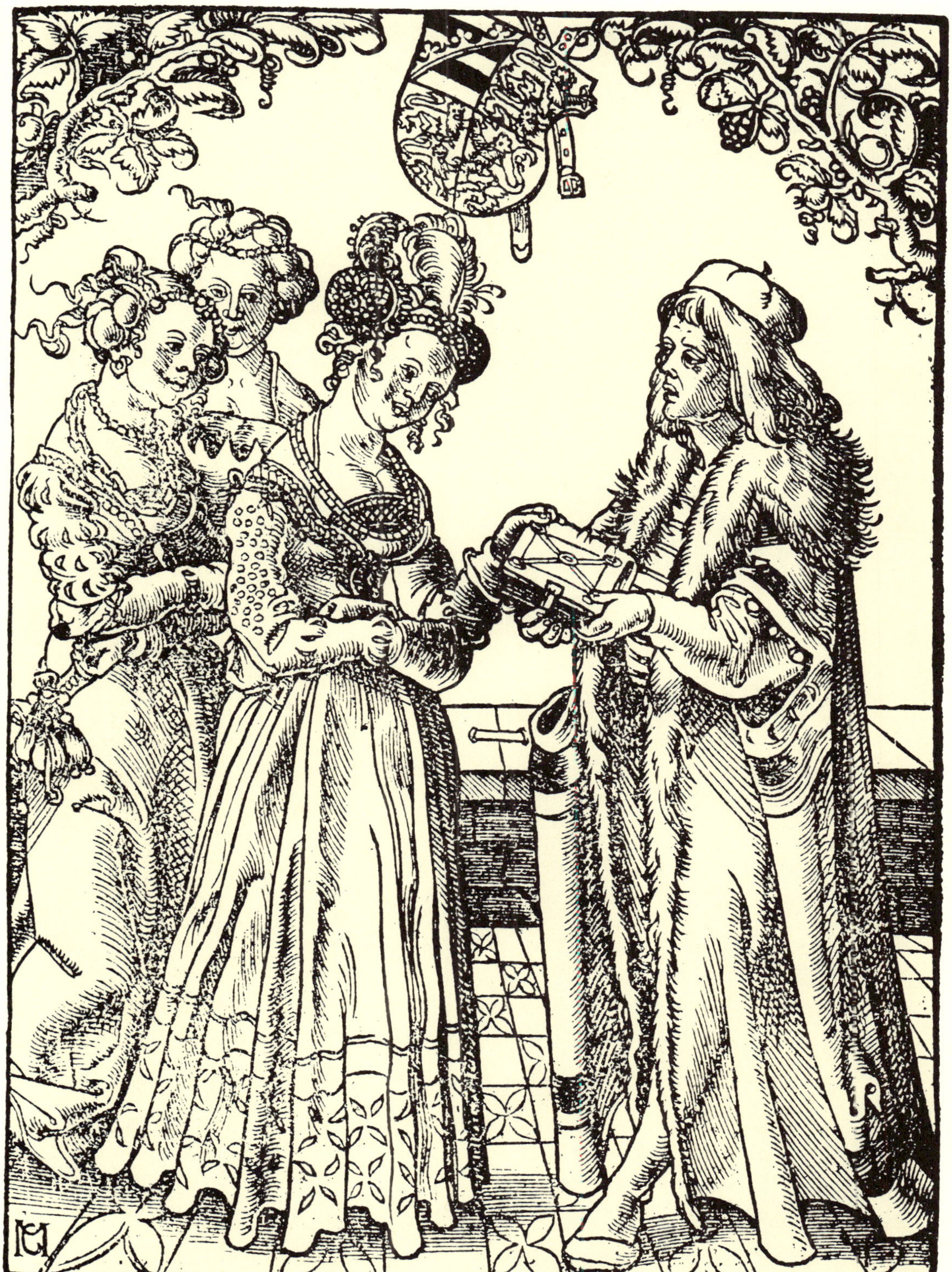

Fig. 20. No. 13. Rösslin. The dedicatory woodcut, attributed to the Frankfurt artist Martin Kaldenbach, shows the author presenting his book to Katherine, Duchess of Brunswick and Lüneburg.

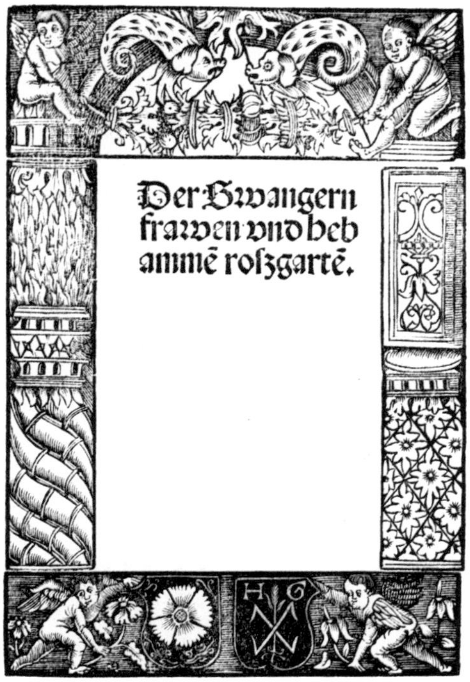

Fig. 21. No. 13B. Rösslin. Title page from the undated second edition (ca. 1515).

Eighteen small woodcut illustrations gave, for the first time, printed figures of the birth chair, positions of the fetus *in utero*, and twins, including Siamese twins. The illustrations of the fetus were derived from those found in manuscripts of works on gynecology by Soranus of Ephesus (I/II cent.) and Moschion (fl. ca. A.D. 500). For more than a century, these woodcuts were reprinted in editions of Rösslin's work or copied in the works of later writers, including Jacob Rueff and Jacques Guillemeau, the latter a pupil of Ambroise Paré (see no. 19).

The full-page dedicatory woodcut, which appears in all three of the earliest editions, shows the author presenting his book to Katherine, Duchess of Brunswick and Lüneburg, to whom he dedicated the volume. It is signed with a monogram of the letters M and C, which have been interpreted as referring to the Frankfurt artist Martin Kaldenbach. A full-page depiction of the lying-in chamber appeared in the first two editions but was omitted from the third. The woodcut title-page border of the first edition is by Hans Baldung Grien.

The first edition of *Rosegarten* was followed by two other, undated editions, one printed by Heinrich Gran of Hagenau, which Benzing dates ca. 1515, and one by Arnt von Aich of Cologne, dated by Benzing ca. 1518.[1] These undated editions were erroneously assigned to 1513 by some older authorities and described as issues rather than as separate editions. They use the same woodcuts as the first edition, except that they have different title-page borders; the third edition not only omits the full-page cut of the delivery room but

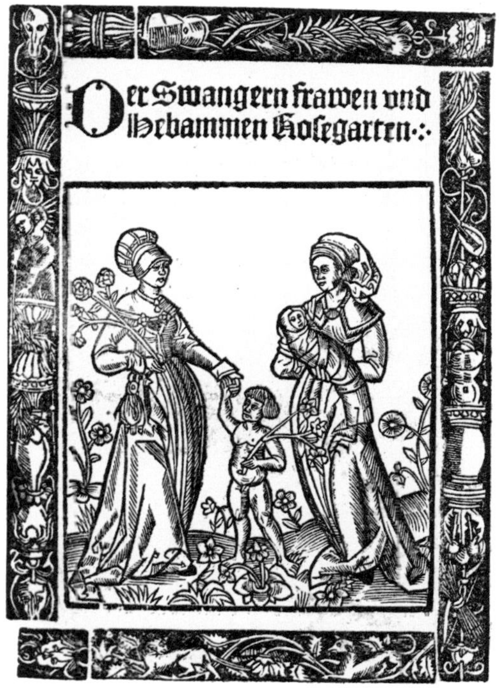

Fig. 22. No. 13c. Rösslin. Title page from the undated third edition (ca. 1518).

adds a title-page woodcut of two women, a baby, and a naked boy. Other German editions of the work appeared in 1522, 1528, 1529, 1530, 1532, and later. A Latin translation was published by Rösslin's son (also named Eucharius) in 1532, with further printings in 1535, 1536, 1538, and subsequently. The first English edition, *The Byrth of Mankynde*, was published in London in 1540; subsequent editions appeared in 1545, 1552, 1565, and thereafter. Rösslin's work became enormously popular and was translated not only into English but also into Dutch, French, Italian, Spanish, Polish, and Czech. It went through more than one hundred editions in various languages; probably no other medical book has been so widely translated and distributed. For nearly two centuries it served as the authoritative treatise on obstetrics throughout Europe.

Eucharius Rösslin was an apothecary of Freiburg im Breisgau in 1493. In 1506 he became physician to the city of Frankfurt am Main, and in 1508 he entered service at the court of Katherine. When he published his *Rosegarten* in 1513 he was working as the *Stadtartz*, or town physician, and supervisor of midwives in Worms. In 1517 he returned to Frankfurt in the same capacity, serving in that post until his death in 1526. His son Eucharius succeeded him as town physician of Frankfurt am Main.

LDL

1. Josef Benzing, "Zu den ersten Ausgaben des 'Rosengarten' von Eucharius Rösslin," *Das Antiquariat* 12 (1956): 57–58.

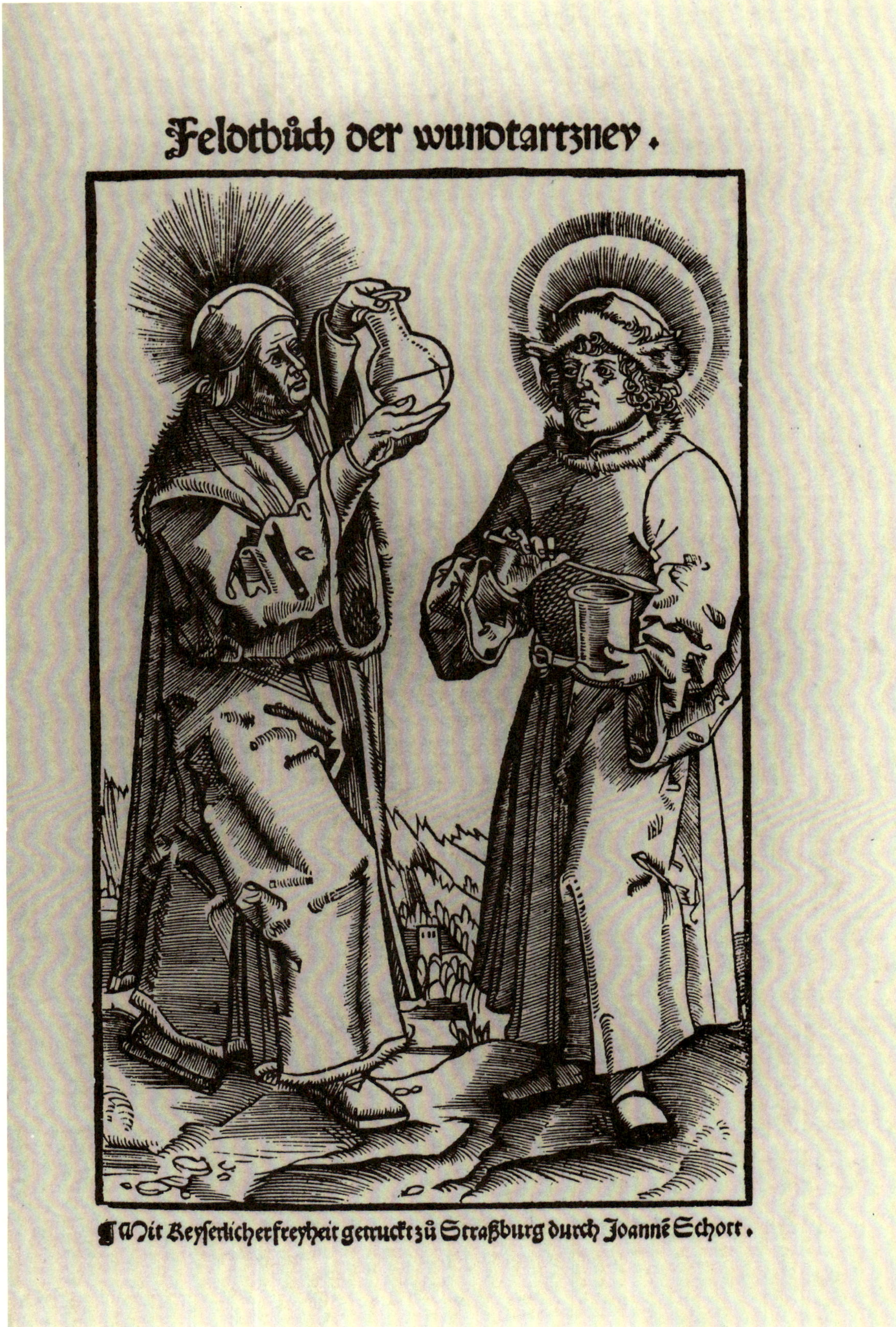

Fig. 23. No. 14. Gersdorff. The woodcut title page.

14

HANS VON GERSDORFF
(ca. 1455–1529)

Feldtbuch der Wundtartzney.

Strassburg: Getruckt durch Joannem Schott, 1517.

2°: π^{4} a–l^{6} m^{6} (m4 + 1,2) n^{6} o^{4} p^{6} q^{8}. 102 leaves, ff. [4] I–LXX [2] LXXI–XCV [1]. 28 woodcuts in text; 2 inserted woodcut plates, printed as broadsides on full sheets, bound as double or folding plates.

Choulant-Frank, pp. 162–66. Durling 2059. GM 5560. Stillwell 387. Waller 3506.

In the same year that Martin Luther posted his Ninety-Five Theses, Gersdorff initiated the reformation of surgery by relating his own extensive experience in his *Feldtbuch der Wundtartzney.* Gersdorff worked as a military surgeon for forty years, and although he was not the first German surgeon to publish a treatise on surgery—that honor goes to Hieronymus Brunschwig, whose *Chirurgia* appeared in 1497 (Goff B–1225)—his was the first to illustrate actual surgical procedures. The *Feldtbuch*'s numerous woodcuts, attributed to the artist Hans Wechtlin, constitute an important feature of the book: many are full-page, and they all enhance the reader's ability to comprehend the nature and details of the operations and instruments described in the text. Among them is the first graphic depiction of an amputation, an illustration that is justly famous. Herrlinger commented that the *Feldtbuch*'s illustrations represent one of the high points of early sixteenth-century medical illustration.[1] In addition to the woodcuts printed with the text, two inserted full sheets depict a skeleton and a viscera man, both with captions and explanations in German verse. These were printed separately by Schott in 1517 and were evidently intended to serve both as independent broadsides and for insertion into the *Feldtbuch,* to which the explanation of the viscera man refers. It is the text accompanying this cut that refers to Hans Wechtlin, thus providing the basis for the general attribution of the woodcuts.

Gersdorff devised a number of surgical instruments, including a tripod screw-elevator for raising depressed skull fragments and machines for reducing fractures and dislocations; many of his instruments are illustrated in the *Feldtbuch.* He was widely experienced in the management of injured limbs, and his two hundred recorded amputations possibly represent the largest total performed by any surgeon of his time. He utilized a tourniquet for amputations and dressed the stumps with moistened bandages, hemostyptics, compresses, and animal bladders tied over the whole. Authorities disagree over whether Gersdorff subscribed to the current belief that gunshot wounds were poisonous, but he appears

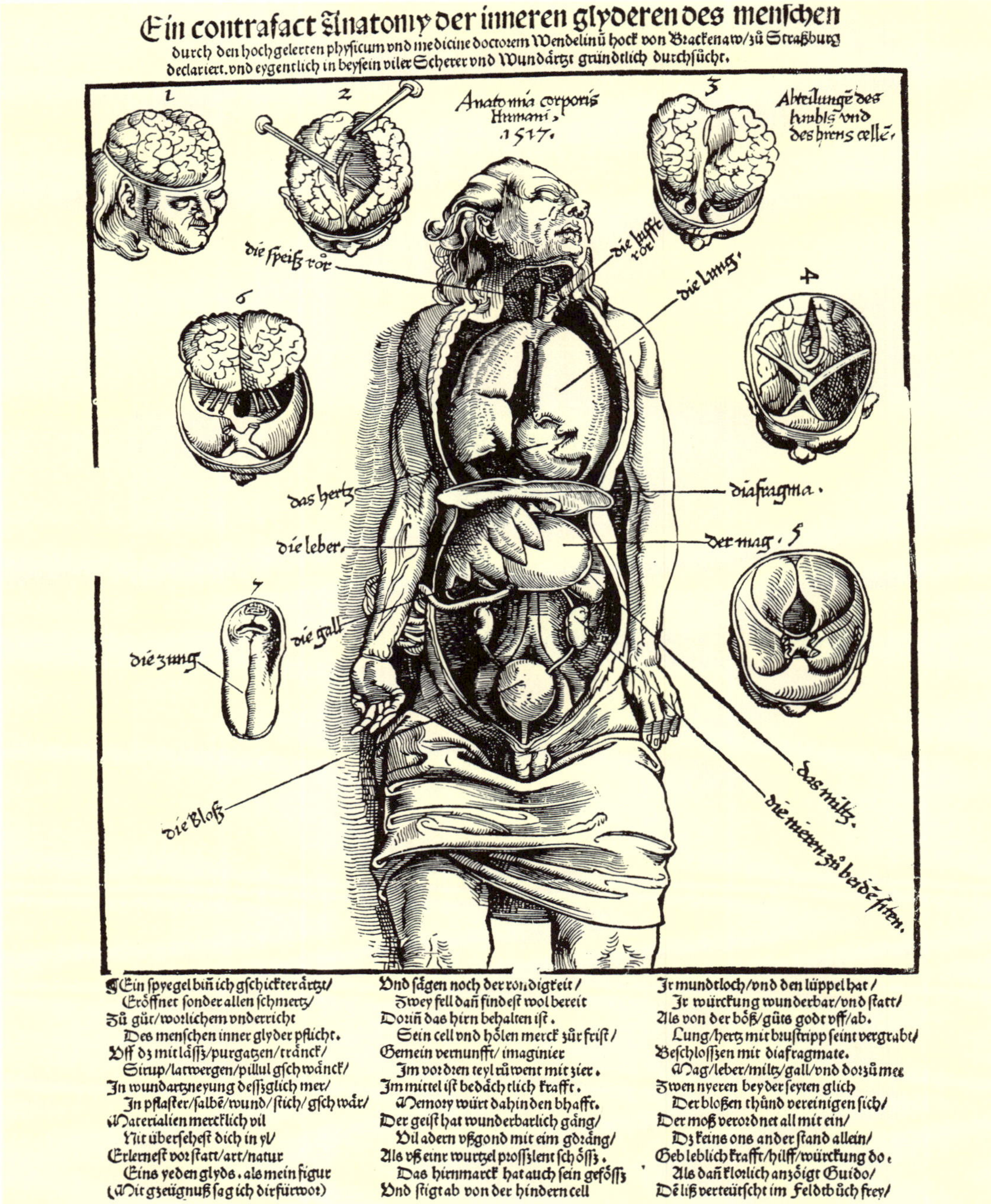

Fig. 24. No. 14. Gersdorff. Diagram of the internal organs, originally published as a fugitive sheet.

to have advocated the use of warm or hot oil in their treatment. The *Feldtbuch*, however, does contain advice that marks the beginning of more gentle treatment of tissue and wounds, as well as a description of the use of an inhaled plant extract to produce sleep. The discussion of the management of a depressed skull fracture shows detailed awareness of the neurological problems associated with this type of injury.

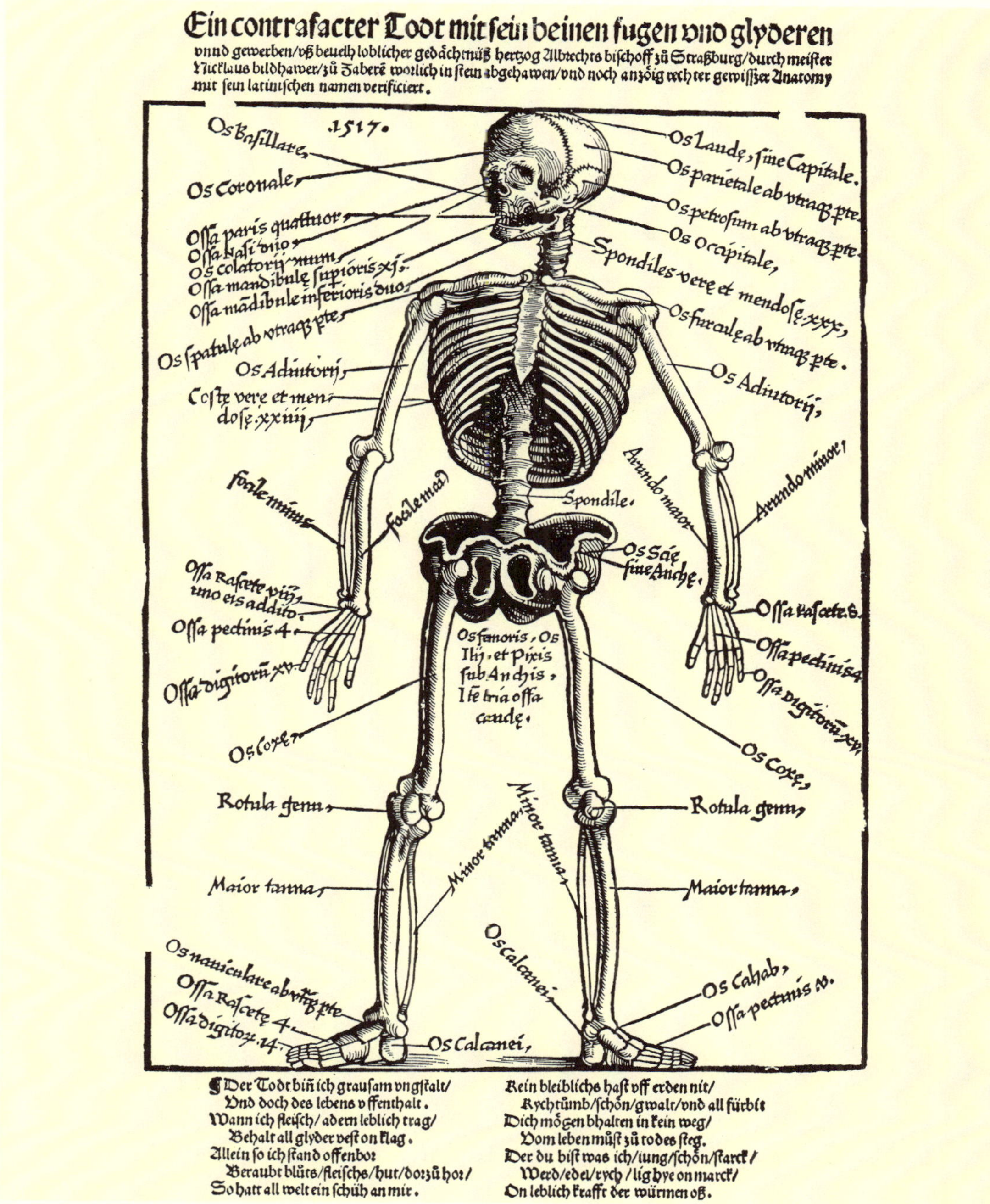

Fig. 25. No. 14. Gersdorff. Diagram of the skeleton, originally published as a fugitive sheet.

Gersdorff's book was quite popular, going through about a dozen editions between the time of its first publication and the early seventeenth century; there were also Latin and Dutch translations.

ESF

1. Robert Herrlinger, *History of Medical Illustration* (London, 1970), p. 142.

See color plate XI.

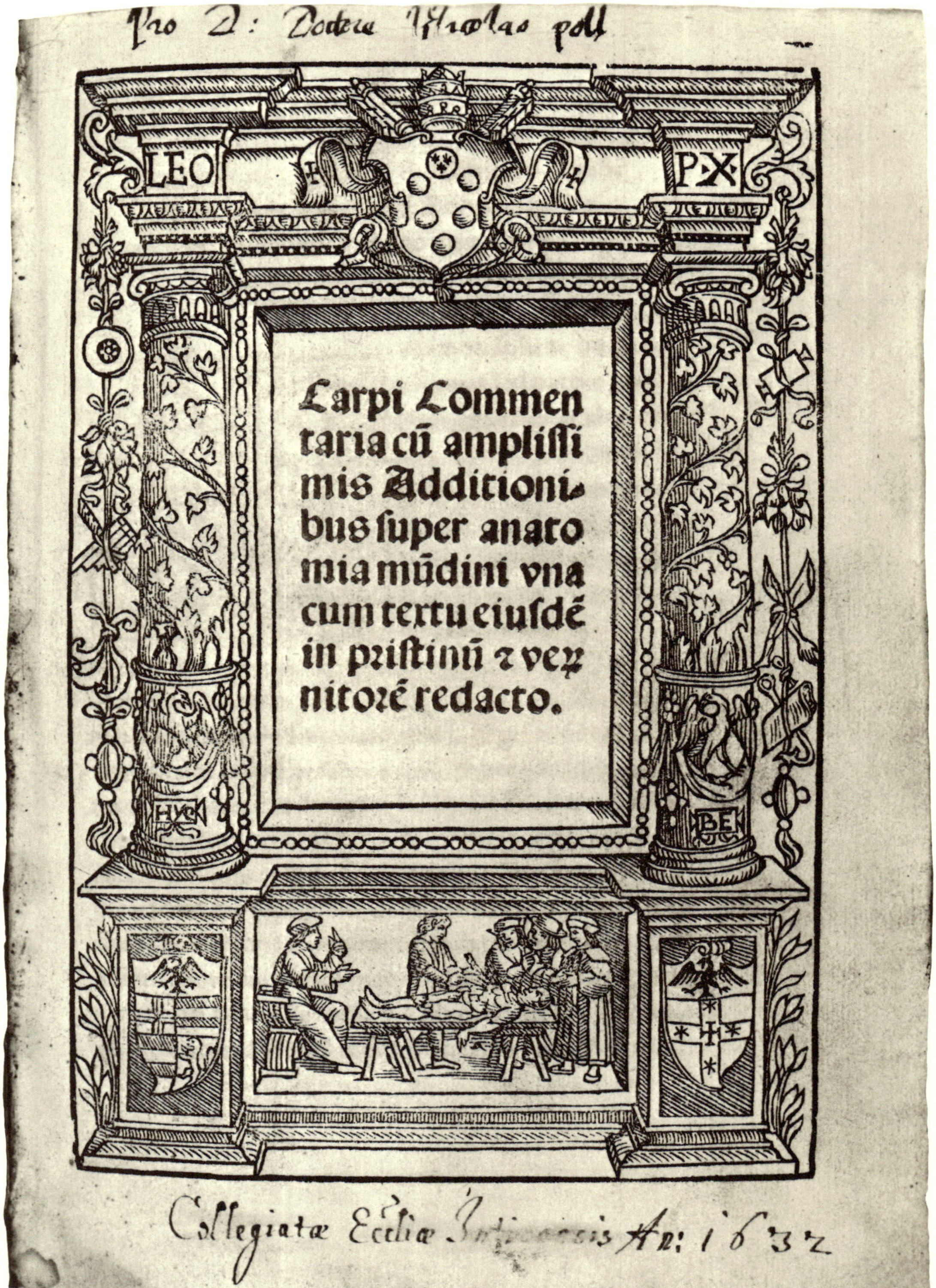

Fig. 26. No. 15. Berengario da Carpi. Nicolaus Pol's copy. "Pro. D: Doctore Nicolao Poll" is inscribed in the upper margin.

15

GIACOMO BERENGARIO DA CARPI
(ca. 1460–1530?)

Commentaria cum amplissimis additionibus super anatomia Mundini.

Bologna: Per Hieronymum de Benedictis, 6 March 1521.

4°: Aa–Zz^4 AAaa–ZZzz^4 AAAaaa–ZZZzzz^4 AAAAaaaa–ZZZZzzzz^4 AAAAAaaaaa–ZZZZZzzzzz^4 AAAAAAaaaaaa–RRRRRRrrrrrr^4. 528 leaves, ff. *I* II–CCCCCXXVIII. Woodcut title border; 21 full-page woodcuts in text.

Choulant-Frank, pp. 136–42. Durling 530. GM 367. Norman 187. Stillwell 310, 598. Wellcome 781.

Berengario, who taught anatomy at Bologna from 1502 to 1527, was the most eminent of the pre-Vesalian anatomists. His *Commentaria* can rightly be considered a starting point of the new anatomy, as it was the first work since the time of Galen to contain a significant amount of anatomical information derived from personal experience and observation. A commentary on the fourteenth-century anatomical text of Mondino de' Luzzi, who had reintroduced human dissection into anatomy, the work contains numerous observations by Berengario himself based on his own dissections. It also includes the first references to the vermiform appendix, the thymus gland, and the sphenoid sinus, as well as Berengario's denial of the presence of the *rete mirabile*, a structure described by Galen and found in some animals but not in humans.

The *Commentaria*'s use of full-page illustrations in which the figures are posed in natural settings and the dissection scene in its title-page border presage the fuller development of these iconographic techniques found in Vesalius's *De humani corporis fabrica* (see no. 18A). The illustrations in the *Commentaria* and in other works by Berengario suggest that he was familiar with the anatomical drawings of Leonardo da Vinci; these may be the only examples of sixteenth- or seventeenth-century anatomical work in which any hint of Leonardo can be found.[1] The woodcut title-page border was designed for the *Commentaria*; it also appeared, with minor variations, in the second edition of Berengario's *Isagogae breves* (1523). The publisher later adapted the border for general use by removing the dissection scene.

The development of Berengario as an anatomist can be seen in his *Isagogae breves*, a condensed version of the *Commentaria* that he published in 1522, with a second edition in 1523. These have a relationship to the *Commentaria* similar to that of Vesalius's *Epitome* to his *Fabrica* (see no. 18B). Many woodcuts of the *Commentaria* were copied, with im-

LXXXII

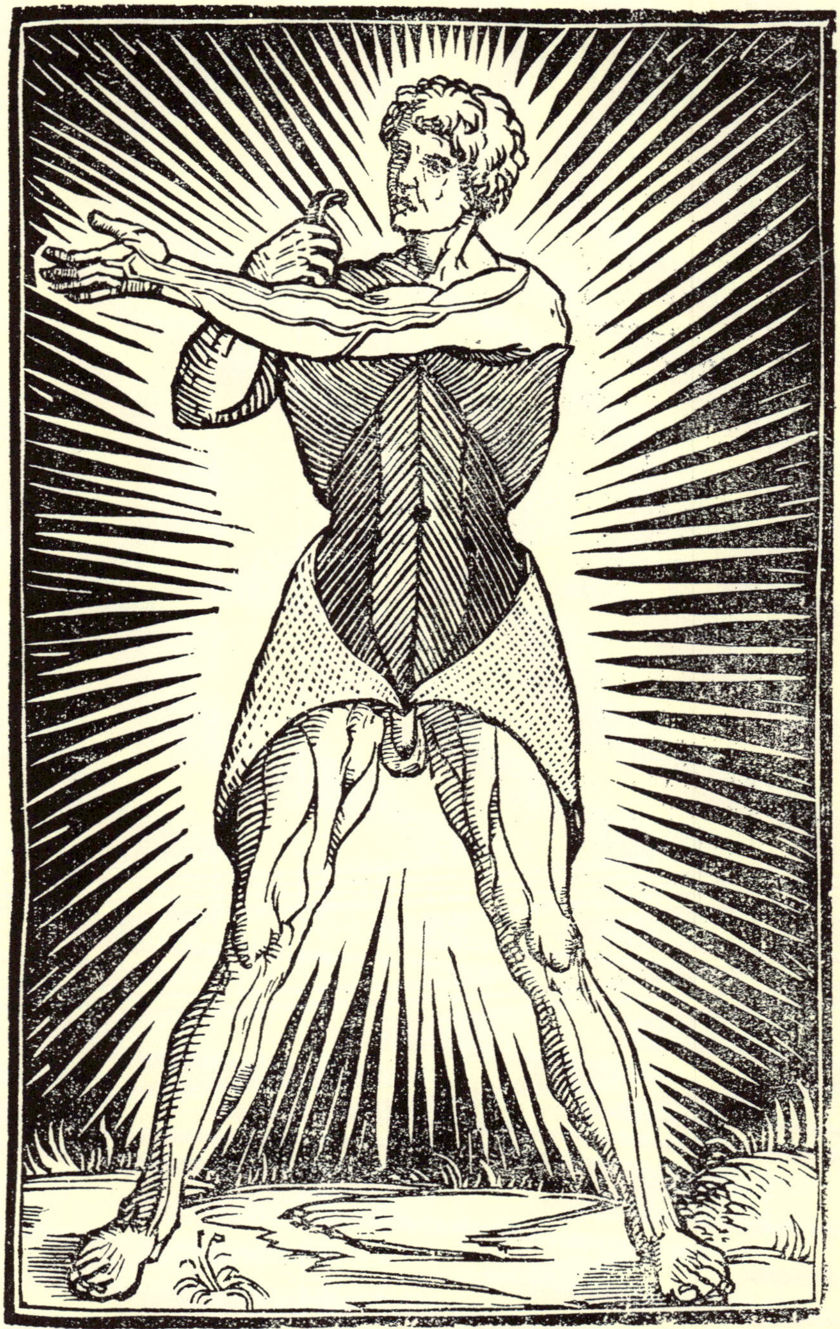

¶In hac fi-
gura hēs du
os muſculos
obliq̄s aſcen
dētes q̄ ſe in
cruciātcū du
ob⁹ deſcēdē
tib⁹i aliafigu
ra poſitis: q
qdē deſcēdē
tes ſūt ſupra
iſtos aſcēdē-
tes / & totus
un⁹ ex p̄dcis
muſculis de
ſcēdētib⁹ ſup̄
poſitis i alia
figura cūcor
da ſua ſupeq
tat obliq̄ mu
ſculū unū ex
iſtis aſcēdēti
b⁹obliq̄:& ſa
ciūt ſimul fi-
gurā .X. lrē
græce: & iſt
o⁊ muſculo
rū ēt ps car-
nea ē a lateri
bus. Cordæ
uero eo⁊ ſūt
in medio uē
tris / q̄ ſūt ēt
dua⁊ pellicu
larū:& habēt
unā pellicu-
lā tm̄ ſupeq-
tantē muſcu
los lūgos: alia v̄o pellicula ē iſra muſculos lūgos: q̄ adheret cordis latitudina
liū muſculo⁊:& iſtæ cordæ ēt terminant̄ i linea/q̄ ē i medio uētris/ ut uid̄s.

Xx ii

Fig. 27. No. 15. Berengario da Carpi. Berengario's use of lifelike poses in anatomical illustration was later developed more fully by Vesalius.

provements, in the *Isagogae* and were further modified in the second edition of this work. The second edition also included an illustration of the brain drawn from actual dissection, in which the cerebral ventricles were accurately shown for the first time. This was a considerable advance over the schematic representation in the medieval tradition that had appeared on the title page of Berengario's work on head injuries, *Tractatus de fractura calve sive cranei*, published in 1518.

ESF

1. Robert Herrlinger, *History of Medical Illustration* (London, 1970), pp. 75, 80–83.

Der grossenn wundartzney/ Das ander Bůch/ Des ergründten vnnd bewerten/ bayder Artzney Doctors Paracelsi/ Von den offnen schäden/ vrsprung vnnd haylung/ Nach der bewärtenn erfarenhayt / ohn irrsale vnnd weytters versůchen.

Geschriben zů dem Großmächtigisten/ Durchleüchtigisten Fürsten vnd Herren/ Herren Ferdinanden von Gottes gnaden Rhömischer/ Vngerischer/ vnnd Böhimischer Künig/ Ertzhertzog zů Osterreich/ vnserm gnädigisten Herren.

Aufgethaylt inn drey Tractaten

Der erst zayget an die alten grund vnd leer/ wie die selbigen auch irrig gehalten vnd gewesen.

Der ander zayget an/ Was der grund vnd vrsprung sey der offnen schäden nach dem natürlichen liecht.

Der dritt zayget an dreyerlay haylung im Vniuersal / vnnd inn zway Particular.

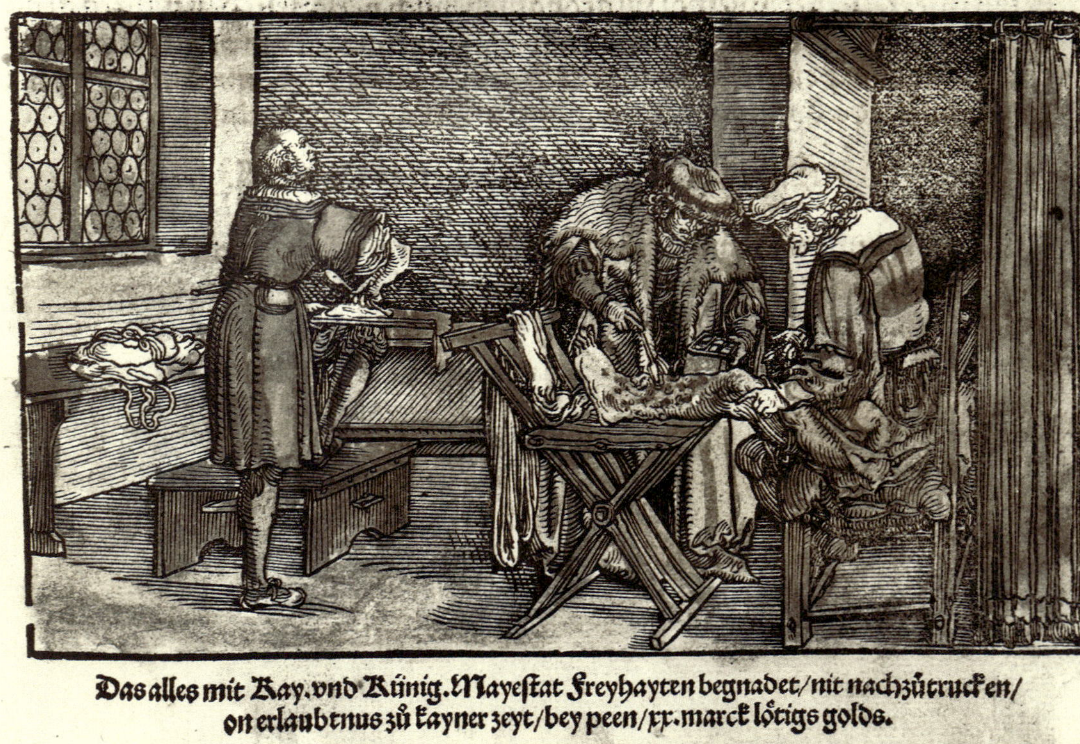

Das alles mit Kay. vnd Künig. Mayestat Freyhayten begnadet/ nit nachzůtrucken/ on erlaubtnus zů kayner zeyt/ bey peen/ xx. marck lötigs golds.

Getruckt zů Augspurg bey Haynrich Stayner/ im jar. M. D. XXXVI.

Fig. 28. No. 16. Paracelsus. Title page of Volume II.

16

PARACELSUS [PHILIPPUS AUREOLUS THEOPHRASTUS BOMBASTUS VON HOHENHEIM] (ca. 1493–1541)

Der grossenn Wundartzney, das erst Buch, des ergründten vnd bewerten, der bayden Artzney, Doctors Paracelsi, von allen Wunden, Stich, Schüß, Bränd, Thierbiß, Baynbrüch, vnd alles was die Wundartzney begreifft. [Vol. II] *Der grossenn Wundartzney, das ander Buch, des ergründten vnnd bewerten, bayder Artzney Doctors Paracelsi.*

Augsburg: Getruckt bey Heynrich Steyner, 1536 (colophons: 28 July 1536; 22 August 1536).

[Vol. I] 2°: A^8 B–K^6 L^8. 70 leaves, ff. [8] I–LXI [1]. Title-page woodcut; 19 woodcuts in text (including 2 repeats).

[Vol. II] 2°: A–K^6 L^8. 68 leaves, ff. [6] I–LX [i.e., LXI] [1]. Title-page woodcut, repeated in text.

Osler 537. PMM 110. cf. Stillwell 467, 868. Sudhoff 15, 16. Waller 7106, 7107.

Philippus Aureolus Theophrastus Bombastus von Hohenheim, also known as Paracelsus, remains one of the most controversial and remarkable personalities of the Renaissance. He has been described as a quack, a magician, an astrologer, and an alchemist, as well as a brilliant physician, prophet, and genius. Sir William Osler called him the "Luther of medicine,"[1] and Fielding Garrison lauded him as "the most original medical thinker of the sixteenth century."[2] He was perhaps all of these. In literature, he has been romanticized by Christopher Marlowe, Goethe, and Robert Browning, among others.

Born in Switzerland, probably in 1493, Paracelsus was the son of a physician, Wilhelm Bombast von Hohenheim, who taught him botany, metallurgy, natural philosophy, and mining. His education was continued by several churchmen, including Johannes Trithemius, Abbot of Spanheim, from whom he is supposed to have learned occultism, astrology, and alchemy. He may have studied medicine at the University of Ferrara with Leoniceno, who emphasized the writings of Hippocrates. Most of his later life he spent as a wanderer, first serving as a military surgeon in Venice, Scandinavia, and the Middle East, and later traveling all over Europe as a physician and lay preacher. He seemed to favor low company, including barbers, midwives, executioners, and gypsies, from whom he learned a great deal about folk medicine. At various times he achieved a reputation for remarkable cures. In 1525 he was summoned for consultation to Basel where he saved the life of the influential humanist and publisher Johannes Froben and impressed the latter's house-guest, Erasmus, with his medical advice. This incident resulted in his appointment as municipal physician and professor of medicine at Basel; however, his rebellious and uncompromising nature soon brought him into conflict with the local professors of medicine, apothecaries, and magistrates, and his stay there was short-lived. Paracelsus has been described as "an angry man [whose] career followed a pattern of initial triumphs followed by losing battles, in the course of which he alienated even his best friends and patrons."[3] He died in Salzburg, where he was buried; thereafter his gravesite was visited by the sick as a shrine.

Paracelsus's writings seem strange to the modern reader—they are often outrageous in tone, include undisguised obscenities, and are dominated by mystical elements, occult forces, astrology, and alchemy. Nonetheless, interspersed among his writings are occasional contributions of scientific value, the chief among these (from a medical point of view) being his introduction of a new concept of disease, based on the idea that each disease is due to a specific external cause, to replace the ancient notion of disease as an internal and idiosyncratic imbalance of humors. Paracelsus's new idea of disease led him to new modes of therapy, using specific agents (often chemically derived) to battle against specific diseases. His followers founded the school of iatrochemistry, which flourished in Europe over the next century. Paracelsus made ether-like preparations that he used as sedatives and narcotics, and he introduced laudanum (tincture of opium) into the pharmacopeia. He advocated the use of minerals as therapeutic agents, including mercury, lead, copper sulfate, and antimony. As a clinician, he was the first to describe congenital syphilis. He also gave the first description of cretinism, which he linked with goiter, and this in turn he connected to the mineral content of water. He studied the diseases of miners and metallurgists and wrote the first monograph on an occupational disease. Forty years before Johann Weyer (see no. 20), he described the clinical manifestations of epilepsy, mania, and hysteria in a manner that was not improved on until Philippe Pinel (see no. 54) and Jean-Étienne-Dominique Esquirol in the nineteenth century. In an age when the mentally ill were viewed as possessed by the devil and burned at the stake, he advocated humane treatment.

Unlike his contemporaries, Paracelsus regarded surgery as no less worthy than medicine, writing on both subjects and signing himself as *Doctor beider Arznei* (doctor of both medicines). As a surgeon, he treated wounds successfully using conservative methods, in contrast to the common practice of cauterization with boiling oil. He was the first to agree with the fourteenth-century French surgeon Henri de Mondeville that wounds must be kept clean, and Garrison described him as "almost the only asepsist between Mondeville and Lister."[4] *Der grossenn Wundartzney* was Paracelsus's first book on surgical technique. In it he gave these instructions to surgeons:

You should know what it is which heals a wound because without this knowledge you cannot use any medicine correctly. You should know that it is the nature of flesh, of the body, of the blood vessels, of the limbs to have within themselves an inborn balsam that heals all wounds, stab wounds or any other sort. It is the balsam in the limb that heals a fracture, the balsam that resides naturally in the flesh that heals flesh. So with every limb it should be understood that it carries its own healing in itself which heals it when it is wounded. Every surgeon therefore should know that it is not he who heals the wound but the balsam in the part that heals it. If he thinks he heals it, he fools himself, and does not know his art. To be a good surgeon, you should protect and shield the natural balsam from ever-present, external enemies, so that they do not destroy the balsam nor poison or damage it but permit it to work and act under your protection. If a wound is open and unprotected, it is evident that it cannot heal. The good surgeon affords this protection by suitable dressings under which in peace and quiet, nature heals the wound, makes grow the flesh, veins and all that has been injured. For what makes flesh, fat, grease, blood and bone marrow grow? Not man, not food, only nature has the growing and developmental powers which make the body whole. Through food and drink this strength is preserved. Rain and the earth do not make wood, only the tree can make wood, but without rain and earth, the tree dies.[5]

Paracelsus was a voluminous writer on both medical and theological subjects, but his controversial views and antagonistic personality alienated publishers, and only a few of his books appeared during his lifetime. One of these was *Der grossenn Wundarzney*, the printing of which Paracelsus supervised after he had disavowed a previous, inaccurate edition of Book I, printed earlier in 1536 by Hans Varnier at Ulm. Most of Paracelsus's medical writings were published by his followers, beginning about twenty-five years after his death, and they were collected into ten quarto volumes as early as 1589–91. The most important modern edition is the fourteen-volume *Sämtliche Werke . . .* , edited by Karl Sudhoff and Wilhelm Mathiessen (Munich and Berlin, 1922–33).

HFN

1. William Osler, *The Evolution of Modern Medicine* (New Haven, 1921), p. 135.
2. Fielding H. Garrison, *An Introduction to the History of Medicine*, 4th ed. (Philadelphia, 1929), p. 204.
3. Walter Pagel, "Paracelsus," in *Dictionary of Scientific Biography*, vol. 10 (New York, 1974), p. 305.
4. Garrison, p. 206.
5. This translation is taken from Leo M. Zimmerman and Ilza Veith, *Great Ideas in the History of Surgery* (Baltimore, 1961), p. 177.

See color plate XII.

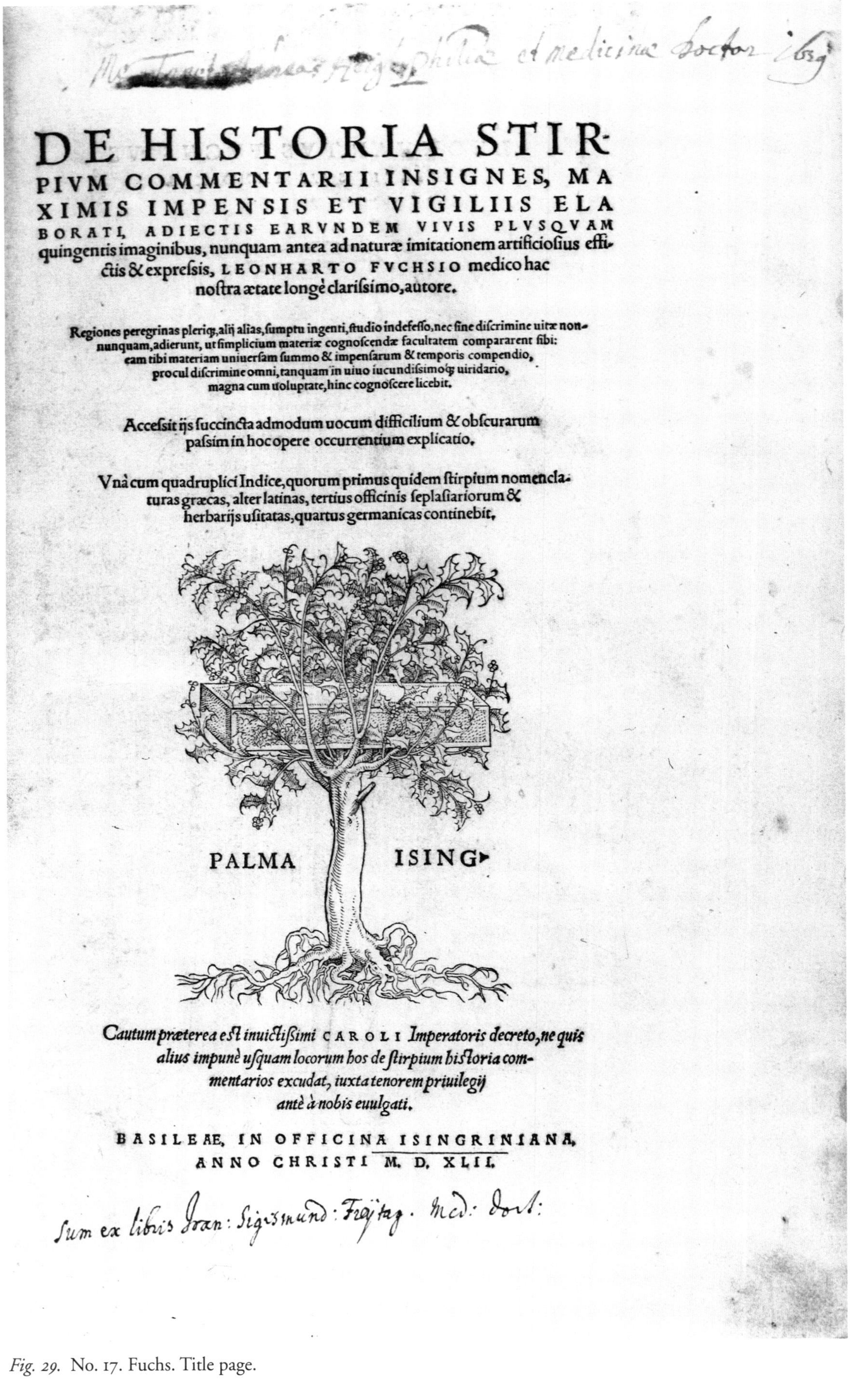
Mr [redacted] philiæ et medicinæ doctor 1639

DE HISTORIA STIRPIVM COMMENTARII INSIGNES, MAXIMIS IMPENSIS ET VIGILIIS ELABORATI, ADIECTIS EARVNDEM VIVIS PLVSQVAM quingentis imaginibus, nunquam antea ad naturæ imitationem artificiosius effictis & expressis, LEONHARTO FVCHSIO medico hac nostra ætate longè clarissimo, autore.

Regiones peregrinas pleriq;, alij alias, sumptu ingenti, studio indefesso, nec sine discrimine uitæ nonnunquam, adierunt, ut simplicium materiæ cognoscendæ facultatem compararent sibi: eam tibi materiam uniuersam summo & impensarum & temporis compendio, procul discrimine omni, tanquam in uiuo iucundissimoq; uiridario, magna cum uoluptate, hinc cognoscere licebit.

Accessit ijs succincta admodum uocum difficilium & obscurarum passim in hoc opere occurrentium explicatio.

Vnà cum quadruplici Indice, quorum primus quidem stirpium nomenclaturas græcas, alter latinas, tertius officinis seplasiariorum & herbarijs usitatas, quartus germanicas continebit.

PALMA ISING.

Cautum præterea est inuictissimi CAROLI *Imperatoris decreto, ne quis alius impunè usquam locorum hos de stirpium historia commentarios excudat, iuxta tenorem priuilegij antè à nobis euulgati.*

BASILEAE, IN OFFICINA ISINGRINIANA, ANNO CHRISTI M. D. XLII.

Sum ex libris Joan: Sigismund: Freytag. Med: doct:

Fig. 29. No. 17. Fuchs. Title page.

17

LEONHART FUCHS
(1501–1566)

De historia stirpium commentarii insignes.

Basel: In officina Isingriniana, 1542.

2°: α^6 β^8 A–Z^6 a–z^6 aa–zz^6 aaa–fff^6. 464 leaves, pp. [28] 1–33 35–60 [1] 61–896 [4]. Woodcut portraits of Fuchs and three artists, 509 full-page and 2 smaller woodcuts of plants, all in text.

Adams F–1099. Durling 1675. GM 1808. *Heirs of Hippocrates* 243. Horblit 33b. Hunt 48. Norman 846. PMM 69. Stillwell 372, 640. Waller 11512. Wellcome 2438.

Although illustrated herbals had had a long tradition, in manuscript and in printed form, the sixteenth century saw considerable advances in both the realism and the aesthetics of botanical illustration. Of all the fine herbals that appeared then, Leonhart Fuch's *De historia stirpium*, a splendid folio with 511 beautiful woodcuts of plants, was one of the most outstanding.

The content and purpose of this book, one of the greatest of all herbals, is well expressed in a complete English translation of its title:

> Notable commentaries on the history of plants, prepared with great expense and diligence by Leonhart Fuchs, a physician by far the most distinguished in this our age, and adorned with more than five hundred lifelike pictures in imitation of nature, never hitherto drawn and printed with greater art.
>
> Many others have visited foreign lands, some here, some there, at huge cost, with tireless effort, and sometimes not without peril to their lives, in order to acquire intimate knowledge of the substance of simples; all this substance you will be pleased to learn from this book, as in a living pleasure garden, at a great saving of money and time, far from any peril. Added to this is a concise explanation of the difficult and obscure words that occur here and there in this work; along with a fourfold index, containing (1) the Greek names of the plants, (2) the Latin names, (3) those used in the shops of druggists and by herb-gatherers, (4) the German names.
>
> Furthermore by the decree of Charles, invincible emperor, warning is given that no other person goes without punishment who anywhere in the world prints these commentaries on the history of plants, just as was said in the privilege previously made known by us.

Fuchs, who was born in Bavaria, studied medicine at the University of Ingolstadt. A Renaissance humanist, philologist, Greek and Latin scholar, administrator, professor, and author, he enjoyed considerable repute as a physician. In addition to his herbal that went through thirty-five editions during his lifetime (including German, Dutch, French, and Spanish translations), Fuchs also published about twenty books on medical subjects, including commentaries on Hippocrates and Galen, and an anatomy based on that of Vesalius. He taught medicine at the University of Tübingen from 1535 until his death, was rector of the same university several times, and wrote the statutes of the medical faculty there. In addition to his many writings and teaching responsibilities, he also had a private medical practice and raised a family of ten children.

In all his writings, including the text of the herbal, Fuchs relied on ancient authorities, but he also railed against the botanical ignorance of the medical men of his day, writing that it was "almost impossible to find even one in a hundred who has any accurate knowledge of even a few plants." The herbal was intended to improve the knowledge of *materia medica* among practitioners, and Fuchs's preface stressed the accuracy of its illustrations, which have been characterized as "represent[ing] the high-water mark of that type of botanical drawing which seeks to express the individual character and habit of each species, treating the plant broadly as a whole."[1] To create the illustrations, Fuchs employed three artists, Albrecht Meyer, who drew the plants from nature, Heinrich Füllmaurer, who transferred the drawings to the blocks, and Veit Rudolf Speckle, who did the wood cutting. Their work is justly memorialized by the inclusion of their portraits at the end of the book.

Of all the books authored by Fuchs, *De historia stirpium* was unquestionably his greatest achievement. The methodical layout, the organization of the subject matter, the spacious design, and the number, size, and beauty of the illustrations have caused the herbal to appeal to botanists and bibliophiles alike. That it was intended to be the first volume of three (the other two were subsequently written but never published) points out the grandiose concept and magnitude of the work. Scholars today consider the herbal to be one of the significant landmarks of pre-Linnaean herbal-botanical literature.

FGM

Fuchs's herbal exists in both hand-colored and uncolored versions. While some colored copies may have been painted by their owners after purchase, as was sometimes done in books of this nature, there is sufficient evidence to show that copies were also colored for the publisher Isingrin, who presumably made use of the artist's original drawings. Such "original colored" copies possess many features in common—for example, the illustration of the rose has the left shoot bearing white flowers and the right shoot red flowers, and the plum tree shows yellow fruits on the left, blue fruits in the center, and reddish fruits on the right—and it is these features that permit one to distinguish between original colored copies and those colored later by private owners. The coloring in the colored copies issued by the publisher accords well with Fuchs's descriptions in the text, which suggests that Fuchs had some control over the painting.[2]

HFN

1. Agnes Arber, *Herbals: Their Origin and Evolution*, 3d ed. (Cambridge, 1986), p. 212.
2. See W. T. Stearn, "The Use of Bibliography in Natural History," in *Bibliography and Natural History*, ed. T. R. Buchman (Lawrence, Kansas, 1966), pp. 1–20; and Agnes Arber, "The Colouring of Sixteenth-Century Herbals," *Nature* 145 (25 May 1940): 803; reprinted in *Herbals: Their Origin and Evolution* (3d ed.), pp. 315–18.

See color plates XIII *and* XIV.

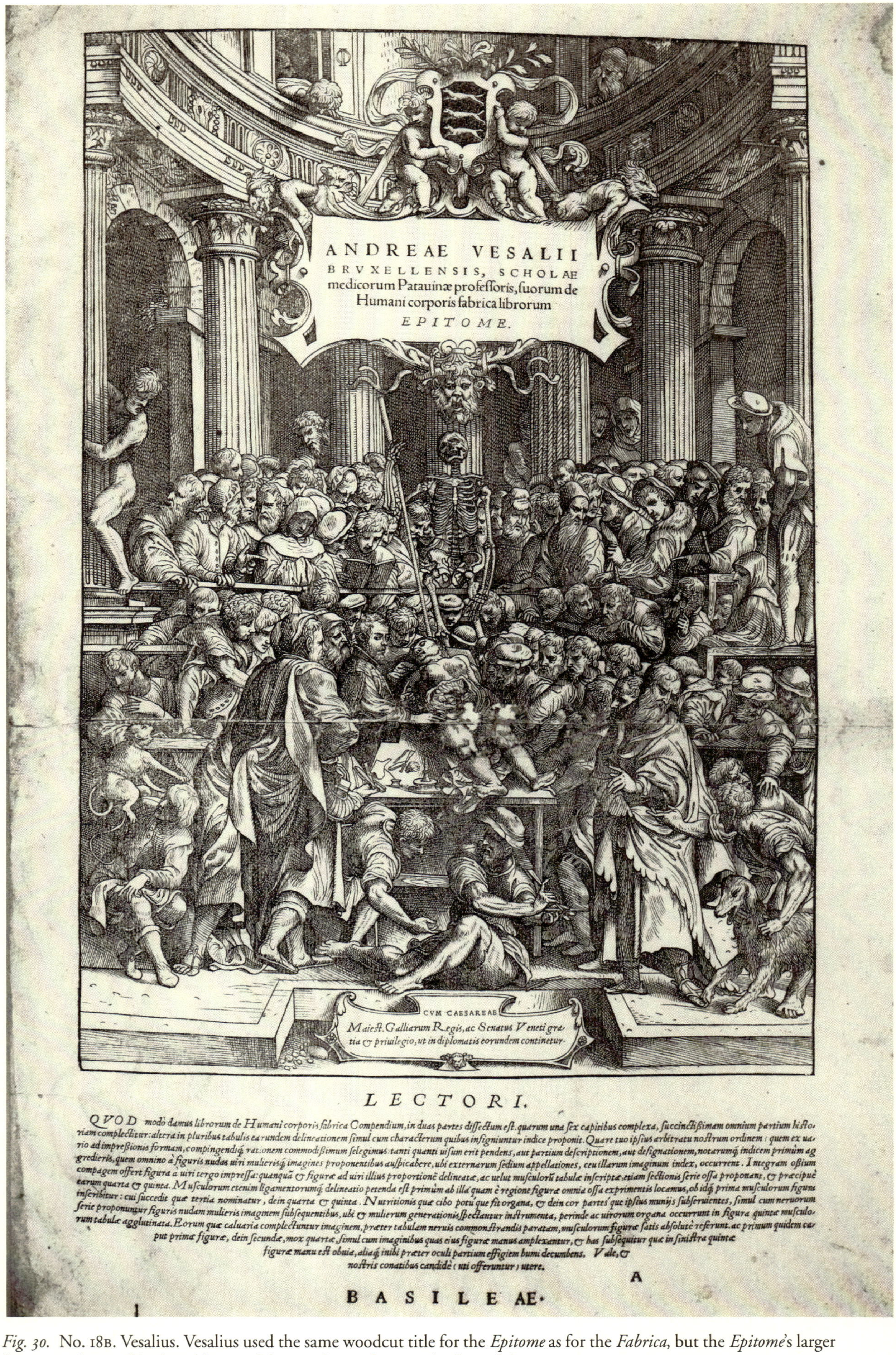

ANDREAE VESALII BRVXELLENSIS, SCHOLAE medicorum Patauinæ professoris, suorum de Humani corporis fabrica librorum EPITOME.

CVM CAESAREAE Maiest. Galliarum Regis, ac Senatus Veneti gratia & priuilegio, ut in diplomatis eorundem continetur.

LECTORI.

QVOD modò damus librorum de Humani corporis fabrica Compendium, in duas partes dissectum est. quarum una sex capitibus complexa, succinctißimam omnium partium historiam complectitur: altera in pluribus tabulis earundem delineationem simul cum characterum quibus insigniuntur indice proponit. Quare tuo ipsius arbitratu nostrum ordinem (quem ex uario ad impreßionis formam, compingendiq; rationem commodißimum selegimus) tanti quanti uisum erit pendens, aut partium descriptionem, aut designationem, notarumq; indicem primùm aggredieris, quem omnino à figuris nudas uiri mulierisq; imagines proponentibus auspicabere, ubi externarum sedium appellationes, ceu illarum imaginum index, occurrent. Integram oßium compagem offert figura à uiri tergo impressa: quanquā & figuræ ad uiri illius proportionē delineatæ, ac uelut musculorū tabulæ inscriptæ, etiam sectionis serie ossa proponant, & præcipuè earum quarta & quinta. Musculorum etenim ligamentorumq; delineatio petenda est primùm ab illa quam è regione figuræ omnia ossa exprimentis locamus, ob idq; prima musculorum figura inscribitur: cui succedit quæ tertia nominatur, dein quarta & quinta. Nutritionis quæ cibo potúque fit organa, & dein cor partes que ipsius munijs subseruientes, simul cum neruorum serie proponuntur figuris nudam mulieris imaginem subsequentibus, ubi & mulierum generationis spectantur instrumenta, perinde ac uirorum organa occurrunt in figura quintæ musculorum tabulæ agglutinata. Eorum quæ caluaria complectuntur imaginem, præter tabulam neruis commonstrandis paratam, musculorum figuræ satis absolutè referunt. ac primum quidem caput primæ figuræ, dein secundæ, mox quartæ, simul cum imaginibus quas eius figuræ manus amplexantur, & has subsequitur quæ in sinistra quintæ figuræ manu est obuia, aliaq; inibi præter oculi partium effigiem humi decumbens. Vale, & nostris conatibus candidè (uti offeruntur) utere.

A

BASILEAE.

Fig. 30. No. 18B. Vesalius. Vesalius used the same woodcut title for the *Epitome* as for the *Fabrica*, but the *Epitome*'s larger format made possible the addition of thirteen lines of text at the foot of the page.

18

ANDREAS VESALIUS
(1514–1564)

A] *De humani corporis fabrica libri septem.*

Basel: Ex officina Ioannis Oporini, June 1543.

2°: *^{6} A–Z^{6} a–l^{6} m^{6} (m2 + 1, 2) n–o^{6} p^{4} (p3 + 1) q–z^{6} Aa–Ll^{6} Mm^{8}. 357 leaves, pp. [12] *1* 2–312 213–313 313 [2] 315–391 492–659 [i.e., 663] [37]. Woodcut title, portrait, and text illustrations. The first added leaf in quire m and the added leaf in quire p are oversized plates, printed in broadside format on full sheets, which may be bound either as double or as folding plates; they are signed and paginated, m2(1) on both sides as 'm3' = p. 313, and p3(1) as 'p4' = pp. 353–354; m2(2), an inserted half sheet, is signed 'm3' and contains figures to be cut out and applied as overlays to the figure on m2(1).

Adams V–603. Choulant-Frank, pp. 178–80. Cushing VI. A. –1. Durling 4577. GM 375. *Heirs of Hippocrates* 281. Horblit 98. Norman 2137. Osler 567. PMM 71. Stillwell 710. Waller 9899. Wellcome 6560.

B] *De humani corporis fabrica librorum epitome.*

Basel: Ex officina Ioannis Oporini, June 1543.

1°: A–M [N–O]. 14 leaves. Woodcut title, portrait, and text illustrations.

Adams V–607. Choulant-Frank, pp. 180–81. Cushing VI. B. –1. Durling 4581. GM 376. *Heirs of Hippocrates* 291. Osler 571. Stillwell 711. Waller 9908. Wellcome 6565.

With *De humani corporis fabrica*, published when he was only twenty-nine years old, Vesalius revolutionized not only the science of anatomy but also how it was taught. Throughout this encyclopedic work on the structure and workings of the human body, Vesalius provided a fuller and more detailed description of human anatomy than any of his predecessors, correcting errors in the traditional anatomical teachings of Galen (whose observations were based on primate rather than human dissection), and arguing that knowledge of human anatomy was to be learned only from human sources. Even more revolutionary than his criticism of Galen and other medieval authorities was Vesalius's assertion that anatomical dissection must be performed by the physician himself—a direct contradiction of the medieval doctrine that dissection was a task to be performed by menials while the physician lectured from the traditional authorities. Only through actual dissection, Vesalius argued, could the physician learn human anatomy in sufficient detail. This "hands-on" principle remained Vesalius's most lasting contribution to anatomy. It is graphically represented in the *Fabrica*'s woodcut title page, which shows Vesalius with his right hand in an opened cadaver, conducting an anatomical demonstration.[1]

The *Fabrica* also broke new ground in its unprecedented blending of scientific exposition, art, and typography. How innovative Vesalius's publishing ideas were may be seen if one compares the *Fabrica* with Berengario da Carpi's *Commentaria* (1521) (see no. 15). It is likely that Vesalius obtained the idea for his title page from the crude representation of a dissection scene on the title page of Berengario's *Commentaria*, and similarly, Berengario began the tradition, now associated with Vesalius, of placing the dissected muscle men within a landscape background. Yet Berengario's relatively crude woodcuts, though considerably advanced from medieval anatomy, still represent a bridge between medieval art and science and the much more detailed and precisely finished Renaissance style of the Vesalian woodcuts, which mark the beginning of modern anatomy. Berengario's illustrations and those in earlier anatomical works tended to be placed rather haphazardly, with little or no relationship to the text. In contrast, Vesalius sent his woodblocks to the printer with precise instructions as to placement within the text and with exact marginal references that established a direct relationship of text to illustrations, or even details within illustrations. (The series of historiated initials, in which putti and dwarfed men humorously perform some of the more grisly actions associated with dissection, have been called pictorial footnotes to the text.)

The *Fabrica*'s magnificent title page and the spectacular series of more than two hundred anatomical woodcuts (full-page and smaller) spread throughout the book remain the most famous series of anatomical illustrations ever published. Because Vesalius published no clues as to their authorship, and no manuscripts, archives, or demonstrably authentic original drawings for the work exist, the source of the woodcuts has always excited the curiosity and speculation of art historians, historians of medicine, and bibliographers. A contemporary reference in Vasari is probably the source of the traditional attribution of the woodcuts to a Flemish associate of Titian, Jan Stephan van Calcar (ca. 1499–1546/50), who drew and possibly engraved the three woodcuts of skeletons in Vesalius's first series of anatomical charts, *Tabulae anatomicae sex* (1538).[2] Calcar is the only named artist definitely known to have worked with Vesalius. Nevertheless, there is no reliable basis for attributing the illustrations in the *Fabrica* to him or any other particular artist. Since we lack any evidence about them other than their style and the understanding that they were cut in Venice, the *Fabrica* woodcuts may be attributed to an unknown artist or artists of the school of Titian. Vesalius commissioned the illustrations and supervised their production. It is also possible that he personally drew some of the lesser illustrations for the *Fabrica*, as it is known that he made the drawings for the first three of the *Tabulae anatomicae sex*. Remarkably, most of the woodblocks for the *Fabrica* survived into this century, preserved in Munich until their destruction in World War II.

Various scholars, including Harvey Cushing, Vesalius's bibliographer, have criticized the woodcut portrait of Vesalius, first published in the *Fabrica*, for its seemingly disproportionate representation of Vesalius's body parts: the head appears too large for the chest, and the arms too short. However, Vesalius's concern with the accurate depiction of the human body, as demonstrated in his attention to the illustrations of the *Fabrica*, and the fact that he reused this portrait both in the 1555 edition of the *Fabrica* and in his letter on the China root (1546), suggest that the portrait reflects his true proportions and that Vesalius may have been somewhat dwarfed. The portrait of Vesalius published in his works is the only reliable extant portrait of him; the many other portraits which have been thought to depict him were derived either from this single portrait or from the imaginations of the artists.[3]

The impressive typography of *De humani corporis fabrica* was the work of Johannes Oporinus of Basel, one of the most widely learned and iconoclastic of the so-called "scholar-printers," whose success with this book apparently caused Vesalius to entrust to him all of his later publications. A 1984 census of the *Fabrica* located 132 copies of the first edition.[4] Five of these, including the Rosenwald copy in the Library of Congress, represent a variant issue, in that they contain a version of the introductory quire with different settings of type from those found in the majority of copies of the first edition. It has been proposed that these variant leaves indicate a state issued prior to the other extant copies; however, the fact that the variant leaves employ the French-style italic font used in the second edition of 1555, as well as a typographic design more closely related to the second edition, suggests that the variant copies consist of an experimental printing done between the first and second editions.

De humani corporis fabrica may be the only masterwork in the history of medicine and science that was published simultaneously with a synopsis prepared by the author. Vesalius designed his *De humani corporis fabrica librorum epitome* to serve as a more affordable outline key to the encyclopedic and expensive *Fabrica*. In its dedication Vesalius stated: "I have made [the *Epitome*] to be as it were a foot-path beside the larger book, and as an index of what is set forth in it." However, unlike the *Fabrica*, which begins with the skeletal system and works outward, the *Epitome*'s approach to anatomy is topographical: that is, the muscles are first discussed, followed by a combined study of the vessels, nervous system, and viscera. The various parts of the anatomy are illustrated in nine woodcuts, divided into two skeletal, four muscular, and two circulatory charts, plus a neurological chart. The skeletal, muscular, and one of the circulatory plates are similar, but not identical, to plates found in the *Fabrica*: the *Epitome*'s plates are some sixty millimeters taller, the figures are in slightly different attitudes, and less space is devoted to background scenery (leaf K duplicates the *Fabrica*'s thinking skeleton, but the inscription on the pedestal has been changed). The remaining circulatory plate and the neurological plate are reproduced, with different texts, on the two folding plates found in the *Fabrica*: the illustration on leaf M of the *Epitome* appears on leaf p3(1) of the *Fabrica*, and the plate on *Epitome* leaf [N] (minus the accompanying organs) appears on *Fabrica* leaf m2(1).[5] In addition to these nine anatomical plates, the *Epitome* includes two woodcuts of a nude male

Fig. 31. No. 18B. Vesalius. The male and female figures in the *Epitome.*

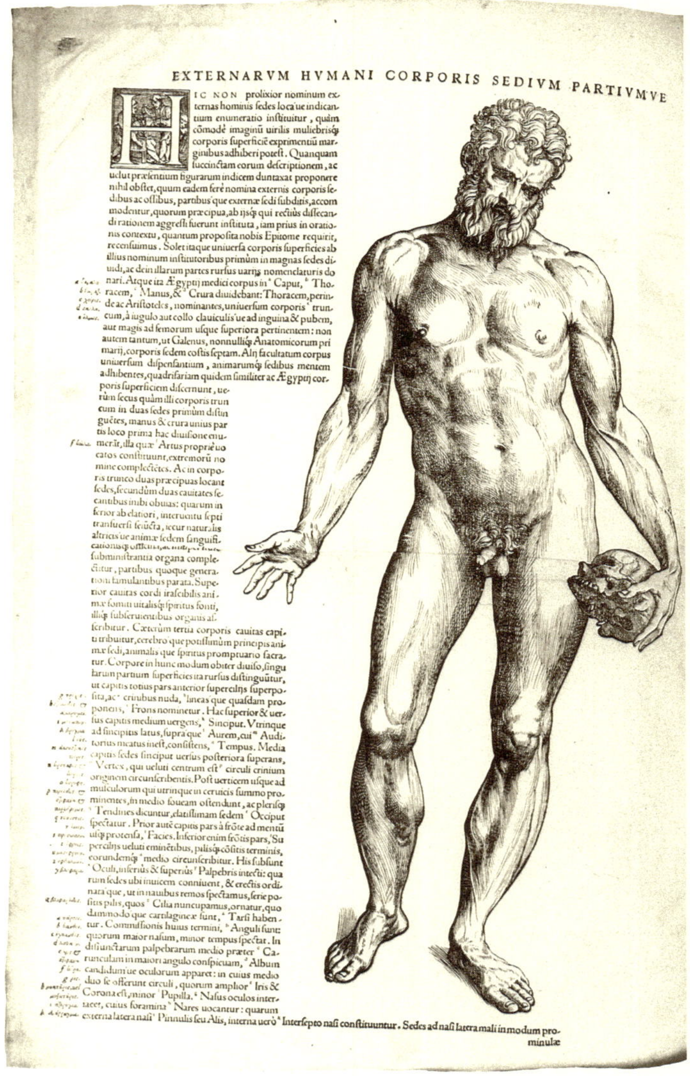

and a nude female figure, accompanied by long descriptions of the surface regions of the body; nothing like them appears in the *Fabrica.* The *Epitome's* title-page woodcut and portrait of Vesalius are from the same blocks used in the *Fabrica.*

Published in a larger format than the *Fabrica,* in the form of separate sheets to be used for wall charts, and not necessarily bound, the *Epitome* is considerably rarer than the *Fabrica* today. Many copies of the *Epitome* are incomplete, and the last two, unsigned sheets ([N] and [O]), printed with individual parts of the body to be cut out and used as overlays for other figures, are especially rare.

JMN

1. Because it was then legal only to dissect the cadavers of executed criminals, and these cadavers were always in short supply, Vesalius urged physicians to take their own initiative in obtaining material for dissection. The *Fabrica* contains

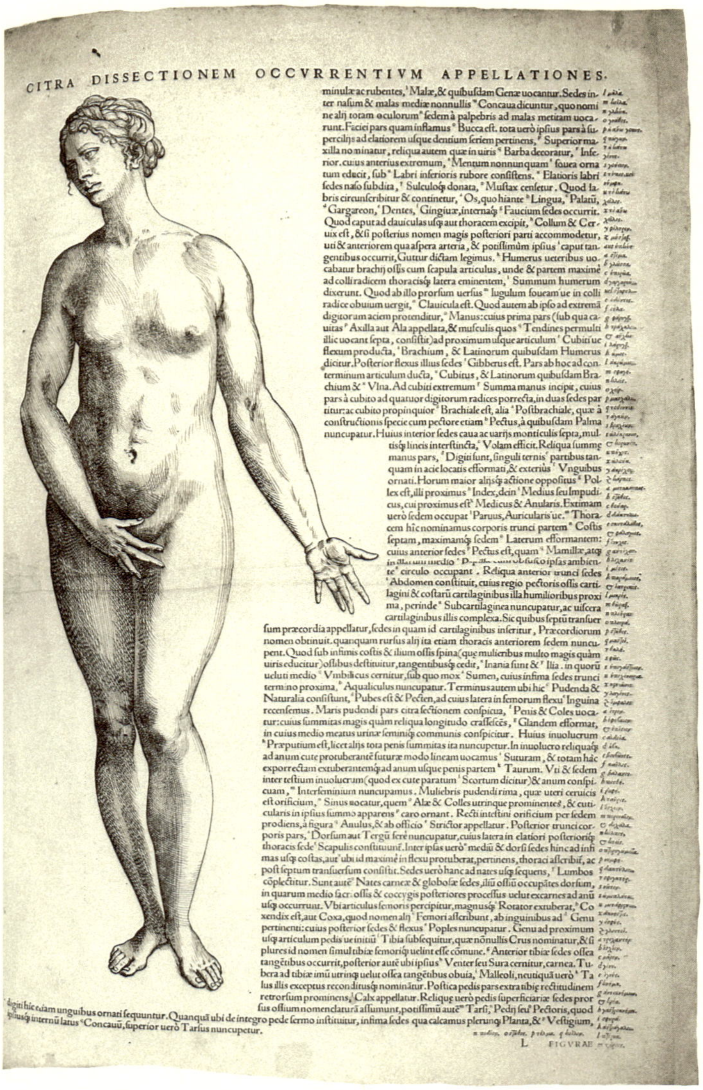

several amusing and unrepentant anecdotes of how students had robbed graves to obtain cadavers, especially those of women, since female criminals were rarely executed in those days.

2. Giorgio Vasari, *Le vite de' piu eccellenti pittori, scultori, e architettori*, 2d ed. (Florence, 1568), p. 408.

3. Marion Harry Spielmann, *The Iconography of Andreas Vesalius (André Vésale), Anatomist and Physician, 1514–1564* (London, 1925).

4. Michael Horowitz and Jack Collins, "A Census of Copies of the First Edition of Andreas Vesalius' *De humani corporis fabrica* (1543), with a Note on the Recently Discovered Variant Issue," *Journal of the History of Medicine and Allied Sciences* 39 (1984): 198–221.

5. According to Cushing, these two woodcuts were originally made for the *Epitome* and were inserted into the *Fabrica* as an afterthought (see Harvey Cushing, *A Bio-Bibliography of Andreas Vesalius* [New York, 1943], p. 109).

See color plates XV, XVI, and XVII.

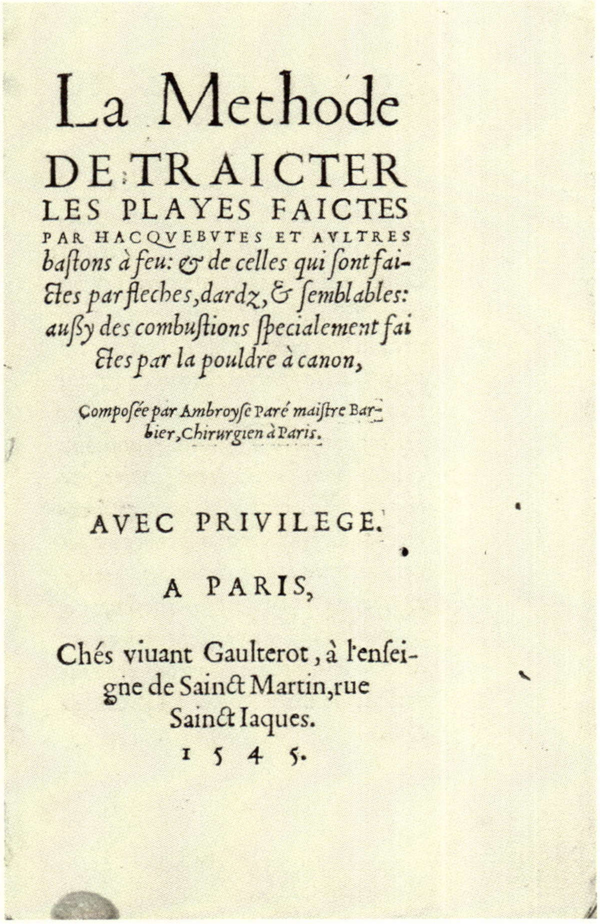

La Methode
DE TRAICTER
LES PLAYES FAICTES
PAR HACQVEBVTES ET AVLTRES
baſtons à feu: & de celles qui ſont faictes par fleches, dardz, & ſemblables: auſsy des combuſtions ſpecialement faictes par la pouldre à canon,

Compoſée par Ambroyſe Paré maiſtre Barbier, Chirurgien à Paris.

AVEC PRIVILEGE.

A PARIS,

Chés viuant Gaulterot, à l'enſeigne de Sainct Martin, rue Sainct Iaques.
1 5 4 5.

Fig. 32. No. 19A. Paré. Title page.

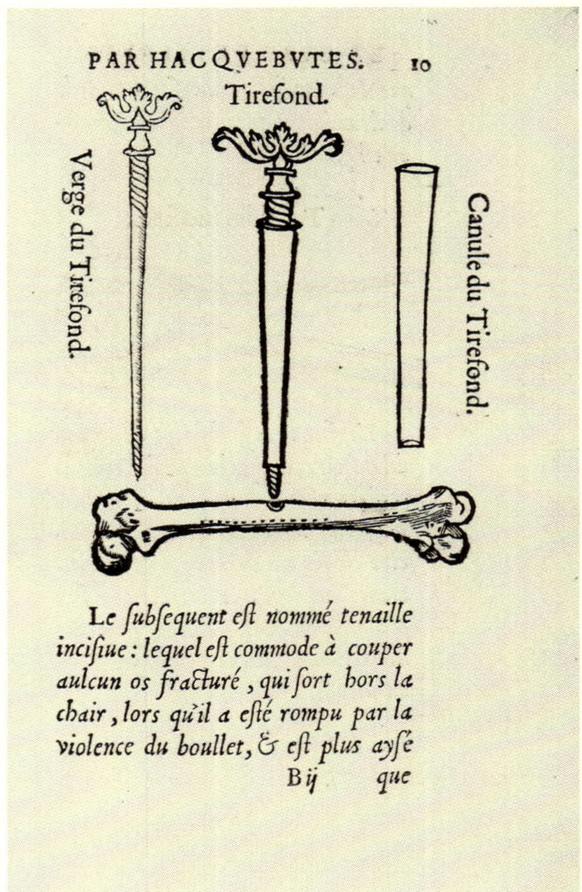

PAR HACQVEBVTES. 10

Le ſubſequent eſt nommé tenaille inciſiue: lequel eſt commode à couper aulcun os fracturé, qui ſort hors la chair, lors qu'il a eſté rompu par la violence du boullet, & eſt plus ayſé
B ij que

Fig. 33. No. 19A. Paré. Surgical instruments.

19

AMBROISE PARÉ
(1510–1590)

A] *La methode de traicter les playes faictes par hacquebutes et aultres bastons à feu.*

Paris: Chés viuant Gaulterot, 1545.

8°: A–H8 I4. 68 leaves, ff. *1* 2–64 [4]. 23 woodcuts in text.

Adams P–317. Doe 1. EFDT 66. GM 2139. Stillwell 471. Waller 7152.

B] *La maniere de traicter les playes faictes tant par hacquebutes, que par fleches; & les accidentz d'icelles, comme fractures & caries des os, gangrene & mortification.*

Paris: Par la vefue Iean de Brie, 1551 (colophon: 10 March 1552).

8°: aa8 A–K8 L12. 100 leaves, ff. [8] 1–80 [12]. Woodcut title-page border; 42 woodcuts in text.

Doe 2. Waller 7153.

Paré's first work, written when he was still a young and unknown military barber-surgeon, was the earliest treatise to be devoted solely to the treatment of gunshot wounds. It was a revolutionary work from the standpoint of the treatment it recommended, as well as for the emphasis Paré placed on experience and observation in place of tradition and dogma. It was widely believed in Paré's day that gunshot wounds were poisoned, and the accepted treatment for such wounds was to cauterize them with boiling oil. *La methode de traicter les playes* dramatically recounts Paré's experience in departing from this standard treatment, a departure necessitated by a lack of the proper supplies. His surprise at seeing wounds do well without the traditional treatment—and, more important, his ability to extrapolate from this observation the general principle of gentle wound treatment—rank among the greatest of surgical observations.

The second edition of Paré's treatise, published seven years after the first, was extensively revised and enlarged by the author, who stated that it might thus fairly be called a new work. The illustrations were recut after those in the first edition, with the addition of new ones. The second edition was dedicated to King Henri II of France (1547–59), and the woodcut title border incorporates the devices publicly used by the king to honor his mistress Diane de Poitiers—the interlaced "HD" monogram and three interlaced crescents. Janet Doe, Paré's bibliographer, states that "with this book Paré [began] to show an

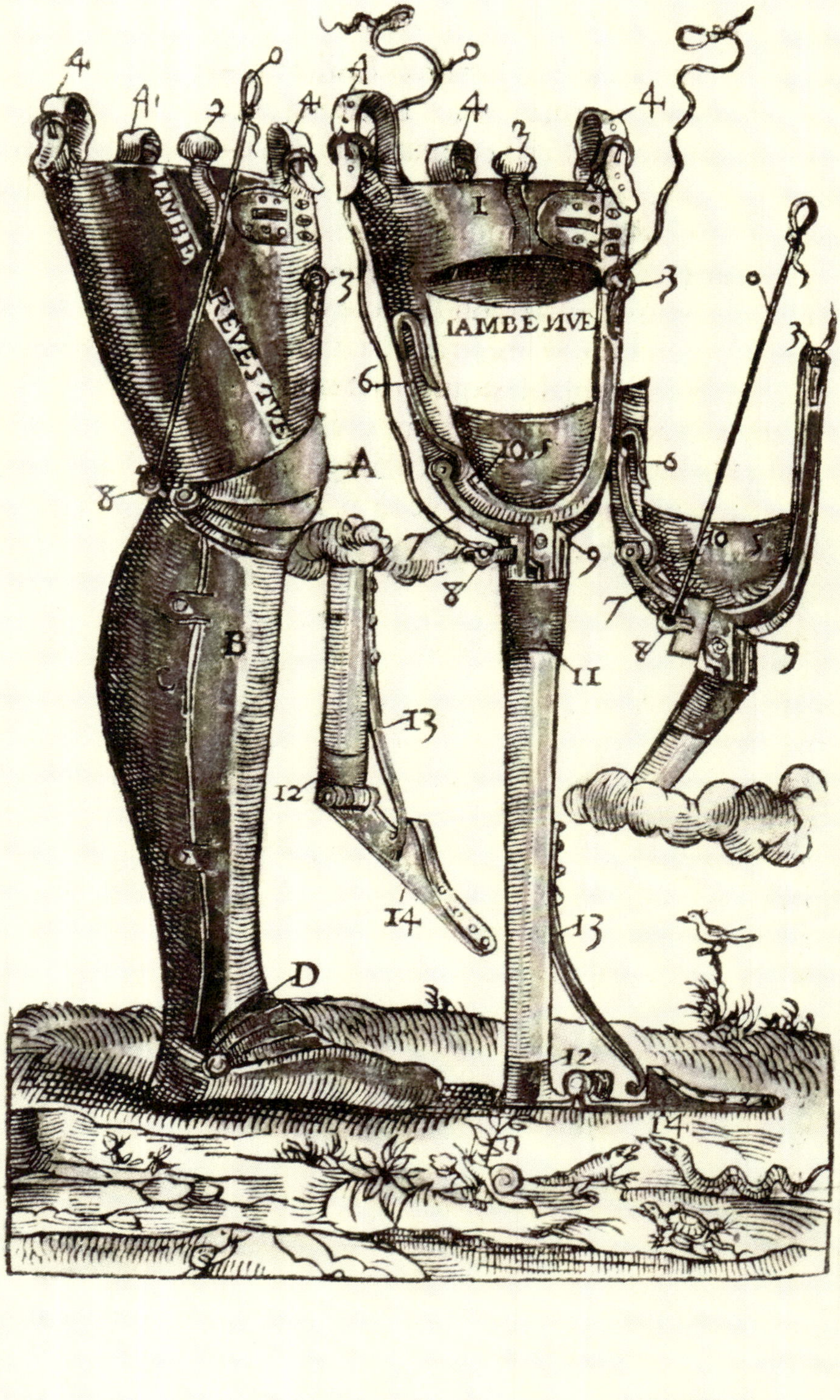

Fig. 34. No. 19B. Paré. Orthopedic prostheses.

interest in the outward appearance of his publications," attributing this interest to his "desire to make as splendid as possible this book he was dedicating to the king."[1] The book may have had something to do with Paré's success at court; in 1552 he was appointed the king's surgeon, a position in which he served several monarchs.

ESF

It is not generally recognized that Paré was the first great surgeon to adopt the ideas of Paracelsus, the sixteenth-century German iconoclast who is now regarded as a founder of chemical medicine (see no. 16). Paré belonged to a small philosophical society in Paris, founded in 1571, which discussed Paracelsian doctrine, prepared Paracelsian medicines, and carried out alchemical experiments. In his *Deux livres de chirurgie* (1573), Paré quoted Paracelsus's remark on the inborn balsam that heals all wounds (*Der grossenn Wundartzney*, 1536). In the *Deux livres de chirurgie*, Paré attributed this idea to Paracelsus, and he referred to it again in later treatises; however, in these later works he dropped all references to the theory's source. This may have been for political reasons: Paracelsus was a controversial figure, and the Paris faculty of medicine, whose approbation Paré needed, was at the time very much embroiled in debates over the use of chemical medicines. It is also possible that Paré's increasing success and connection with the French royal family made it necessary for him to distance himself from the French Paracelsians.

SA

1. Janet Doe, *A Bibliography of the Works of Ambroise Paré* (Chicago, 1937), p. 33.

See color plates XVIII *and* XIX.

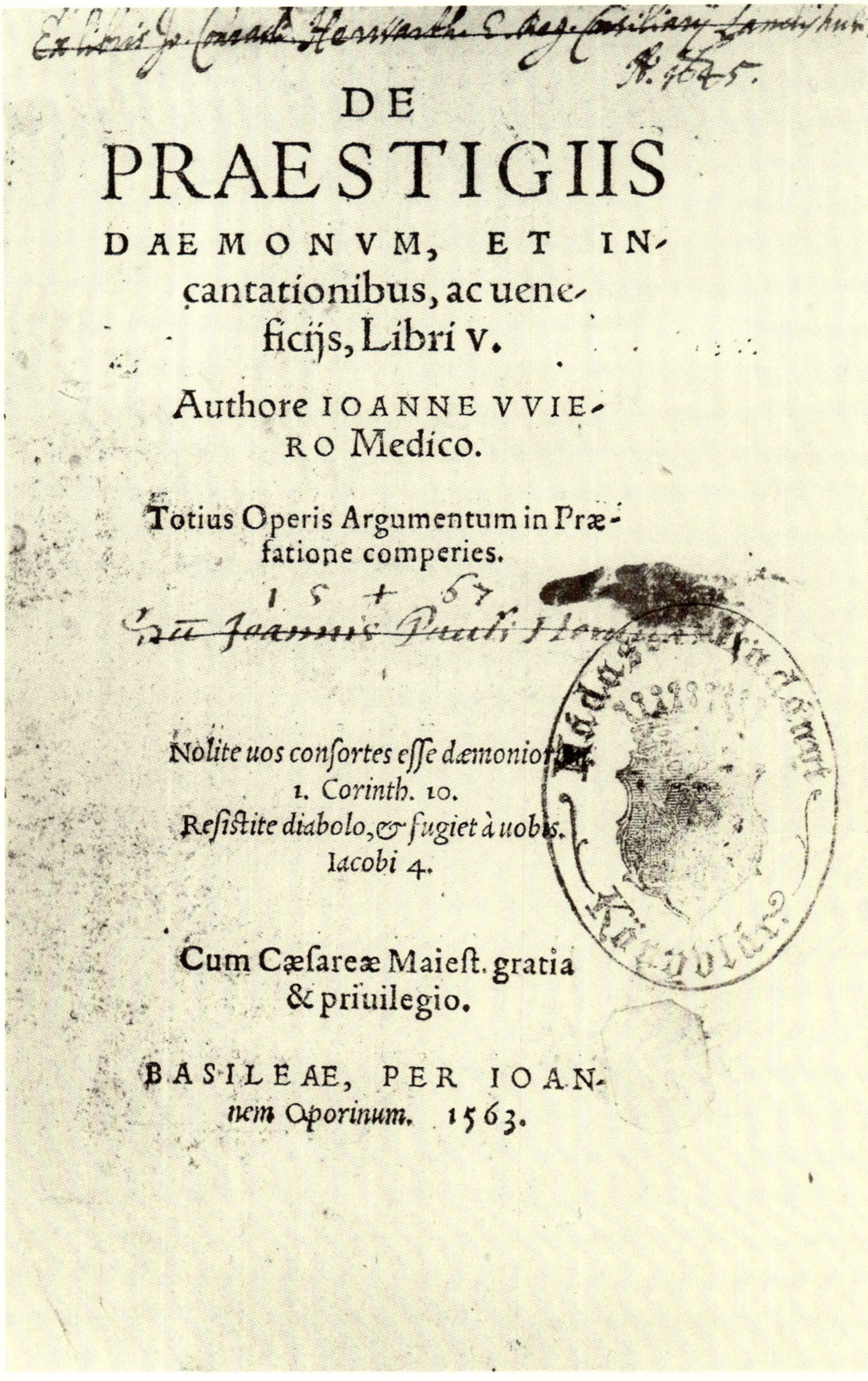

DE
PRAESTIGIIS
DAEMONVM, ET IN-
cantationibus, ac uene-
ficijs, Libri V.

Authore IOANNE VVIE-
RO Medico.

Totius Operis Argumentum in Præ-
fatione comperies.

Nolite uos consortes esse dæmoniorum.
1. Corinth. 10.
Resistite diabolo, & fugiet à uobis.
Iacobi 4.

Cum Cæsareæ Maiest. gratia
& priuilegio.

BASILEAE, PER IOAN-
nem Oporinum. 1563.

Fig. 35. No. 20. Weyer. Title page.

20

JOHANN WEYER [WIER]
(1515–1588)

De praestigiis daemonum, et incantationibus, ac ueneficijs, libri V.

Basel: Per Ioannem Oporinum, 1563.

8°: a–z^8 A–G^8. 240 leaves, pp. *1–3* 4–479 [1].

Adams W–144. Durling 4734. GM 4916. Norman 2209.

Johann Weyer, born in 1515 to a middle-class family in a small town on the border between the Netherlands and Germany, grew up in an atmosphere influenced by the *devotio moderna* and Erasmus's lifelong goal of returning the Church to early Christian ideals without a schism. From age fifteen to nineteen he was apprenticed to Cornelius Agrippa of Nettesheim, an extremely learned man well versed in occult sciences and "natural magic," whose thought combined aspects of mysticism and skepticism. He later studied at the medical schools of Paris and Orléans, where he obtained a medical degree in 1537. In 1550, after several years of practice, Weyer was appointed court physician to Duke William V of Jülich, Berg and Cleves. The Duke, an enlightened man, carried on a program of Erasmian reforms in his domain and maintained a tolerant attitude toward followers of various religious denominations. Weyer found this atmosphere congenial to his open-minded personality and remained there for the rest of his life.

In *De praestigiis daemonum*, Weyer approached the subject of witchcraft from four different viewpoints: theological, philosophical, medical, and legal. Although extremely well versed in ancient, patristic, and medieval literature, he did not engage in philosophical and theological subtleties; rather his book shows evidence of an inquisitive mind, good clinical knowledge, a distinct professional attitude, and a dispassionate approach to medical matters, among which he also included witchcraft. The book contains more than sixty reports of cases of alleged witchcraft or of unusual mental phenomena observed directly by Weyer, related personally to him in oral or written form, or known to him in various ways.

Contrary to the received opinion of his day, which held that witchcraft was evidence of demonic possession, Weyer believed the basic cause of witchcraft to be a disturbance of the imagination, that faculty traditionally regarded as the interface between bodily and mental functions. He described most of those accused of witchcraft as poor, gullible old women who had fallen into this reckless credulity because of "their being circumvented by fraud, constrained by force, compelled by fear, induced by error, and deceived by ignorance." Weyer brought a serene, rational approach to the investigation of each case, establishing and confirming the facts, providing a firsthand assessment of the situation through description of the person's appearance, behavior, speech, ideation, and emotional traits, and following these with the formulation of a concrete and sensible plan of treatment, often based on what we would now describe as psychological principles. In some cases he succeeded, with the Duke's approval, in liberating women accused of witchcraft, saving them from torture and possibly death.

In the last period of his life Weyer's enlightened approach lost ground. As a result of increasing Spanish influence in the Low Countries and the progress of the Counter-Reformation after the Council of Trent, the Duke (who, in the meantime had suffered a cerebral vascular accident, resulting in some mental symptoms) consented to have trials for witchcraft resumed. Weyer himself remained a highly respected figure, although it is not clear whether his retirement in 1578 was forced or voluntary. During his lifetime, his book continued to appear in Latin editions (1564, 1566, 1568, 1577, 1583), in German translation (1565, 1567, 1575, 1578), and in French (1567, 1579). These later editions and translations show no trace of the inner turmoil their author must have endured as a result of the continuous opposition of ecclesiastical authorities and contemporary writers—there are only occasional references to Jean Bodin, a well-known jurisprudent and political philosopher, who in 1580 published *Demonomanie des sorciers*, containing an appendix pointedly directed against Weyer's position on witchcraft.

During the late sixteenth and seventeenth centuries, belief declined in the role of supernatural factors in daily events, and there was increasing acceptance of the notion of fixed laws in science. As a result, witchcraft was gradually relegated to the realm of superstition, and Weyer's work fell into obscurity. He remained forgotten until the end of the nineteenth century when, after Jean-Martin Charcot's dramatic presentation of hysteria as a functional nervous disorder, the French translation of Weyer's book was reprinted in Paris in 1885.[1] This happened to be the very year in which Sigmund Freud (see no. 87) was in Paris attending Charcot's lectures; he must have known of this publication and probably read it. More than twenty years later, in 1907, when asked to name the ten most important books ever published, Freud listed Weyer's work after those of Copernicus and Darwin;[2] however, Freud's comment passed unnoticed and the book was forgotten again until its rediscovery by the psychoanalyst and medical historian Gregory Zilboorg. Zilboorg considered Weyer the founder of modern psychiatry, but from today's historical perspective on the development of psychiatry, it is more properly said that he was a great precursor of modern psychiatry.[3] An English translation of *De praestigiis daemonum* was published in 1991.[4]

GM

1. The new edition, in two volumes, reprinted the French text that had been published in 1579 under the title *Histoires, disputes et discours, des illusions et impostures des diables.*

2. Sigmund Freud, *Letters*, ed. Ernst L. Freud, trans. Tania and James Stern (New York, 1960), p. 269.

3. Gregory Zilboorg, *The Medical Man and the Witch during the Renaissance* (Baltimore, 1935), pp. 109–207; Zilboorg, *A History of Medical Psychology* (New York, 1941), p. 226.

4. George Mora, ed., *Witches, Devils, and Doctors in the Renaissance: Johann Weyer, De Praestigiis Daemonum* (Binghamton, N.Y., 1991).

BARTHOLOMAEI

EVSTACHII

SANCTOSEVERINATIS MEDICI
AC PHILOSOPHI
OPVSCVLA ANATOMICA.

Quorum numerum & argumenta auersa pagina indicabit.

Cum Priuilegijs Summi Pont. Illustriss. Senatus Veneti, Sereniss. Francorum Regis, & Catolicæ ac Cæsareæ Maiestatis.

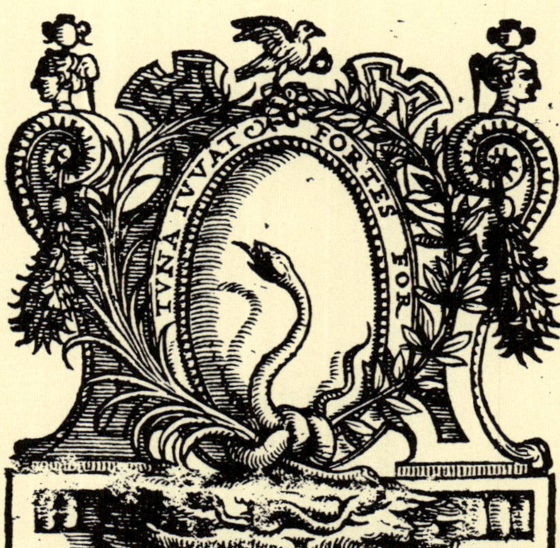

VENETIIS,

M D LXIIII.

Vincentius Luchinus excudebat.

Fig. 36. No. 21. Eustachi. Title page.

21

BARTOLOMEO EUSTACHI
(ca. 1500/10–1574)

Opuscula anatomica.

Venice: Vincentius Luchinus excudebat, 1564.

4°: $*^{6}$, α–β^{8} κ^{4}, $*^{4}$ A–Z^{4} Aa–Ii^{4} Kk^{2} Ll–Ss^{4}, a–h^{4} I–N^{4}, A–V^{4} X^{2}. 326 leaves, pp. [12], [40], 1 [1] 2–4 [1] 5–8 [1] 9–12 [1] 13–15 [1] 16–17 [1] 18 [1] 19 [1] 20–323 [1], [8] 1–95 [1], [164]. Tab. Prima-Octava: 8 engravings, printed on recto or verso of letterpress pages 1, 4, 9, 12, 15, 18, 19, 20, but not included in the pagination.

Adams E–1103. Choulant-Frank, pp. 200–1. Durling 1408. GM 801, 1093, 1139, 1228, 1538, 3668. *Heirs of Hippocrates* 322. Norman 739. Wellcome 2091.

In 1562 and 1563 Eustachi wrote a series of anatomical treatises on the kidneys (*De renum structura*), the organs of hearing (*De auditus organis*), the venous system (*De vena quae azygos graecis dicitur*), and the teeth (*De dentibus*), which he published together under the title *Opuscula anatomica.* The treatise on the kidney, the first work devoted specifically to that organ, showed a detailed knowledge surpassing that of any earlier work; it contained the first account of the adrenal (suprarenal) gland and a correct determination of the relative levels of the kidneys. The treatise on the ear provided the first postclassical account of the Eustachian tube, while the work on the azygos vein contained the first description of the thoracic duct and of the *valvula venae cavae* in the right ventricle of the heart, the so-called "Eustachian valve." In his treatise on dentistry Eustachi was the first to study the teeth in any great detail: basing his work on the dissection of fetuses and stillborn infants, he gave an important description of the first and second dentitions, described the hard outer tissue and soft inner structure of the teeth, and attempted an explanation of the problem (not yet completely solved) of the sensitivity of the tooth's hard structure. *De dentibus* may also have been issued separately; it bears its own title leaf dated 1563 and has a separate index.

The engraved plates illustrating the *Opuscula anatomica* were the first eight in a series of forty-seven anatomical plates engraved by Giulio de' Musi after drawings by Eustachi and his relative, Pier Matteo Pini, an artist. These were prepared in 1552 to illustrate a projected book entitled *De dissensionibus ac controversiis anatomicis*, the text of which was lost after Eustachi's death. Had the full series of plates been published at the time of their completion, Eustachi would have ranked with Vesalius as a founder of modern anatomy. As it happened, only the first eight plates were issued during Eustachi's lifetime, while the

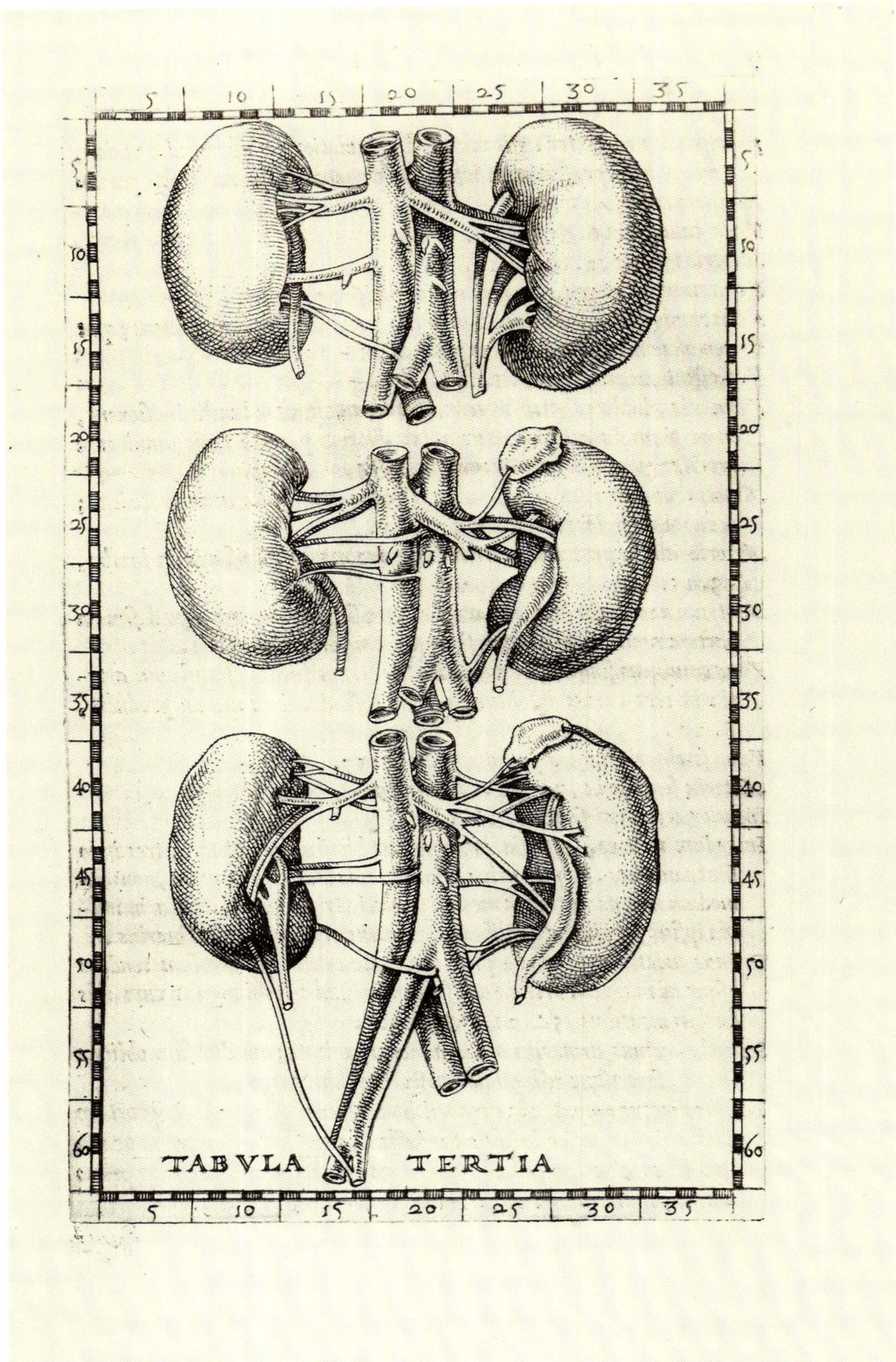

Fig. 37. No. 21. Eustachi. This plate illustrates Eustachi's use of numbered coordinates for locating any part of the anatomical image.

remaining thirty-nine were lost for over a century after his death; after a long search, the missing plates were discovered in the hands of a descendant of Pier Matteo Fini and were published by Giovanni Maria Lancisi, physician to Pope Clement XI (1700–21).[1] Eustachi's plates are strikingly modern, produced without the conventional sixteenth-century decorative accompaniment, and framed on three sides by numbered rules providing coordinates by which any part of the image can be located. The images are generic figures, composites of many anatomical observations, and are mathematically as well as representationally exact.

JMN

1. Bartolomeo Eustachi, *Tabulae anatomicae* (Rome, 1714).

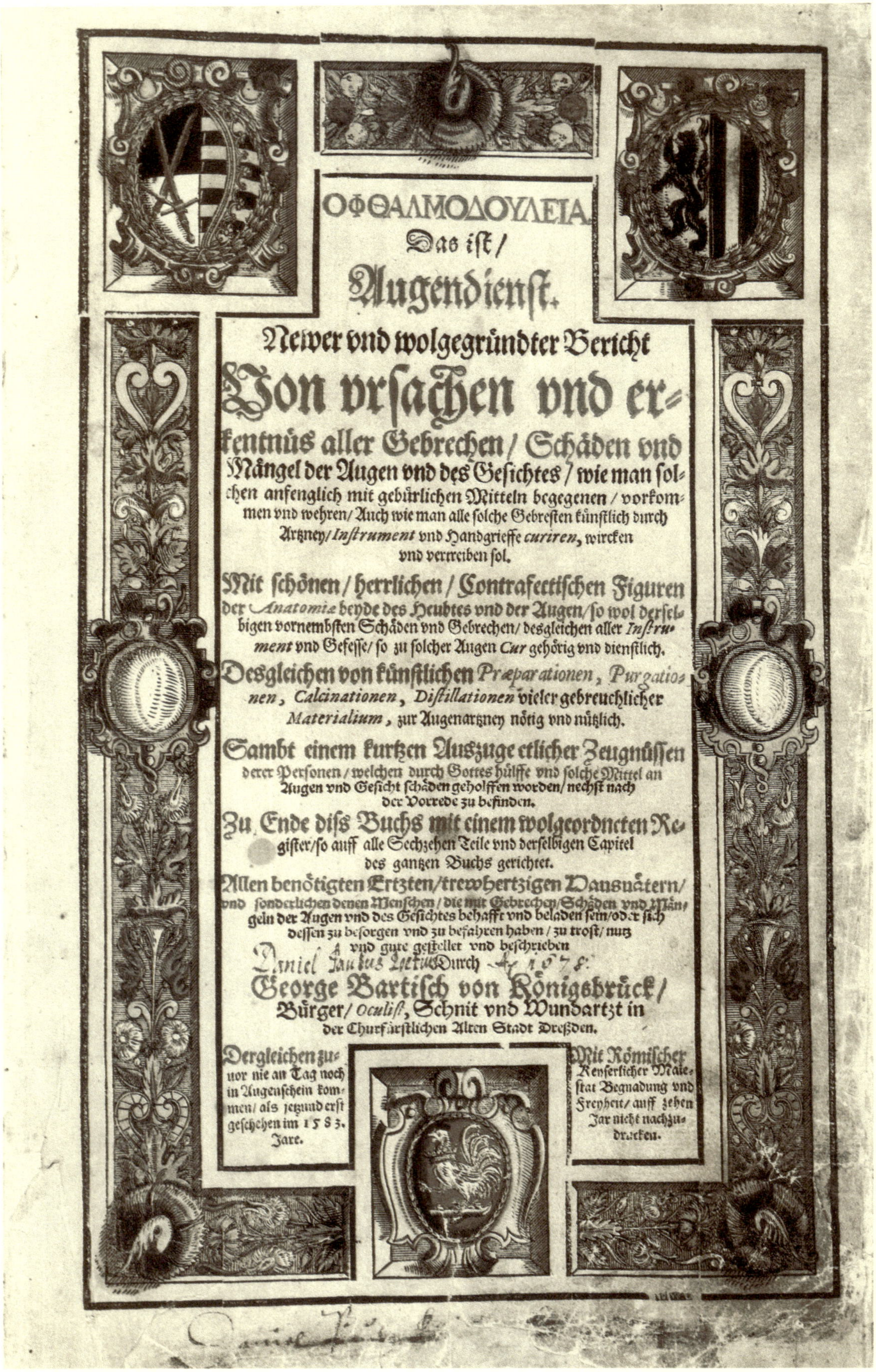

ΟΦΘΑΛΜΟΔΟΥΛΕΙΑ.

Das ist/

Augendienst.

Newer vnd wolgegründter Bericht

Von vrsachen vnd erkentnüs aller Gebrechen/ Schäden vnd Mängel der Augen vnd des Gesichtes/ wie man solchen anfenglich mit gebürlichen Mitteln begegenen/ vorkommen vnd wehren/ Auch wie man alle solche Gebresten künstlich durch Artzney/ *Instrument* vnd Handgrieffe *curiren*, wircken vnd vertreiben sol.

Mit schönen/ herrlichen/ Contrafectischen Figuren der *Anatomiæ* beyde des Heubtes vnd der Augen/ so wol derselbigen vornembsten Schäden vnd Gebrechen/ desgleichen aller *Instrument* vnd Gefesse/ so zu solcher Augen *Cur* gehörig vnd dienstlich.

Desgleichen von künstlichen *Præparationen*, *Purgationen*, *Calcinationen*, *Distillationen* vieler gebreuchlicher *Materialium*, zur Augenartzney nötig vnd nützlich.

Sambt einem kurtzen Auszuge etlicher Zeugnüssen derer Personen/ welchen durch Gottes hülffe vnd solche Mittel an Augen vnd Gesicht schäden geholffen worden/ nechst nach der Vorrede zu befinden.

Zu Ende dises Buchs mit einem wolgeordneten Register/ so auff alle Sechzehen Teile vnd derselbigen Capitel des gantzen Buchs gerichtet.

Allen benötigten Ertzten/ trewhertzigen Hausvätern/ vnd sonderlichen denen Menschen/ die mit Gebrechen/ Schäden vnd Mängeln der Augen vnd des Gesichtes behafft vnd beladen sein/ oder sich dessen zu besorgen vnd zu befahren haben/ zu trost/ nutz vnd gute gestellet vnd beschrieben

Durch

George Bartisch von Königsbrück/ Bürger/ *Oculist*, Schnit vnd Wundartzt in der Churfürstlichen Alten Stadt Dreßden.

Dergleichen zuvor nie an Tag noch in Augenschein kommen/ als jetzund erst geschehen im 1583. Jare.

Mit Römischer Keyserlicher Maiestat Begnadung vnd Freyheit/ auff zehen Jar nicht nachzudrucken.

Fig. 38. No. 22. Bartisch. Title page, with hand-colored woodcut borders.

22

GEORG BARTISCH

(1535–1606)

Οφθαλμοδουλεια. *Das ist, Augendienst. Newer vnd wolgegründter Bericht von Vrsachen vnd Erkentnüs aller Gebrechen, Schäden vnd Mängel der Augen vnd des Gesichtes.*

Dresden: Gedruckt durch Matthes Stöckel, 1583.

2°: A–D^6 E^4 A–Z^6 a–x^6 y^8 z^4 Aa^6. 310 leaves, ff. [28] 1–274 [8]. Title printed in red and black. Woodcut title border (repeated), 4 lesser borders; in text, woodcut arms of Duke Augustus of Saxony and of the city of Dresden; 91 woodcuts in text (including repeats), most full-page, including one with 5 overlay flaps (f. 5r) and one with 6 overlay flaps (f. 8v).

Choulant-Frank, p. 234. Durling 479. GM 5817. *Heirs of Hippocrates* 369. Norman 125. Waller 756. Wellcome 697.

Georg Bartisch is considered the founder of modern ophthalmology. *Ophthalmoduleia* or *Augendienst* ("the care of the eyes") was the first modern work on eye surgery. It was also the first work to establish a subspecialty within the domain of surgery, and its title in both Greek and German forms established the phrases by which ophthalmology (*Augenheilkunde*) became known.

Bartisch rose from obscure beginnings to the position of court oculist in Dresden. He was famous for his facility in dealing with cataracts, and his book describes his method of couching, in which he employed a silver needle and kept patients immobilized for seven days. Bartisch was the first to extirpate the bulbus in cancer of the eye; this was accomplished by scooping the eye out with one sweep of an instrument resembling a spoon with knife-sharp edges. He was also a pioneer in the principle of postoperative care. He opposed the use of eyeglasses, although his book contains an illustration of an individual wearing spectacles. Instead of glasses or the many clever operations he could devise, Bartisch often recommended drugs, lotions, pastes, and washes, and stressed attention to diet and personal hygiene.

Augendienst was dedicated to Duke Augustus I of Saxony, whom Bartisch served as court oculist. The book's text, in twelve parts, and its woodcut illustrations combine to give a comprehensive view of Renaissance eye surgery. The woodcuts constitute one of the most remarkable features of the publication: they total ninety-one, including some repetitions, and they are believed to have been executed by Hans Hewamaul after Bartisch's own drawings. Two of the illustrations are presented with overlays showing anatomical parts lying successively one under the other; Bartisch was the first to illustrate the brain and the eye in this manner. The book was printed at Bartisch's own expense and was widely used for the next century. It was reprinted in 1686 with the illustrations redrawn to include seventeenth-century costumes.

DMA/ESF

Several copies of Bartisch's work are known in which the woodcuts have been colored by a contemporary hand, possibly under the author's supervision. One such belongs to the Putti Collection at the Rizzoli Institute, Bologna, Italy,[1] and another to the Karolinska Institute, Stockholm, Sweden.[2] The latter may have been presented originally to Peter Vok Orsini of Rosenberg (1539–1611), the wealthiest and most powerful Bohemian nobleman of his day, who formed one of the most famous libraries assembled north of the Alps in the sixteenth century. The Karolinska Institute copy has been compared to the one presented to Duke Augustus I of Saxony, formerly in the Dresden State Library but missing since 1945. In both of these copies all the cuts are hand-colored, and both were bound by Jakob Krause, the greatest German bookbinder of the Renaissance.

HFN

1. Illustrated in Roberto Margotta, *The Story of Medicine* (New York, 1968).
2. Ove Hagelin, *Rare and Important Medical Books in the Library of the Karolinska Institute: An Illustrated and Annotated Catalogue* (Stockholm, 1992).

See color plate XX.

23

GASPARE TAGLIACOZZI
(1545–1599)

De curtorum chirurgia per insitionem, libri duo.

Venice: Apud Gasparem Bindonum iuniorem, 1597.

2°: †^{6} ††^{8} A–H^{6} Aa–Hh^{6} Aaa–Ddd^{6} a–b^{6} c^{4}. 150 leaves, pp. [28] 1–94 [2], 1–95 [1], *1–3* 4–47 [33]. Additional engraved title page; 24 woodcuts in text, including 22 full-page woodcuts with keys on opposite pages.

Durling 4310. GM 5734. *Heirs of Hippocrates* 379. Norman 2048. Waller 9451. Wellcome 6210.

Although Western writers beginning with Celsus (see no. 4) had discussed aspects of plastic operations, Tagliacozzi was the first medical author to devote a book entirely to what he called "The surgery of mutilations through grafting," a type of surgery that came to be called "plastic surgery" in the nineteenth century.[1] The role of *De curtorum chirurgia* in the development of this field of surgery was twofold. First, it made available to the medical world surgical procedures, chiefly for the repair of mutilated noses and ears, that had been developed over generations by the Branca and Vianeo families of Sicily and Calabria, and it added to these operations improvements made in the light of the best medical knowledge of Tagliacozzi's day. Second, the work attempted to explode the erroneous beliefs surrounding the subject of plastic operations and to combat the prejudices resulting from these misconceptions. Despite Tagliacozzi's efforts, however, his contemporaries refused to adopt his methods, possibly for fear of complications, or possibly because the Catholic Church regarded plastic operations as meddling with the work of God (after Tagliacozzi's death, the Church had his body exhumed and reburied in unconsecrated ground). Tagliacozzi's work remained virtually forgotten until the revival of plastic surgery by Joseph Constantine Carpue and Carl Ferdinand von Graefe in the early nineteenth century.

The series of twenty-two full-page woodcuts in Book III of *De curtorum chirurgia* depict Tagliacozzi's instruments and the individual steps of various facial reconstructive operations through the postoperative stage, including the famous "Italian" method of rhinoplasty that uses a graft from the patient's arm. Tagliacozzi, who was a professor of medicine at Bologna, went to great expense to have these illustrations prepared, as he indicated in a letter of 16 July 1596 to the Senators of Bologna.[2] The artist who created them remains anonymous, although he may have been one of the many artists patronized by Vincenzo Gonzaga, Duke of Mantua, to whom Tagliacozzi dedicated the work.

There are two issues of *De curtorum chirurgia.* The majority of copies, printed on or-

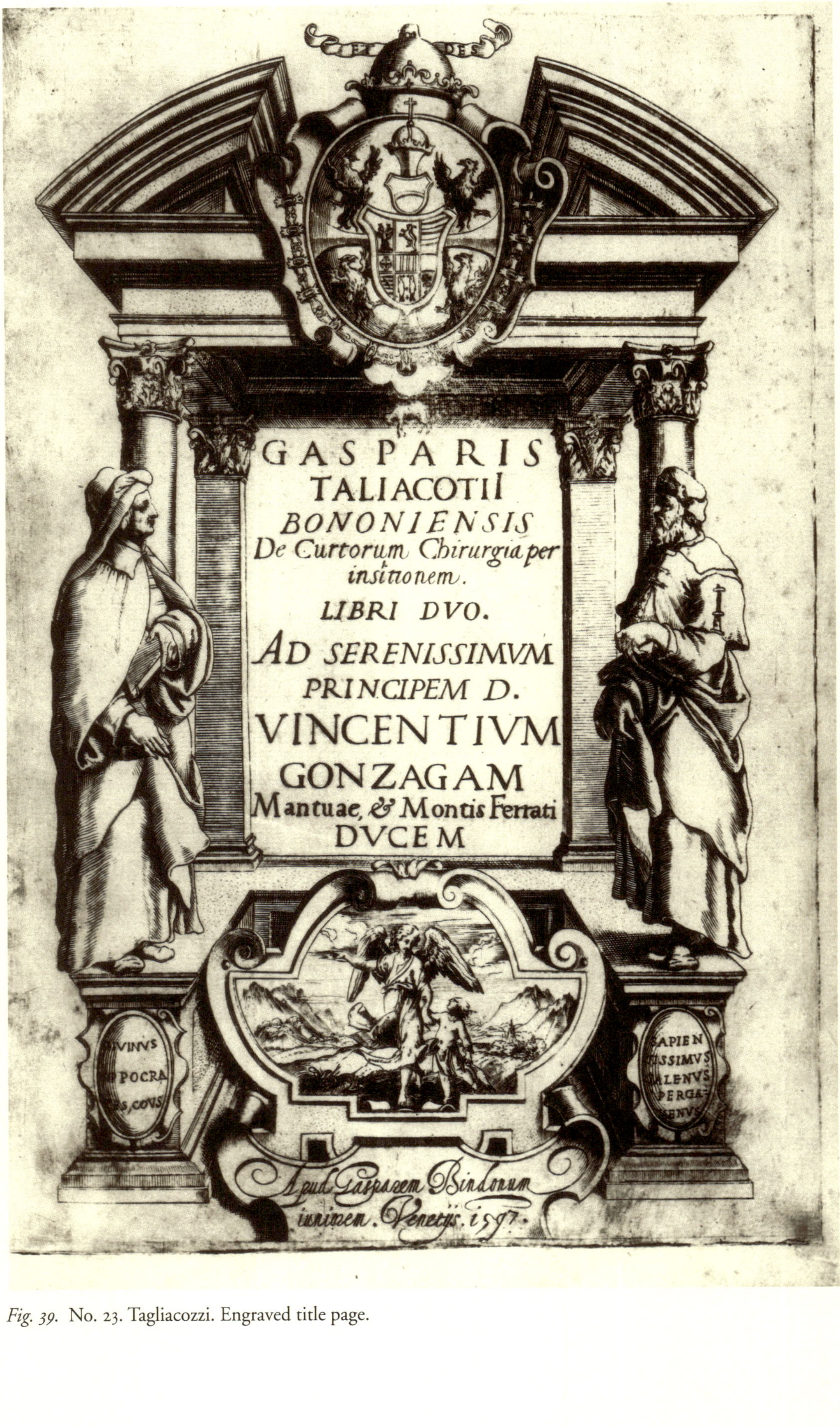

Fig. 39. No. 23. Tagliacozzi. Engraved title page.

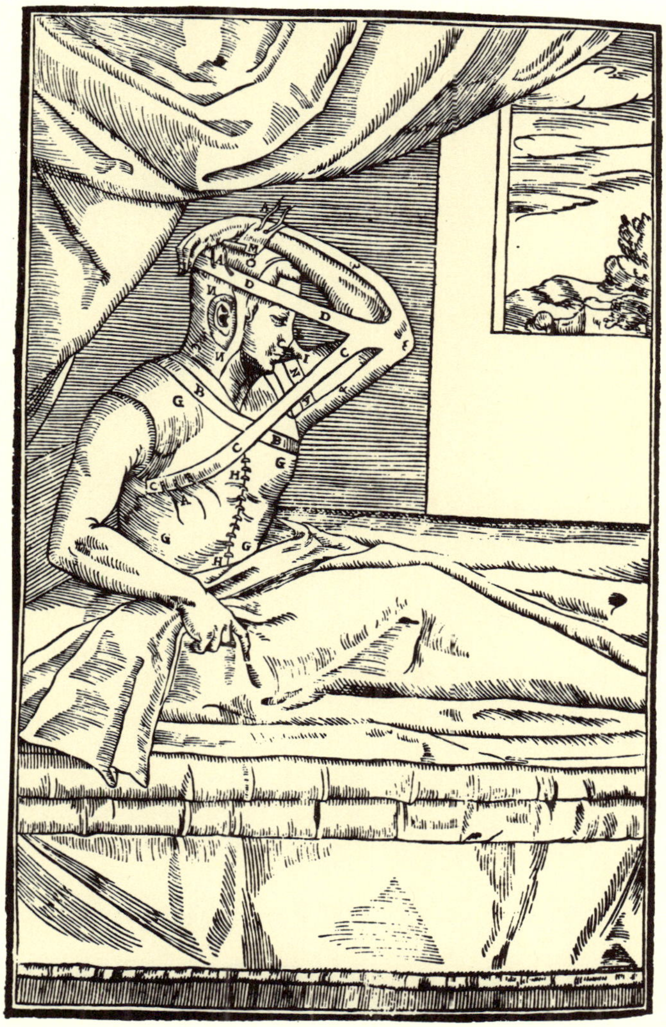

Fig. 40. No. 23. Tagliacozzi. The "Italian" operation for rhinoplasty.

dinary paper, have an imprimatur on the verso of the title page. Other copies, which lack the imprimatur, are printed on large and thick paper that can be distinguished by its watermarks. These copies were undoubtedly intended as presentation copies.[3] A pirated edition was issued by Roberto Meietti in Venice in 1597, the year of the original publication, and the work was reprinted the following year in Frankfurt.

JMN

1. The term "plastic surgery" was coined by Eduard Zeis in his *Handbuch der plastischen Chirurgie* (Berlin, 1838).

2. Reprinted in Martha Teach Gnudi and Jerome Pierce Webster, *The Life and Times of Gaspare Tagliacozzi, Surgeon of Bologna, 1545–1599* (New York, 1950), p. 175.

3. Ibid., pp. 189–90.

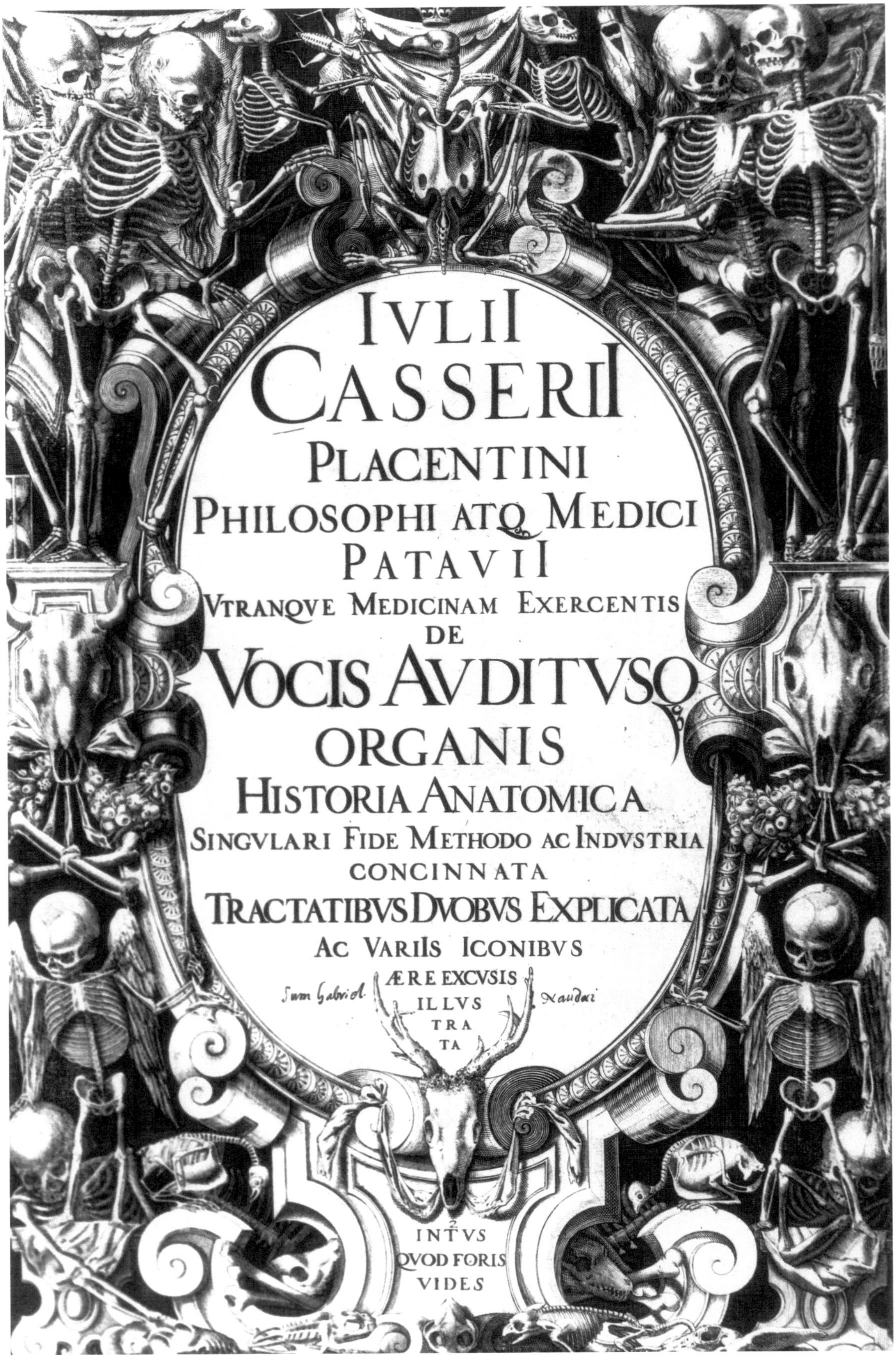

Fig. 41. No. 24. Casserio. This elaborate engraved title, attributed to Jacopo Ligozzi, may be unique in the history of iconography in its use of dissected putti. Gabriel Naudé's signature appears in the lower part of the central cartouche.

24

GIULIO CASSERIO

(ca. 1552–1616)

De vocis auditusque organis historia anatomica singulari fide methodo ac industria concinnata tractatibus duobus explicata ac variis iconibus aere excusis illustrata.

Ferrara: Excudebat Victorius Baldinus, 1601 (colophon, part I); Excudebat Victorius Baldinus, Sumptibus Vnitorum Patavii, 1600 (colophon, part II).

2°: a–b^{6}, a–c^{4} d^{6}, A–Z^{4} Aa^{4}, A–Q^{4}. 190 leaves, pp. [24], [36], 1–191 [1], 1–126 [2]. Engraved title and 2 engraved portraits, conjugate with text leaves; Tab. prima, II–XXII, Tab. prima, II–XII: 34 full-page engraved plates, all printed on rectos or versos of letterpress pages and included in the pagination.

Choulant-Frank, p. 223. GM 286. *Heirs of Hippocrates* 397. Krivatsy 2199. Norman 410. Waller 1809. Wellcome 1333.

Casserio (Casseri, Casserius), sometimes called Placentinus after his birthplace, Piacenza, was outstanding in the field of gross anatomy. A student of Girolamo Fabrici (see no. 27B), Casserio remained under the influence of his teacher, first as his domestic servant, then his secretary, later as an assistant lecturer, and finally as his successor at Padua (the successor died three years before the teacher). Casserio was more a gifted craftsman than a great thinker. His skill in dissecting surpassed Fabrici's, but his detailed descriptions were not as good as those of his teacher.

De vocis auditusque organis consists of two treatises, the first on the vocal organs and the second on the structure of the ear. Each treatise is further divided into three sections: anatomy, function, and physiology. The first book, on the vocal apparatus, contains comparative investigations of the vocal organs of the cicada, grasshopper, and similar insects, as well as the first accurate description of the laryngeal muscles and nerves. The second book, on the structure of the ear, contains the first clear description of the ossicles, comparative studies of the auditory ossicles of various animals, and anatomical descriptions of the inner ear that were far more accurate than any given before, as well as a detailed account of the external ear muscles. Although he made no new discoveries, Casserio's comparative studies of the anatomy of the larynx and of the ear, especially the ossicles and muscles of the middle ear in animals, were probably the first of their kind.

The complete work was published in 1601. A total of thirty-seven copperplate engravings were used to illustrate it, including the engraved title page, a bust of Duke Ranuccio Farnese of Parma (to whom the work was dedicated), a bust of Casserio, twenty-

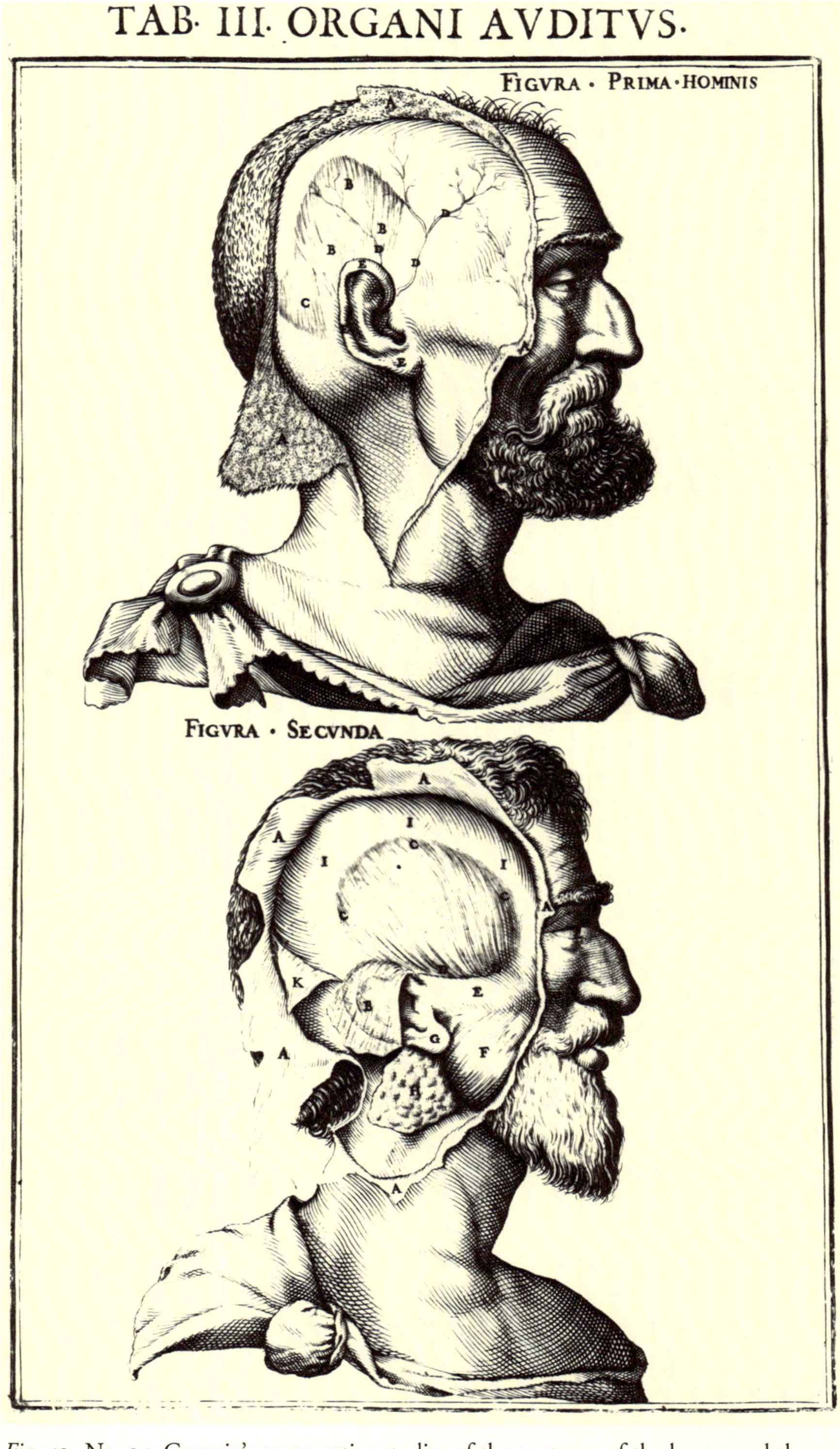

Fig. 42. No. 24. Casserio's comparative studies of the anatomy of the larynx and the ear were probably the first of their kind.

two plates of the vocal organs, and twelve plates of the ear. The engraved title, most recently attributed to Jacopo Ligozzi, may be unique in the history of iconography in its use of dissected putti. An English translation of Casserio's treatise on the larynx, i.e., chapters 1–8 of the first treatise of *De vocis auditusque organis,* was published in 1969.[1]

DGP

1. Giulio Casserio, "The Larynx, Organ of Voice," trans. Malcolm H. Hast and Erling B. Holtsmark, in *Acta oto-laryngologica,* suppl. 261 (Uppsala, 1969).

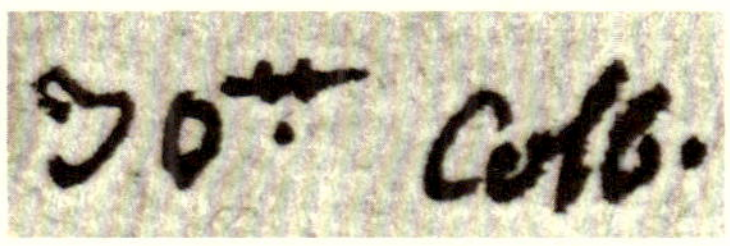

Fig. 43. Jean-Baptiste Colbert's abbreviated signature in his copy of Casserio.

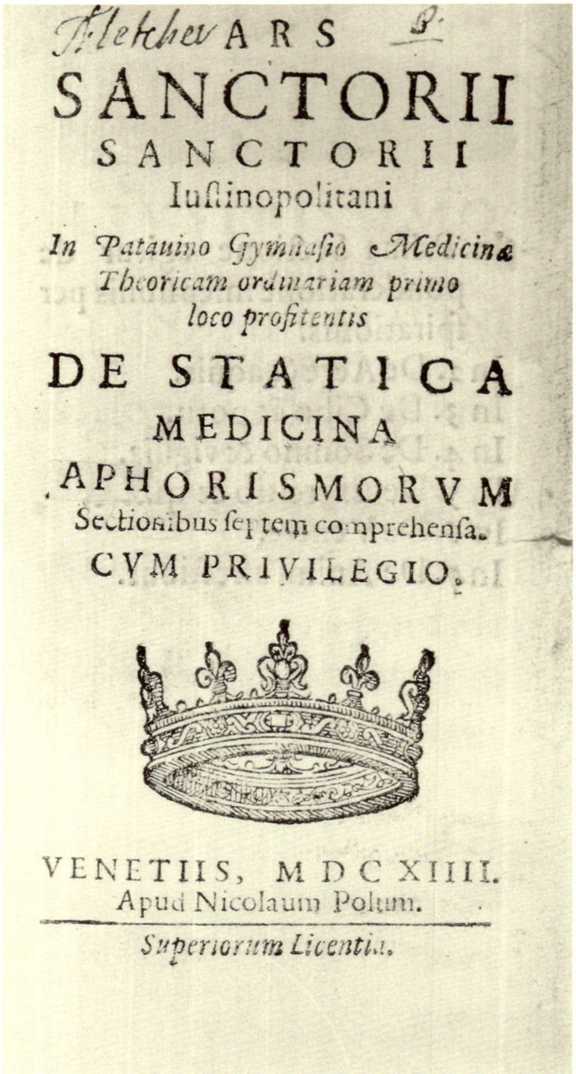

Fletcher ARS
SANCTORII
SANCTORII
Iustinopolitani
In Patauino Gymnasio Medicinæ Theoricam ordinariam primo loco profitentis
DE STATICA
MEDICINA
APHORISMORVM
Sectionibus septem comprehensa.
CVM PRIVILEGIO.

VENETIIS, M D C XIIII.
Apud Nicolaum Polum.

Superiorum Licentia.

Fig. 44. No. 25. Santorio. Title page.

25

SANTORIO SANTORIO
(1561–1636)

Ars Sanctorii Sanctorii . . . de statica medicina aphorismorum sectionibus septem comprehensa.

Venice: Apud Nicolaum Polum, 1614.

12°: a^{12} A–G^{12}. 96 leaves, ff. [12] 1–84.

GM 573. Norman 1890. Wellcome 5760.

The slow process by which Hippocratic and Galenic medicine was modified and finally abandoned is well illustrated in the career and writings of Santorio. While remaining faithful to many of the key assumptions and doctrines of classical medicine, Santorio nuanced and updated them sufficiently to position physiology within the compass of the new iatrophysics of the seventeenth century.

The son of a Venetian nobleman, Santorio was educated at Padua and later taught there. His family's connections and social standing brought him into close contact with such eminent intellectuals and scientists as Paolo Sarpi, Girolamo Fabrici (see no. 27B), Giambattista della Porta, and Galileo; he even sent the last-named a copy of his most important work, *De statica medicina*, in 1615. Cautious, even conservative, *De statica medicina* nevertheless broke enough new ground to be widely esteemed and praised by contemporaries. In the seventeenth and eighteenth centuries, Santorio was frequently associated with Harvey (see no. 27A) as one of the founders of the new medicine.

Santorio made two related and fundamental contributions to seventeenth-century medicine. He was foremost among physicians of his time in introducing quantitative techniques and experimentation into biology. The "static medicine" Santorio described and developed was essentially Hippocratic and was founded on a conception of health as the proper balance of the bodily humors, health being defined as an equilibrium and pathology as a disequilibrium. In Santorio's view, however, this balance was expressed not only in terms of kind but of degree as well—static medicine therefore required exact methods of detection, description, and measurement of degree with respect to what the body consumes and expels. Part of Santorio's originality here was in verifying his hypothesis that much of what is eliminated by the organism is discharged through the skin and lungs and that the relationship between these and visible excretions is a function of various factors, including age, diet, and activity.

Santorio's other basic contribution was intimately related to the first: the invention of a variety of instruments with which to carry out his program of quantitative medicine. Among the many devices credited to him are a thermometer, a hygrometer, a trocar, and special instruments for measuring the pulse rate and for removing bladder stones. Santorio demonstrated that proper instrumentation is as important to medicine as Galileo had shown it is to physics and astronomy. In so doing, Santorio helped shift the emphasis in medical research from anatomy to physiology, from the description of structure to the documentation of function, process, and change.

Santorio's work was quite popular, going through many editions and translations. The first English translation, by Abiah Cole, was published in 1663. The Leiden edition of 1642 appears to be the first to contain the famous illustration of Santorio's weighing chair, a suspended seat counterbalanced by weights that enabled him to measure the amount of respiration through the skin.

MTR

26

GASPARE ASELLI
(1581–1625)

De lactibus siue lacteis venis quarto vasorum mesaraicorum genere novo inuento . . . dissertatio.

Milan: Apud Ioannem Baptistum Bidellium, 1627.

4°: †4 †4 A–K4 †4. 52 leaves, pp. [16] 1–79 [9]. Engraved title and engraved author portrait by Cesare Bassano, both conjugate with text leaves; Tab. I–IIII: 4 folding chiaroscuro woodcuts printed in black, dark red, and light red.

Choulant-Frank, pp. 240–41. GM 1094. *Heirs of Hippocrates* 453. Krivatsy 446. Norman 76. Osler 1846. Waller 502. Wellcome 6837.

Among the last to continue the preeminent northern Italian traditions of anatomy and physiology, Aselli studied medicine at the University of Padua with Giambattista Carcano Leone, himself a pupil of Gabriele Falloppio. He subsequently obtained a position with the Spanish army in Milan that allowed him sufficient leisure for research. The context in which Aselli studied and experimented was one of considerable intellectual excitement, and although he died young, he was nonetheless able to make some important contributions to the history of medicine.

In 1622, while performing vivisection on a dog, Aselli chanced upon the lacteal vessels, which had gone virtually unnoticed since Galen and Erasistratus reported their documentation by Hippocrates and Aristotle. Aselli's achievement was not only to have "rediscovered" these vessels but to have clarified their nature and function. However, Aselli's *De lactibus siue lacteis venis* is important also as a landmark in the history of anatomical illustration: it may well be the first publication to use colored illustrations in the service of scientific clarity. The four chiaroscuro woodcut charts that accompany the text use color—black, dark red, light red, and the natural white of the paper—to distinguish more precisely the different types of vessels from one another.

Although *De lactibus siue lacteis venis* probably had no influence on Harvey (see no. 27A), its findings were confirmed later in the seventeenth century by such anatomists as Nicolaas Tulp, Guerner Rolfinck, and Johann Vesling. Aselli's work also significantly influenced Jean Pecquet's vascular researches (see no. 28A).

MTR

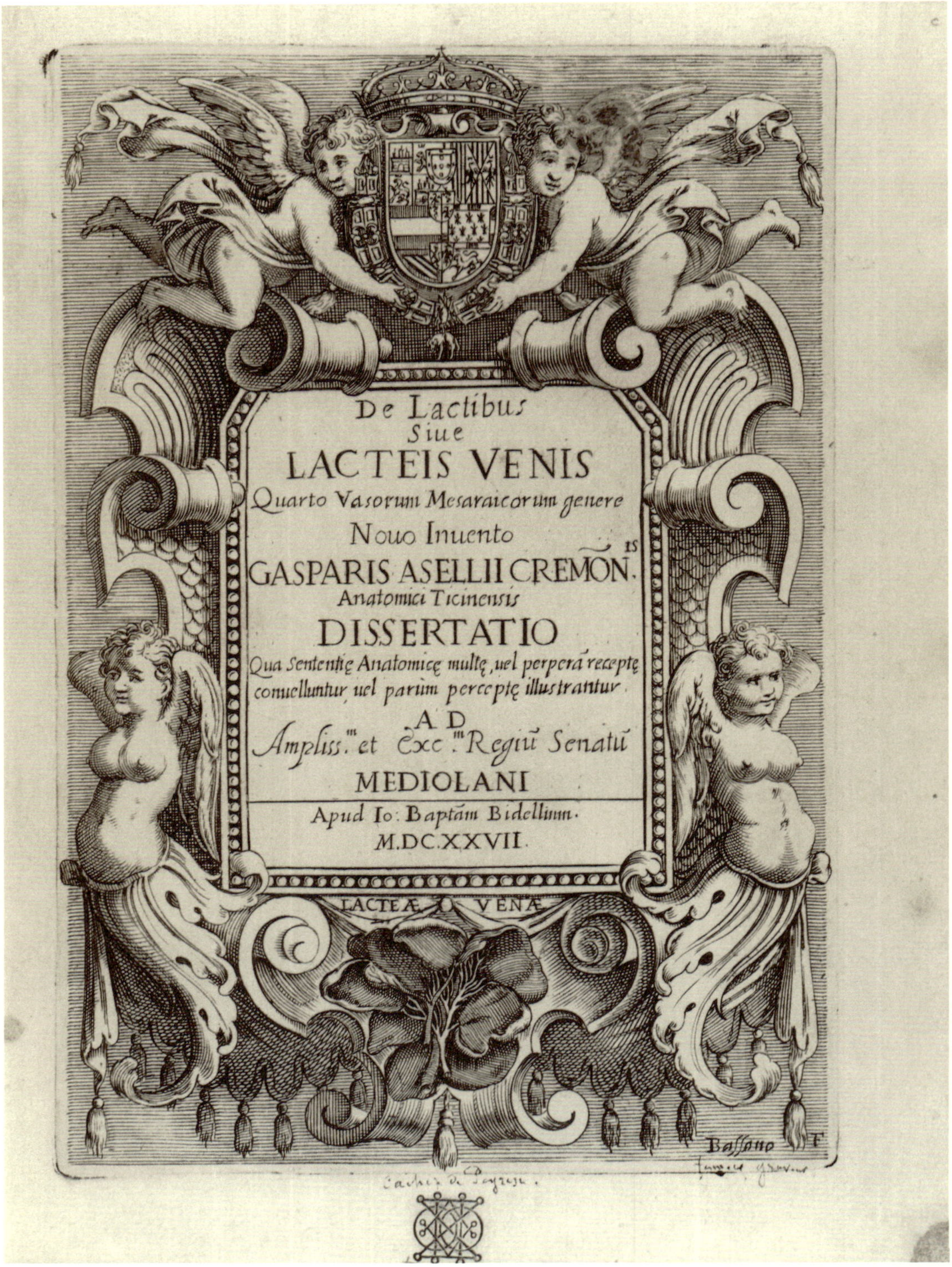
De Lactibus
Siue
LACTEIS VENIS
Quarto Vasorum Mesaraicorum genere
Nouo Inuento
GASPARIS ASELLII CREMONIS
Anatomici Ticinensis
DISSERTATIO
Qua Sententię Anatomicę multę, uel perperā receptę
conuelluntur, uel parūm perceptę illustrantur.
AD
Ampliss.m et Exc.m Regiū Senatū
MEDIOLANI
Apud Io: Baptam Bidellium.
M.DC.XXVII.
LACTEÆ VENÆ
Bassano F

Fig. 45. No. 26. Aselli. The engraved title. The elaborate cipher of Aselli's contemporary, Nicolas-Claude Fabri de Peiresc, who owned this copy, appears at the foot of the page. It is built up from the initials of his name in Greek letters.

The color-printed woodcuts illustrating the first edition of *De lactibus siue lacteis venis* have been attributed to Caesare Bassano, who engraved the title and the portrait of Aselli for this edition and who was also a wood-engraver, or to Bassano's associate Domenico Falcini. Preparatory drawings and proofs for the plates are preserved at the College of Physicians of Philadelphia.[1]

Aselli's work was reprinted in Basel in 1628, in Leiden in 1640, and in Amsterdam in 1645 (the last in Adriaan van de Spiegel's *Opera quae extant omnia*). In all of these later editions, the illustrations were reduced in size and printed in black only from copperplate engravings.

[ED.]

1. Thomas A. Horrocks, "A Selection of Treasures from the Historical Collections of the Library of the College of Physicians of Philadelphia," *Transactions and Studies of the College of Physicians of Philadelphia*, series 5, 9 (1987): 13.

See color plate XXI.

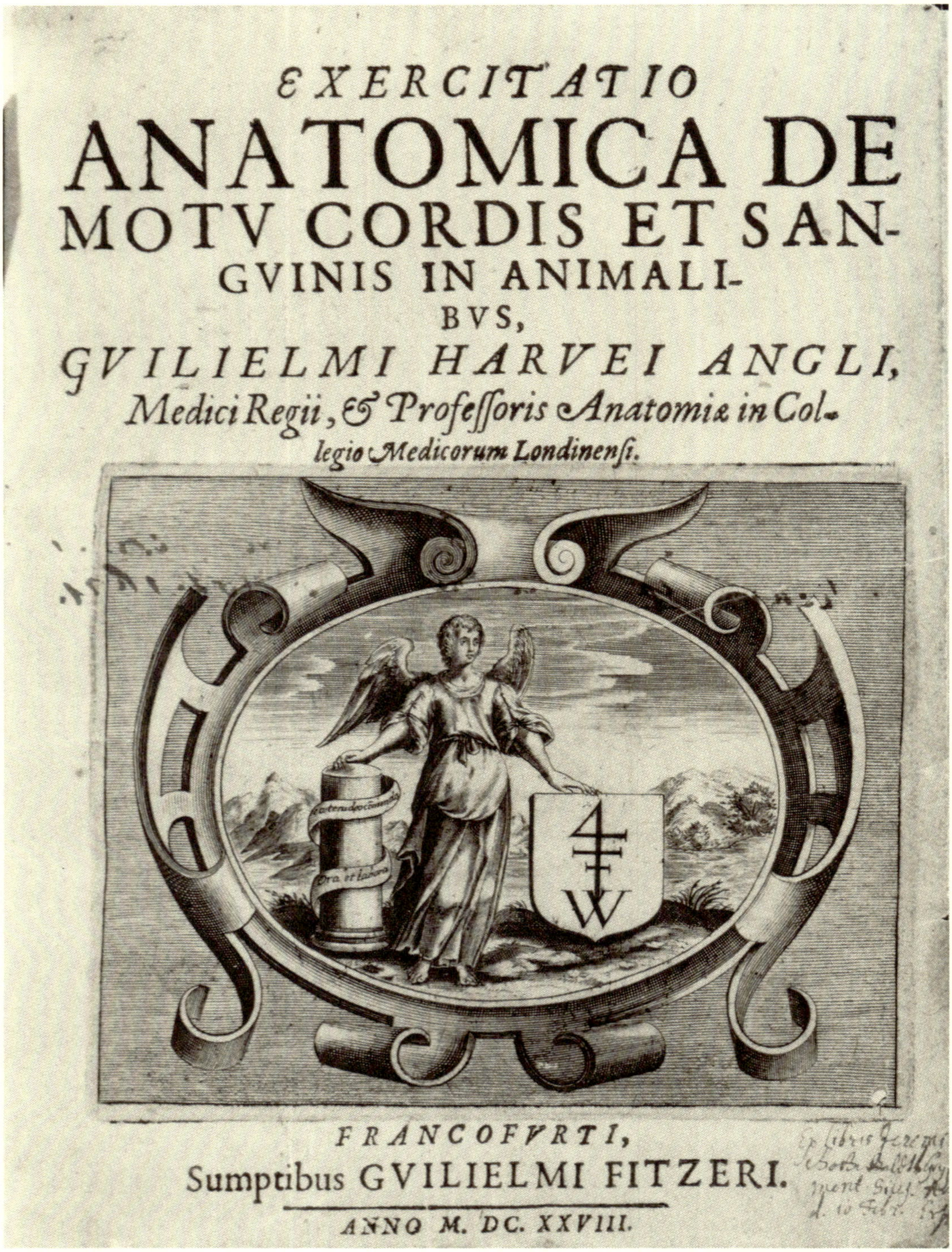
EXERCITATIO
ANATOMICA DE
MOTV CORDIS ET SAN-
GVINIS IN ANIMALI-
BVS,
GVILIELMI HARVEI ANGLI,
Medici Regii, & Professoris Anatomiæ in Col-
legio Medicorum Londinensi.

FRANCOFVRTI,
Sumptibus GVILIELMI FITZERI.
ANNO M. DC. XXVIII.

Fig. 46. No. 27A. Harvey. Title page.

27

WILLIAM HARVEY
(1578–1657)

A] *Exercitatio anatomica de motu cordis et sanguinis in animalibus.*

Frankfurt: Sumptibus Guilielmi Fitzeri, 1628.

4°: A–I4 K2. 38 leaves, pp. *1–2* 3–72 [4]. Engraved title vignette; 2 engraved plates. Quire K, the errata, is not found in all copies.

GM 759. *Heirs of Hippocrates* 416. Horblit 46. Keynes 1. Krivatsy 5328. Norman 1006. Osler 692. PMM 127. Waller 4088. Wellcome 3069.

B] GIROLAMO FABRICI (ca. 1533–1619). *De venarum ostiolis.*

Padua: Ex typographia Laurentij Pasquati, 1603.

2°: π1 A4 B–C2 D4. 13 leaves, pp. [2] 1–23 [1]. Tab. I–VIII: 7 full-page engraved plates and 1 double engraved plate (Tab. II), printed on rectos or versos of letterpress pages.

GM 757. Krivatsy 3831. Norman 750. Waller 2886.

Of all books in the history of medicine, none has interested scholars more than William Harvey's *De motu cordis.* Fielding Garrison claimed that Harvey's "work has exerted a profounder influence upon modern medicine than that of any other man save Vesalius."[1]

Born in Folkestone, Kent, England, in 1578, Harvey studied at Cambridge and at the University of Padua in Italy, where he was a pupil of Girolamo Fabrici. He began practicing in London in 1602. Harvey's pioneering physiological observations, gathered from dissections and animal experiments, were first reflected in his Lumleian lectures at the Royal College of Physicians of London in 1616; these included a summary of his early thoughts on the movements of the heart and blood. Harvey continued his researches and in 1628 published *De motu cordis,* which included his revolutionary theory of the circulation of the blood.

The most significant and certainly the most famous of Harvey's observations was his claim that blood moved around the body in a circle—propelled by the heart through the arteries and returning to this central organ through the veins. As important as this single discovery was, however, Harvey's book also has a broader significance as an influential example of the value of the experimental method. It was, in the opinion of the historian H. P. Bayon, "the first record of a complete biological investigation" in which a problem was defined, methods to solve it expounded, and the results reported.[2]

Although Galen's teachings had come under increasing scrutiny during the Renaissance, his influence still remained strong nearly fifteen hundred years after his death. Harvey's explanation of the circulation rejected Galen's views on the motion of the blood; it is not surprising, therefore, that Harvey's theory was not immediately embraced by his contemporaries. Indeed, for several years after the publication of *De motu cordis* he confronted verbal challenges, printed refutations, and a dramatic decline in his medical practice. By his death in 1657, however, Harvey's contemporaries generally acknowledged the correctness of his theory and its significance.

Harvey's book, a small quarto of seventy-two pages, was published in Frankfurt, the center of the European book trade. Almost all copies were printed on thin paper that has become brittle and brown, although Keynes's bibliography of Harvey records five copies printed on fine, thick paper.[3] Fewer than seventy copies of the first edition are known to have survived. The last signature, K, containing the errata, is found in only a few copies and can be assumed to have been added to only part of the edition.

Girolamo Fabrici was born in Aquapendente, Italy—hence the Latin form of his name, Hieronymus Fabricius ab Aquapendente—and received his medical degree from the University of Padua. A pupil of the gifted anatomist Falloppio, who himself had studied under Vesalius, Fabrici taught anatomy and surgery at Padua after his mentor's death. A prolific author, he published many works detailing his discoveries and observations, including two treatises on embryology and two on the anatomy of the speech organs. His best-known and most important medical work is his classic monograph on the venous valves, *De venarum ostiolis*, published in Padua in 1603 and reissued with four other works in 1625 under the general title *Opera anatomica*. This tract, published originally as an unbound folio pamphlet consisting of twenty-three pages of text and eight engraved plates, has been described as one of the rarest and most beautiful works in the history of anatomical illustration.[4] Among its plates is the well-known depiction of the surface anatomy of the veins of the forearm that William Harvey adapted to illustrate his *De motu cordis*. Although Fabrici did not fully appreciate the functional significance of the venous valves, his work was a crucial precursor of Harvey's discovery. As Harvey told the British physicist and chemist Robert Boyle, it was his recognition of the significance of Fabrici's observations and his own realization of the function of the venous valves that led him to conceptualize the circulation of the blood.

WBF

Fabrici had several of his early treatises—*De locutione* (1603), *De brutorum loquela* (1603), and *De formato foetu* (1604)—published in the same sumptuous format as *De venarum ostiolis*, according to a plan he announced in the dedication of this work to the students of the German nation at the University of Padua:

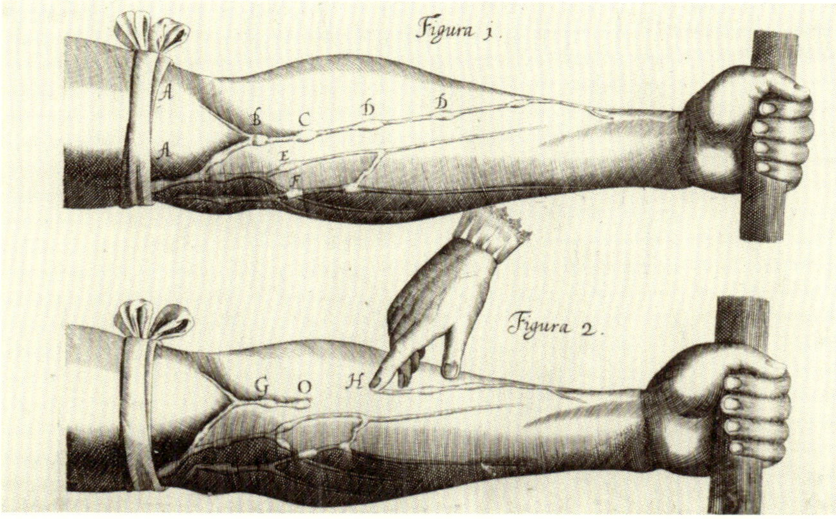

Fig. 47. No. 27A. Harvey. Engraved plate from *De motu cordis*, showing the venous valves.

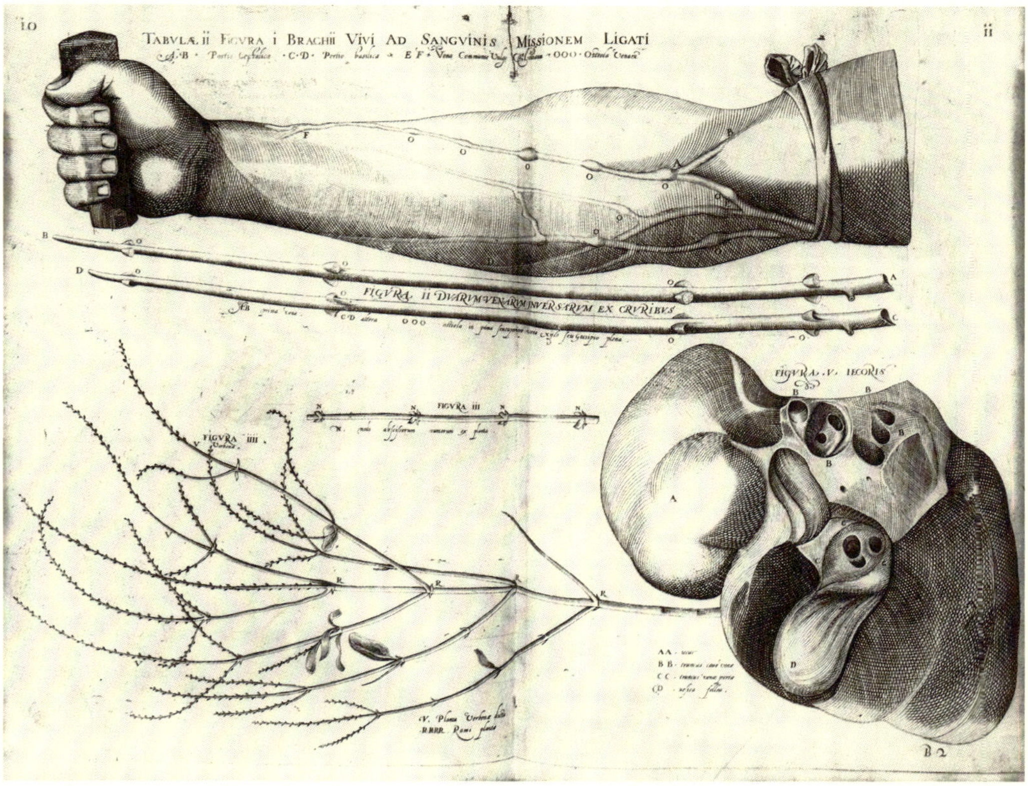

Fig. 48. No. 27B. Fabrici. Engraved plate from *De venarum ostiolis*, showing the venous valves. Harvey adapted this plate for his *De motu cordis*.

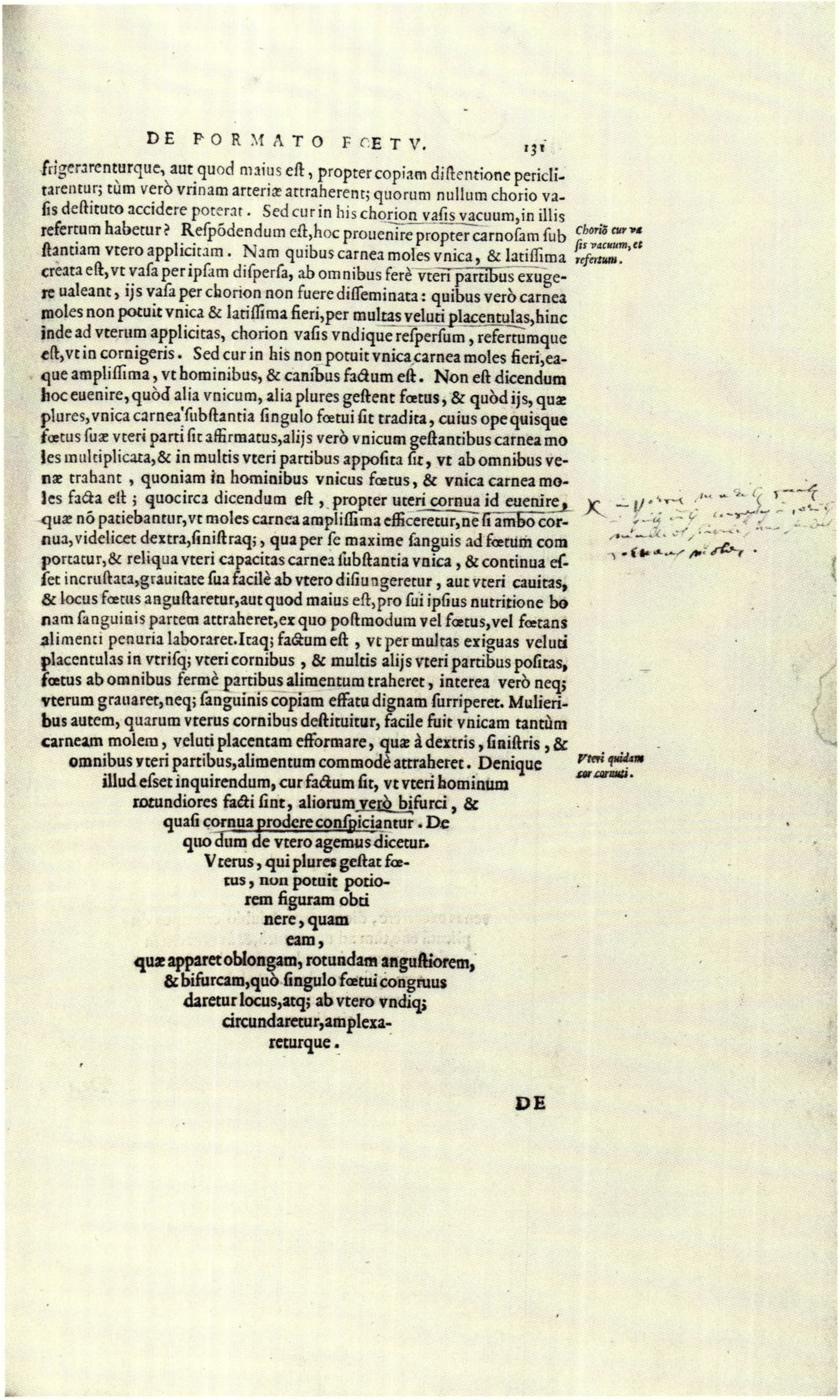

frigerarenturque, aut quod maius est, propter copiam distentione pericli-tarentur; tùm verò vrinam arteriæ attraherent; quorum nullum chorio va-sis destituto accidere poterat. Sed cur in his chorion vasis vacuum, in illis refertum habetur? Respōdendum est, hoc prouenire propter carnosam sub stantiam vtero applicitam. Nam quibus carnea moles vnica, & latissima creata est, vt vasa per ipsam dispersa, ab omnibus ferè vteri partibus exuge-re ualeant, ijs vasa per chorion non fuere disseminata: quibus verò carnea moles non potuit vnica & latissima fieri, per multas veluti placentulas, hinc inde ad vterum applicitas, chorion vasis vndique respersum, refertumque est, vt in cornigeris. Sed cur in his non potuit vnica carnea moles fieri, ea-que amplissima, vt hominibus, & canibus factum est. Non est dicendum hoc euenire, quòd alia vnicum, alia plures gestent fœtus, & quòd ijs, quæ plures, vnica carnea substantia singulo fœtui sit tradita, cuius ope quisque fœtus suæ vteri parti sit affirmatus, alijs verò vnicum gestantibus carnea mo les multiplicata, & in multis vteri partibus apposita sit, vt ab omnibus ve-næ trahant, quoniam in hominibus vnicus fœtus, & vnica carnea mo-les facta est; quocirca dicendum est, propter uteri cornua id euenire, quæ nō patiebantur, vt moles carnea amplissima efficeretur, ne si ambo cor-nua, videlicet dextra, sinistraq;, qua per se maxime sanguis ad fœtum com portatur, & reliqua vteri capacitas carnea substantia vnica, & continua es-set incrustata, grauitate sua facilè ab vtero disiungeretur, aut vteri cauitas, & locus fœtus angustaretur, aut quod maius est, pro sui ipsius nutritione bo nam sanguinis partem attraheret, ex quo postmodum vel fœtus, vel fœtans alimenti penuria laboraret. Itaq; factum est, vt per multas exiguas veluti placentulas in vtrisq; vteri cornibus, & multis alijs vteri partibus positas, fœtus ab omnibus fermè partibus alimentum traheret, interea verò neq; vterum grauaret, neq; sanguinis copiam effatu dignam surriperet. Mulieri-bus autem, quarum vterus cornibus destituitur, facile fuit vnicam tantùm carneam molem, veluti placentam efformare, quæ à dextris, sinistris, & omnibus vteri partibus, alimentum commodè attraheret. Denique illud esset inquirendum, cur factum sit, vt vteri hominum rotundiores facti sint, aliorum verò bifurci, & quasi cornua prodere conspiciantur. De quo dum de vtero agemus dicetur.

Choriō cur va sis vacuum, et refertum.

Vteri quidam cor cornuti.

Vterus, qui plures gestat fœtus, non potuit potiorem figuram obtinere, quam eam, quæ apparet oblongam, rotundam angustiorem, & bifurcam, quò singulo fœtui congruus daretur locus, atq; ab vtero vndiq; circundaretur, amplexareturque.

DE

Fig. 49. No. 27B. Harvey's copy of Fabrici's *Opera anatomica* (1625), with his annotations. This volume includes Fabrici's *De venarum ostiolis* (1603), which contained his observations on the venous valves. Harvey's recognition of the significance of Fabrici's observations on the venous valves was a prerequisite for his discovery of the circulation of the blood.

> I have also made it so that you, who await most eagerly of all these anatomical works of mine, may also be the first to learn that this pamphlet is that which shows the printer both the size of the page and the type of print of all the remaining pamphlets, and of that large work, which we are compiling on the structure of the animal as a whole. From this form no departure is allowed. The remaining pamphlets will be printed to this pattern, and thus young students, who have procured these pamphlets one by one on publication, and have arranged them in orderly sequence, will be able finally to put them all into one volume and bind them properly together without any unnecessary loss of text or money.

After Fabrici's death his treatise *De formatione ovi et pulli* (1621) was published with a type page of the same size but on different paper, and some of the earlier works may have been reprinted. Then in 1625 combinations of these pamphlets were brought together and published in Padua by Antonio Meglietti, who entitled his collection *Opera anatomica*, and by Roberto Meglietti, who called his *Opera physica anatomica.* Copies of these collections, of which Antonio Meglietti's is more common, vary as to whether the parts have individual title pages, whether the general title page lists *De venarum ostiolis* among the contents, and whether this treatise is actually present in the volume.[5] In general, it appears that only a limited number of copies of *De venarum ostiolis* were available for reissue in 1625, and this suggests that those copies found in the collected editions of 1625 were remainders from the original printing of 1603.

[ED.]

1. Fielding H. Garrison, *An Introduction to the History of Medicine*, 4th ed. (Philadelphia, 1929), p. 246.
2. H. P. Bayon, "William Harvey, Physician and Biologist: His Precursors, Opponents and Successors," *Annals of Science* 3 (1938): 62.
3. Geoffrey Keynes, *A Bibliography of the Writings of Dr. William Harvey 1578–1657*, 3d ed., revised by Gweneth Whitteridge and Christine English (Winchester, 1989), pp. 30–35.
4. K. J. Franklin, ed., *De venarum ostiolis 1603 of Hieronymus Fabricius of Aquapendente (1533?–1619)* (Springfield, Ill., 1933), p. 33.
5. Ibid., pp. 31–36; Howard B. Adelmann, ed., *The Embryological Treatises of Hieronymus Fabricius of Aquapendente* (Ithaca, 1942), pp. 122–27.

IOANNIS

PECQVETI

DIEPÆI

EXPERIMENTA NOVA

ANATOMICA,

QVIBVS INCOGNITVM HACTENVS Chyli RECEPTACULUM, & ab eo per Thoracem in ramos usque Subclavios VASA LACTEA deteguntur.

EIVSDEM

DISSERTATIO ANATOMICA DE CIRCVLATIONE SANGVINIS, ET CHYLI MOTU.

Accedunt Clarissimorum Virorum perelegantes ad Authorem Epistolæ.

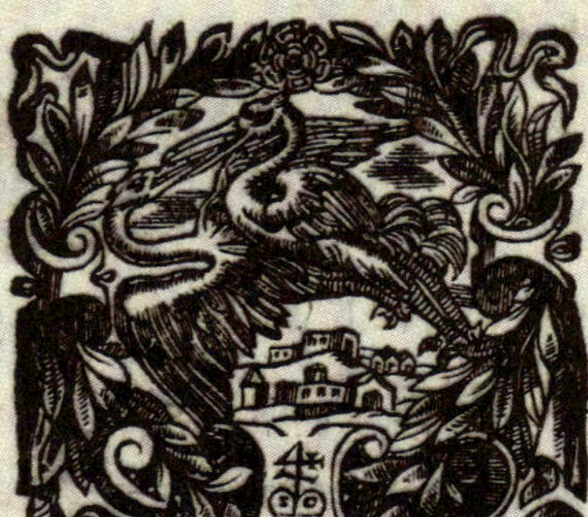

PARISIIS,

Apud { SEBASTIANVM CRAMOISY, Regis & Reginæ Regentis Architypographum, ET GABRIELEM CRAMOISY. } viâ Iacobæâ, sub Ciconiis.

M. DC. LI.

CVM PRIVILEGIO REGIS.

Fig. 50. No. 28A. Pecquet. Title page.

28

JEAN PECQUET
(1622–1674)

A] *Experimenta nova anatomica, quibus incognitum hactenus chyli receptaculum, & ab eo per thoracem in ramos usque subclavios vasa lactea deteguntur . . . Dissertatio anatomica de circulatione sanguinis, et chyli motu.*

Paris: Apud Sebastianum Cramoisy, et Gabrielem Cramoisy, 1651.

4°: ā^4 ē^2 A–N^4 O^2. 60 leaves, pp. [12] 1–108. 1 full-page engraved illustration in text; 5 smaller engraved figures in text.

GM 1095. *Heirs of Hippocrates* 543. Krivatsy 8757. Norman 1676. Waller 7278.

B] THOMAS BARTHOLIN (1616–1680). *Vasa lymphatica, nuper Hafniae in animantibus inventa, et hepatis exsequiae.*

Copenhagen: Sumptibus Georgii Holst, Typis Petri Hakii, 1653.

4°: π–2π^2 A–G^4 H^2. 34 leaves, pp. [8] *1* 2–58 [2]. 1 engraved illustration, conjugate with letterpress "Figurae explicatio."

GM 1097. Waller 750. Wellcome II, p. 107.

C] OLOF RUDBECK (1630–1702). *Nova exercitatio anatomica, exhibens ductus hepaticos aquosos, & vasa glandularum serosa, nunc primum inventa, aeneisque figuris delineata.*

Västerås: Excudebat Eucharius Lauringerus, 1653.

4°: A–F^4. 24 leaves. Tab. I–II: 2 engraved plates after drawings by Rudbeck, the first signed "sculpsit Magn. Celsius."

GM 1098. Norman 1855. Waller 8283.

Bartholin, Pecquet, and Rudbeck matured professionally in a scientific world that had been transformed decisively by Harvey's work on the circulation of the blood (see no. 27A). Harvey's discoveries defined the preferred directions of research for anatomists and physiologists beginning their careers in the mid-seventeenth century, and it is no accident that those who chose to follow his lead cultivated similar fields and eventually made overlapping discoveries. Thus Bartholin in Denmark, Pecquet in France, and Rudbeck in

Sweden are linked both by the common nature of their research in lymphatics and by the similarity of the conclusions—independently arrived at—they were able to draw from that research. Whether Pecquet or Rudbeck first identified the thoracic duct, or whether Bartholin or Rudbeck first described the lymphatic system, is finally less important than the testimony these disputes over priority give to the broader consensus across Europe as to the nature and direction of anatomical and physiological research after Harvey.

Of these three men, Rudbeck was the youngest and probably the most versatile. His work relates to that of both Pecquet and Bartholin. Conducting his research in relative isolation at the University of Uppsala, the precocious Rudbeck carried out a series of dissections and vivisections between 1650 and 1652 that led him to discover, first, the thoracic duct, through which the liver transmits chyle to the veins, and then the lymphatic system itself. His *Nova exercitatio anatomica* (1653) brought him to the attention of the wider community of doctors and scientists in Europe, among whom was a colleague to the south, at the University of Copenhagen, Thomas Bartholin.

The oldest and most accomplished scientist of the three, Bartholin was a member of a family famous for gifted savants. After a peripatetic education that took him to Leiden, Paris, Montpellier, Padua, and Basel over the course of a decade, Bartholin was given the chair in anatomy at Copenhagen. There he too confirmed the existence of the thoracic duct, and through a series of dissections, identified the human lymphatic system at about the same time as did Rudbeck. Like Rudbeck's *Nova exercitatio*, Bartholin's *Vasa lymphatica* appeared in 1653 and occasioned an ultimately unresolvable dispute over who "really discovered" the lymphatic system.

Pecquet's contribution to the field was more limited but no less important. A protégé of the powerful Fouquet family in Paris, Pecquet studied medicine at Montpellier at mid-century, the same time when Bartholin and Rudbeck were conducting their own researches. However, Pecquet's truly important work appears to have been done previously and announced in his *Experimenta nova anatomica* (1651). In Paris, he had worked with a small group of Harveyites at the Jardin du Roi, since Harvey's theories had been rejected at the University of Paris, and there his vivisections of dogs allowed him to observe the process of digestion and ultimately to identify the thoracic duct.

Behind the indisputably important work of Pecquet, Bartholin, and Rudbeck stand not only the epochal revelations of Harvey but also the discoveries of Gaspare Aselli (see no. 26), Francis Glisson (see no. 29), Johann Vesling, and others, which cumulatively defined the nature and functioning of the lymphatic system and laid the foundations of the new science of human anatomy and physiology.

MTR

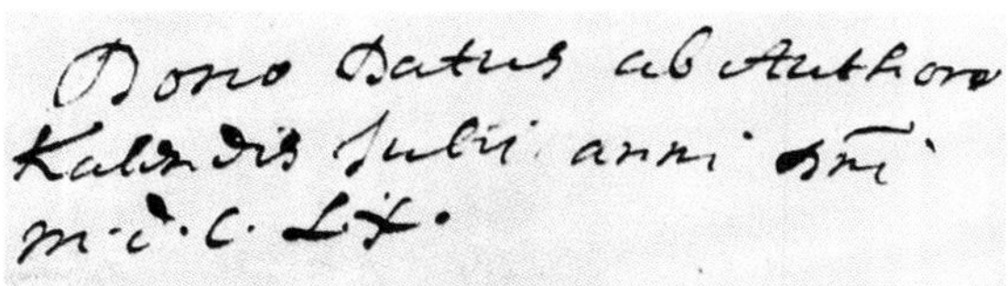

Fig. 51. No. 28A. Pecquet. Presentation inscription.

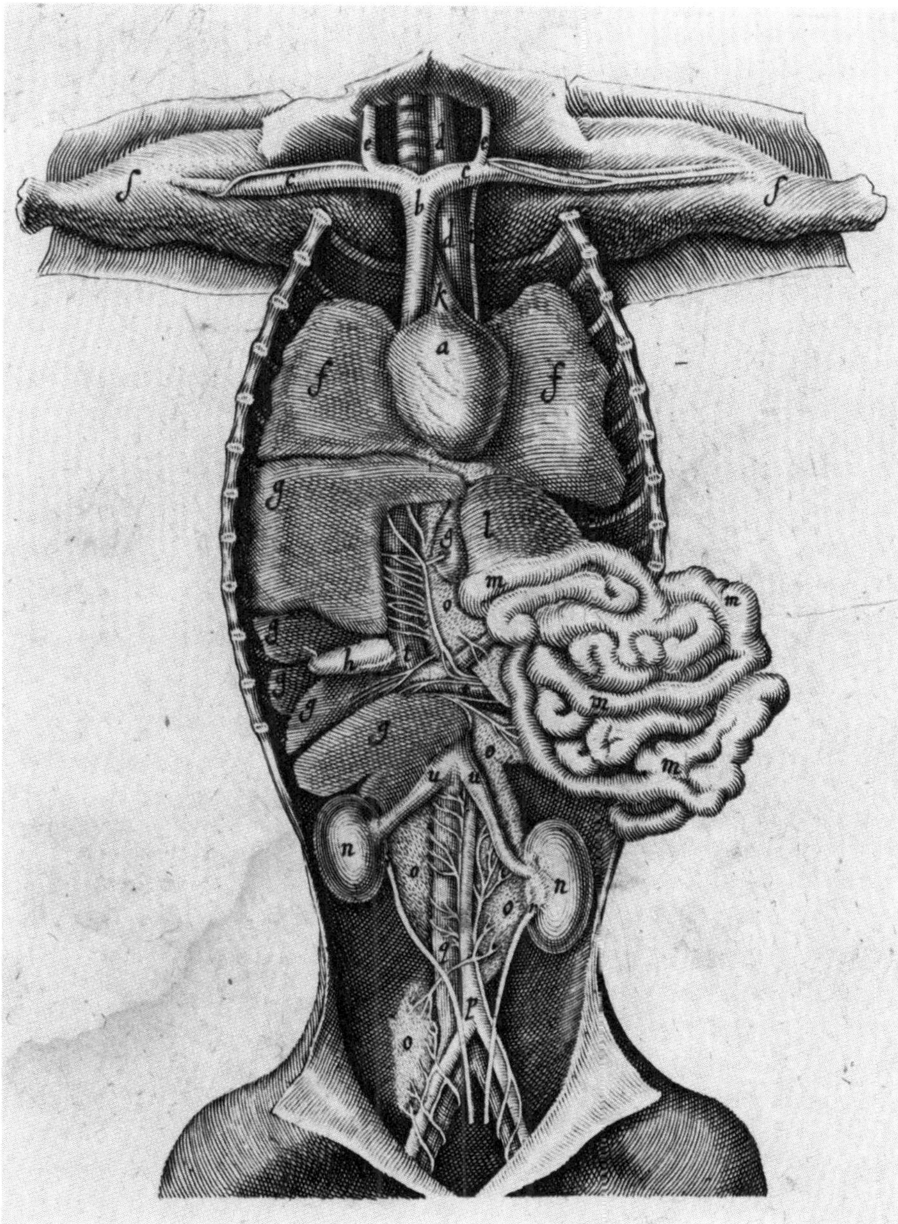

Fig. 52. No. 28B. Bartholin. Engraved plate from *Vasa lymphatica.*

FRANCISCI GLISSONII

In Inclyta

Cantabrigiæ Academia

Medicinæ Professoris publici,

& Collegii *Londinensis* Socii,

ANATOMIA HEPATIS.

Cui præmittuntur

Quædam ad rem Anatomicam

universè spectantia.

ET

Ad calcem Operis subjiciuntur nonnulla de

Lymphæ-ductibus nuper repertis.

Nulla est disciplina, aut ars, quæ singulari consummata sit ingenio. Columella.

LONDINI,

Typis *Du-Gardianis*, Impensis *Octaviani Pullein*, apud quem extant venales. *M.DC.LIV.*

Fig. 53. No. 29. Glisson. Title page.

29

FRANCIS GLISSON
(1597–1677)

Anatomia hepatis. Cui praemittuntur quaedam ad rem anatomicam universe spectantia.

London: Typis Du-Gardianis, Impensis Octaviani Pullein, 1654.

8°: a–c⁸ B–Z⁸ Aa–Gg⁸ Hh⁴. 260 leaves, pp. [48] 1–458 [14]. 2 folding engraved plates; 1 engraved illustration in text; 10 small woodcut illustrations in text.

GM 972. *Heirs of Hippocrates* 472. Krivatsy 4818. Norman 911. Wellcome III, p. 126. Wing G853.

Educated at Cambridge, where he later served as Regius professor of physic, Glisson contributed to the extraordinary ferment in medicine and the life sciences that occurred in the two English universities in the seventeenth century. Like his colleague and friend William Harvey (see no. 27A), Glisson epitomized the English style of biological research: he was theoretically conservative and nondogmatic; and at the same time he was committed to a rigorous program of experimentation, precise observation, and accurate description.

Although connected with Cambridge for most of his life, Glisson made London and the Royal College of Physicians his real professional home. At the college he shared in a community of research interests and projects, the most notable being a pioneering investigation of rickets, a disease believed by many to have been new to England in the seventeenth century. Glisson and his colleagues produced the major treatise on rickets, *De rachitide* (1650), which incorporated Harvey's new theory of the circulation of the blood.

Glisson's classic work on the liver, *Anatomia hepatis*, was based on dissections that he had carried out over a decade earlier. It made fundamental contributions to understanding the physiology of the abdominal organs, in that it delineated the structure and function of the liver, and identified and described the fibrous tissue encasing the liver (Glisson's capsule). It also introduced Glisson's important concept of "irritability," in which he argued that irritation was the organism's way of recognizing substances to be expelled.

Glisson made important and far-reaching contributions to the understanding of the anatomy and physiology of the digestive organs, as well as to the theory and practice of general anatomy. Although presented in a difficult, archaic, scholastic manner, Glisson's works, particularly the *Anatomia hepatis*, remapped and reconceived physiology very much in the spirit of Harvey.

MTR

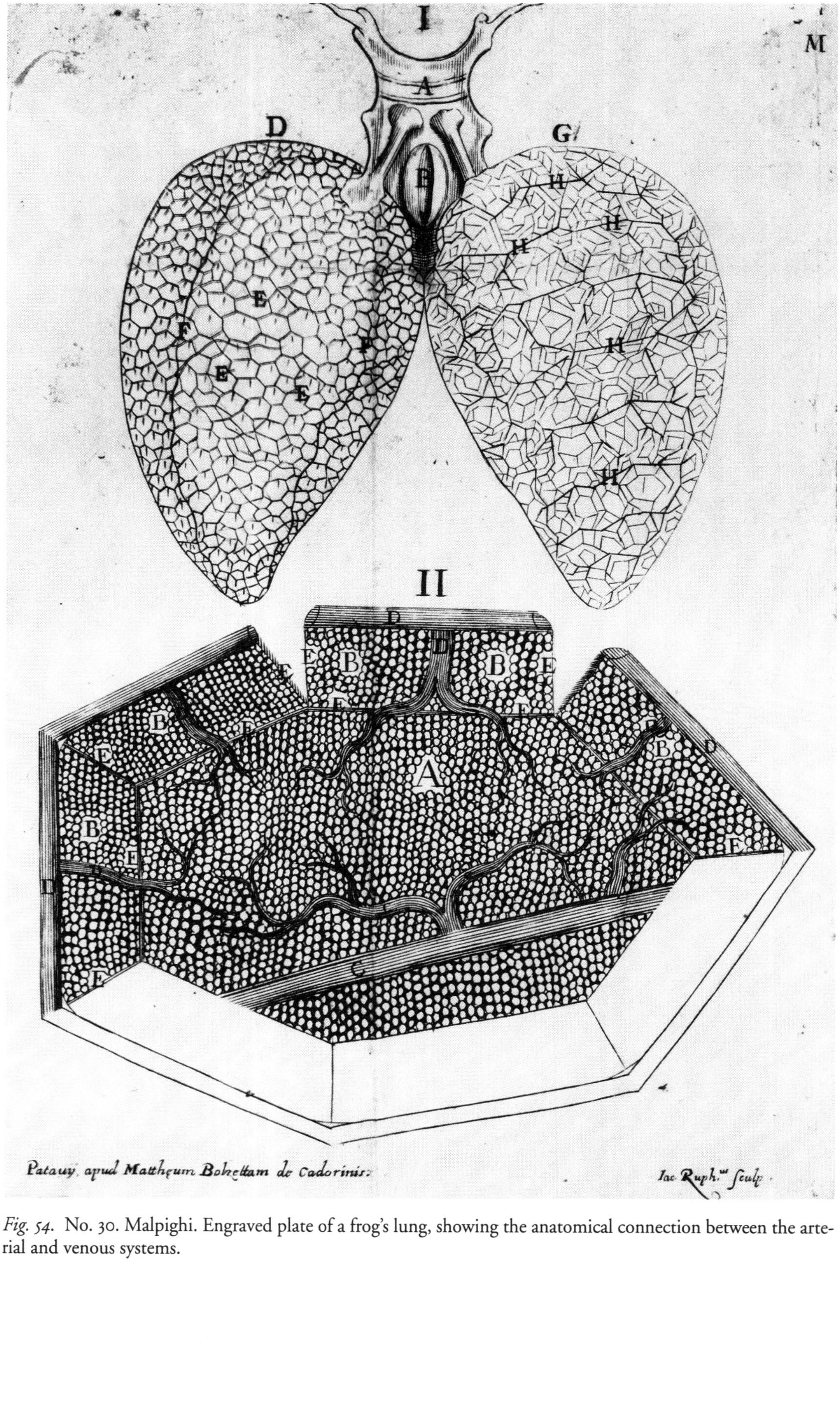

Fig. 54. No. 30. Malpighi. Engraved plate of a frog's lung, showing the anatomical connection between the arterial and venous systems.

30

MARCELLO MALPIGHI
(1628–1694)

A] *De pulmonibus observatio anatomica.*

Bologna, 1661.

8°: A–B⁸. 16 leaves, pp. 1–32. 1 folding engraved plate, signed "Iac. Ruphus sculp."

B] *De pulmonibus observationes anatomicae.*

Bologna: Typis Ioannis Baptistae Ferronij, 1661.

2°: A^8, A^6. 14 leaves, pp. *1–2* 3–14 [2], *1–2* 3–9 [3]. 1 inserted engraved plate; 1 engraving in text.

Frati 10. GM 760. Waller 6197.

Marcello Malpighi was born near Bologna, Italy, in 1628, the year William Harvey published his landmark *De motu cordis* (see no. 27A). Malpighi's greatest scientific contribution was his demonstration, in 1661, of capillary circulation in the lung, which provided the "missing link" in Harvey's theory of the circulation of the blood—an anatomical connection between the arterial and venous circulations.

Malpighi studied at the University of Bologna but was strongly influenced by Giovanni Alfonso Borelli, with whom he taught briefly at the University of Pisa. A pioneering microscopist, Malpighi used this instrument to study the lung, and in the course of his studies he identified the capillary circulation in the expanded lung of a living frog. With the recognition of a vascular passage connecting the arterial and venous circulations, rational opposition to Harvey's theory was no longer possible.

Malpighi informed his friend and mentor Borelli of his discovery of the capillary circulation in the lung in letters published in Bologna in 1661.

WBF

Malpighi's first epistle, in which he argued that the lungs are composed of inflatable membranes, was printed at the urging of Borelli, who acknowledged receipt of a copy in February 1661. It was after this, during further study of the lungs, that Malpighi discovered the capillaries and their function of connecting the arteries and veins, a discovery he announced to Borelli in May 1661. When the letter describing the second discovery was printed at Bologna by Giovanni Battista Ferroni, the text of the first letter was reprinted in the same format. Borelli acknowledged receipt of the two letters on 2 July 1661.

[ED.]

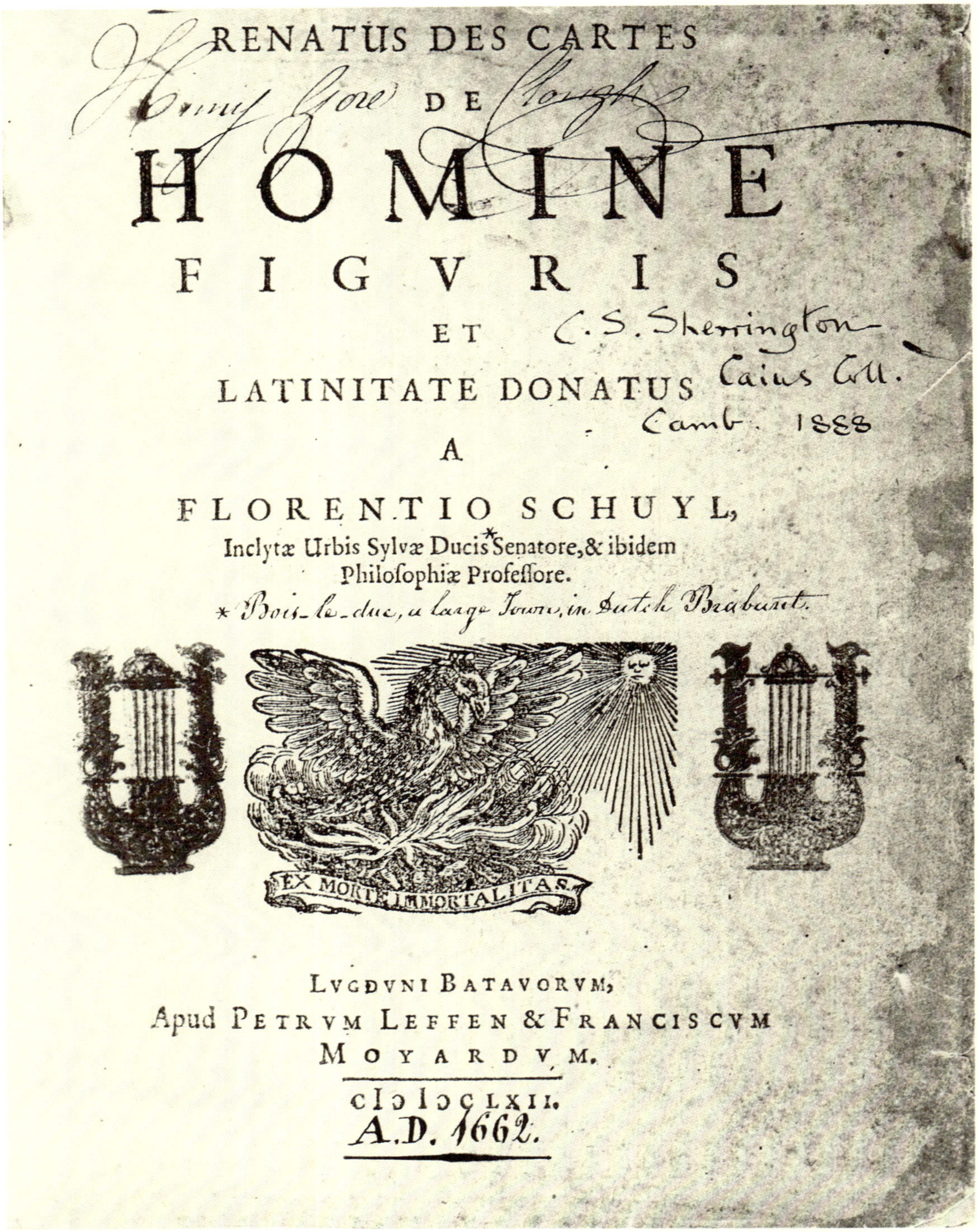

RENATUS DES CARTES

DE

HOMINE

FIGVRIS

ET

LATINITATE DONATUS

A

FLORENTIO SCHUYL,

Inclytæ Urbis Sylvæ Ducis* Senatore, & ibidem
Philosophiæ Professore.

C. S. Sherrington
Caius Coll.
Camb. 1888

* Bois-le-duc, a large Town, in Dutch Brabant.

EX MORTE IMMORTALITAS

LVGDVNI BATAVORVM,
Apud PETRVM LEFFEN & FRANCISCVM MOYARDVM.

CIↃIↃCLXII.
A.D. 1662.

Fig. 55. No. 31. Descartes. Title page.

31

RENÉ DESCARTES
(1596–1650)

De homine figuris et latinitate donatus a Florentio Schuyl.

Leiden: Apud Petrum Leffen & Franciscum Moyardum, 1662.

4°: a–d⁴ e² A–P⁴ Q². 80 leaves, pp. [36] 1–112 111–121 [i.e., 123] [1]. 10 engraved plates, including 2 with lift-up flaps; 33 engravings in text; 23 woodcuts in text.

GM 574. Krivatsy 3120. Norman 627. Osler 931. Wellcome II, p. 453.

Descartes's *De homine* is at once audacious and curiously hesitant—audacious because it stakes out a radically new and bold approach to man and nature; hesitant because it is couched in hypothetical language and presented as a fiction, an innocent thought-experiment. Descartes was by temperament a cautious radical. In the wake of the trial and condemnation of Galileo by the Church in 1633, he was so reluctant to make public his new system of human physiology that *De homine* was issued only posthumously. It first appeared in 1662 in a Latin translation by the Dutch Cartesian Florentius Schuyl. Claude Clerselier, Descartes's literary executor, published the original French manuscript text two years later.

The boldness of *De homine* rests less with its empirical descriptions of the human body than with its philosophical orientation to man as a natural being. It is the first work in the history of science and medicine to construct a unified system of human physiology that presents man as a purely material and mechanical being: man as *machine de terre.* In conceptualizing man as a machine, Descartes helped emancipate the study of human physiology from religious and cultural constraints and validated a clinical and experimental approach to anatomy and physiology.

De homine is an integral part of Descartes's philosophical synthesis. His fundamental concern was to establish the conditions for certain knowledge and so to make the world rationally intelligible. He found in mathematics and geometry paradigms for philosophical thinking and criteria for truth; he saw in mechanism an explanatory model of great power and simplicity. A strict dualist, Descartes divided the world into *res extensa* and *res cogitans. Res extensa,* or extension, comprised the totality of the material world; its sole properties were size, shape, and motion. The atomistic world it constituted behaved like a well-made machine, operating according to rationally comprehensible laws. *Res cogitans,* on the other hand, pertained solely to man as a thinking, spiritual being and had no other

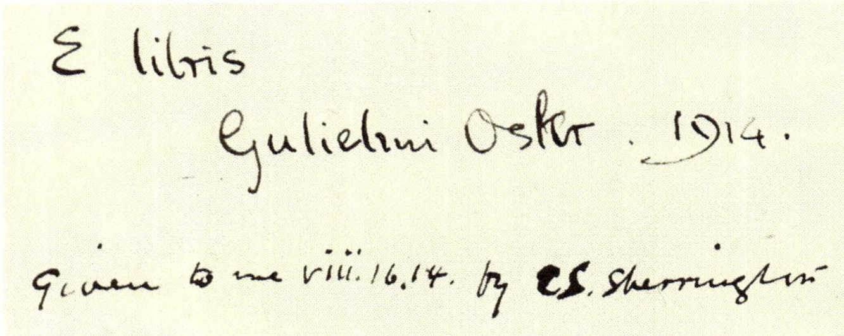

Fig. 56. No. 31. Descartes. The ownership inscriptions of Osler and Sherrington.

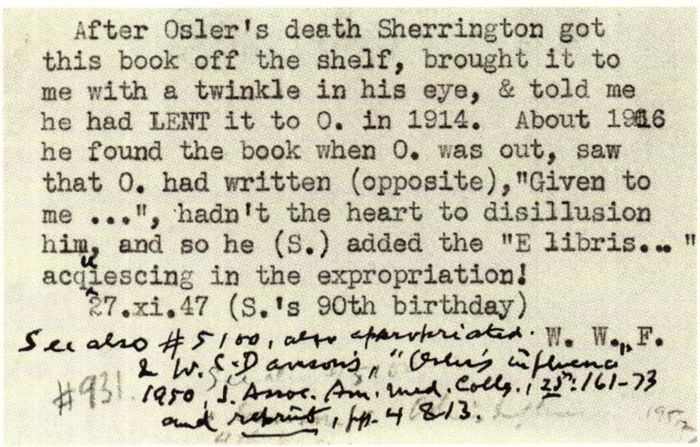

After Osler's death Sherrington got this book off the shelf, brought it to me with a twinkle in his eye, & told me he had LENT it to O. in 1914. About 1916 he found the book when O. was out, saw that O. had written (opposite),"Given to me ...", hadn't the heart to disillusion him, and so he (S.) added the "E libris... " acquiescing in the expropriation!
27.xi.47 (S.'s 90th birthday)
See also #5100, also appropriated. W. W., F.
& W. G. Dawson's, "Osler's influence" 1950, J. Assoc. Am. Med. Colls., 25: 161-73 and reprint, pp. 4 & 13.
#931

Fig. 57. No. 31. Descartes. W. W. Francis's note explaining how this copy came to be in Osler's library.

role, no other locus in the world. Thus, Descartes emptied nature of all vestiges of vitalism and occult forces—life was understandable as extension operating according to natural laws. Man's body, in turn, could be seen simply as extension, and *De homine* described a rationally coherent, though empirically flawed, physiology.

Descartes was not hostile to observation and empirical science—indeed, he performed a substantial number of experiments and dissections in preparation for his treatise—but his physiology remained stubbornly Galenic and Aristotelian. He was attracted, for example, to Harvey's theory of the circulation of the blood (see no. 27A) but not to Harvey's revisionist views on the function of the heart as a pump propelling blood through the body. His descriptions of the brain and the nervous system are characteristic of their time, and his theory of the pineal gland operating as a sort of switchboard in transmitting sensation is reminiscent of the classical *sensorium commune*. The mechanical model served him better when it came to describing and explaining involuntary muscle behavior, and his theory of reflexes represents a significant departure from the past.

In spite of its weaknesses as empirical science, *De homine* had a far-reaching and profound impact as an explanatory system. It helped establish a program for future physiological research, and influential figures such as Thomas Bartholin (see no. 28B), Nicholas Steno, Robert Hooke, Jan Swammerdam, and Giovanni Borelli came under its sway. *De homine* remains important as a model, a fruitful and productive hypothesis. This is, perhaps, what Descartes himself intended.

Descartes's bibliographer A. J. Guibert notes two states of the title page: one with the imprint "Apud Petrum Leffen & Franciscum Moyardum" and a woodcut printer's device of a phoenix rising from the flames, with the motto *Ex morte immortalia*; the other with the names of the publishers reversed and a device showing an angel under a laurel tree, with the motto *Insigne maxime laurus*. He does not establish any priority of issue.[1]

MTR

1. A. J. Guibert, *Bibliographie des oeuvres de René Descartes publiées au XVIIe siècle* (Paris, 1976), pp. 196–98.

CEREBRI ANATOME:

CUI ACCESSIT

NERVORUM DESCRIPTIO

ET USUS.

STUDIO

THOMÆ WILLIS, ex *Æde Chriſti Oxon*. M. D. & in iſta Celeberrima Academia Naturalis Philoſophiæ Profeſſoris *Sidleiani*.

LONDINI,

Typis *Ja. Fleſher*, Impenſis *Jo. Martyn* & *Ja. Alleſtry* apud inſigne Campanæ in Cœmeterio *D. Pauli*. MDCLXIV.

Fig. 58. No. 32A. Willis. Title page of the quarto edition.

32

THOMAS WILLIS
(1621–1675)

A] *Cerebri anatome: cui accessit nervorum descriptio et usus.*

London: Typis Ja. Flesher, Impensis Jo. Martyn & Ja. Allestry, 1664.

4º: A4 a–d4 B–O4 P4 (P1 + 1) Q–Z4 Aa–Zz4 Aaa–Mmm4. 249 leaves, pp. [40] 1–106 [2] 107–456. Fig. I–VI [1] VII–VIII [1], Tab. VIIII–XIII: 15 engraved plates.

GM 1378. *Heirs of Hippocrates* 538. Krivatsy 13009. Norman 2243. Waller 10315. Wing W2824.

B] *Cerebri anatome: cui accessit nervorum descriptio et usus.*

London: Typis Tho. Roycroft, Impensis Jo. Martyn & Ja. Allestry, 1664.

8º: A8 a8 (–a8) B–D8 E8 (E4 + 1 [=a8]) F–Q8. 136 leaves, pp. [30] 1–56 [2] 57–240. Fig. I–VI [1] VII–VIII [1], Tab. VIIII–XIII: 15 engraved plates.

Krivatsy 13010. Osler 4249. Waller 10314. Wing W2823.

Thomas Willis was one of a number of remarkable scientists and doctors who flourished at Oxford in the mid-seventeenth century. Dispersed among the colleges of Oxford, these talented investigators coalesced into a loosely organized "club" or invisible college that helped define and disseminate a new experimental philosophy and that served as the informal prototype of the Royal Society. The legacy of William Harvey (see no. 27A) was crucial to science and medicine in Oxford, and anatomical investigations were central to programs of research in these subjects; as a physician and one of the charter members of the Oxford club, Willis played a leading role in shaping those programs. His *Cerebri anatome* remapped the brain and described the cranial, spinal, and involuntary nervous systems so accurately and thoroughly that it remained the standard work in its field until well into the nineteenth century. Willis himself was probably the first to use the term "neurology."

Of modest origins, Willis enjoyed a highly successful career as a physician. The unyielding Anglicanism and royalist sympathies he maintained during the Civil War and Commonwealth served him well at the Restoration (1660), when he was named Sedleian professor of natural philosophy at Oxford. His lectures on neurology attracted a galaxy of famous auditors, including Robert Hooke, John Locke, Edmund King, Thomas Millington, and Christopher Wren. But he was even better known as a physician. By the time of the publication of *Cerebri anatome* he was thought to be the highest-paid person in the

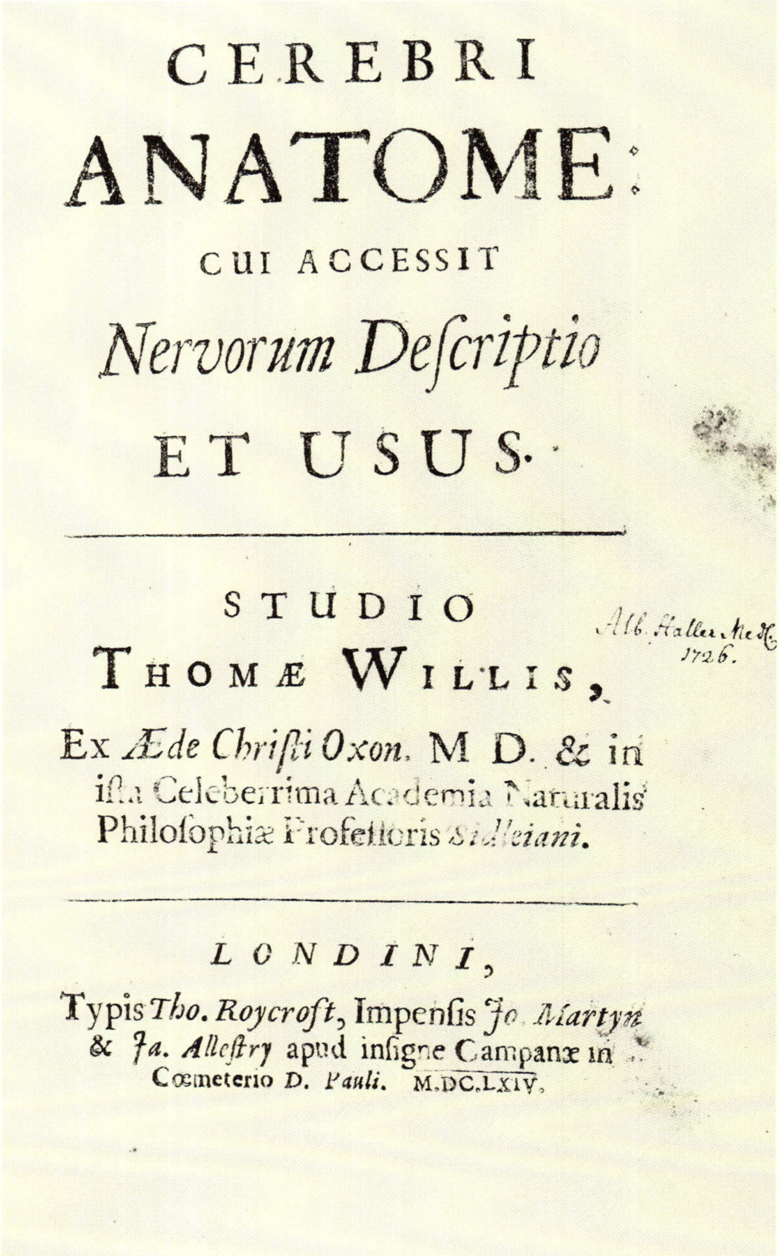
CEREBRI
ANATOME:
CUI ACCESSIT
Nervorum Descriptio
ET USUS.

STUDIO
THOMÆ WILLIS,
Ex *Æde Christi Oxon.* M D. & in
ista Celeberrima Academia Naturalis
Philosophiæ Professoris *Sidleiani.*

LONDINI,
Typis *Tho. Roycroft*, Impensis *Jo. Martyn*
& *Ja. Allestry* apud insigne Campanæ in
Cœmeterio *D. Pauli.* M.DC.LXIV.

Fig. 59. No. 32B. Willis. Title page of the octavo edition. Albrecht von Haller's signature appears in the outer margin.

city of Oxford (at £300 per annum), and in 1667 he moved to London, where he established a large and lucrative medical practice. His contemporary fame sufficed to earn him a final resting place in Westminster Abbey.

Cerebri anatome was the product of two years of intense anatomical investigation by Willis and his collaborator, Richard Lower (see no. 34), during which they performed scores of dissections of fish, birds, and mammals to gain as full a comparative view as possible of the topography and functions of the brain and nervous system. Willis described and classified ten pairs of cranial nerves in considerable detail and undertook to explain their physiological roles. Like most doctors and scientists of his day, Willis believed that the nerves transmitted vitalistic animal spirits throughout the body. He placed the origin of animal spirits in the cerebral and cerebellar cortices and made important contributions to neurology through his observations on the localization of mental functions in the brain. Willis associated voluntary motor action with the corpus striatum or cerebrum and involuntary functions with the cerebellum. His observations on cerebral blood circulation have stood the test of time, and even though he did not really discover the "circle of Willis"—beautifully drawn for these editions by Christopher Wren—his description of the arteries of the brain was fuller and functionally more complete than any before it.

Cerebri anatome joins the mechanistic and corpuscular physiology of René Descartes (see no. 31) and Pierre Gassendi with the new experimentalism of the seventeenth century. While many of its speculations about neurophysiology have been eclipsed, they inspired significant further research. As descriptive anatomy the work remains a singular example of rigor and exactitude.

Cerebri anatome, like many of Willis's works, was published in both quarto and octavo editions, the quarto edition appearing a few weeks before the cheaper octavo edition. The illustrations, which are unsigned, were drawn by Richard Lower and Christopher Wren (whose early achievements as a scientist have been largely eclipsed by his later fame as an architect), and they were probably engraved by David Loggan. The same plates were used for both editions: the copperplates were engraved with the pagination of the quarto edition and this was corrected in manuscript for the octavo publication.

MTR

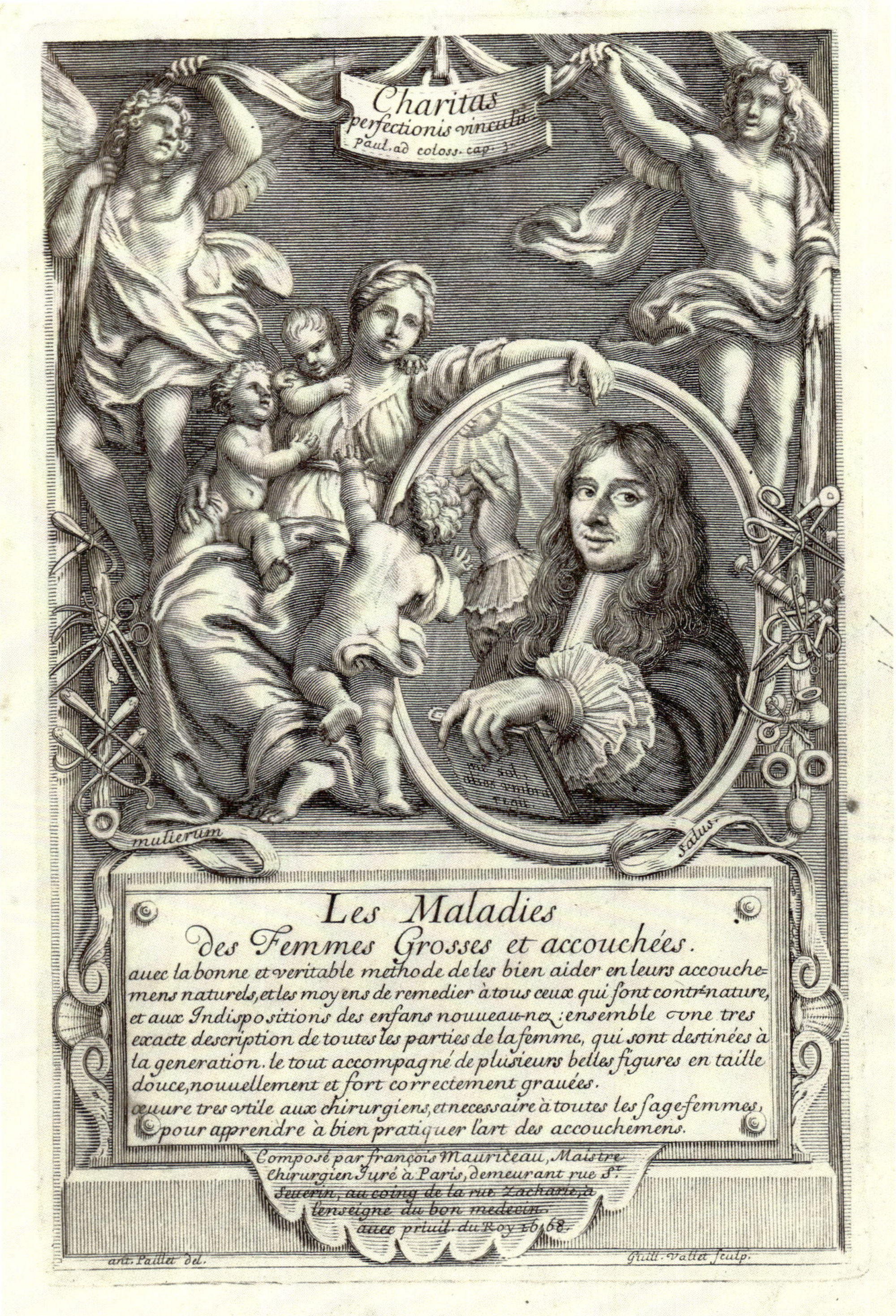
Charitas
perfectionis vinculu
paul. ad coloss. cap. 3
mulierum
salus
Les Maladies
des Femmes Grosses et accouchées.
auec la bonne et veritable methode de les bien aider en leurs accouche-
mens naturels, et les moyens de remedier à tous ceux qui sont contre nature,
et aux Indispositions des enfans nouueau-nez; ensemble vne tres
exacte description de toutes les parties de la femme, qui sont destinées à
la generation. le tout accompagné de plusieurs belles figures en taille
douce, nouuellement et fort correctement grauées.
œuure tres vtile aux chirurgiens, et necessaire à toutes les sage-femmes,
pour apprendre à bien pratiquer l'art des accouchemens.
Composé par françois Mauriceau, Maistre
Chirurgien Iuré à Paris, demeurant rue S.t
Seuerin, au coing de la rue Zacharie, à
lenseigne du bon medecin.
auec priuil. du Roy 1668.
ant. Paillet del.
Guill. Vallet sculp.

Fig. 60. No. 33. Mauriceau. Engraved title page, showing a variant form of the title.

33

FRANÇOIS MAURICEAU
(1637–1709)

Des maladies des femmes grosses et accouchées. Avec la bonne et veritable méthode de les bien aider en leurs accouchemens naturels, & les moyens de remedier à tous ceux qui sont contre-nature, & aux indispositions des enfans nouveau-nés.

Paris: Chez Iean Henault, Iean d'Houry, Robert de Ninville, Iean Baptiste Coignard, 1668.

4°: $\bar{a}^4$ $\bar{e}^4$ $\bar{\imath}^4$ A–Z^4 Aa–Zz^4 AAa–XXx^4. 280 leaves, pp. [24] 1–536. Additional engraved title page by Guillaume Vallet after Antoine Paillet; 30 engraved illustrations in text.

EFDT 107. GM 6147. Krivatsy 7588. Norman 1461.

Perhaps the first obstetric text in the modern sense, Mauriceau's *Maladies des femmes grosses et accouchées* established obstetrics as a science and as a separate medical specialty. Through its various translations, it exercised a dominant influence on seventeenth-century obstetrical practice.

Following the introduction, which describes anatomic landmarks, the work is divided into three sections dealing with diseases and abnormalities from conception to the end of pregnancy, normal childbirth, and the care of the mother and newborn infant, including the choice of a suitable wet nurse. Among the important new ideas presented in Mauriceau's work were the delivery of women in bed rather than in the obstetric chair, treatment of the various gestational periods, and discussions of many difficult cases. He also presented an analysis of the mechanism of labor and maintained that during labor the uterus is the active agent while the fetus plays a passive role. He gave the earliest account of the prevention of congenital syphilis by antisyphilitic treatment during pregnancy. He was also the first to refer to tubal pregnancy, complications of prolapse of the umbilical cord, and epidemic puerperal fever.

Mauriceau practiced podalic version but condemned both cephalic version and cesarean section. He gave rules for the management of placenta previa and advanced the concept of primary repair of perineal lacerations. Mauriceau discredited the observation of Ambroise Paré (see no. 19) and others that the pubic bones separated during childbirth. He also denied that the uterus contains two cavities and that the amniotic fluid is an ac-

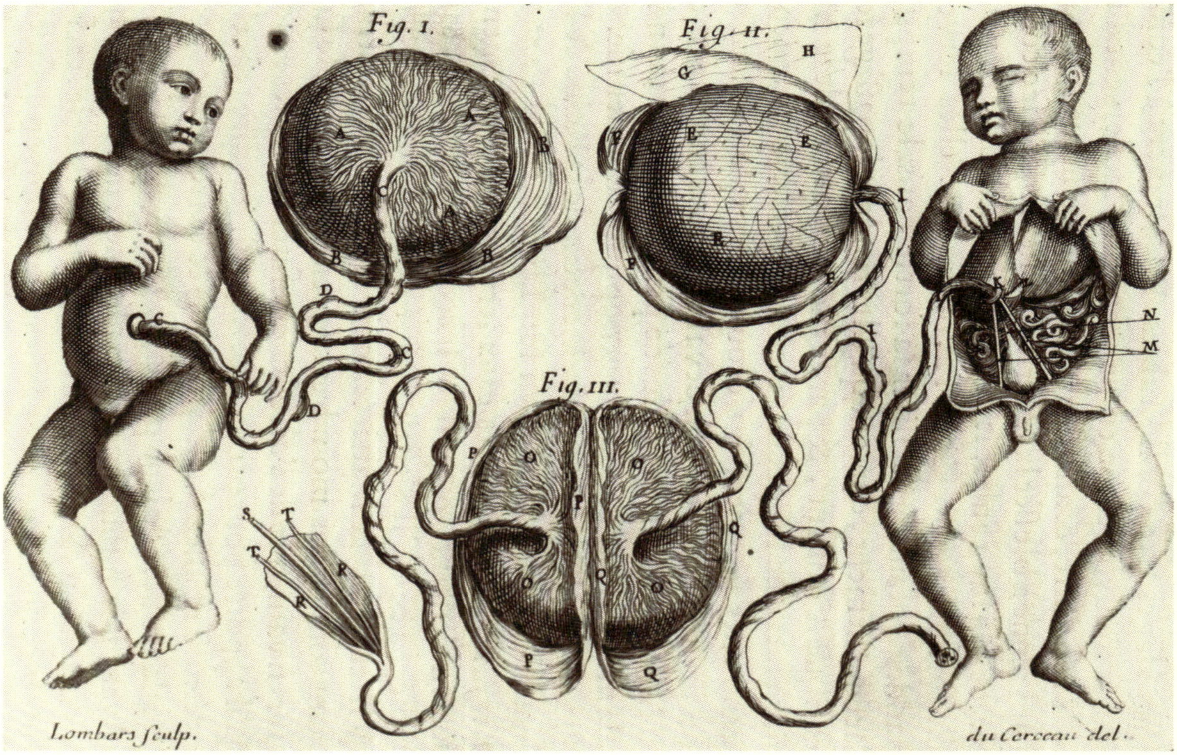

Fig. 61. No. 33. Mauriceau. Engraved plate from *Des maladies des femmes grosses et accouchées*, showing the fetus, placenta, umbilical cord, and uterus.

cumulation of menstrual blood or milk. He argued against the common misconceptions that a child born at seven months' gestation had a greater chance of survival than one born at eight months and that a woman can give birth to only two children at a time because of the presence of two breasts. In the third edition (1681) he first described management of the aftercoming head in breech delivery with the aid of an index finger in the infant's mouth, a technique now called the "Mauriceau-Smellie-Viet" maneuver.

Mauriceau's book went through three more editions in his lifetime (1675, 1681, 1694) and was translated into English (1673), German (1680), Latin (1681; by the author), Dutch (1683), and Italian (1684). The English translation was prepared by Hugh Chamberlen the elder (b. 1630), of the famous Huguenot family that succeeded in maintaining a monopoly on the use of the obstetric forceps for nearly two centuries.

LDL

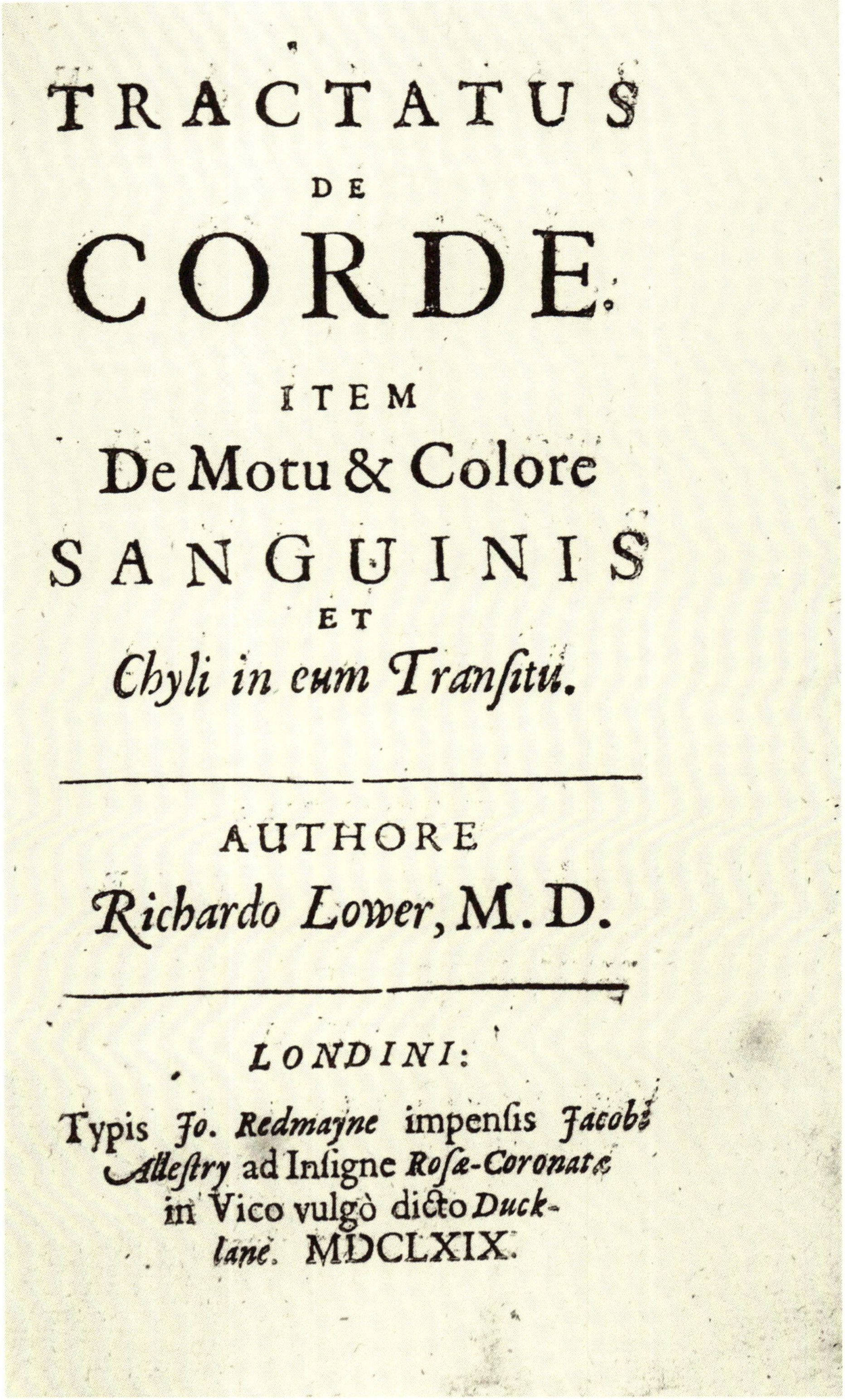

TRACTATUS
DE
CORDE.
ITEM
De Motu & Colore
SANGUINIS
ET
Chyli in eum Transitu.

AUTHORE
Richardo Lower, M.D.

LONDINI:
Typis *Jo. Redmayne* impensis *Jacobi Allestry* ad Insigne *Rosæ-Coronatæ* in Vico vulgò dicto *Duck-lane*. MDCLXIX.

Fig. 62. No. 34. Lower. Title page.

34

RICHARD LOWER
(1631–1691)

Tractatus de corde. Item de motu & colore sanguinis et chyli in eum transitu.

London: Typis Jo. Redmayne impensis Jacobi Allestry, 1669.

8°: A–Q^8. 128 leaves, pp. [16] 1–220 [20]. In some copies, A6 is replaced by a cancellans. Tab. 1–7: 7 folding engraved plates.

Fulton 4. GM 761. Krivatsy 7157. Norman 1397. PMM 149. Waller 6046. Wellcome III, p. 552. Wing L3310.

Lower's *Tractatus de corde* is the most important contribution to circulatory physiology after William Harvey's *De motu cordis* (see no. 27A), published three years before Lower's birth. Nobel laureate André Cournand considered Lower's book to be one of the most important texts in the history of physiology because of the nature of its observations, the rigor of its experimental design and demonstrations, and its simple and convincing form of presentation.

Born into an affluent Cornish family in 1631, Lower received undergraduate and medical degrees from Oxford, where he came under the influence of Thomas Willis (see no. 32), Robert Boyle, and Robert Hooke. Lower entered medical practice in London in 1666 and continued experiments he had begun in Oxford on the motion and color of the blood and on transfusion. His observations on these subjects were summarized in *Tractatus de corde.*

Lower made important observations on the structure of cardiac muscle, the quantity of blood in the vascular system, the velocity of blood flow, and the effects of aeration of blood as it passed through the lungs. He was impressed by the complex arrangement of the muscular fibers in the heart and felt their unique arrangement was responsible for the contraction of the ventricular cavities in systole that propelled blood into the vascular system. In a series of experiments performed with Robert Hooke, Lower showed that the red color of arterial blood was due to its contact with "fresh air" in the lungs. His book also contained observations on the technique and safety of blood transfusion, a technique he pioneered.

Lower's book received praise from British and Continental physicians and scientists and helped establish its author's reputation as the leading investigator, after William Harvey, of the anatomy and physiology of the circulation of the blood. When he died in 1691 Lower was hailed as one of England's greatest contributors to medical science.

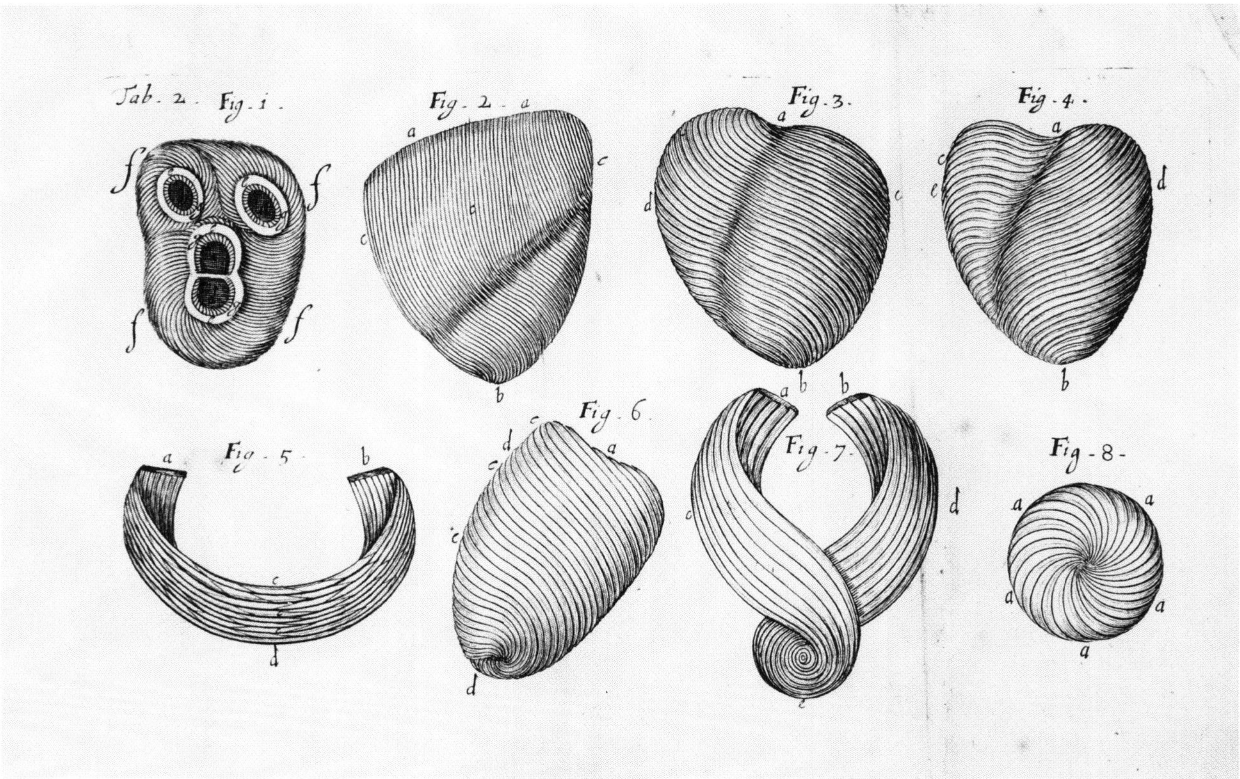

Fig. 63. No. 34. Lower. Engraved plate from *Tractatus de corde,* showing the arrangement of fibers in cardiac muscle.

There are two issues of Lower's book. The first has the original leaf A6, with the catchword "Im-"; in the second the cancellans A6 has the catchword "quic-". The reason for the change, according to John F. Fulton, was "to modify (very slightly) a scurrilous remark that [Lower] had originally made concerning the Irishman O'Meara."[1]

WBF

1. John F. Fulton, *Two Oxford Physiologists: Richard Lower 1631–1691; John Mayow 1643–1679* (Oxford, 1935), p. 17.

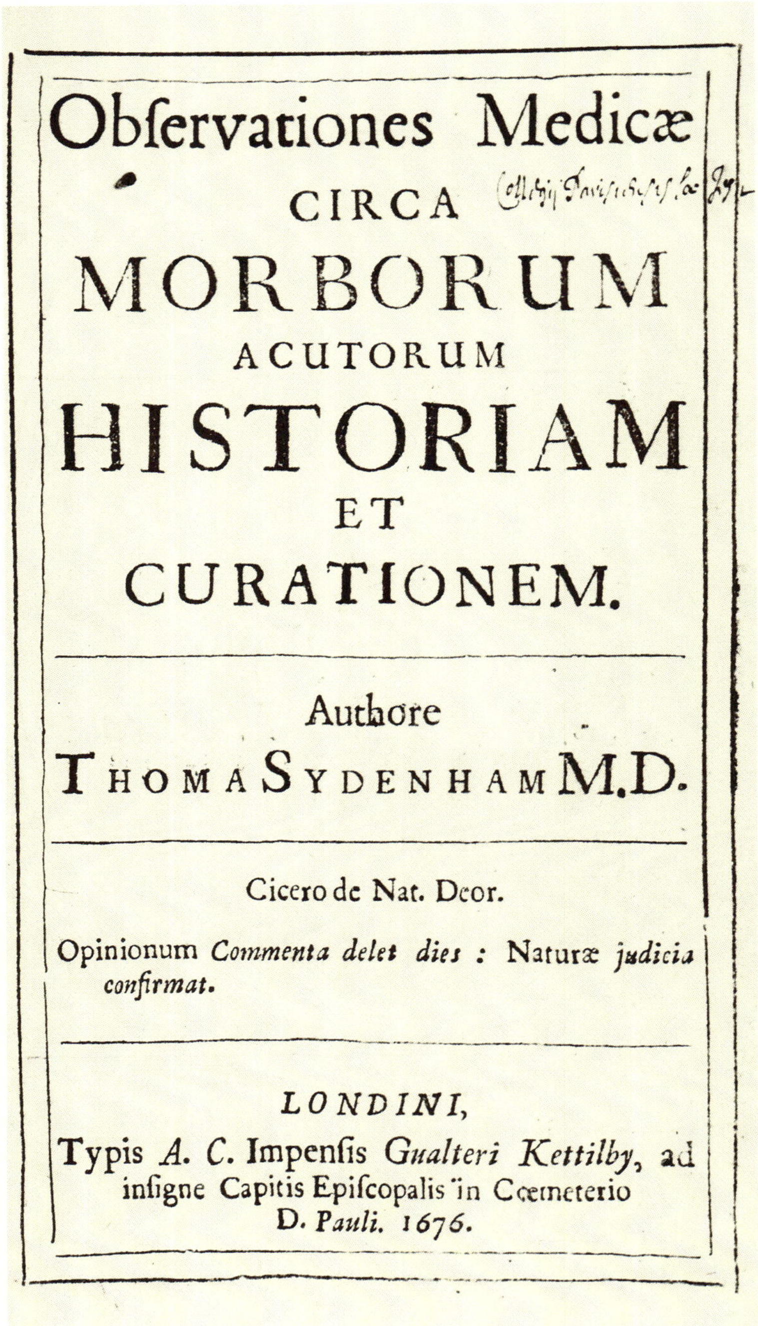

Obſervationes Medicæ
CIRCA
MORBORUM
ACUTORUM
HISTORIAM
ET
CURATIONEM.

Authore
THOMA SYDENHAM M.D.

Cicero de Nat. Deor.

Opinionum *Commenta delet dies* : Naturæ *judicia confirmat.*

LONDINI,
Typis *A. C.* Impenſis *Gualteri Kettilby*, ad inſigne Capitis Epiſcopalis in Cœmeterio D. *Pauli.* 1676.

Fig. 64. No. 35. Sydenham. Title page.

35

THOMAS SYDENHAM
(1624–1689)

Observationes medicae circa morborum acutorum historiam et curationem.

London: Typis A. C. Impensis Gualteri Kettilby, 1676.

8°: A^8(–A1) a–b^8 c^4 B–Z^8 Aa–Hh^8. 267 leaves, pp. [54] 1–425 [55]. Frontispiece portrait (replacing A1) engraved by Abraham Bloteling after the painting by Mary Beale.

GM 2198. *Heirs of Hippocrates* 549. Krivatsy 11627. Norman 2038. Osler 994. Waller 9402. Wing S6314.

If the case of Descartes confirms the adage that good philosophy does not always make for good science, the career of Thomas Sydenham suggests that good clinical medicine and good medical science may not always go hand in hand—at least, that was Sydenham's own prejudice. To his contemporaries and to posterity of the eighteenth and nineteenth centuries, Sydenham was renowned as a clinician and healer, a superb patient's doctor whom Herman Boerhaave (see no. 39) dubbed the "English Hippocrates"; at the same time, Sydenham distanced himself from the scientific medicine of his day and deliberately remained aloof from the fellowship of science in seventeenth-century England. In spite of his mid-century studies at Oxford (then a center of the new science), his friendship with Robert Boyle, and his relationship with John Locke (who served as his amanuensis), Sydenham eschewed universities and academic medicine in favor of clinical practice. Anatomy, dissections, and microscopy had little to offer him: how would studying the dead—insensate, inanimate—help relieve the sufferings of the living? In place of the science of cadavers, Sydenham proposed the careful observation of patients; in place of pure knowledge, he valued results. What counted in medicine, finally, was the efficacy of the treatment, the *curatio*. His most important work, the *Observationes medicae*, summarizes his method and its applications.

Sydenham, who came from a Puritan family in Dorset, supported Parliament during the Civil War and became a protégé of Cromwell during the Commonwealth. Periods of military service interrupted his studies at Oxford, though his appetite for university life seemed small in any event. He won his degrees in odd ways. He was evidently made a bachelor of medicine in 1648 by fiat of the Earl of Pembroke, Chancellor of Oxford, without ever having taken a degree in the arts. In 1655 Cromwell helped set him up in medical practice in Westminster, where he remained for the rest of his life. There is some irony in

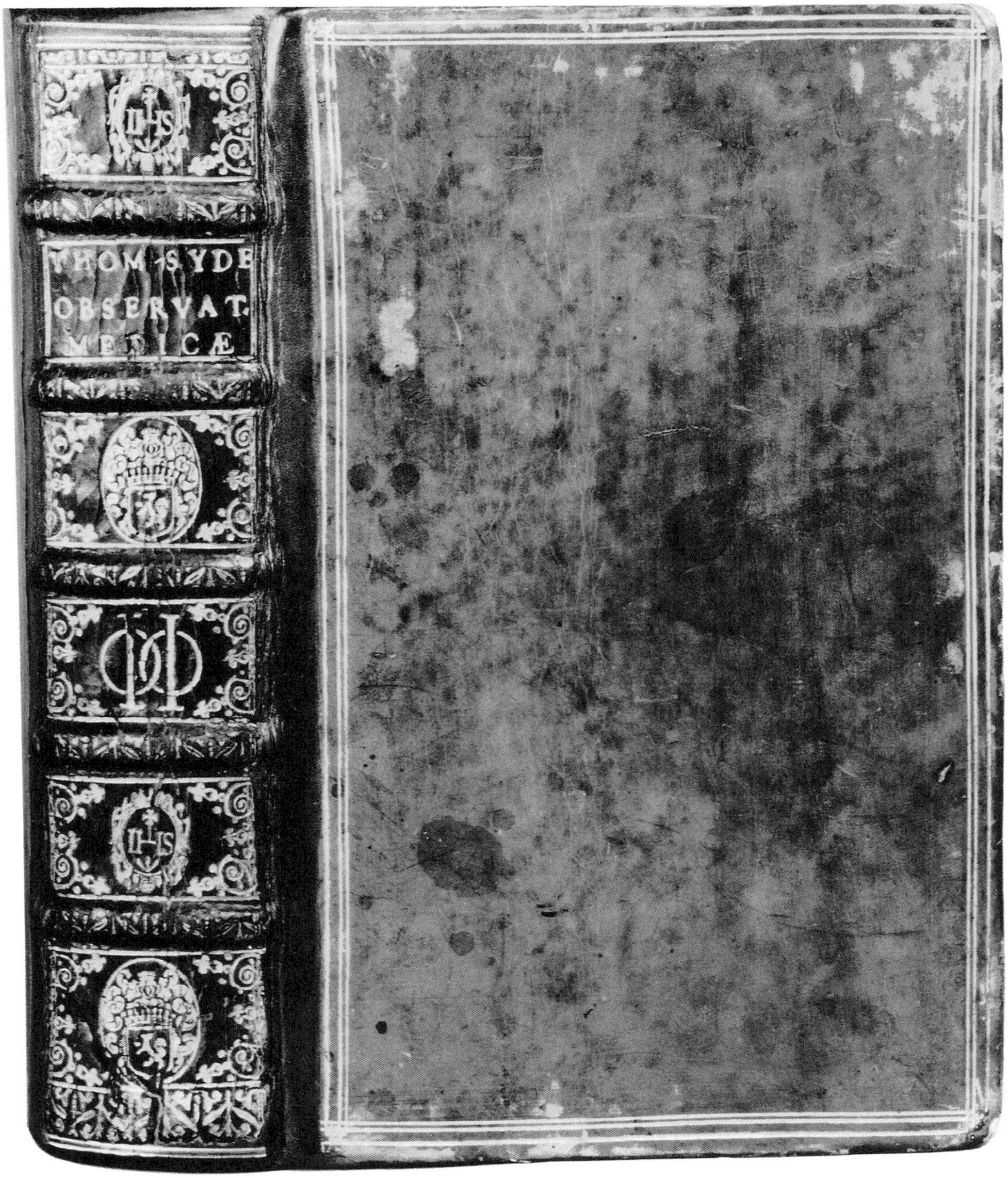

Fig. 65. No. 35. Sydenham. Binding of the copy that once belonged to Nicolas Fouquet and Joseph-Ignace Guillotin. Fouquet's cipher appears in the fourth spine panel from the top.

the fact that Sydenham did not actually receive an M.D. degree until 1676, the year of the publication of *Observationes medicae.* Since he was a Puritan, public life was closed to him after the Restoration, and he never joined the Royal Society. He styled himself a Baconian, and his work is filled with glowing references to the philosopher; in contrast, there are no indications of his ever having read William Harvey (see no. 27A). Sydenham's religious sympathies do not seem to have interfered with his medical practice, which flourished until he succumbed to the gout.

Observationes medicae draws on the extensive observations Sydenham was able to make during and subsequent to the Great Plague of 1666. The work builds on his earlier *Methodus curandi febres* (1666), and some assert that it is really the "third edition" of the *Methodus. Observationes medicae* represents the first major effort to create a nosology of disease. Sydenham's insight was that diseases could be understood and organized like plants: that is, they could be individually identified and classified, with each species of disease having its own natural history. In this, Sydenham shared the broader taxonomic interest of seventeenth-century science and medicine, imposing on diseases the same rigorous, methodical analysis and description that others were applying to the natural world in general. He took disease seriously as a natural phenomenon, an event in nature, and described it accordingly. *Observationes medicae* also reflects Sydenham's belief in the deep curative power of nature and his conviction that disease—especially fever—is nature's way of ridding the organism of morbific matter.

For all its emphasis on empirical observation and the need to understand the life cycles of particular diseases as keys to successful treatment, Sydenham's treatise rests solidly on the humoral medicine of Hippocrates and Galen. However, the importance of the *Observationes medicae* lies in its author's pathfinding methodology, not in the theory that undergirds the work. Sydenham's contribution to medicine remains the methodical empiricism of his clinical orientation rather than the actual clinical results he was able to achieve.

MTR

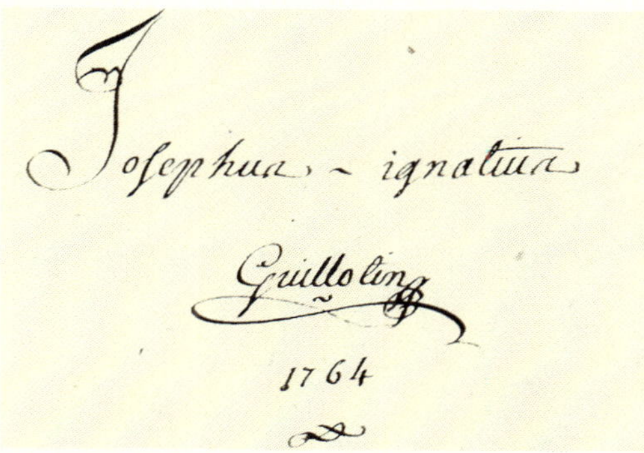

Fig. 66. No. 35. Sydenham. Ownership signature of Joseph-Ignace Guillotin (1738–1814). In the early years of the French Revolution, Guillotin was responsible for reviving the decapitation machine that now bears his name.

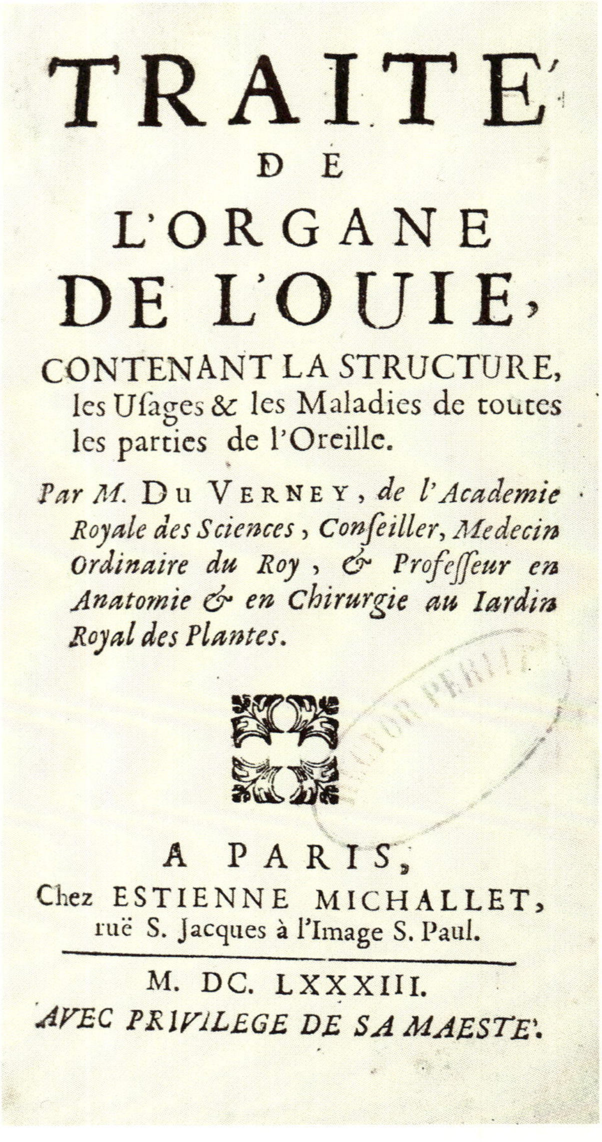

TRAITÉ DE L'ORGANE DE L'OUIE,

CONTENANT LA STRUCTURE, les Usages & les Maladies de toutes les parties de l'Oreille.

Par M. DU VERNEY, *de l'Academie Royale des Sciences, Conseiller, Medecin Ordinaire du Roy, & Professeur en Anatomie & en Chirurgie au Iardin Royal des Plantes.*

A PARIS,
Chez ESTIENNE MICHALLET, ruë S. Jacques à l'Image S. Paul.

M. DC. LXXXIII.
AVEC PRIVILEGE DE SA MAESTÉ.

Fig. 67. No. 36. Duverney. Title page.

36

GUICHARD JOSEPH DUVERNEY
(1648–1730)

Traité de l'organe de l'ouie, contenant la structure, les usages & les maladies de toutes les parties de l'oreille.

Paris: Chez Estienne Michallet, 1683.

12°: ā[12] A–I[12]. 120 leaves, pp. [24] 1–210 [6]. Pl. I–XVI; 16 folding engraved plates, each with letterpress "explication" printed on the same sheet.

GM 1545. *Heirs of Hippocrates* 664. Krivatsy 3590. Norman 674. Waller 2670. Wellcome II, p. 506.

During the seventeenth century the trend among anatomists was to concentrate on specific organs, pursuing investigations and descriptions of their minute details. It may have been for this reason that Guichard Joseph Duverney studied the ear, a structure that had received only limited attention previously.

Duverney was born in Feurs-en-Forez, France, on the banks of the Loire River, the son of the village doctor. After studying medicine at Avignon, he moved to Paris at age nineteen to establish himself as an anatomist. Elected to the Royal Academy of Sciences in 1674, he was appointed professor of anatomy at the Jardin du roi in 1679.

In his *Traité de l'organe de l'ouie*, Duverney used a three-part format to discuss the anatomy of the ear, the physiology of hearing, and the pathology of the hearing organ. In the anatomical section Duverney gave a clear description of the external auditory canal and was the first to depict the arteries, veins, and nerve branches of the auricle. He was also the first to show that the osseous part of the external canal originated from the tympanic bone and that the tympanic ring is incomplete superiorly. Duverney presented the first detailed description of the ossicles of the middle ear and the first account of the relationship of the communication between the tympanic cavity and the cells of the mastoid. He divided the labyrinth or inner ear into three parts: (1) the posterior part, containing the semicircular canals; (2) the front part or cochlea; and (3) the vestibule, an area between the other two parts. The first in-depth description of the osseous labyrinth was included in this book, as well as an outstanding section in which Duverney thoroughly described the embryological anatomy of the ear in a fetus and compared it to the anatomy of the adult ear. He found a number of interesting points, most notably that the ossicles and labyrinth of the fetal and adult ear are of the same size.

In his section on the pathology of the hearing organ, Duverney was first to dispute the

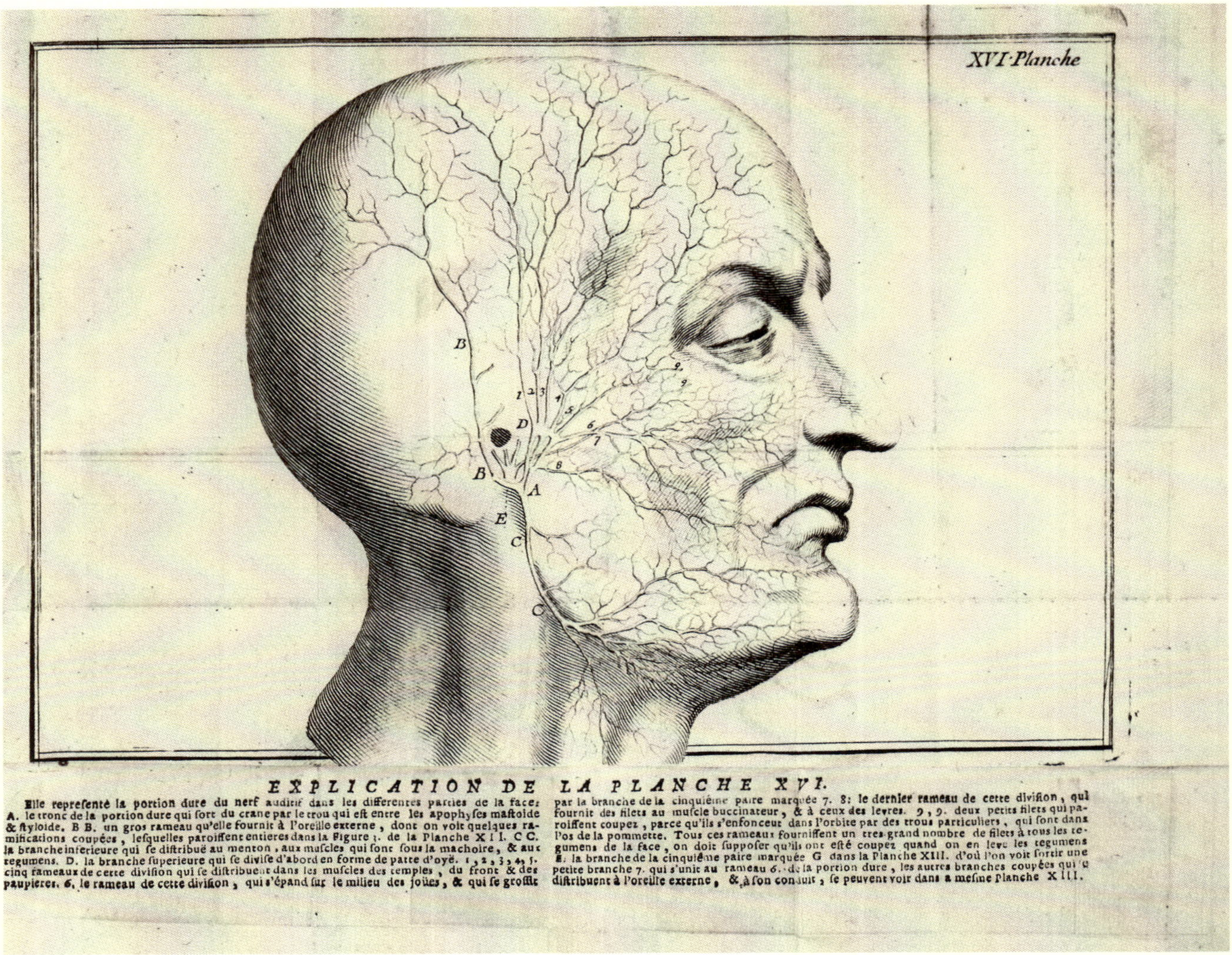

Fig. 68. No. 36. Duverney. Engraved plate from *Traité de l'organe de l'ouie*, illustrating the auditory nerve.

generally accepted, centuries-old opinion that otorrhea originated from the brain and showed that the meatus of the internal auditory canal was closed by the auditory nerve. He also classified diseases of the ear according to the anatomical structures affected. In the section on the physiology of hearing, Duverney presented a vividly detailed explanation of the hearing mechanism. Although he had no knowledge of the microscopic structure of the hearing organ, he nonetheless gave a version of a resonance theory two centuries before Hermann von Helmholtz (see no. 65). His most valuable theories were that sound was conducted by the bones of the skull and that the labyrinth played a role in the perception of different tones.

Traité de l'organe de l'ouie was published in 1683. It was illustrated with sixteen engraved plates that are unsigned but traditionally attributed to Sebastien Le Clerc (1637–1714). Latin translations appeared in 1684 and 1730, and in 1737 John Marshall's English translation was published.

DGP

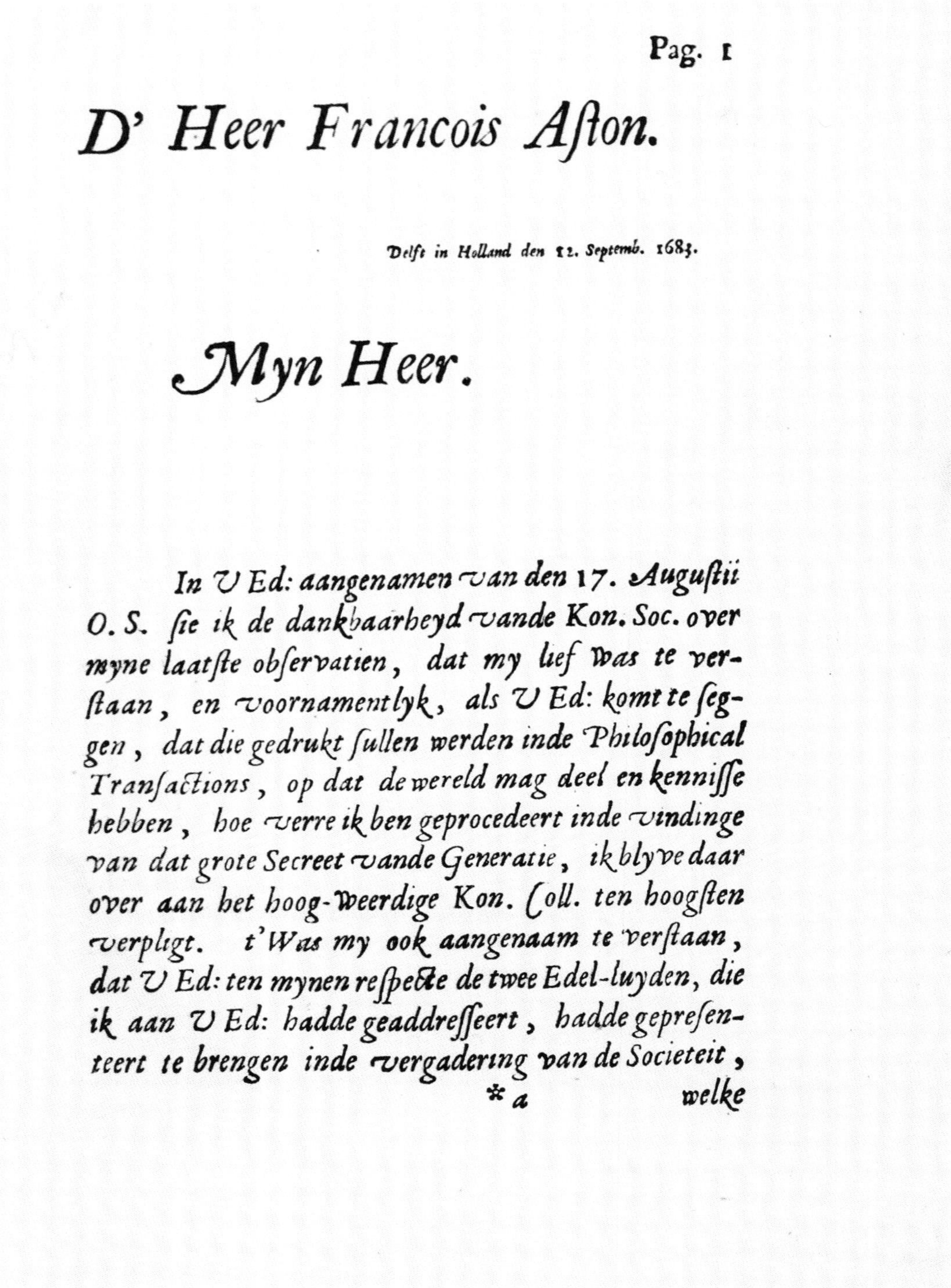

Pag. 1

D' Heer Francois Aston.

Delft in Holland den 12. Septemb. 1683.

Myn Heer.

In U Ed: aangenamen van den 17. Augustii O. S. sie ik de dankbaarheyd vande Kon. Soc. over myne laatste observatien, dat my lief was te verstaan, en voornamentlyk, als U Ed: komt te seggen, dat die gedrukt sullen werden inde Philosophical Transactions, op dat de wereld mag deel en kennisse hebben, hoe verre ik ben geprocedeert inde vindinge van dat grote Secreet vande Generatie, ik blyve daar over aan het hoog-weerdige Kon. Coll. ten hoogsten verpligt. t'Was my ook aangenaam te verstaan, dat U Ed: ten mynen respecte de twee Edel-luyden, die ik aan U Ed: hadde geaddresseert, hadde gepresenteert te brengen inde vergadering van de Societeit,

* a   *welke*

Fig. 69. No. 37. Leeuwenhoek. First page of Letter 39, which contains the first description of bacteria.

37

ANTONI VAN LEEUWENHOEK
(1632–1723)

Ondervindingen en beschouwingen der onsigbare geschapene waarheden, waar in gehandeld werd vande eyerstok.

Leiden: By Daniel van Gaesbeeck, 1684.

4°: π1 A–E² [F]1, *a–*e². 22 leaves, pp. [2] 1–21 [1], 1–19 [1]. 8 engravings in text.

Dobell 2. cf. GM 2464.1. Norman 1303. cf. PMM 166. Waller 10887.2. Wellcome III, p. 476.

Antoni van Leeuwenhoek, who lacked formal university training in the sciences, philosophy, or languages, surely ranks among the greatest autodidacts in the history of science and medicine. Born into a comfortable middle-class Dutch family, he passed his long life almost entirely in Delft. There he had two careers: the first as a civil servant, the second as a microscopist of international renown. His career in the service of the city of Delft brought him a pension at the age of thirty-nine, and this allowed him to devote himself full-time to observing and describing the "little worlds" he encountered through his microscopes. Although a man of limited theoretical skills, he was a consummately acute observer, and for fifty years he patiently and painstakingly documented the hidden realms of nature in a way no one had done before him. Like the great Dutch artists of the seventeenth century, he had a profound interest in and talent for representing the natural world around him.

Leeuwenhoek was the best lens grinder of his day, and while he did not invent the microscope, he perfected it sufficiently to permit him to conduct a long series of observations. He also developed a system of micrometry for measuring and bringing some order to his observations. With encouragement and assistance from Reinier de Graaf, his friend and colleague in Delft, Leeuwenhoek and his work were brought to the attention of the Royal Society in London as early as 1673. During the next forty years, letters by Leeuwenhoek to the Royal Society appeared regularly in its *Philosophical Transactions.* These in turn became the chief means by which the results of his work were recorded and disseminated, since he wrote no monographs and trained no students.

It is not without reason that Leeuwenhoek is often referred to as "the father of microbiology." Early in his career as a scientist, he observed what he described as animalcules or "little animals" in water, and from then on he described in considerable detail a spectrum

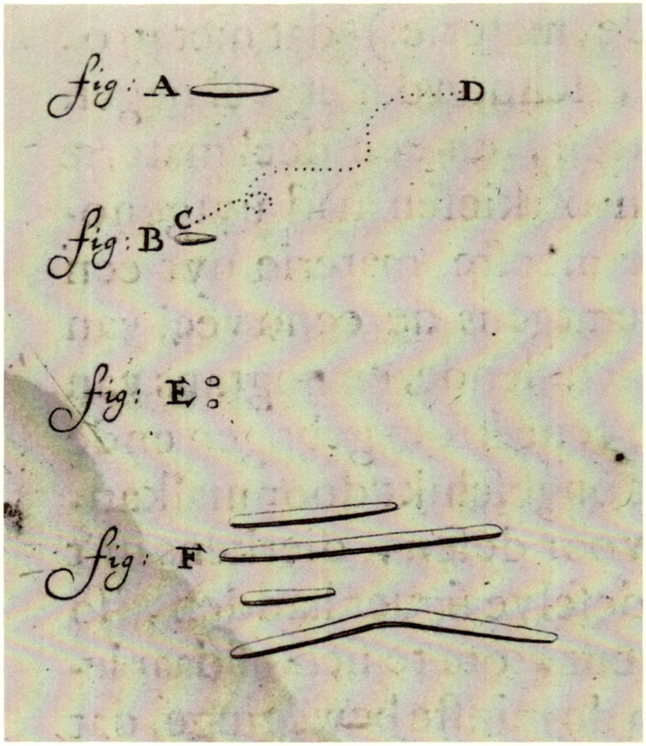

Fig. 70. No. 37. Leeuwenhoek. The first illustration of bacteria.

of microorganisms never before detected, including bacteria, protozoa, and rotifers. Leeuwenhoek thought that these organisms were quite literally "little animals" and thus identical in nature and structure to all other animals—a view that might seem naive in retrospect, but one that was grounded in the then widely held belief in the uniformity of nature. This belief allowed him to avoid being distracted by theoretical concerns for which he had little appetite or aptitude.

There were few areas that Leeuwenhoek did not investigate with his instruments. He dissected and studied dozens of species of insects and genera of plants and trees and helped clarify a variety of anatomical issues. He made patient and important observations of nerves and of blood and discovered (independently of Malpighi; see no. 30) red blood cells and intestinal capillaries. In his own day, however, it was principally his work on sexual reproduction that caught the attention of contemporaries. Leeuwenhoek was the first to observe and record the spermatozoa, not only of humans but also of other mammals, as well as those of birds, fish, reptiles, and mollusks. An ardent opponent of spontaneous generation theories of reproduction, he was a committed preformationist and believed that the sperm itself was a "little man." Since the sperm moved and the egg did not, and since motility was associated with life, Leeuwenhoek attributed the generative capacity solely to the sperm, regarding the egg as primarily a source of nutrients and sustenance—this in opposition to Harvey, who regarded the egg as the source of all new life. The controversy between the animalculists and ovists persisted until the late nineteenth century, when Wilhelm Hertwig showed that fertilization consists of the union of sperm and egg nuclei.

In a more general sense, it was not only Leeuwenhoek's particular discoveries that were crucial for early modern science and medicine. The cumulative impact of his investigations with the microscope helped to make the instrument an integral part of biological and medical research.

MTR

Leeuwenhoek communicated all of his scientific observations in letters, 165 of which were published during his lifetime in two numbered, chronological sequences, 28–146 and I–XLVI. Most of the letters were addressed to the Royal Society in London, which published abstracts of 120 of them, in English or Latin, in volumes VIII (1673) to XXXIII (1723) of the *Philosophical Transactions.* Letters 1–27 were not published separately, but many were abstracted in the *Philosophical Transactions.*[1] Leeuwenhoek's letters were written in Dutch and appeared in both Dutch and Latin editions. The Latin translations were made by others, as Leeuwenhoek had no knowledge of that language.

Letter 37, addressed to Christopher Wren, and Letter 39 (written 12 September 1683), which contains Leeuwenhoek's famous description of bacteria, were published together in 1684.

HFN

1. Clifford Dobell, *Antony van Leeuwenhoek and His "Little Animals"* (London, 1932), pp. 305, 356–59, 390–91.

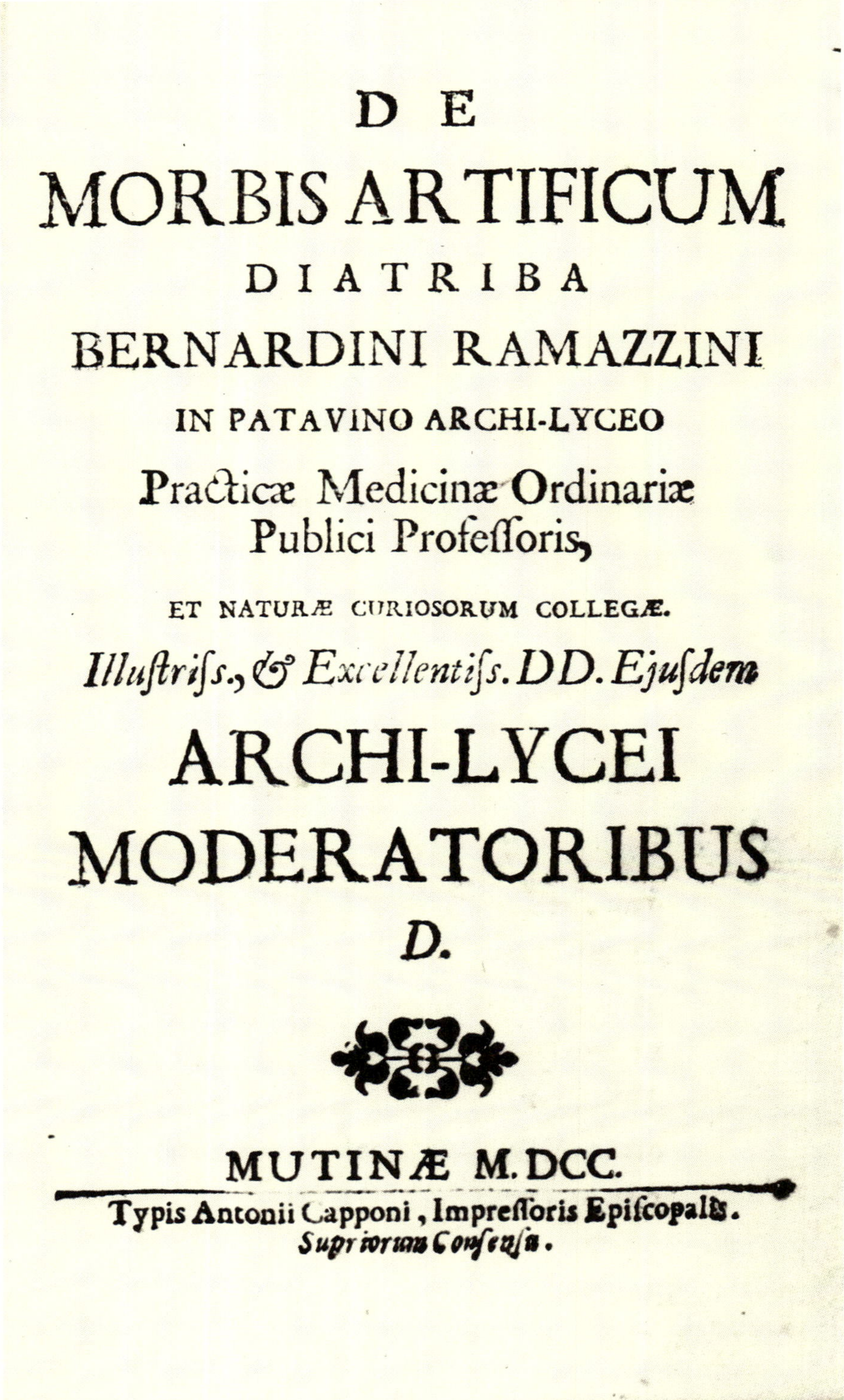

D E

MORBIS ARTIFICUM

DIATRIBA

BERNARDINI RAMAZZINI

IN PATAVINO ARCHI-LYCEO

Practicæ Medicinæ Ordinariæ
Publici Professoris,

ET NATURÆ CURIOSORUM COLLEGÆ.

Illustriss., & Excellentiss. DD. Ejusdem

ARCHI-LYCEI
MODERATORIBUS

D.

MUTINÆ M.DCC.

Typis Antonii Capponi, Impressoris Episcopalis.
Superiorum Consensu.

Fig. 71. No. 38. Ramazzini. Title page.

38

BERNARDINO RAMAZZINI

(1633–1714)

De morbis artificum diatriba.

Modena: Typis Antonii Capponi, 1700.

8°: π4 A–Y8 Z4. 184 leaves, pp. *i–iv* v–viii 1–360.

GM 2121. *Heirs of Hippocrates* 592. Krivatsy 9366. Norman 1776. Osler 3760. PMM 170. Waller 7727.

With his book on occupational diseases, Bernardino Ramazzini founded a new medical discipline: industrial hygiene. Apart from books on the diseases of miners by Paracelsus (see no. 16) and a few others, very little had previously been published on this subject. Ramazzini made a special study of the effect of labor on health, particularly among his many working-class patients. He based his book primarily on his own cases and observations, augmented by scattered descriptions compiled from the works of other authors.

Two main classes of occupational diseases were identified. "First, [those caused by] the noxious quality of the matter that goes through [the workers'] hands which by breathing out noxive steams and thin particles offensive to human nature, give rise to particular diseases." Ramazzini described the diseases of metalworkers, with the symptoms of the different types of metal poisoning, pneumoconiosis in miners, silicosis in stonemasons, and poisoning from lead, mercury, and antimony in painters, apothecaries, chemists, surgeons, and others. "In the next place [are diseases caused by] certain violent and disorderly postures of the body, by which the natural structure is so undermin'd, as gradually to make way for grievous distempers." Those affected by this latter category included blacksmiths, bricklayers, tailors, and those in sedentary occupations.

Ramazzini gave clear, clinical descriptions of occupational diseases, but the emphasis of his book was on prevention rather than cure. He lamented, as did many later writers on industrial hygiene, the lack of interest of so many employers in the health of their workmen, in spite of the obvious benefits to themselves of a fit work force. He was equally critical of the attitude of the many workmen who were reluctant to take preventive measures when these involved changing old habits. Ramazzini's work remained the leading textbook of occupational medicine until the early nineteenth century, when the working world on which it was based was changed forever by the Industrial Revolution. An English translation appeared in 1705, and the work was translated into French and Italian during the eighteenth century. A new English translation was published in 1940.

RDG

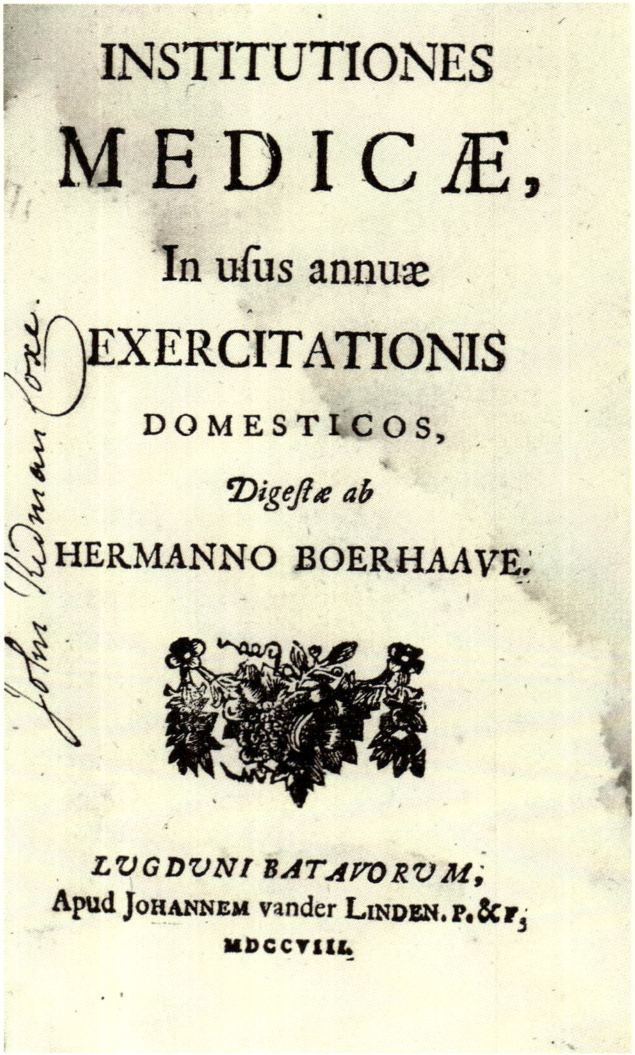

INSTITUTIONES
MEDICÆ,
In uſus annuæ
EXERCITATIONIS
DOMESTICOS,
Digeſtæ ab
HERMANNO BOERHAAVE.

LUGDUNI BATAVORUM,
Apud JOHANNEM vander LINDEN. P. & F.
MDCCVIII.

Fig. 72. No. 39. Boerhaave. Title page. The John Redman Coxe copy, with Coxe's signature in the left margin.

39

HERMAN BOERHAAVE
(1668–1738)

Institutiones medicae, in usus annuae exercitationis domesticos.

Leiden: Apud Johannem vander Linden, 1708.

12°: *2 A–K12 L6. 128 leaves, pp. [4] 1–250 [2]. One woodcut in text.

Blake, p. 53. GM 581. *Heirs of Hippocrates* 749. Lindeboom 40. Norman 255. Waller 1200. Wellcome II, p. 188.

Boerhaave's *Institutiones medicae*, originally intended for the use of his medical students, was one of the earliest textbooks of physiology. More than any other work, it established the teaching of physiology as a modern academic discipline. Boerhaave's extraordinary grasp of medicine, chemistry, and physics, and his ability to bring all the sciences to the service of the patient brought him great fame as a teacher of medicine, and his *Institutiones medicae* had an enormous influence in systematizing the study of physiology in all the major European medical schools. During his lifetime the book went through five revised editions in Latin, was reprinted many times in all major European countries, and was translated into all the important European languages. After the author's death, editions were issued by the French physician Julien Offray de La Mettrie and by Boerhaave's brilliant pupil Albrecht von Haller, who became the first professor of anatomy, surgery, and botany at the University of Göttingen, where he passed on his master's teachings.

The *Institutiones medicae* was divided into five sections: physiology, pathology, semeiotica, hygiene, and therapeutics, with the first part on physiology taking up over half the text.[1] "It is notable that this is the only part that is furnished with footnotes on almost every page. . . . Apparently the author considered that physiology was a most important but much-neglected subject in the medical course. So the physiological part is not only the most extensive but also the best-documented part of the *Institutiones*."[2] The work summarized the general ideas about physiology and pathology current in Boerhaave's time, and "represents a serious attempt to establish knowledge of the functions of organs as a basis of pathology. The approach to pathology is not morphological but, as it should be, physiological."[3]

By the time of Boerhaave's retirement he held three chairs at the University of Leiden, which he had made into Europe's leading center for medical education. Students came to

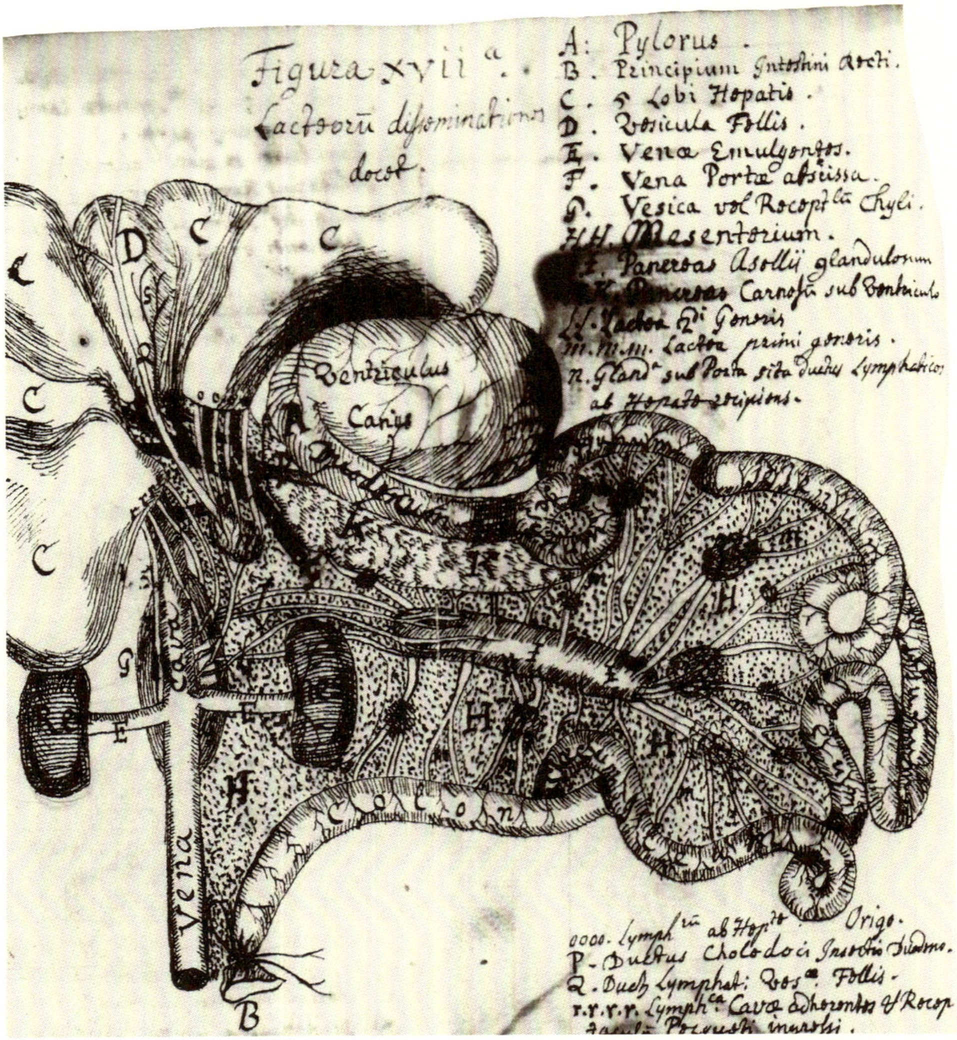

Fig. 73. No. 39. Boerhaave. Interleaved pen-and-ink drawing from the John Redman Coxe copy.

Leiden from many different countries, returning with textbooks by their professor to teach his methods at home, so that Boerhaave's academic system, both in style and in organization, survived through his pupils long after his death. The most remarkable example of his influence was in the medical school at Edinburgh. Alexander Monro *primus*, Edinburgh's first professor of anatomy, was his pupil, and Andrew St. Clair, who gave a course of lectures commenting on the *Institutiones*, was the first to hold Edinburgh's chair of the Institutes of Medicine, the name of which was taken directly from the title of Boerhaave's work. At one moment, in 1726, the whole medical faculty at Edinburgh consisted of Boerhaave's pupils following his teaching. "Through his pupils he is the real founder of the Edinburgh Medical School, and through it of the best medical teaching in the English-speaking countries of the world."[4]

RDG

1. G. A. Lindeboom, *Herman Boerhaave: The Man and His Work* (London, 1968), pp. 71–73.
2. Ibid., p. 74.
3. Ibid.
4. Charles Singer, *A Short History of Medicine*, 2d ed. (New York, 1962), p. 150; John F. Fulton, "The Influence of Boerhaave's *Institutiones Medicae* on Modern Physiology," *Nederl. tijdschrift voor geneeskunde* 82, no. 40 (1 October 1928): 4860–66.

See color plate XXII.

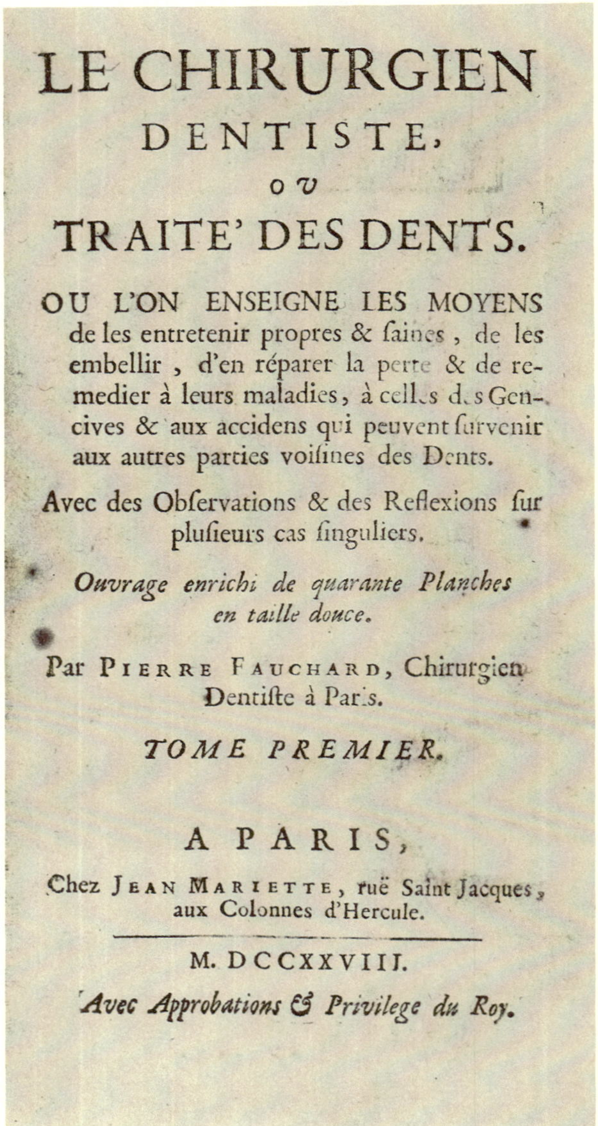

LE CHIRURGIEN
DENTISTE,
OU
TRAITE' DES DENTS.

OU L'ON ENSEIGNE LES MOYENS de les entretenir propres & ſaines, de les embellir, d'en réparer la perte & de remedier à leurs maladies, à celles des Gencives & aux accidens qui peuvent ſurvenir aux autres parties voiſines des Dents.

Avec des Obſervations & des Reflexions ſur pluſieurs cas ſinguliers.

Ouvrage enrichi de quarante Planches en taille douce.

Par PIERRE FAUCHARD, Chirurgien Dentiſte à Paris.

TOME PREMIER.

A PARIS,
Chez JEAN MARIETTE, ruë Saint Jacques, aux Colonnes d'Hercule.

M. DCCXXVIII.

Avec Approbations & Privilege du Roy.

Fig. 74. No. 40. Fauchard. Title page.

40

PIERRE FAUCHARD
(1678–1761)

Le chirurgien dentiste, ou traité des dents.

Paris: Chez Jean Mariette, 1728.

[Vol. I] 12°: a^{12} b^{8} c^{4} A–$Z^{8/4}$ Aa–$Rr^{4/8}$ Ss^{4}. 268 leaves, pp. [48] *1* 2–456 [32]. Frontispiece portrait of Fauchard engraved by J. B. Scotin after J. Le Bel; Pl. première, 2me – 8me: 8 engraved plates, the first signed "P. Belhomme delineavit. I.B. Scotin sculpsit."

[Vol. II] 12°: π1 $\tilde{a}^{4}$ A^{8} B^{4} C^{8} D^{4} (±D2) E–$Z^{8/4}$ Aa–$Gg^{4/8}$ Gg^{4} Hh^{2}. 191 leaves, pp. [10] *1* 2–346 [26]. Pl. 9me – 40me: 32 engraved plates.

Blake, p. 144. EFDT 142. GM 3671. Norman 768. PMM 186. Waller 10620. Wellcome III, p. 12.

Toward the end of the seventeenth century, dentistry, which had previously been considered a part of surgery, was beginning to emerge as a distinct specialty. The eventual separation of the two disciplines was inevitable, but dentistry was not sufficiently advanced as a science until the publication of *Le chirurgien dentiste* by the Parisian dental surgeon Pierre Fauchard marked the beginning of a new epoch in the history of dental treatment. Indeed, Fauchard's treatise was the first scientific work on the subject and the first to use the word "dentiste" to describe the profession. The second edition of 1746 was revised and considerably enlarged by the author, and it included a description of pyorrhea alveolaris, a common affliction of the gums. A third edition appeared in 1786, after Fauchard's death. The work was translated into German in 1733, but there was no English edition until 1946.

Fauchard recognized that there was much ignorance of dentistry in the medical profession, even among eminent surgeons, and very little literature on the subject, partly because it was the custom of practitioners to withhold information concerning their own successful methods and remedies. Fauchard realized the limitations of this practice and the enormous benefit of disseminating such knowledge and experience as were available. There was much that was good in dental practice at the time, and in his book he collected and arranged in a single work the whole of contemporary knowledge, giving it a solid scientific basis. Because of this, Fauchard is universally regarded by dental historians as the founder of modern dentistry—indeed, no single individual has had a more profound influence on the development of dentistry. In the first years of the eighteenth century France was the leading country in the dental art, closely followed by Germany, and the state of dental practice in Fauchard's time can be inferred from his writing.

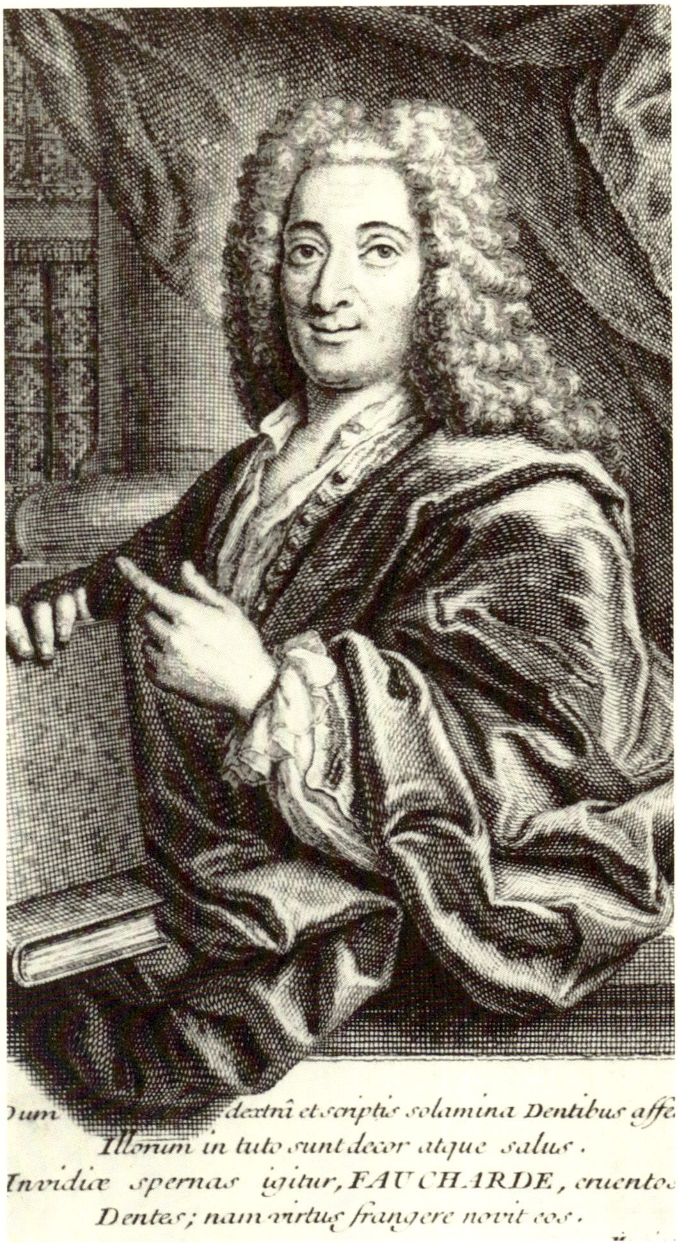
um dextrâ et scriptis solamina Dentibus affe
Illorum in tuto sunt decor atque salus.
Invidiæ spernas igitur, FAUCHARDE, cruento
Dentes; nam virtus frangere novit eos.

Fig. 75. No. 40. Fauchard. Engraved frontispiece portrait.

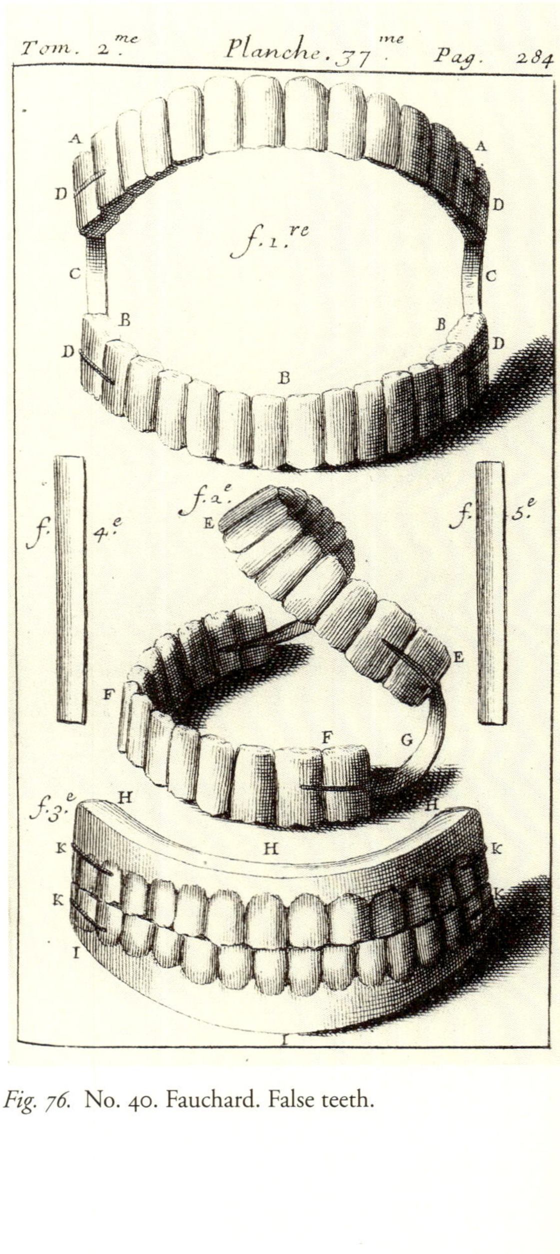

Fig. 76. No. 40. Fauchard. False teeth.

Le chirurgien dentiste discussed every aspect of dentistry with extraordinary thoroughness, and the book was profusely illustrated. In the first volume Fauchard gave a good description of the anatomy of the teeth, set forth rules for their cleaning and preservation, commented that neglect of the teeth is the chief cause of their decay, and devoted a chapter to tartar. He classified dental maladies into three groups and identified more than one hundred morbid conditions. The second volume was entirely devoted to operative dentistry, orthodontics, and in particular prosthetics, the branch of dentistry concerned with false teeth, bridgework, and the like. As a result of Fauchard's comprehensive treatment of his subject, his book became the first worthwhile textbook of dentistry.

NP

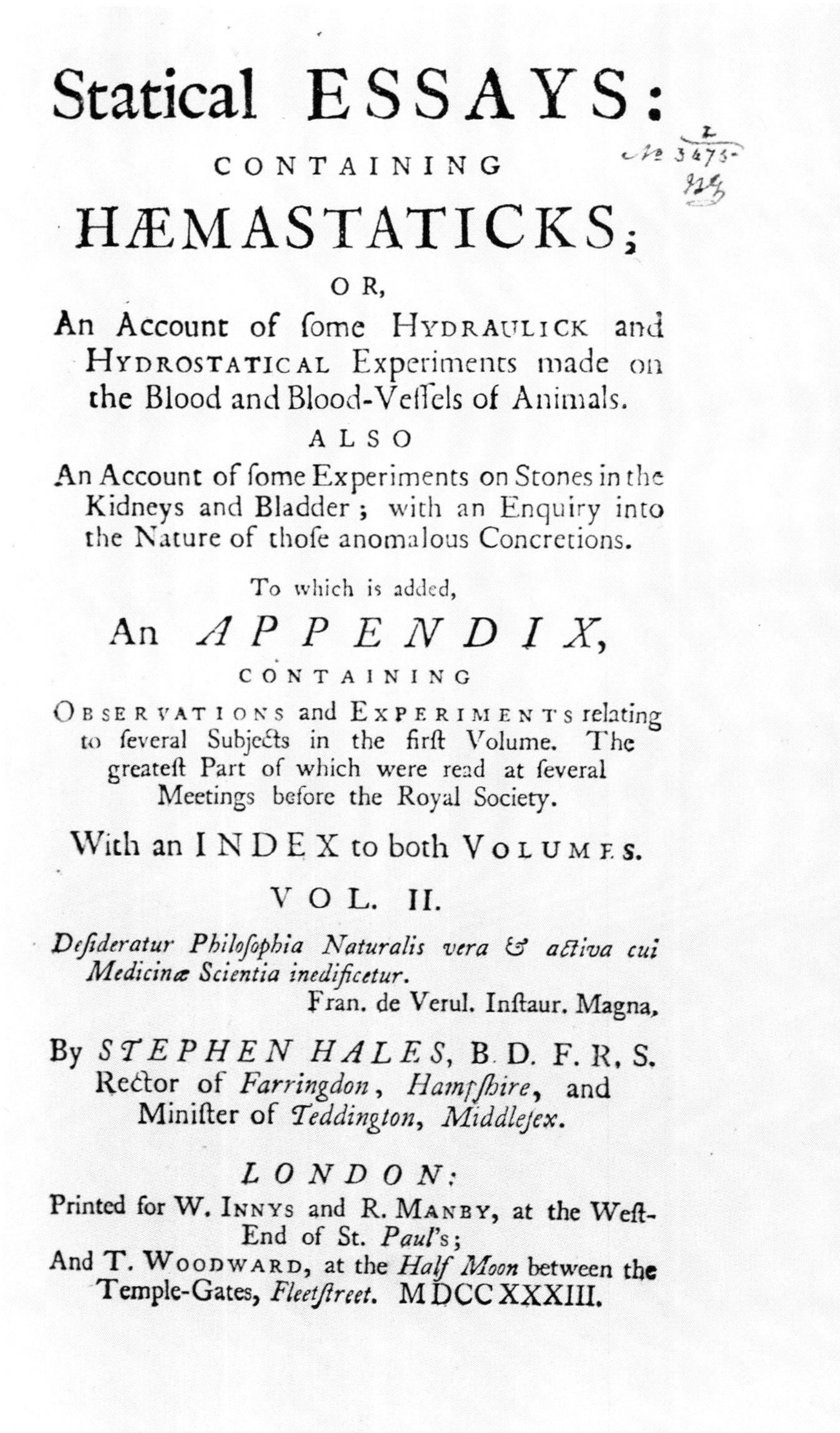

Statical ESSAYS:

CONTAINING

HÆMASTATICKS;

OR,

An Account of ſome HYDRAULICK and HYDROSTATICAL Experiments made on the Blood and Blood-Veſſels of Animals.

ALSO

An Account of ſome Experiments on Stones in the Kidneys and Bladder; with an Enquiry into the Nature of thoſe anomalous Concretions.

To which is added,

An *APPENDIX*,

CONTAINING

OBSERVATIONS and EXPERIMENTS relating to ſeveral Subjects in the firſt Volume. The greateſt Part of which were read at ſeveral Meetings before the Royal Society.

With an INDEX to both VOLUMES.

VOL. II.

Deſideratur Philoſophia Naturalis vera & activa cui Medicinæ Scientia inedificetur.

Fran. de Verul. Inſtaur. Magna,

By *STEPHEN HALES*, B. D. F. R. S.
Rector of *Farringdon*, *Hampſhire*, and
Miniſter of *Teddington*, *Middleſex*.

LONDON:

Printed for W. INNYS and R. MANBY, at the Weſt-End of St. *Paul's*;
And T. WOODWARD, at the *Half Moon* between the Temple-Gates, *Fleetſtreet*. MDCCXXXIII.

Fig. 77. No. 41. Hales. Title page of *Haemastaticks*, published as Volume II of Hales's *Statical Essays.*

41

STEPHEN HALES
(1677–1761)

Statical Essays: Containing Haemastaticks; or, An Account of Some Hydraulick and Hydrostatical Experiments Made on the Blood and Blood-Vessels of Animals.

London: Printed for W. Innys and R. Manby, and T. Woodward, 1733.

8°: A^8 $a–b^8$ $B–Z^8$ Aa^8 $Bb–Cc^4$. 216 leaves, pp. *i–v* vi–xxii [26] 1–361 [23].

Blake, p. 194. GM 765. *Heirs of Hippocrates* 784. Horblit 45b. Norman 970. Osler 1081. PMM 189. Waller 11527. Wellcome III, p. 194.

The most significant of Stephen Hales's many scientific contributions was his pioneering study of hemodynamics, published in 1733 in his monograph *Statical Essays: Containing Haemastaticks.* Hales was born in 1677 in Bekesbourne, Kent, England, and received a M.A. degree from Cambridge in 1703. Although he studied for the clergy at Cambridge, his interest in science was stimulated in the intellectually fertile atmosphere of the university.

In 1709 he moved to Teddington, a village on the Thames between Twickenham and Hampton Court, where he combined his work as a parish priest with experiments on a wide variety of subjects. His pioneering study of plants, *Vegetable Staticks,* appeared in 1727. Six years later, in the companion volume *Haemastaticks,* Hales recounted two decades of experiments in which he studied the dynamics of the circulation of the blood. The book includes descriptions of Hales's attempts to evaluate (and quantify where possible) blood flow, blood pressure, and the velocity of blood in circulation. He was the first to employ a manometer to measure blood pressure in animals.

In addition to measuring blood pressure in the resting state, Hales repeated his measurements to assess the effect on blood pressure of bleeding, respiration, and exertion. Adapting techniques developed a few years earlier by James Keill, Hales estimated the ventricular volume, the velocity of blood flow, and cardiac output. A subject of special interest to him was the influence on blood pressure of constriction or dilation of the small blood vessels. His observations and comments reflect a remarkably sophisticated understanding of the interrelationships among blood flow, pressure, and resistance.

Hales's observations on hemodynamics influenced other eighteenth-century scientists, including Robert Whytt and Albrecht von Haller. Physiologists William Hamilton and Dickinson Richards claimed that his "broad concept of blood pressure, blood flow, blood velocity, and their relations, and quantitative measurements or calculations of each . . . oriented all future work."[1] Hales's lasting influence reflects the significance of his innovative experiments and observations.

WBF

Hales's work is regarded as one of the greatest contributions to our knowledge of the vascular system after that of Harvey (see no. 27A). In *Haemastaticks*, he described his invention of the manometer, with which he was first able to measure blood pressure. This instrument was the forerunner of the blood pressure cuff as eventually developed by Samuel Siegfried von Basch (1881) and Scipione Riva-Rocci (1896) and effectively put to use by Nikolai Korotkov (1905). It was the last who introduced the modern method of applying the stethoscope to the brachial artery during blood pressure examinations with the sphygmomanometer for the purpose of investigating sounds made by the blood after the release of the pressure cuff.

HFN

1. William F. Hamilton and Dickinson W. Richards, "The Output of the Heart," in *Circulation of the Blood: Men and Ideas*, ed. Alfred P. Fishman and Dickinson W. Richards (New York, 1964), p. 84.

42

NICOLAS ANDRY
(1658–1742)

L'orthopédie ou l'art de prevenir et de corriger dans les enfans, les difformités du corps.

Paris: Chez la veuve Alix; Lambert & Durand, 1741.

[Vol. I] 12°: π^2 a–h$^{8/4}$ i1 A–Z$^{8/4}$ Aa–Ee$^{4/8}$ Ff^6. 225 leaves, pp. [4] i–cxviij [i.e. xcviij] *1* 2–345 [3]. Engraved frontispiece by J. Guélard after A. Humblot; 13 engraved plates.

[Vol. II] 12°: π1 a^4 (–a4) A–Z$^{8/4}$ Aa–Ee$^{4/8}$ Ff^6 Gg^8 Hh^4 (–Hh4) A–D$^{8/4}$. 213 leaves, pp. [2] i–v [1] *1* 2–365 [5], 1–47 [1]. 1 engraved plate.

Blake, p. 15. GM 4301. *Heirs of Hippocrates* 697. Norman 55. Waller 418. Wellcome II, p. 45.

Andry coined the term *orthopaedia* from the Greek words for "straight" (*orthos*) and "child" (*pais*) and in doing so named the science of orthopedics. His book was the first monograph on the subject, and the emblematic engraving it contains of a tree with a crooked trunk tied to a straight post has been adopted as a symbol of orthopedics.

Andry grasped the crucial principles that the muscles in balance are the molders of the body in childhood and that weakness in a muscle, resulting in a muscle imbalance, can result in the onset of a deformity during growth. He therefore recommended that the offending muscle be subjected to a course of exercise, by which deformities could be prevented or cured. His methods were simple but ingenious, based on observation and on the principle that deformities that are due to one form of movement or habit can be undone by a movement or habit of the opposite kind. For example, he observed that a corpulent man or a pregnant woman walks with a straight back; therefore, if a youth stoops, he should be made to carry a burden in front of his body. Andry devised balancing and gymnastic exercises and encouraged childhood games. He also used massage, cold applications, and what we now call orthopedic beds. For established deformities, he resorted to the use of mechanical aids. He also believed that deformities in children were caused by ill-fitting or restrictive clothing and by unnatural postures enforced by badly designed children's furniture. He thus paid great attention to the adoption of proper posture, which he regarded as being of the utmost importance. Later in the eighteenth century, Jean Pierre David was to show the value of rest in the body's own repair system, but Andry demonstrated that exercise as well as rest had an appropriate place in the treatment of physical problems.

NP

L'ORTHOPÉDIE

OU

L'ART

DE PREVENIR ET DE CORRIGER

DANS LES ENFANS,

LES DIFFORMITÉS DU CORPS.

LE TOUT PAR DES MOYENS A LA PORTE'E des Peres & des Meres, & des Perſonnes qui ont des Enfans à élever.

PAR M. ANDRY, CONSEILLER DU ROY, Lecteur & Profeſſeur en Médecine au College Royal, Docteur-Regent, & ancien Doyen de la Faculté de Médecine de Paris, &c.

Avec Figures.

TOME PREMIER.

A PARIS, RUE SAINT JACQUES.

Chez { La Veuve ALIX, au-deſſus de la ruë des Noyers, au Griffon.
LAMBERT & DURAND, à la Sageſſe, & à Saint Landry. }

M. DCC. XLI.

AVEC APPROBATIONS ET PRIVILEGE DU ROY.

Fig. 78. No. 42. Andry. Title page.

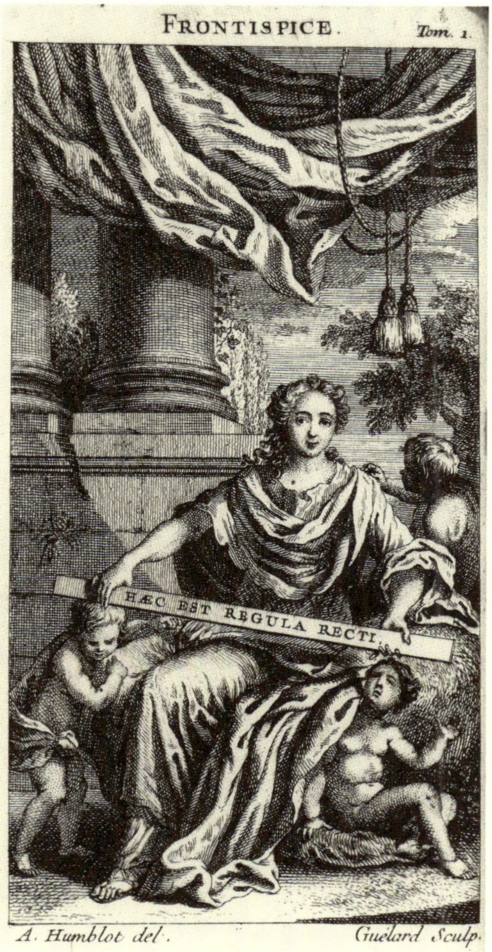

Fig. 79. No. 42. Andry. Engraved allegorical frontispiece.

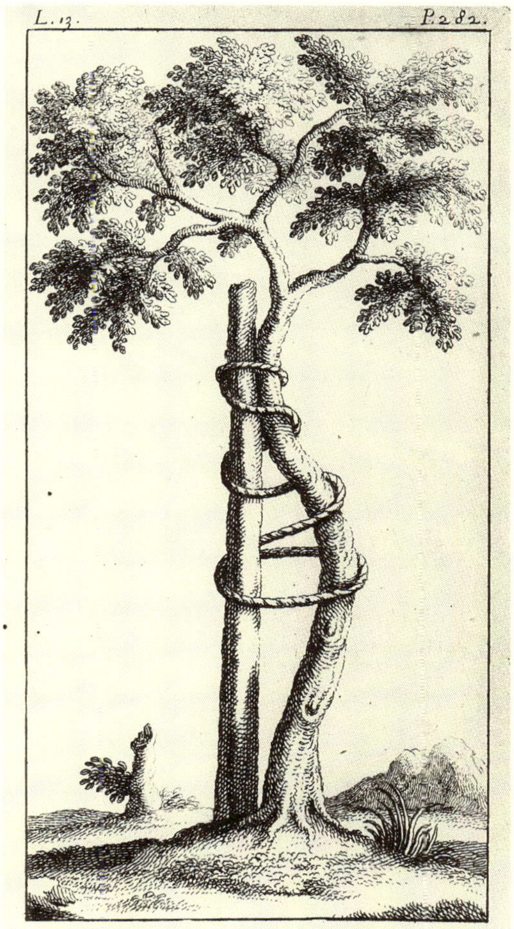

Fig. 80. No. 42. Andry's famous "crooked tree" is now a universally recognized symbol of orthopedics.

A

TREATISE

ON THE

Theory and Practice

OF

MIDWIFERY.

By W. SMELLIE, M. D.

LONDON:

Printed for D. WILSON, at Plato's Head, near Round-Court, in the Strand.

MDCCLII.

Fig. 81. No. 43A. Title page of Smellie's initial volume on midwifery.

43

WILLIAM SMELLIE
(1697–1763)

A] *A Treatise on the Theory and Practice of Midwifery.*

London: Printed for D. Wilson, 1752.

8°: a^8 B–Z^8 Aa–Gg^8. 240 leaves, pp. [2] *i* ii–xiv, *i* ii–lxxii *73* 74–454 [10].

[Vol. II] *A Collection of Cases and Observations in Midwifery.*

London: Printed for D. Wilson and T. Durham, 1754.

8°: A–Z^8 Aa–Kk^8. 264 leaves, pp. *i–ii* iii–xvi *1* 2–512.

[Vol. III] *A Collection of Preternatural Cases and Observations in Midwifery.*

London: Printed for D. Wilson, and T. Durham, 1764.

8°: A^4 B–Z^8 Aa–Mm^8 Nn^4. 280 leaves, pp. *i–iii* iv–viii *1* 2–544 [8].

Blake, p. 421. GM 6154. *Heirs of Hippocrates* 825. Norman 1954. Waller 9013.

B] *A Sett of Anatomical Tables, with Explanations, and an Abridgment, of the Practice of Midwifery, with a View to Illustrate a Treatise on That Subject, and Collection of Cases.*

London, 1754.

1°: 22 leaves. 39 engraved plates by Charles Grignon after Jan van Rymsdyck and Pieter Camper.

Blake, p. 420. GM 6154.1. *Heirs of Hippocrates* 826. Norman 1955. Waller 9012.

Smellie, the foremost obstetrician of the eighteenth century, described more accurately than any previous writer the mechanical relation of the fetal head to the mother's pelvis during parturition. He introduced the English lock on the obstetrical forceps, and coincidentally with André Levret of Paris, added the pelvic curve. He was the first to rotate the fetal head with forceps and to use them on the aftercoming head of a breech delivery. Smellie was the first to lay down rules for the safe use of the forceps; these remain valid today. He also invented several important obstetric instruments.

Smellie's *Treatise on the Theory and Practice of Midwifery* was the first important textbook of obstetrics written by a Briton. Based on 1,150 deliveries, it is a general discussion of normal obstetrics, as well as of pathological problems. *A Collection of Cases and Observations . . .* (1754) and *A Collection of Preternatural Cases and Observations . . .* (1764) were presented as Volumes II and III of the *Treatise.* They consist largely of case histories collected from Smellie's extensive practice. Smellie began compiling the last volume in his retirement in Lanark, Scotland, and following his death it was completed by his friend, the novelist and physician Tobias Smollett (1721–71), who also practiced midwifery. The last five leaves of the *Treatise* consist of Smellie's advertisement for the forthcoming atlas of plates.

The *Sett of Anatomical Tables,* published two years after the first volume of the *Treatise,* was intended as a supplement to the text to illustrate as accurately as possible the female pelvis and the fetus. The plates in this classic of obstetrical illustration are far superior to any that had appeared before. They give everywhere a masterly representation, true to nature, of the relations of the parts of mother and child, and have perhaps contributed more to spreading correct ideas of labor than all the books that have ever been written on the subject. Of the thirty-nine plates, twenty-six were based on drawings by the Dutch comparative anatomist Jan van Rymsdyck. Eleven other plates were by one of Smellie's students from Holland, Dr. Pieter Camper, and Smellie himself is believed to have drawn the illustrations for the other two plates. All were beautifully engraved by Charles Grignon. Among the plates is the first illustration of a rachitic pelvis.

Smellie was born in Lanarkshire, Scotland. Following an apprenticeship with a local apothecary-physician, naval service, and general practice, he moved to London where he taught obstetrics in his own home. Smellie used mannequins fabricated from pelvic and fetal bones covered with leather to demonstrate obstetrics scientifically. He became a popular teacher, giving over 280 courses of midwifery to more than nine hundred pupils, among whom was William Hunter, brother of John Hunter (see no. 52).

LDL

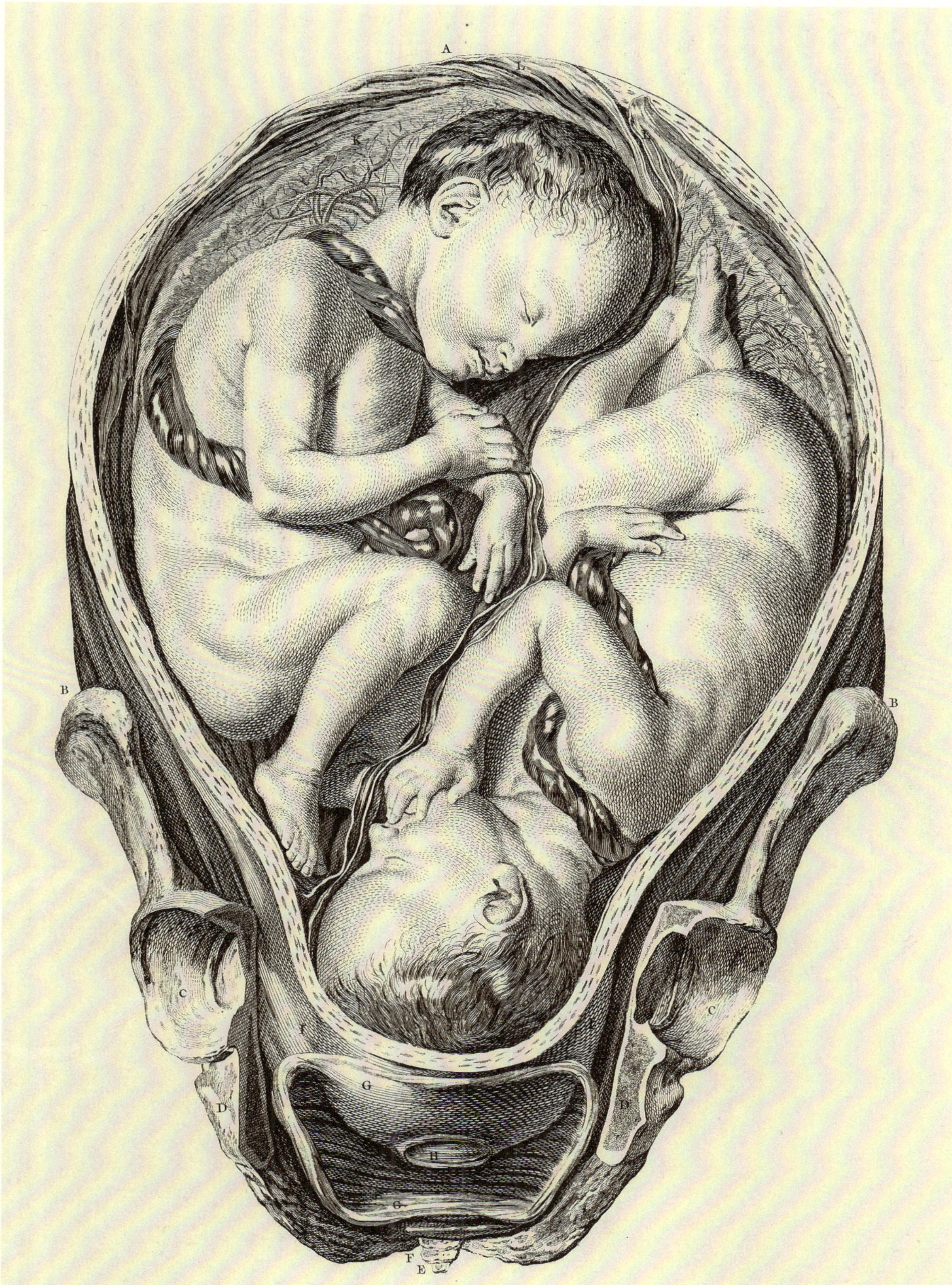

Fig. 82. No. 43B. Smellie. Twins *in utero*, from *A Sett of Anatomical Tables.*

A

TREATISE

OF THE

SCURVY.

IN THREE PARTS.

CONTAINING

An inquiry into the Nature, Cauſes, and Cure, of that Diſeaſe.

Together with

A Critical and Chronological View of what has been publiſhed on the ſubject.

By *JAMES LIND*, M. D.

Fellow of the Royal College of Phyſicians in *Edinburgh*.

EDINBURGH:

Printed by SANDS, MURRAY, and COCHRAN.

For A. KINCAID & A. DONALDSON.

MDCCLIII.

Fig. 83. No. 44. Lind. Title page of a copy with the variant imprint.

44

JAMES LIND
(1716–1794)

A Treatise of the Scurvy. In Three Parts. Containing an Inquiry into the Nature, Causes, and Cure, of that Disease. Together with a Critical and Chronological View of What Has Been Published on the Subject.
Edinburgh: Printed by Sands, Murray and Cochran, For A. Millar, London, 1753.

8°: [a]^4 b^4 A–Z^4 Aa–Zz^4 3A–3L^4. 236 leaves, pp. *i–v* vi–xv [1] *1* 2–456.

Blake, p. 272. GM 3713. Norman 1354.

A century before the absence of vitamin C in the diet was identified as the cause of scurvy, this disease, so long endemic among seamen, had largely disappeared. This was mainly due to the work of James Lind and to the publication in 1753 of his *Treatise of the Scurvy*, in which he drew upon his own experiences as a naval doctor to give a clear, clinical account of the disease and to demonstrate conclusively by experiment that orange and lemon juice were the only known effective cure.

Lind's controlled experiment was remarkable for its time.

> On the 20th of May 1747, I selected twelve patients in the scurvy, on board the "Salisbury" at sea. Their cases were as similar as I could have them. . . . They lay together in one place . . . and had one diet common to all. . . . Two of these were ordered each a quart of Cyder a-day. Two others took twenty-five drops of *elixir vitriol*, three times a-day, upon an empty stomach. . . . Two others took two spoonfuls of vinegar three times a-day. . . . Two of the worse patients . . . were put under a course of sea-water. Of this they drank half a pint every day. . . . Two others had each two oranges and one lemon given them every day. . . . The two remaining patients, took the bigness of a nutmeg three times a-day of an electuary recommended by an hospital-surgeon, made of garlic, mustard-seed, *rad. raphan.* [horse radish], balsam of Peru, and gum myrrh; using for common drink, barley-water well acidulated with tamarinds.[1]

Those on oranges and lemons were substantially cured in six days; those on cider improved slowly; the other remedies, standard in their time, were useless. However, in spite of this conclusive experiment, and the success of the antiscorbutics, based on Lind's suggestions, that were used during Cook's second voyage in 1774, it was not until 1795 that Lind's follower Gilbert Blane persuaded the Admiralty to issue citrus juices to ships' crews. This led to the rapid disappearance of scurvy at sea.

In addition to his own classic account of scurvy, Lind's book included selections on the disease from the writings of his predecessors. Among these, he drew attention to and commented on Johannes Bachstrom's *Observationes circa scorbutum* (1734). Bachstrom was the first to state categorically that scurvy was caused by a deficiency in the diet of fresh fruit and vegetables; Lind, however, was unable to concur with Bachstrom's hypothesis. Some of the difficulties Lind had in fully accepting this view were not resolved until the discovery of vitamins.

There are three issues of the first edition of *A Treatise of the Scurvy*: one with the imprint as given above; another, also dated 1753, with the imprint "Printed by Sands, Murray and Cochran, For A. Kincaid & A. Donaldson"; and a later issue of the first imprint that has the date 1754 on the title page. A second edition was published in 1757 and a third in 1772; in the latter the word *of* in the title was changed to *on*. French editions appeared in 1756 and 1783, an Italian translation in 1766, and a German version in 1775.[2]

RDG

1. James Lind, *A Treatise of the Scurvy* (Edinburgh, 1753), pp. 191–93.
2. Louis H. Roddis, *James Lind: Founder of Nautical Medicine* (New York, 1950), pp. 158–59, 161–62.

45

LEOPOLD AUENBRUGGER

(1722–1809)

Inventum novum ex percussione thoracis humani ut signo abstrusos interni pectoris morbos detegendi.

Vienna: Typis Joannis Thomae Trattner, 1761.

8°: A–F⁸. 48 leaves, pp. *1–11* 12–95 [1].

Bishop 1. Blake, p. 23. GM 2672. *Heirs of Hippocrates* 954. Norman 81. Osler 1863. Waller 519. Wellcome II, p. 70.

With the introduction of percussion of the chest, which offered a new and dependable method of diagnosing diseases of the heart and lungs in living persons, Leopold Auenbrugger made the first advance in physical diagnosis since the age of Hippocrates. The son of an innkeeper, Auenbrugger had learned as a boy how to establish the level of wine in a cask by thumping the barrel—"casks as long as they are empty are resonant everywhere, but when they are filled lose their resonance in proportion as the volume of air they contain is diminished."[1] Applying the same technique to the human chest, he noticed that different sounds—tympanitic, dull, or obscure—were produced when there was underlying disease of the heart or lungs in the interior of the chest. He verified his diagnoses by experiments on cadavers and by postmortems. After seven years of research, he published his results in 1761, in a small book of ninety-five pages; the English translation of its Latin title is "A new discovery, in which percussion of the human thorax is used to discover signs of hidden diseases of the chest." The book remains one of the classics of medicine, anticipating the later developments in physical diagnosis of René Théophile Laennec and Wilhelm Roentgen in the nineteenth century (see nos. 57 and 83) and Willem Einthoven and Godfrey Hounsfield in the twentieth (see nos. 89 and 100).

Auenbrugger had studied medicine at the University of Vienna under Gerhard van Swieten and Anton de Haen, disciples of Herman Boerhaave (see no. 39), who had emphasized the importance of bedside observation. However, both of these men ignored Auenbrugger's contribution, and the significance of his discovery was largely overlooked by the medical community. An early French translation of his work by Rozière de la Chassagne (1770) was buried at the end of Rozière's own treatise on pulmonary diseases and so attracted little notice,[2] and although Maximilian Stoll, de Haen's successor at Vienna, discussed percussion favorably in his lectures and publications, his early death cut short this support. In the late 1790s, however, the French physician Jean-Nicolas Corvisart learned of Auenbrugger's methods through Stoll's writings, particularly his *Aphorismi de cognoscendis et curandis febribus* (1786). After practicing percussion for several years, Corvisart was inspired to translate Auenbrugger's book in 1808,[3] a year before Auenbrugger's death; this led to the widespread acceptance of percussion as a diagnostic tool.

Two issues of Auenbrugger's book were printed in 1761, the first with leaf $F8^{v}$ blank and the second with errata on this page. A second edition was printed in 1763. In addition to the French translations, the book appeared in English in 1824 and in German in 1843.

HFN

1. Quoted in Ralph H. Major, *Classic Descriptions of Disease* (Springfield, Ill., 1932), p. 525.

2. Rozière de la Chassagne, *Manuel des pulmoniques* (Paris, 1770).

3. J.-N. Corvisart, *Nouvelle méthode pour reconnaître les maladies internes de la poitrine par la percussion de cette cavité* (Paris, 1808).

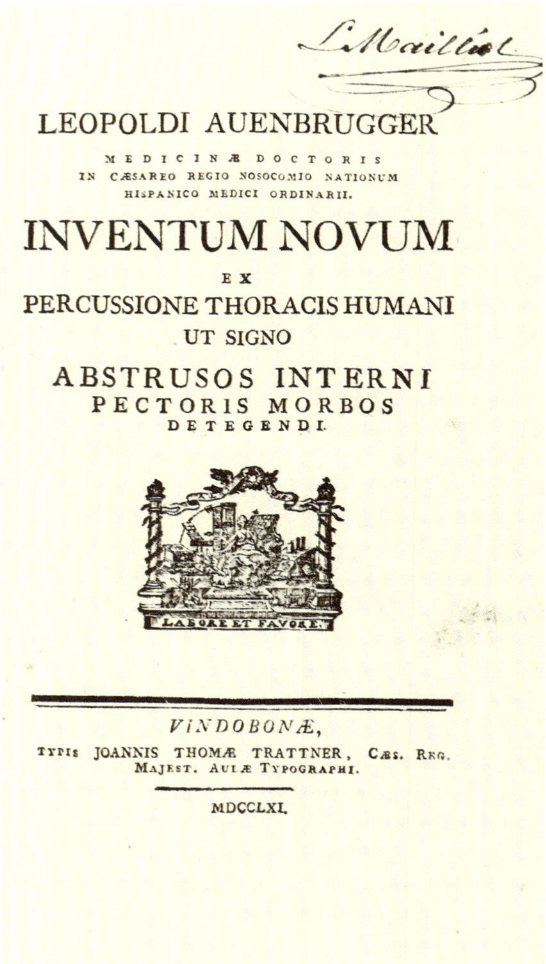
LEOPOLDI AUENBRUGGER

MEDICINÆ DOCTORIS
IN CÆSAREO REGIO NOSOCOMIO NATIONUM
HISPANICO MEDICI ORDINARII.

INVENTUM NOVUM
EX
PERCUSSIONE THORACIS HUMANI
UT SIGNO
ABSTRUSOS INTERNI
PECTORIS MORBOS
DETEGENDI.

LABORE ET FAVORE.

VINDOBONÆ,
TYPIS JOANNIS THOMÆ TRATTNER, CÆS. REG.
MAJEST. AULÆ TYPOGRAPHI.

MDCCLXI.

Fig. 84. No. 45. Auenbrugger. Title page.

46

GIOVANNI BATTISTA MORGAGNI
(1682–1771)

De sedibus, et causis morborum per anatomen indagatis libri quinque.
Venice: Ex typographia Remondiniana, 1761.

[Vol. I] 2°: [a]^4 b–m^4 A–Z^4 Aa–Nn^4 Oo^6. 198 leaves, pp. *I–VIII* IX–XCVI *1–2* 3–298 [2]. Title printed in red and black. Engraved frontispiece portrait by Jean Renard after Giovanni Volpato; engraved title vignette.

[Vol. II] 2°: A–Z^4 Aa–Zz^4 Aaa–Iii^4 Kkk^6. 226 leaves, pp. *1–2* 3–452. Engraved title vignette.

Blake, p. 312. GM 2276. *Heirs of Hippocrates* 792. Norman 1547. Osler 1178. PMM 206. Waller 6672. Zanelli, p. 144.

After Antonio Benivieni (see no. 12), Giovanni Battista Morgagni is considered the founder of pathological anatomy. His *De sedibus*, regarded as one of the most important books in the history of medicine, established a new era in medical research.

Morgagni was a teacher of anatomy at Padua from 1716 until his death in 1771. In his day the standard compilation of pathological case histories was Théophile Bonet's *Sepulchretum*, a huge work published in 1679; Bonet, however, made no attempt to analyze his findings and Morgagni found them unsatisfactory. The concept for Morgagni's book was provided by Marcello Malpighi (see no. 30), in whose tradition Morgagni had been schooled, and it is implicit in the title, "The seats and causes of diseases investigated through anatomy." Morgagni regarded the body as a collection of harmonious parts, many deep in the recesses of the body and discernible only through the microscope. He reasoned that failure of one of these parts was both the seat and cause of disease and that anatomical investigation would reveal the point of failure. Morgagni therefore set about compiling case histories and analyzing them. His methodical analysis and classification of symptoms systematized a branch of medicine hitherto studied in isolation and without method. He compared clinical symptoms with postmortem findings and in this way may be said to have laid the foundations of pathological anatomy. He drew not only on his own records, compiled during his long career, but also on existing literature and the records of his predecessors, in particular those of his teacher Antonio Maria Valsalva, whose posthumous papers Morgagni edited. The case histories included in the book therefore represent the work of an entire school of anatomists, from Malpighi to Morgagni himself.

There is hardly a phase of pathological anatomy observable with the naked eye that

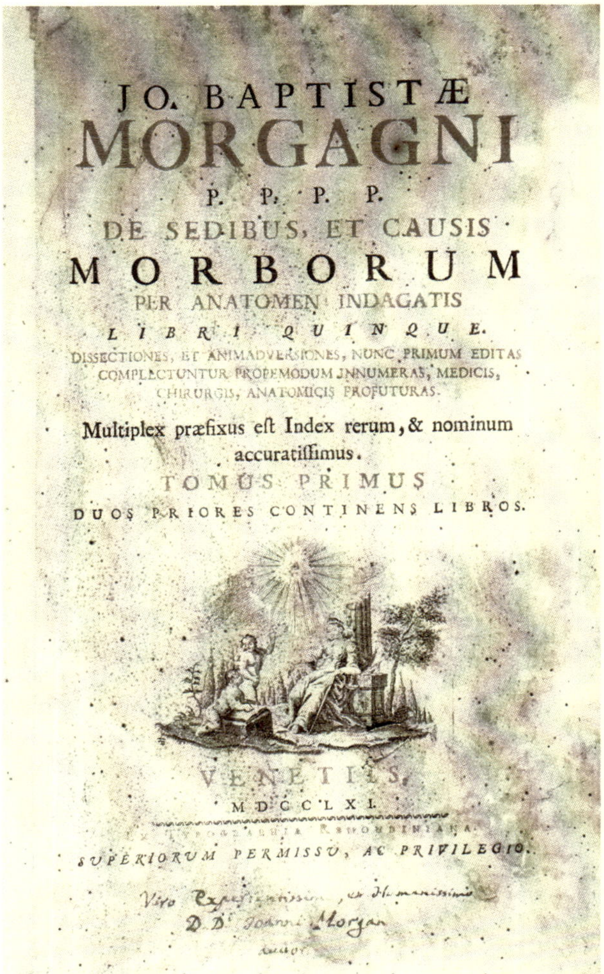

JO. BAPTISTÆ
MORGAGNI
P. P. P. P.
DE SEDIBUS, ET CAUSIS
MORBORUM
PER ANATOMEN INDAGATIS
LIBRI QUINQUE.
DISSECTIONES, ET ANIMADVERSIONES, NUNC PRIMUM EDITAS
COMPLECTUNTUR PROPEMODUM INNUMERAS, MEDICIS,
CHIRURGIS, ANATOMICIS PROFUTURAS.
Multiplex præfixus eſt Index rerum, & nominum
accuratiſſimus.
TOMUS PRIMUS
DUOS PRIORES CONTINENS LIBROS.
VENETIIS,
MDCCLXI.
SUPERIORUM PERMISSU, AC PRIVILEGIO.
Viro Expertissimo, et Humanissimo
D. D. Joanni Morgan
Auctor

Fig. 85. No. 46. Morgagni. Title pages of the set inscribed by Morgagni to his American namesake, Dr. John Morgan.

Morgagni did not cover in these two folio volumes. In accounts of about seven hundred necropsies, mostly by Morgagni, there are excellent descriptions of cancers, particularly of the pancreas, stomach, and rectum, and of renal calculi, cirrhosis of the liver, and atrophied kidneys. There is also an unmistakable description of typhoid fever. It is, though, in Morgagni's contribution to the pathology of the vascular system that the value of his method is best shown. Apoplexy was a subject of particular interest, and his descriptions of aneurysms are outstanding. On the other hand, it is interesting to note that the descriptions of pulmonary tuberculosis are unusually weak, as Morgagni understood the concept of contagion and refrained from exposing himself to unnecessary risk by dissecting the bodies of victims of certain highly infectious diseases.

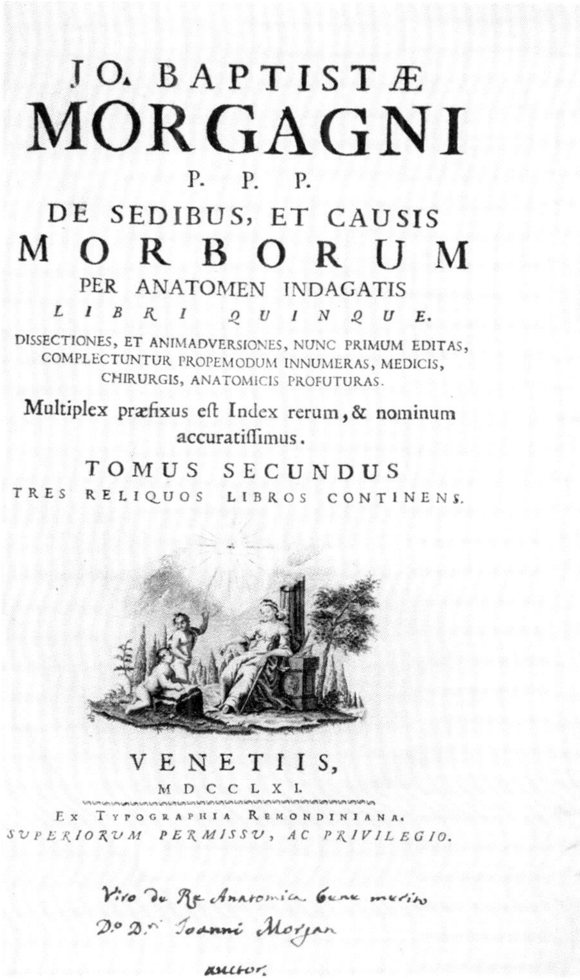

JO. BAPTISTÆ
MORGAGNI
P. P. P.
DE SEDIBUS, ET CAUSIS
MORBORUM
PER ANATOMEN INDAGATIS
LIBRI QUINQUE.
DISSECTIONES, ET ANIMADVERSIONES, NUNC PRIMUM EDITAS, COMPLECTUNTUR PROPEMODUM INNUMERAS, MEDICIS, CHIRURGIS, ANATOMICIS PROFUTURAS.
Multiplex præfixus eſt Index rerum, & nominum accuratiſſimus.
TOMUS SECUNDUS
TRES RELIQUOS LIBROS CONTINENS.

VENETIIS,
MDCCLXI.
Ex Typographia Remondiniana.
SUPERIORUM PERMISSU, AC PRIVILEGIO.

Viro de Re Anatomica bene merito
D.o D.ri Joanni Morgan
auctor.

The first issue of *De sedibus* had the title page of Volume I printed in red and black. In a second issue, also of 1761, the title page was printed entirely in black, and there exists at least one copy of the first edition with the imprint, Venice: Ex Typographia Remondiniana, 1762. The work was reprinted in Naples in 1762 and at Padua in 1765, as well as subsequently. A three-volume English translation by Benjamin Alexander appeared in 1769, a German translation in 1771–76, a French translation in 1821–24, and an Italian version in 1823–29.

NP

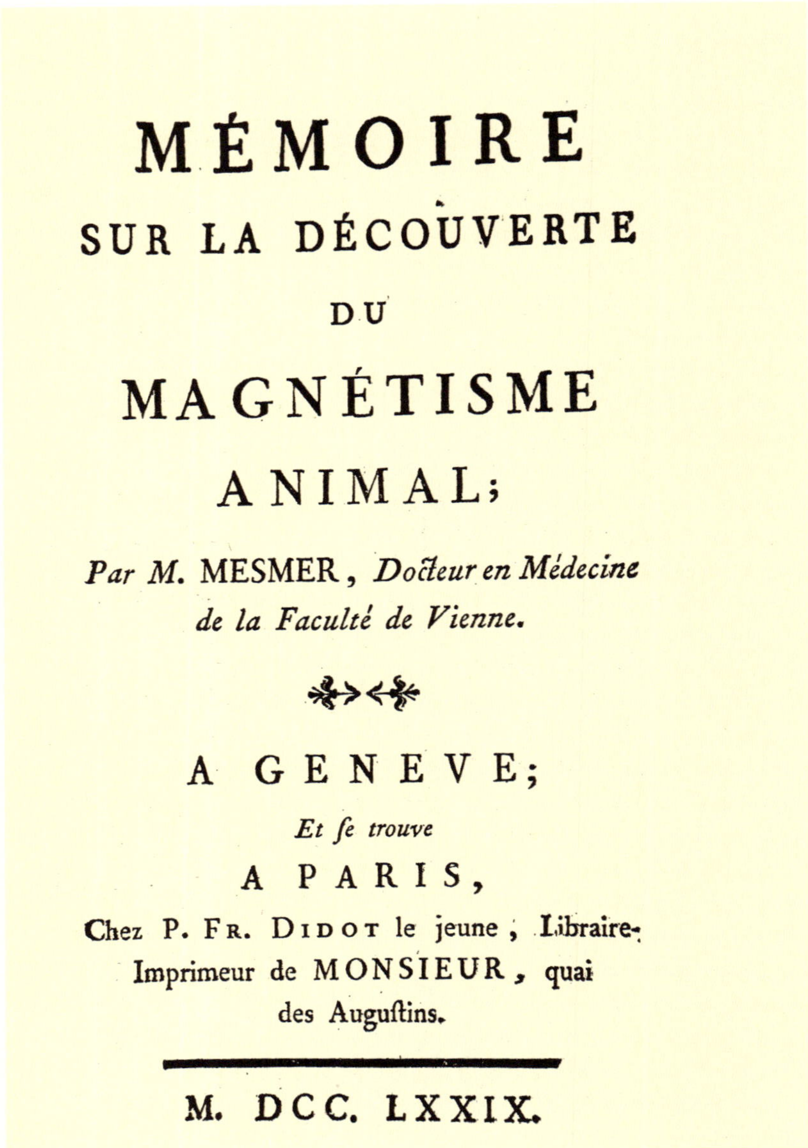

MÉMOIRE
SUR LA DÉCOUVERTE
DU
MAGNÉTISME
ANIMAL;

Par M. MESMER, *Docteur en Médecine de la Faculté de Vienne.*

A GENEVE;
Et se trouve
A PARIS,
Chez P. FR. DIDOT le jeune, Libraire-Imprimeur de MONSIEUR, quai des Augustins.

M. DCC. LXXIX.

Fig. 86. No. 47. Mesmer. Title page.

47

FRANZ ANTON MESMER
(1734–1815)

Mémoire sur la découverte du magnétisme animal.

Geneva & Paris: Chez P. Fr. Didot le jeune, 1779.

8°: π4 A–E8 F4. 48 leaves, pp. [2] *i–iii* iv–vi *1* 2–85 [3].

Blake, p. 302. EFDT 171. GM 4992.1. *Heirs of Hippocrates* 1013. Norman M4. PMM 225. Waller 6505.

The basis of Mesmer's fame has been described as the creative function of an erroneous idea. In his doctoral thesis in medicine at the University of Vienna, *Dissertatio physico-medica de planetarum influxu* (1766), Mesmer revived the ancient doctrine of the influence exerted by the gravitational forces of the sun, moon, and planets on human well-being. He believed that health was the result of harmony between the bodily organs and planetary gravitation (a force he called "animal gravitation"); disease was then a disharmony, and the purpose of treatment was to restore harmony or equilibrium. In 1775, inspired by the experiments of the Jesuit astronomer Maximilian Hell, Mesmer began to use magnets in his treatment of patients, producing in them first a trance or somnambulic state in which they were neither asleep nor awake, and then convulsions or a crisis that led to a cure. Accordingly, he now attempted to explain his treatment as due to "animal magnetism" in contrast to "mineral magnetism." He later found that he did not need the magnet to obtain these results but could produce them merely by touch.

Mesmer's practice and the claims he made aroused so much controversy and criticism in the medical community of Vienna that he decided in 1778 to move to Paris. Arriving on the eve of the French Revolution, he quickly captured the imagination of the Parisian public to the exclusion of nearly everything else; in fact, it has been shown that in France in the decade before the beginning of the French Revolution more literature was generated on mesmerism than on any other single topic.[1] In 1779 Mesmer published his *Mémoire sur la découverte du magnétisme animal*, his manifesto on the subject of animal magnetism, containing twenty-seven propositions that supposedly accounted for the cures he effected, as well as case histories of some of the patients he had treated successfully in Vienna. Another version of the work in duodecimo format, with different pagination, possibly a piracy, was also published in 1779. A second edition appeared in 1781, and a German translation also in 1781. An English translation was not published until 1948.

Mesmer's activities and the excitement they produced aroused the concern of the

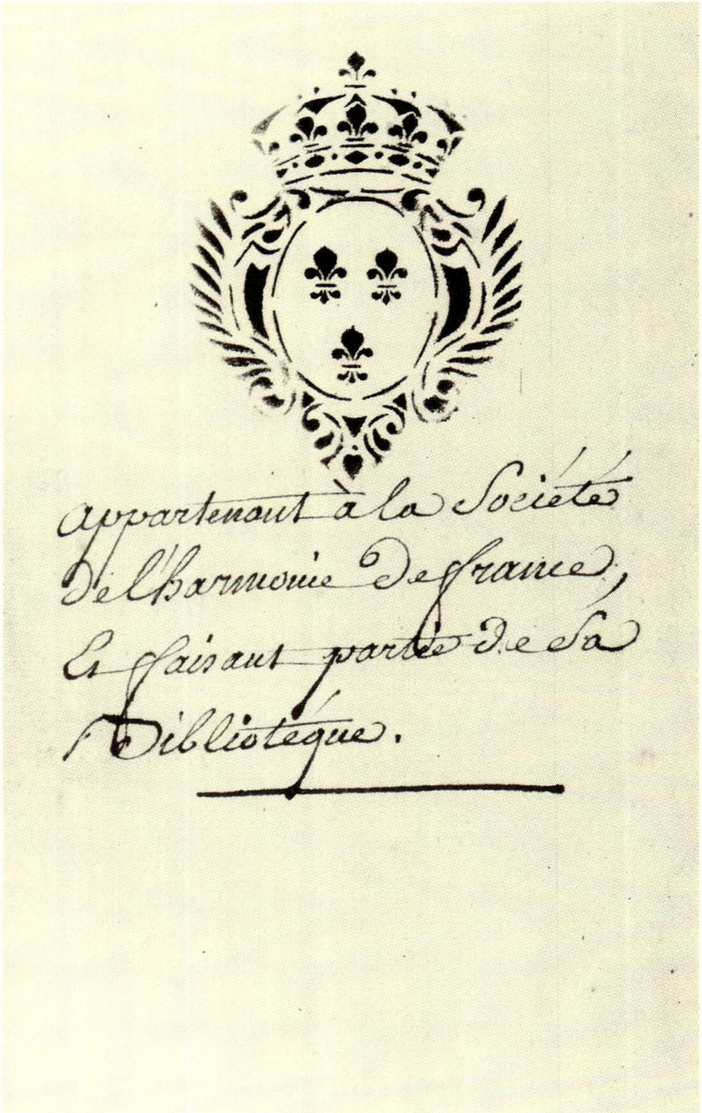

Fig. 87. No. 47. Mesmer. The Society of Harmony's ownership stamp and inscription.

Parisian medical community, which in 1784 prevailed upon the king of France to appoint a royal commission to investigate Mesmer's work. The commission, which included such scientific notables as Benjamin Franklin, the chemist Antoine Lavoisier, and Dr. Joseph-Ignace Guillotin, found no evidence of the physical magnetic force claimed by Mesmer; rather, its members attributed all the phenomena they witnessed to the effects of the imagination. Ironically, Mesmer refused to credit the agency of the mind in any of his cures and insisted upon a physical explanation throughout the remainder of his life.

Mesmer left France about 1789, spending the rest of his life in obscurity; however, his many followers or "magnetists" continued their practice for several decades. In 1841 the English surgeon James Braid began an investigation of mesmeric phenomena after attending a popular demonstration of mesmerism and reported his observations in a book entitled *Neurypnology; or, The Rationale of Nervous Sleep, Considered in Relation with Animal Magnetism* (1843). It was Braid who coined the terms "hypnosis," "hypnotism," and "hypnotize," from the Greek *hypnos*, meaning sleep. His work established the fact that subjects in hypnosis were very susceptible to suggestion and that this was the basis of its therapeutic potential. In 1866 a French physician, A. A. Liébeault, stressed the fact that suggestibility was the most important feature of the hypnotic state, an idea also advocated by Liébeault's disciple Hippolyte Bernheim. Sigmund Freud (see no. 87), a student of Bernheim, treated his patients with hypnosis and suggestion and then used hypnosis to recover forgotten memories, eventually developing from hypnosis the techniques of free association and psychoanalysis.

HFN

1. Robert Darnton, "Mesmer, Franz Anton," in *Dictionary of Scientific Biography*, vol. 9 (New York, 1974), p. 327.

A

TREATISE

ON

THE DISEASES OF CHILDREN,

WITH DIRECTIONS

FOR THE MANAGEMENT OF INFANTS

FROM THE BIRTH;

ESPECIALLY

Such as are brought up *by Hand.*

By MICHAEL UNDERWOOD, M. D.

LICENTIATE in MIDWIFERY

OF THE

Royal College *of* PHYSICIANS in LONDON,

AND

PRACTITIONER at the BRITISH LYING-IN HOSPITAL.

Ornari Res ipsa negat, contenta doceri. HOR.

LONDON,

Printed for J. MATHEWS, No. 18, Strand.

MDCCLXXXIV.

Fig. 88. No. 48. Underwood. Title page.

48

MICHAEL UNDERWOOD
(1736–1820)

A Treatise on the Diseases of Children, with Directions for the Management of Infants from the Birth; Especially Such as are Brought Up by Hand.

London: Printed for J. Mathews, 1784.

8°: a^{6} A–S^{8}. 150 leaves, pp. *i–iii* iv–xii *1* 2–288.

Blake, p. 463. GM 6326. *Heirs of Hippocrates* 1024. Norman 2121. Osler 4144.

Michael Underwood was the most advanced pediatrician of his day. He studied surgery and midwifery (a field that then included both obstetrics and pediatrics) in both London and Paris. In 1779 he was appointed surgeon to the British Lying-In Hospital, and in 1784 he became one of the few physicians licensed in midwifery by the Royal College of Physicians. His distinction was such that he was called upon to treat many notables, and in 1796 he attended the Princess of Wales at the birth of Princess Charlotte, the first legitimate grandchild of King George III.

Underwood's influential *Treatise on the Diseases of Children* (1784) remained an important pediatric text for over sixty years and initiated the modern study of the diseases of childhood. The single-volume first edition, addressed to both the medical profession and the laity, provided the first description of sclerema neonatorum ("Underwood's disease"), as well as accounts of some forty "new disorders" of children. The book discussed pediatric luxations and fractures, subjects that had been neglected for two hundred years, and included a pioneering essay on infant psychology. Most significant, however, was Underwood's discussion of artificial infant feeding, a practice that originated in his century. His formulation of boiled cow's milk diluted with barley water was the closest approximation to mother's milk at that time and was certainly more appropriate for infant feeding than the boiled bread, beer, and other unsuitable foodstuffs that had previously been recommended.[1]

A total of seven editions of Underwood's book were published during his lifetime, each directed more and more toward the medical profession. The second edition (1789), a two-volume work, gave the first account of poliomyelitis, and for this Underwood is now recognized as one of the founders of pediatric neurology. In the fourth edition (1799), a three-volume work, he gave the first description of congenital heart disease, which makes him one of the pioneers of pediatric cardiology. The last edition during his lifetime was published in 1819. Posthumous editions appeared in 1827 (ed. S. Merriman), 1835 (ed. Marshall Hall), and 1846 (ed. H. Davies). American editions were published in 1793, 1806, 1841, and 1842; French editions in 1786 and 1823; and a German edition in 1848.

HFN

1. Fielding H. Garrison, *An Introduction to the History of Medicine*, 4th ed. (Philadelphia, 1929), p. 402.

See color plate XXIII.

49

WILLIAM WITHERING
(1741–1799)

An Account of the Foxglove, and Some of Its Medical Uses: With Practical Remarks on Dropsy, and Other Diseases.

Birmingham: Printed by M. Swinney; For G. G. J. and J. Robinson, London, 1785.

8°: a^4 b^8 A–N^8. 116 leaves, pp. [2] *i–v* vi–xx [2] *1* 2–207 [1]. 1 folding engraved plate, which occurs in three states: (1) uncolored, with the two lower leaves pointing left, signed by the artist J. Sowerby; (2) a hand-colored version of this plate; and (3) a reverse of this image, hand-colored, with the two lower leaves pointing right.

Blake, p. 493. GM 1836. *Heirs of Hippocrates* 1039. Hunt 676. Norman 2255. Osler 4261. Waller 10378.

William Withering, the son of an apothecary, was born in Wellington, Shropshire, England, in 1741. He received his medical degree from the University of Edinburgh, then the world's leading center for medical training. After a tour of the Continent he returned to England to practice medicine in a village near his birthplace. In 1775 he moved to Birmingham seeking a more lucrative practice and more intellectual stimulation from colleagues who shared his scientific interests.

Withering first recognized the therapeutic value of foxglove (*Digitalis purpurea*) in 1775, when he identified it as the active ingredient in a folk remedy that contained nearly two dozen herbs. He used digitalis for a decade before publishing his experience in 1785 in *An Account of the Foxglove, and Some of its Medical Uses*, in which he described the effects of administering *Digitalis purpurea* to more than 150 patients. Based on his administration of various doses of the drug, Withering concluded that digitalis could produce dramatic improvement in the signs and symptoms of dropsy or heart failure. It was not a benign drug, however—many patients developed side effects, some individuals had seizures or syncopal attacks, and a few died after receiving digitalis. Withering was most impressed by digitalis's effectiveness as a diuretic, and he also recognized its remarkable effect on the action of the heart. In some patients the heartbeat slowed dramatically with administration of the drug.

Withering supplemented his own observations on the effects of digitalis with reports and testimonials from other physicians and apothecaries who used the drug, and they in turn learned much about its administration from Withering's monograph. The book was

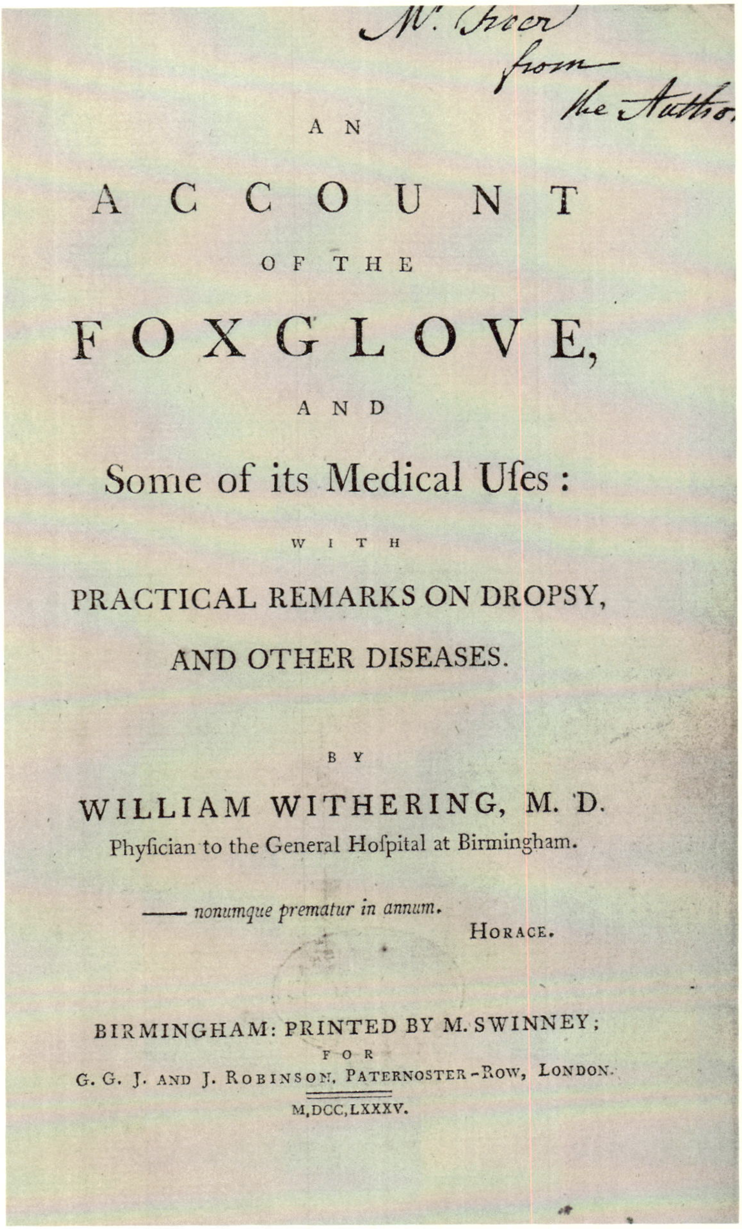

Mr. Freer from the Author.

AN

ACCOUNT

OF THE

FOXGLOVE,

AND

Some of its Medical Ufes:

WITH

PRACTICAL REMARKS ON DROPSY,

AND OTHER DISEASES.

BY

WILLIAM WITHERING, M. D.

Phyfician to the General Hofpital at Birmingham.

—— *nonumque prematur in annum.*

HORACE.

BIRMINGHAM: PRINTED BY M. SWINNEY;

FOR

G. G. J. AND J. ROBINSON, PATERNOSTER-ROW, LONDON.

M,DCC,LXXXV.

Fig. 89. No. 49. Withering. Title page. Presentation copy to Mr. Freer, who contributed a case history to Withering's book.

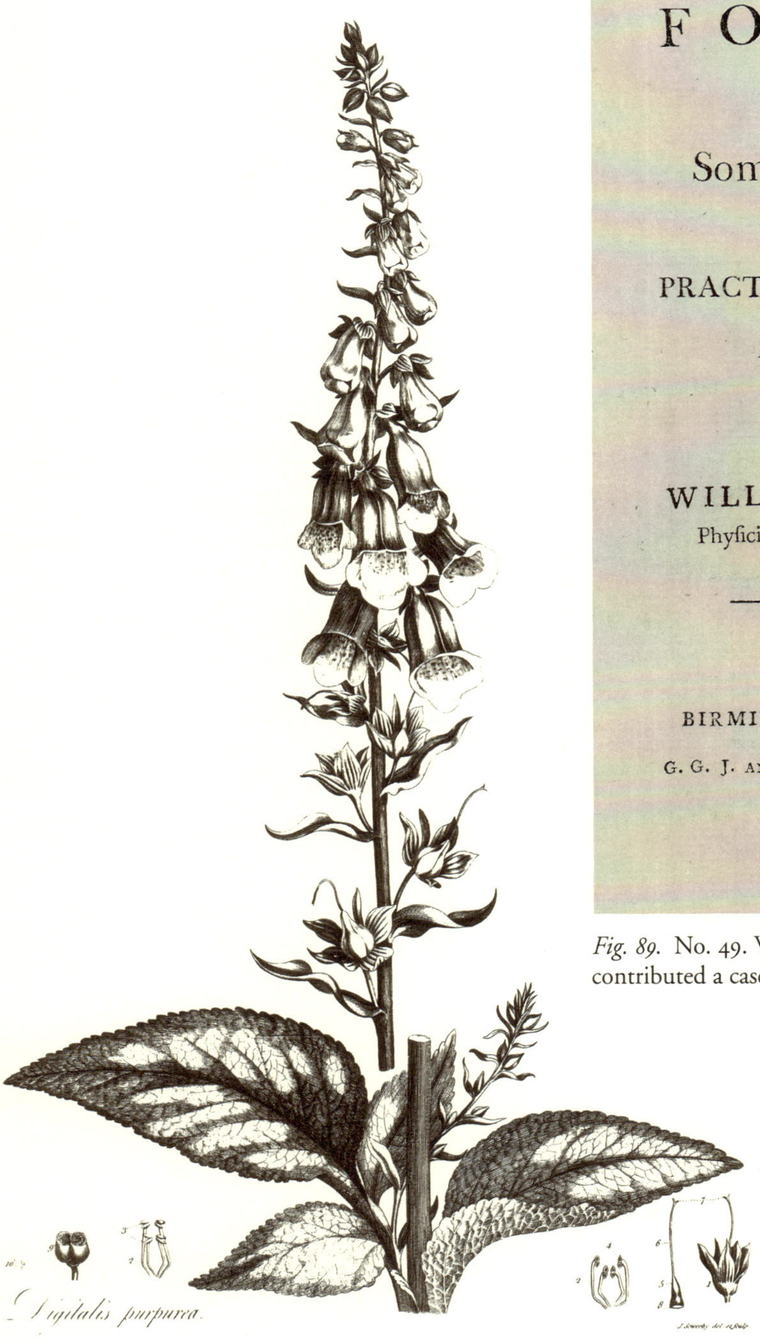

Fig. 90. No. 49. Withering. The folding plate of the foxglove plant in its uncolored state.

more than the narrative of the introduction of a new drug into medical practice; it represented one of the earliest examples of clinical research.

WBF

On page xxi of *An Account of the Foxglove*, Withering stated that "the figure of the Foxglove, facing the Title Page, is copied by the permission and under the inspection of Mr. [William] Curtis, from his admirable work, entitled *Flora Londinensis* [1777]." This copied figure, a mirror image of the foxglove in Curtis's work, was signed by the artist and engraver, James Sowerby, a contributor to *Flora Londinensis* who may also have been responsible for the unsigned original published in that work. The Sowerby plate exists in two versions, uncolored and hand-colored; the few known presentation copies of Withering's work all have this plate uncolored, which has led some bibliographers to conclude that copies with uncolored plates are of the earliest issue. Copies with uncolored plates sold for four shillings while those with colored plates cost five shillings[1]; it may be that Withering gave his friends copies with uncolored plates to save a shilling! Some copies of *An Account of the Foxglove* contain the original plate from *Flora Londinensis* instead of Sowerby's signed version—since Withering's work remained in print at least until 1798, it is possible that the publisher ran out of Sowerby's plates before exhausting the edition and had to substitute plates from Curtis's publication in late-selling copies. At least one bibliographer, however, has argued that the publisher began with a supply of *Flora Londinensis* plates and that the plate was reengraved only after these were exhausted.[2] The *Flora Londinensis* plate may be distinguished from Sowerby's plate by the following characteristics: the *Flora Londinensis* plate is unsigned, and the two lower leaves on the foxglove stem point to the right.

HFN

1. J. K. Aronson, *An Account of the Foxglove and Its Medical Uses 1785–1985* (London, 1985), p. xxi (n); Patricia C. Want, "Medical Books from 1701 to 1800," in *Thornton's Medical Books, Libraries and Collectors*, 3d ed., ed. Alain Besson (Aldershot, 1990), p. 136.
2. Estelle Brodman, "Two Different Plates in Withering's *Account of the Foxglove*," *Bulletin of the History of Medicine* 17 (1945): 414–17.

See color plates XXIV and XXV.

ALOYSII GALVANI

DE

VIRIBUS ELECTRICITATIS

IN

MOTU MUSCULARI.

COMMENTARIUS.

BONONIÆ

Ex Typographia Inſtituti Scientiarum. 1791.

CUM APPROBATIONE.

Fig. 91. No. 50. Galvani. Title page, second issue of the offprint.

50

LUIGI GALVANI
(1737–1798)

De viribus electricitatis in motu musculari commentarius.
In: *De Bononiensi Scientiarum et Artium Instituto atque Academia Commentarii.* Tomus Septimus.

Bologna: Ex Typographia Instituti Scientiarum, 1791 (imprimatur: 27 March 1791).

[journal volume] 4°: a–h4 A–Z4 Aa–Zz4 Aaa–Ooo4. 272 leaves, pp. *1–6* 7–62 [2], 1–478 [2]. Tab. I–II: 2 folding letterpress tables; [1], Tab. 1–3, [9], Tav. 1–4, [1]: 18 engraved plates (13 folding); 1 folding engraved map; engraved title vignette.

[article] Zzz2r–Ggg1v, pp. 363–418. Tav. 1–4: 4 folding engraved plates.

Fulton & Stanton 1. GM 593. Horblit 37a. Osler 1242.

[offprint, first issue] *De viribus electricitatis in motu musculari commentarius.*

4°: A–G4 H1. 29 leaves, pp. *1–2* 3–58. Tav. 1–4: 4 folding engraved plates by J. Zambelli.

With the half-title only. The type pages from the journal volume were reimposed and renumbered.

Fulton & Stanton 2.

[offprint, second issue] *De viribus electricitatis in motu musculari commentarius.*

Bologna: Ex Typographia Instituti Scientiarum, 1791.

4°: A4 (±A1) B–G4 H1. 29 leaves, pp. *1–2* 3–58. Tav. 1–4: 4 folding engraved plates by J. Zambelli.

Gathering A has been entirely reset.

Fulton & Stanton 3.

Although the existence of electricity has been recognized for many centuries, it was not until the eighteenth century, with the invention of man-made apparatus for its creation, that the study of electricity became a science. That electricity was involved somehow in the function of living tissue had been noted in studies of the activity of electric fishes and eels, but it was Luigi Galvani, professor of anatomy in Bologna, who first carried out systematic experiments demonstrating that muscular contraction could result from an electric current.

Galvani, born in Bologna and trained as a physician, was appointed public lecturer in anatomy in 1762 and first gained fame as a comparative anatomist with his researches on

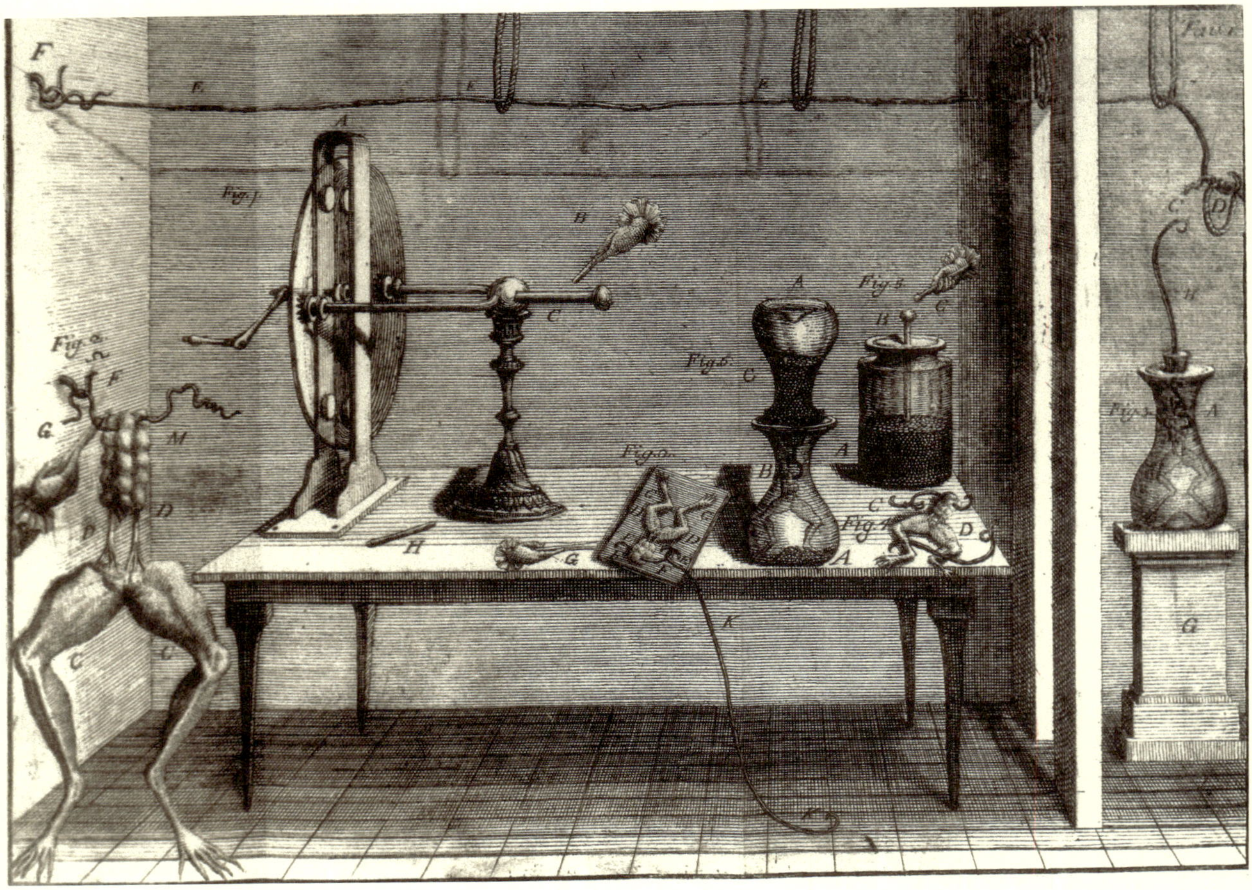

Fig. 92. No. 50. Galvani's experiments with "animal electricity."

the ear. In 1780 he began to study the effect of electric discharge on the nervous system of the frog, using a Leyden jar and an electrostatic machine. One day Galvani prepared a frog and "placed it upon a table on which there was an electric machine. . . . The frog was entirely separated from the conductor of the machine, and indeed was at no small distance away from it."[1] Galvani's assistant by chance touched the frog's exposed crural nerve with the metal blade of a scalpel at the same time that the electric machine was discharging a spark, whereupon the frog's muscles contracted violently. In further investigating this phenomenon, he discovered that muscular contractions could be produced even in the absence of an electrical machine, simply by utilizing two different metals to contact the muscle and its accompanying nerve. From these observations Galvani developed a theory that "animal electricity" originated in animal tissue, and he concluded that muscular activity was the result of the connection, by means of a metal conductor, between negative external charges and positive internal charges. He outlined this theory in "De viribus electricitatis in motu musculari commentarius," published in 1791 both in the *Commentaries of the Academy and Institute of Arts and Sciences of Bologna* and in offprint form.

Galvani's theory was of course erroneous: his results were in fact due to the generation of electricity by two dissimilar metals in a moist environment, a phenomenon fully investigated and reported by Alessandro Volta in the decade following the publication of Galvani's article. Nevertheless, despite the failure of his theory, Galvani's investigations showed that electric currents can produce measurable biologic phenomena, and thus they provided a foundation for the study of electrophysiology.

AEL

1. Quoted in Bern Dibner, *Galvani–Volta* (Norwalk, Conn., 1952), p. 11.

ALOYSII GALVANI

DE VIRIBUS ELECTRICITATIS

IN MOTU MUSCULARI.

COMMENTARIUS.

Fig. 93. No. 50. Galvani. Detail of the half-title from the first issue of the offprint.

THE

MORBID ANATOMY

OF

SOME OF THE MOST IMPORTANT PARTS

OF THE

HUMAN BODY.

BY

MATTHEW BAILLIE, M.D. F.R.S.

FELLOW OF THE ROYAL COLLEGE OF PHYSICIANS, AND PHYSICIAN OF ST. GEORGE'S HOSPITAL.

LONDON:

PRINTED FOR J. JOHNSON, ST. PAUL'S CHURCH-YARD; AND G. NICOL, PALL-MALL.

1793.

Fig. 94. No. 51A. Baillie. Title page of *The Morbid Anatomy.*

51

MATTHEW BAILLIE
(1761–1823)

A] *The Morbid Anatomy of Some of the Most Important Parts of the Human Body.*

London: Printed for J. Johnson, and G. Nicol, 1793.

8°: π^2 a^8 b^6 B–U^8 X^6. 174 leaves, pp. [4] *i* ii–xxviii *1* 2–314 [2].

Blake, p. 27. Crainz I.1. GM 2281. *Heirs of Hippocrates* 1176. Norman 108. Wellcome II, p. 87.

B] *A Series of Engravings, Accompanied with Explanations, Which are Intended to Illustrate the Morbid Anatomy of Some of the Most Important Parts of the Human Body.*

London: Printed by W. Bulmer and Co. for J. Johnson, and G. and W. Nicol, 1803.

4°: π^2 $[A]^4$ B–E^4 F^2 G–H^4 I^2 K1 L–N^4 O^4 (–O4) P–Q^4 R^4 (–R4) S–T^4 U^2 X–Y^4 Z^2 Aa–Kk^4. 121 leaves, pp. [4] *i* ii *3* 4–228 [10]. Pl. 1–6 (fasc. 1), pl. 1–4 V 6 (fasc. 2), pl. 1 II 3 IV 5–7 (fasc. 3), pl. 1–9 (fasc. 4), pl. I–III 4–6 VII (fasc. 5), pl. 1 II–III 4 V 6 VII–VIII (fasc. 6), pl. I–VI (fasc. 7), pl. I–II 3–5 VI–VII 8 (fasc. 8), pl. 1 II–III 4–5 VI 7–8 (fasc. 9), pl. 1–2 III–IV 5–7 VIII (fasc. 10): 73 engraved plates after drawings by William Clift.

Blake, p. 27. Crainz II.1. GM 2282. Norman 109. Osler 1891. Wellcome II, p. 87.

Baillie's two books are rightly taken together. The *Series of Engravings* illustrates many of the specimens described in the unillustrated *Morbid Anatomy*, which for its part gives clinical background for many of the engraved specimens. Each can also be used independently.

Matthew Baillie was a nephew of the Hunter brothers William (1718–83) and John (1728–93; see no. 52), who dominated the medical world of their day in London. All were Scots. Baillie studied anatomy with William who left him £5,000, his house and premises in Great Windmill Street, and the use of his museum (the majority of the specimens illustrated in Baillie's *Series of Engravings* came from William Hunter's collection). Baillie became a very successful physician; he was the last recipient of the gold-headed cane that was originally owned by John Radcliffe (1650–1729) and that passed successively to Richard Mead (1673–1754), Anthony Askew (1722–74), and William Pitcairn (1711–91).[1] After 1799 Baillie devoted himself to clinical practice, becoming physician to King George III.

Baillie is best remembered for his two books, of which the first, *The Morbid Anatomy* (1793), went into ten English and three American editions and was translated into

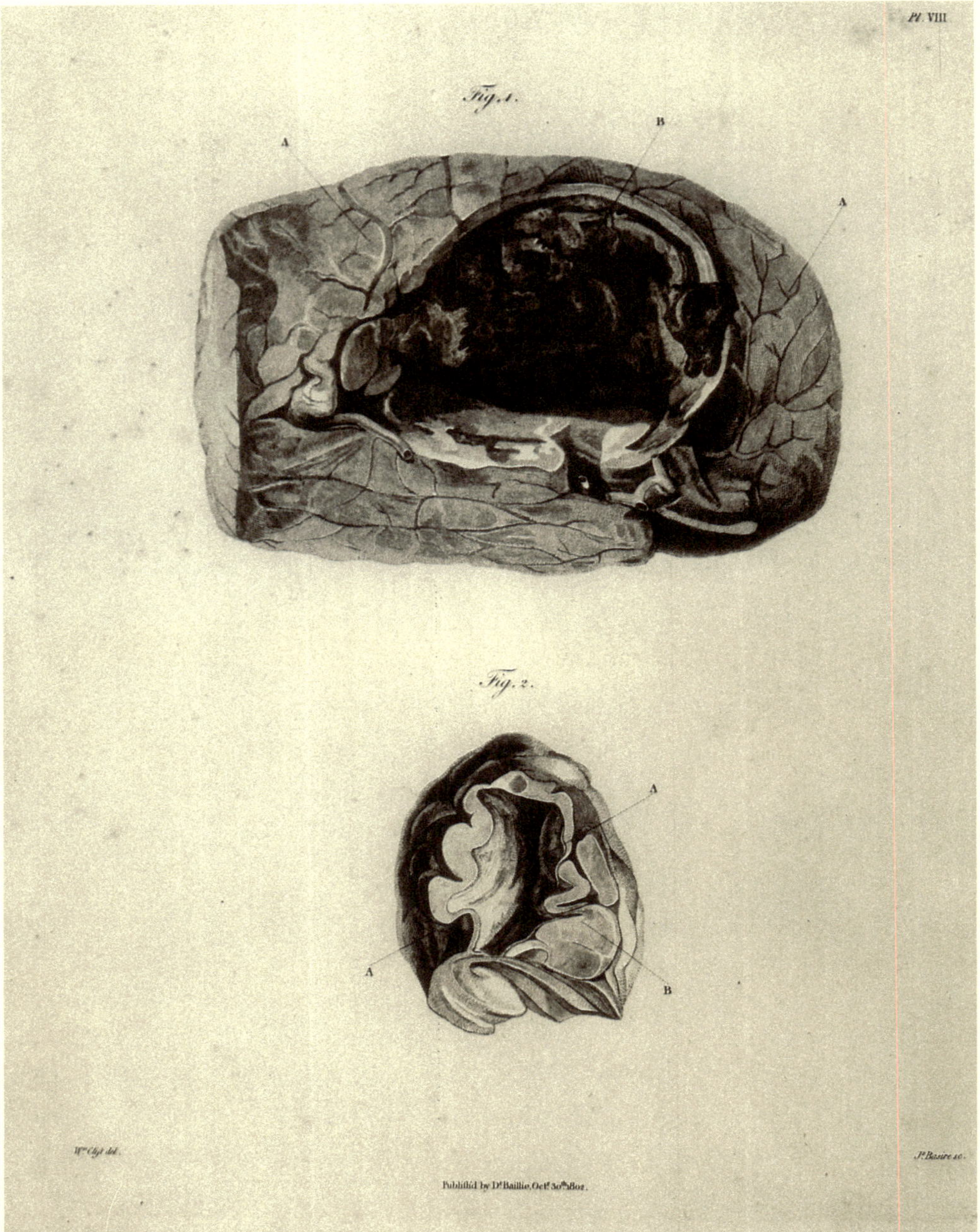

Fig. 95. No. 51B. Baillie. Plate VIII of *A Series of Engravings*, showing the error of the engraver James Basire in keying the illustration.

German, French, Italian, and Russian. This unillustrated text was the first book to treat pathology as an independent science and to deal with disease systematically according to the organs involved. Between 1799 and 1802 Baillie issued, in ten fascicles, his *Series of Engravings*. Copies of this title bound from the original fascicles bear the date 1799 and Fasciculus I on the title page; the complete work was also issued in 1803, with an additional half-title, dedication, and index, and with the first fascicle reprinted in slightly larger type. The drawings from which the engravings were made were done by William Clift (1775–1849),[2] who was paid one guinea per drawing; the engravers William Skelton (1763–1848), James Basire (1769–1822), and James Heath (1757–1834) were paid five guineas per plate. The engraving for Fasc. 10, Plate 8, Fig. 2 contains an error by James Basire, who keyed the lines improperly—his line B does not enter the cavity, which it should do in keeping with the caption. The error may have arisen from Clift's request that his drawing "be engraved with the lower end upward so that the whole will be inverted"—an added difficulty for any engraver.

The descriptions in both works have the simplicity and accuracy characteristic of a good observer; for example, Baillie's account of cholesterol in gallstones: "white splendid matter, like spermaceti or mica." His interpretations are often astonishingly modern; for example: "the most common tubercle of the liver" (cirrhosis) is "commonly produced by a long habit of drinking spirituous liquors"; hydatids of the liver "would seem to be animalcules of a very simple structure"; and polycystic disease of the kidney is referred to as "the spurious hydatid." Since 1849 it has been generally accepted and widely publicized that the specimen of lung depicted in Fasc. 2, Plate 6, Fig. 1 is an example of emphysema and came from the body of Dr. Samuel Johnson. The lung in the plate, however, shows diffuse interstitial fibrosis and not emphysema, and it has been recently proved that it could not have come from Dr. Johnson.[3] It is very likely, however, that Baillie gave a description of Dr. Johnson's emphysematous lung on page 51 of his *Morbid Anatomy*.

HA

1. William Macmichael, *The Gold-Headed Cane: A Facsimile of the Author's 1827 Copy Illustrated and Interleaved with His Own Amendments and Additions*, ed. Thomas Hunt (London, 1968), pp. 152–79.

2. Clift, who had been technical assistant to John Hunter for eighteen months before Hunter's death, became the first Curator of the Hunterian Collection in the Royal College of Surgeons and was made a Fellow of the Royal Society in 1823.

3. Harold D. Attwood, "A Dissertation upon the Lung of the Late Dr Samuel Johnson, the Great Lexicographer," *Lancet*, no. 8469/70 (21/28 Dec. 1985): 1411–13.

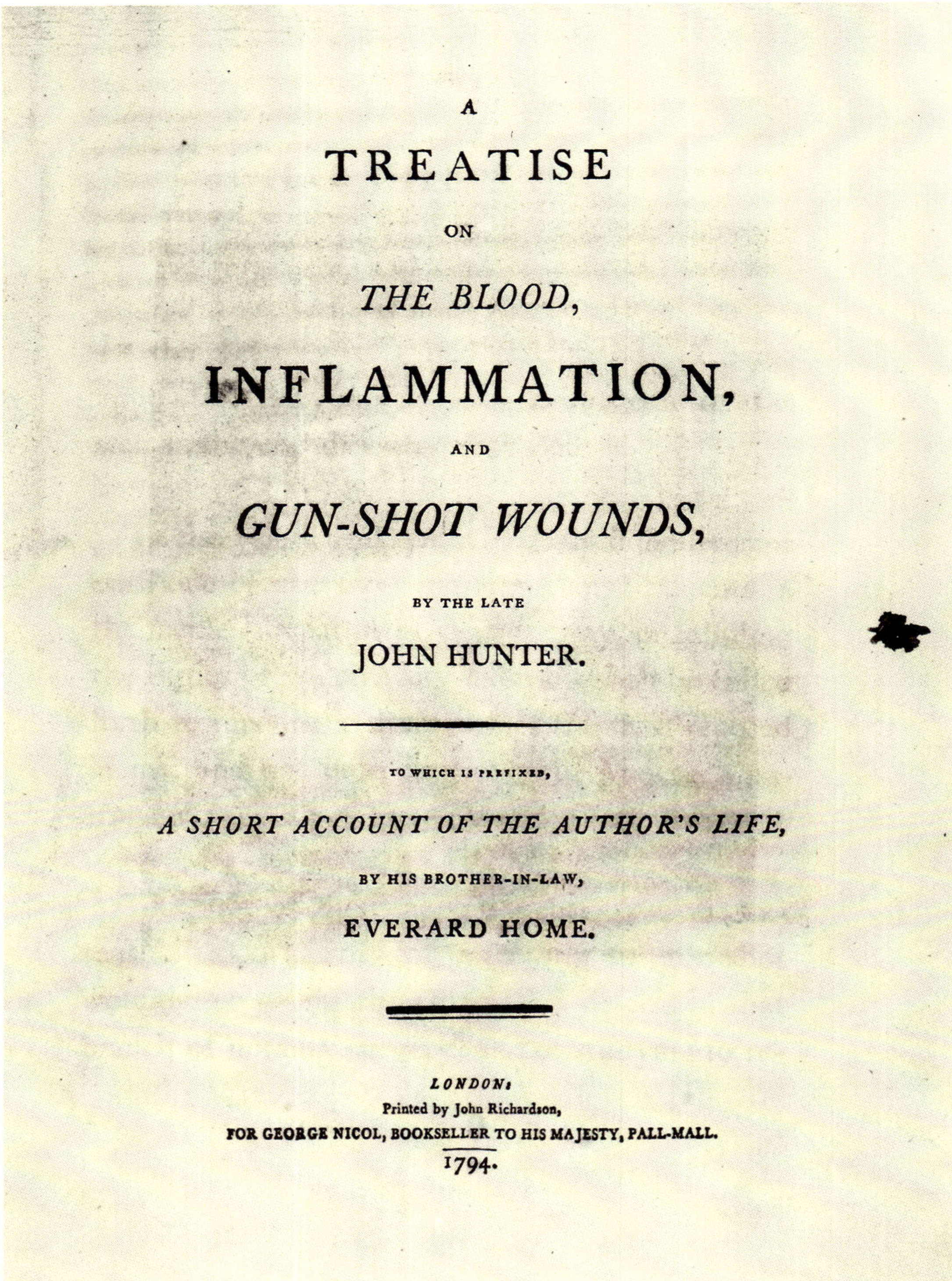

A

TREATISE

ON

THE BLOOD,

INFLAMMATION,

AND

GUN-SHOT WOUNDS,

BY THE LATE

JOHN HUNTER.

TO WHICH IS PREFIXED,

A SHORT ACCOUNT OF THE AUTHOR'S LIFE,

BY HIS BROTHER-IN-LAW,

EVERARD HOME.

LONDON:

Printed by John Richardson,

FOR GEORGE NICOL, BOOKSELLER TO HIS MAJESTY, PALL-MALL.

1794.

Fig. 96. No. 52. Hunter. Title page.

52

JOHN HUNTER
(1728–1793)

A Treatise on the Blood, Inflammation, and Gun-Shot Wounds. . . . To Which is Prefixed, a Short Account of the Author's Life, by His Brother-in-Law, Everard Home.

London: Printed by John Richardson, for George Nicol, 1794.

4°: [a]4 b–h4 i2 B–Z4 Aa–Zz4 3A–3Z4 4A–4D4. 322 leaves, pp. *i–ii* iii–lxvii [1] 1–575 [1]. Engraved frontispiece portrait of Hunter by William Sharp after the painting by Joshua Reynolds; Pl. [1], I–VIII: 9 engraved plates by William Skelton.

Blake, p. 226. GM 2283. *Heirs of Hippocrates* 972. Norman 1122. Osler 1230. Waller 4997. Wellcome III, p. 317.

The younger brother of William Hunter (1718–83), John Hunter came to London from Edinburgh initially as his brother's assistant and later studied under William Cheselden and Percivall Pott. By his natural talents and great industry he became house surgeon at St. George's Hospital in 1756, but his relentless work affected his health, and he was advised to go abroad. He took an appointment with the army and was sent with the British expedition to Belle Isle off the French coast in 1761. While on this service he began to assemble the material for this book, as he had ample opportunity to experience the surgery of gunshot wounds at first hand. After two years' service abroad Hunter returned to London and embarked on a life of unrelenting hard work, teaching, researching, writing, and running his private practice. He died of angina pectoris the year before the publication of his *Treatise*, having revised only a third of the proofs; the work was issued posthumously by his nephew Matthew Baillie (see no. 51) and his brother-in-law Everard Home. Hunter belongs to the select band of physicians whose books contain descriptions of their own fatal illnesses—in Hunter's case the description, drawn from his own notes, was included by Home in the biography included in the book.

Hunter's *Treatise on the Blood, Inflammation and Gun-Shot Wounds* is a work of great magnitude, easily the largest work by a British surgeon to date. His studies on inflammation in particular are fundamental for pathology, as there had been little understanding of the subject before his time. He classified inflammation into three types and was the first to assess and describe three essential factors of wound pathology: first, that an external agent in the air, and not the air itself, is a factor in wound inflammation; second, that a

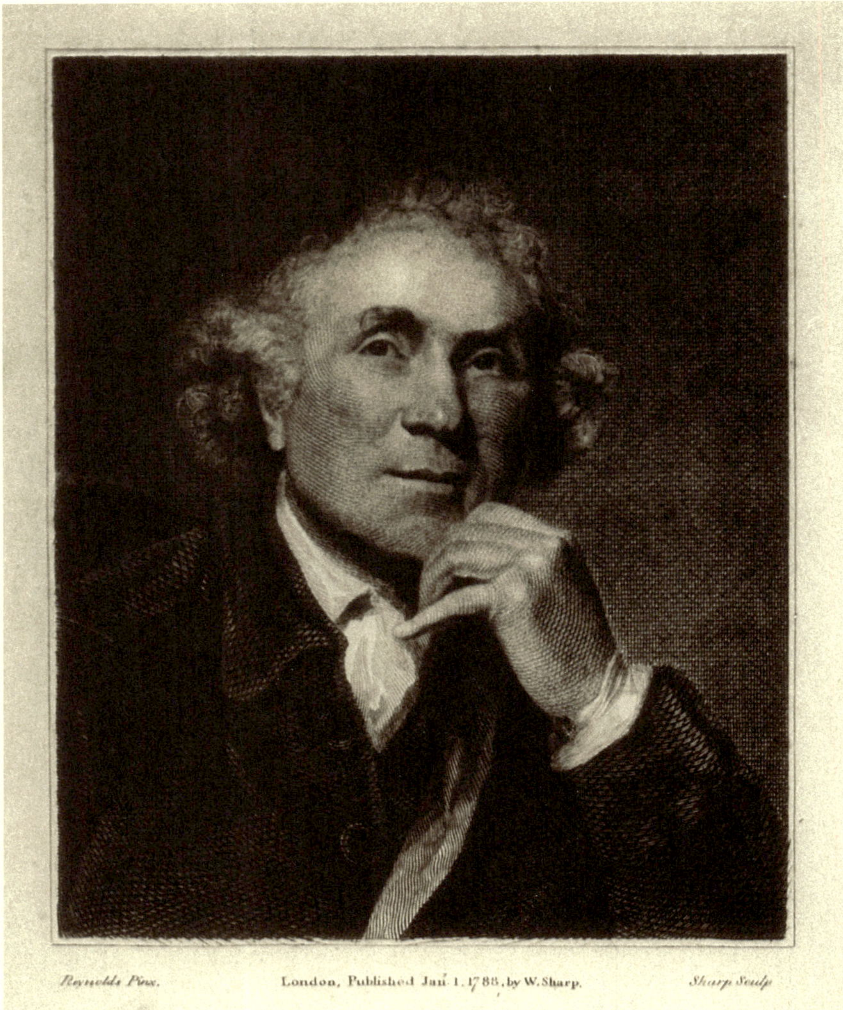

Fig. 97. No. 52. Hunter. Engraved frontispiece portrait, after the painting by Sir Joshua Reynolds.

good blood supply is essential in maintaining the natural defences of the body; and third, that the presence of mortified tissue in a deep wound prevents healing and promotes the onset of sepsis. Hunter was acknowledged by Rudolf Virchow (see no. 69) as the founder of experimental and surgical pathology, and his collection of pathological specimens was at one time the finest in the world. He was also outstanding among eighteenth-century surgeons for orthopedic surgery, and he performed epoch-making studies of the surgical diseases of the vascular system.

Hunter's *Treatise* was the last work printed at his private press, which he established in 1786 at his house on Castle Street in an attempt to prevent the unauthorized publication of cheap and foreign editions of his works. The first edition consisted of 992 copies.

NP

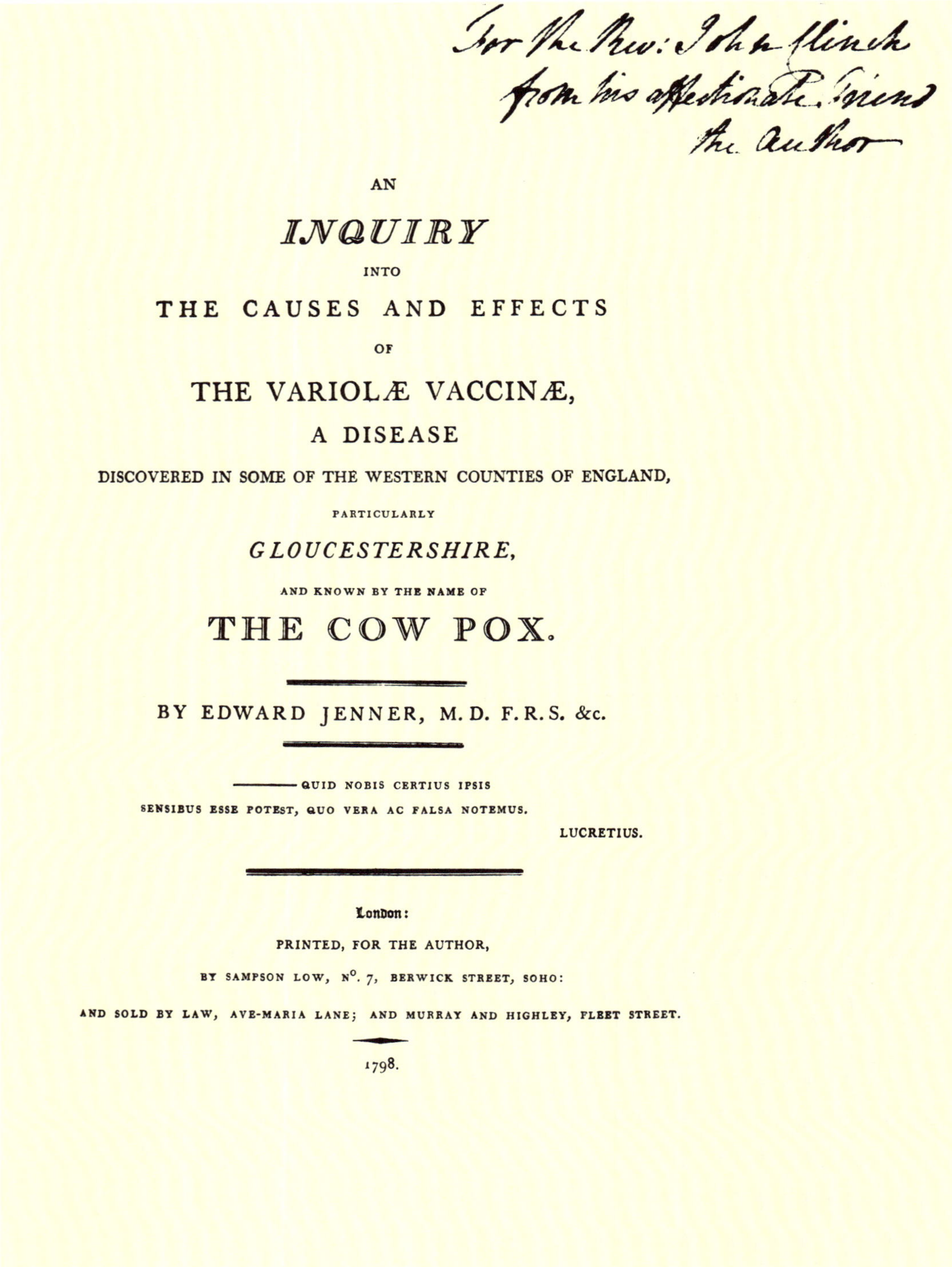

For the Rev: John Clinch
from his affectionate Friend
the Author

AN

INQUIRY

INTO

THE CAUSES AND EFFECTS

OF

THE VARIOLÆ VACCINÆ,

A DISEASE

DISCOVERED IN SOME OF THE WESTERN COUNTIES OF ENGLAND,

PARTICULARLY

GLOUCESTERSHIRE,

AND KNOWN BY THE NAME OF

THE COW POX.

BY EDWARD JENNER, M.D. F.R.S. &c.

——— QUID NOBIS CERTIUS IPSIS
SENSIBUS ESSE POTEST, QUO VERA AC FALSA NOTEMUS.

LUCRETIUS.

London:

PRINTED, FOR THE AUTHOR,

BY SAMPSON LOW, N°. 7, BERWICK STREET, SOHO:

AND SOLD BY LAW, AVE-MARIA LANE; AND MURRAY AND HIGHLEY, FLEET STREET.

1798.

Fig. 98. No. 53. Jenner. Title page. In the upper right corner is Jenner's presentation inscription to his longtime friend, the Rev. John Clinch, who helped promote the practice of vaccination in Canada.

53

EDWARD JENNER

(1749–1823)

An Inquiry into the Causes and Effects of the Variolae Vaccinae, a Disease Discovered in Some of the Western Counties of England, Particularly Gloucestershire, and Known by the Name of the Cow Pox.

London: Printed, for the Author, by Sampson Low, and sold by Law, and Murray and Highley, 1798.

4°: A4(–A4) B–K4 L4(–L4). 42 leaves, pp. [2] *i–iii* iv *1* 2–75 [3]. No. 1–4: 4 engraved plates by William Skelton, after Edward Pearce, printed in sanguine and enhanced with hand-coloring.

Blake, p. 235. GM 5423. *Heirs of Hippocrates* 1086. Horblit 56. LeFanu 23[20]. Norman 1162. Osler 1251. PMM 250. Waller 5136. Wellcome III, p. 351.

Edward Jenner was born in the English town of Berkeley and spent most of his professional life there. As a young man, he was a pupil of and later assistant to the legendary English surgeon John Hunter (see no. 52), who encouraged his interest in natural history. His education with Hunter sharpened his powers of observation and prepared him for the great discovery of his life.

Jenner's medical practice drew him to the treatment of smallpox, a dread disease in his time. It had been known since Antiquity that persons who survived smallpox were later immune to a recurrence, and in 1714 two Greek-Italian physicians, Emanuele Timoni and Jacob Pylarini, published letters in the Royal Society's *Philosophical Transactions* describing to the Western world the practice of variolation, which consists of inoculating a healthy person with material from smallpox pustules in order to confer immunity to the disease. Variolation, which for centuries had been practiced in Asia, Africa, and the Middle East, usually resulted in a mild infection and subsequent immunity; however, it occasionally produced severe reactions, even death, and there was also the ever-present danger of contagion. Despite these drawbacks, as variolation became better known in England, patients demanded it from their physicians, and Jenner soon began to practice it.

Jenner had known from his youth of a local belief that dairymaids who contracted cowpox—a mild illness transmitted from cattle that produced characteristic eruptions on the hands and arms—developed a subsequent immunity to smallpox. This belief was reaffirmed for him when he discovered that his patients who had had cowpox earlier did not respond to variolation. Although he was convinced as early as 1780 that cowpox could be transmitted to healthy persons to protect them from smallpox, he did not put his conviction to the test until sixteen years later when, on 14 May 1796, he inoculated an eight-year-old boy, James Phipps, with cowpox taken from the arm of a milkmaid, Sarah Nelmes, who had contracted the disease from an infected cow. On 1 July 1796 Jenner inoculated Phipps with smallpox and found that it had no effect—the boy was immune.

By 1798 Jenner had assembled twenty-three case reports which he published in a rather thin quarto volume of seventy-five pages. Although *An Inquiry* met initially with some criticism, acclaim was soon widespread, and within a few years vaccination—as the new process was called—was being practiced throughout Europe. It was introduced into the United States by Benjamin Waterhouse, M.D., in 1800, and was practiced by many, including President Thomas Jefferson, who on 14 May 1806 wrote to Rev. George Charles Jenner, Jenner's nephew and assistant, concerning the smallpox vaccination:

> Medicine has never before produced any single improvement of such utility. Harvey's discovery of the circulation of the blood was a beautiful addition to our knowledge of the animal economy; but on a review of the practice of medicine before and since that epoch, I do not see any great amelioration which has been derived from that discovery. You have erased from the calendar of human afflictions one of its greatest. Yours is the comfortable reflection that mankind can never forget that you have lived; future nations will know by history only that the loathsome small-pox has existed, and by you has been extirpated.[1]

Jenner was not only the first to demonstrate experimentally that cowpox produced immunity against smallpox, but he also provided the first proof that a population could be immunized against disease; he was therefore a pioneer not only of immunology, but also of preventive medicine. He introduced the term "virus" to refer to the material that produced cowpox—the initial step toward further specialization of the word—and was the first to describe anaphylaxis, although the word itself was not coined until 1902 by Paul Portier and Charles Richet. The use of smallpox vaccination became worldwide in this century and on 8 May 1980 the World Health Organization announced that the disease had been eradicated from all countries of the earth.

Jenner published the second edition of his *Inquiry* in 1800 and the third in 1801. The book has been reprinted several times, the latest edition a facsimile that appeared in 1984. It has also been translated into Latin, German, French, Italian, Dutch, Portuguese, Russian, and Croatian.

HFN

1. This quotation is taken from Victor Robinson, *Pathfinders in Medicine,* 2d ed. (New York, 1929), p. 214. Robinson believed that this letter had been sent by President Jefferson to Edward Jenner himself; however, Eugene R. Sheridan, senior associate editor of the Jefferson Papers at Princeton University, reports that the letter was in fact sent to Jenner's nephew George Jenner. Jefferson is not known to have sent any letters directly to Edward Jenner.

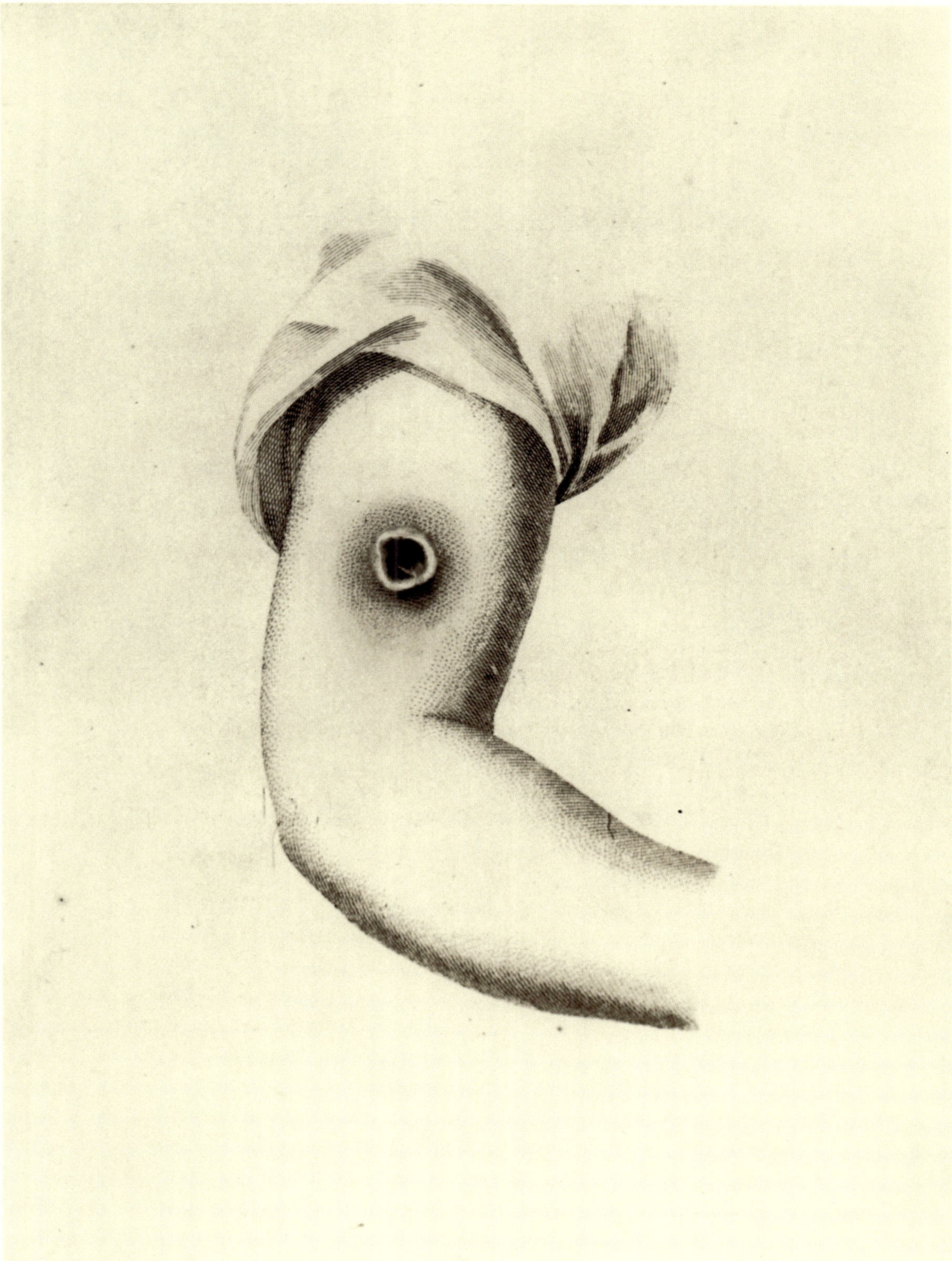

Fig. 99. No. 53. Jenner. The first illustration of vaccination.

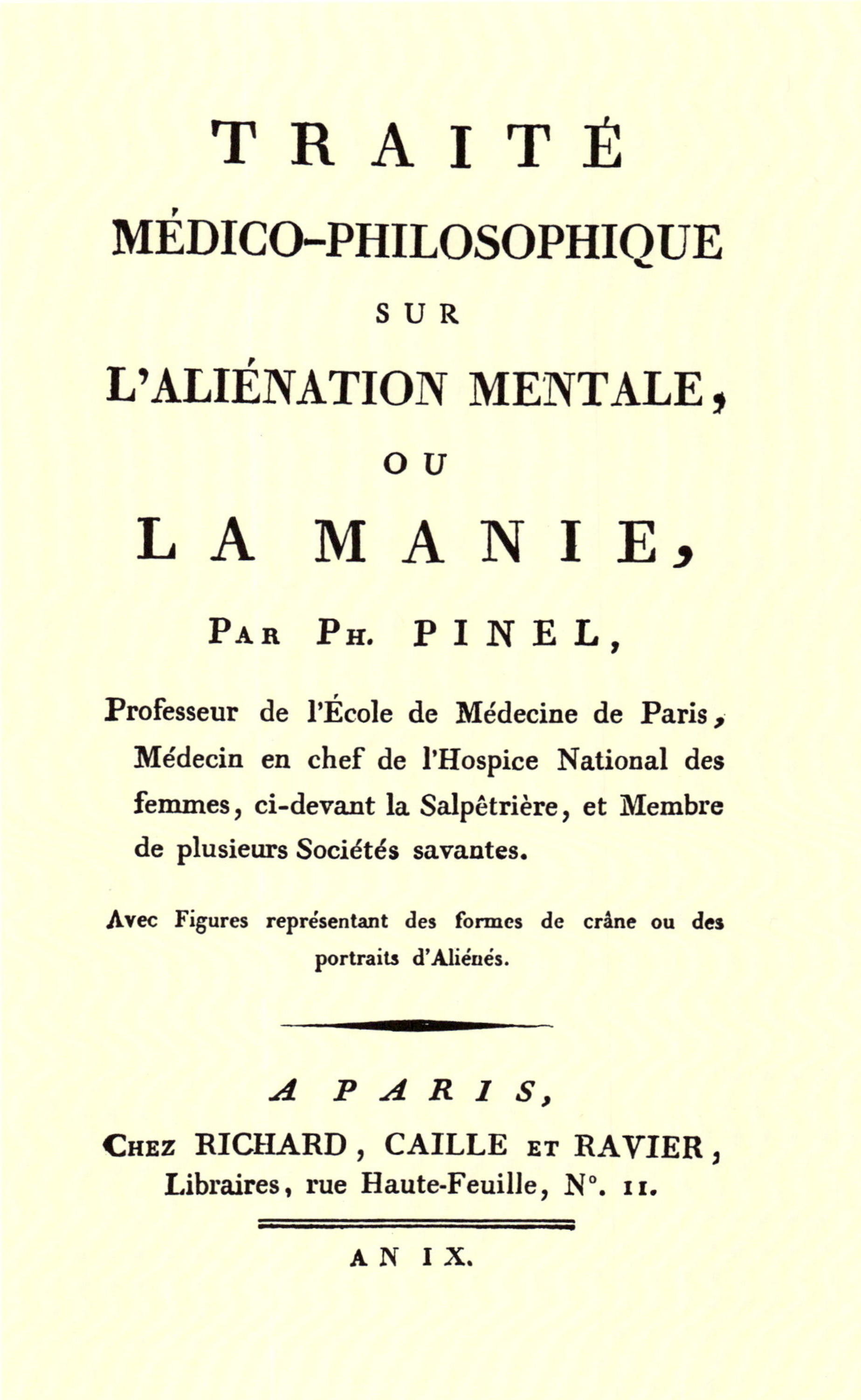

TRAITÉ

MÉDICO-PHILOSOPHIQUE

SUR

L'ALIÉNATION MENTALE,

OU

LA MANIE,

PAR PH. PINEL,

Professeur de l'École de Médecine de Paris, Médecin en chef de l'Hospice National des femmes, ci-devant la Salpêtrière, et Membre de plusieurs Sociétés savantes.

Avec Figures représentant des formes de crâne ou des portraits d'Aliénés.

A PARIS,

CHEZ RICHARD, CAILLE ET RAVIER, Libraires, rue Haute-Feuille, N°. 11.

AN IX.

Fig. 100. No. 54. Pinel. Title page.

54

PHILIPPE PINEL
(1745–1826)

Traité médico-philosophique sur l'aliénation mentale, ou la manie.

Paris: Chez Richard, Caille et Ravier, An IX [1800–01].

8º: a–c⁸ d⁴ A–T⁸ V⁸ (–V8). 187 leaves, pp. *i–v* vi–lvi *1* 2–318. 1 folding letterpress table; Pl. I–II: 2 engraved plates.

EFDT 203. GM 4922. *Heirs of Hippocrates* 1070. Norman 1701. Waller 7456.

Philippe Pinel's *Traité médico-philosophique sur l'aliénation mentale, ou la manie,* which presented the textual foundation of psychiatry, stands as the first great publication of the nineteenth century in clinical medicine, and at the same time as one of the paradigmatic expressions of the medical and scientific revolution that was taking place in the late eighteenth and early nineteenth centuries. A reform movement had begun gathering momentum in Paris during the 1780s, calling for a new approach to medicine based upon observation, experience, new nosologies, and expanded use of autopsies for pathological studies. Pinel was a leader in this movement, helping to reorganize hospitals, establish a new medical curriculum, unify medicine and surgery, and promote hospital-based patient study and direct clinical experience.

In August 1793 Pinel was appointed "physician of the infirmatories" at the Bicêtre, the public hospice for men in Paris that included two hundred mentally ill patients. For nineteen months he made extensive studies of these men, whom he released from the chains that had been used to confine mental patients. In 1795 Pinel left the Bicêtre to assume the position of chief physician at the Salpêtrière, the large Paris hospital for women with mental disorders and chronic illnesses. There he established an advanced psychiatric hospital and the first training program for the new specialty of psychiatry. The principles later described in Pinel's *Traité* were applied at the Salpêtrière, which became the most highly recognized institution in the world at that time for its clinical care and treatment of the mentally ill and for its related teaching and research activities.

In his *Traité,* Pinel departed from past interpretations of mental illness, which placed it within a supernatural or spiritual, rather than a somatic, realm, and accepted the mentally ill as legitimate patients in the domain of medicine. According to Pinel, the manifestations of insanity, including disturbed reason, inappropriate thought, bizarre behavior, and exaggerated passions, represented phenomena of natural history and its pathology that could be studied like those of any other medical or surgical condition. He studied the historical development, treatment, and outcome of mental illnesses, often for years, and if the illnesses resulted in death, he called for autopsies to examine for pathological anatomy. Pinel's system of treatment for mental illness included good hygiene, a favorable environment, activities, work, and the avoidance of drastic physical and medical measures. He introduced a psycho-therapeutic technique called moral therapy, which used a kind and benevolent approach to the patient during interviews.

Pinel had a great interest in nosography, but his classification system for psychiatry was deliberately simple. He described five different species of mental derangement: (1) melancholia, (2) mania without delirium, (3) mania with delirium, (4) dementia, and (5) idiotism. Pinel held that the prime need for psychiatry was to establish an effective typology of insanity, with descriptions of specific disease entities. He believed that traumatic events in a person's life could initiate insanity in one so predisposed, and he illustrated this concept with examples of loss of love, fortune, and other stress-provoking situations such as the turmoil that occurred during the French Revolution.

Apart from his contributions to medicine and psychiatry, Pinel was a remarkable linguist, trained in classical Greek and Latin as well as the contemporary European languages. He cherished a deep respect for Hippocrates and the latter's humanitarian and observational approach to medicine. Pinel was also an intimate member of the main intellectual movement of the period, the Idéologues. The last of the French Philosophes, the Idéologues introduced a practical movement toward a more complex and organic conception of nature, humankind, and society; for them science and experimentation were essential to their encompassing concepts. Pinel's circle of friends included Condillac, Condorcet, Cabanis, Destutt de Tracy, and Benjamin Franklin, as well as many other major physicians and scientists.

A second, enlarged edition of Pinel's *Traité* was published in 1809 with the abbreviated title *Traité médico-philosophique sur l'aliénation mentale.* Translations appeared in German (1801), Spanish (1804), English (1806), and Italian (1830).

GT

55

ROBERT WILLAN
(1757–1812)

On Cutaneous Diseases. Vol. I.

[publication in parts] *Description and Treatment of Cutaneous Diseases* [wrapper title]. (fasc. 1: London: Printed for J. Johnson, 1798) 4°: B–O^4 P^4 (–P4). 55 leaves, pp. *i* ii–xvi *17* 18–110. Pl. I–VII. (fasc. 2: London: Printed for J. Johnson, 1801) 4°: Q–Z^4 2A–2D^4 2E^4 (–2E4). 51 leaves, pp. *111* 112–212. Pl. VIII–XVI XVI* XVII–XIX. (fasc. 3: London: Printed for J. Johnson, 1805) 4°: Ff^4–Zz^4 3A–3E^4. 92 leaves, pp. *213* 214–396. Pl. XX–XXIV. Red printed wrappers.

No separate copies of fasc. 4 are known, but some copies bound up from fasc. 1–3 also include quires 3F–3Z^4 4A–4B^4 (pp. 397–556) and plates XXV–XXXIII.

[complete publication] London: Printed for J. Johnson, 1808.

4°: [A]1 χ1 2χ1 B–Z^4 2A–2D^4 2E^2 Ff–Zz^4 3A–3Z^4 4A–4B^4. 281 leaves, pp. [6] *i* ii–xvi *17* 18–556. Pl. I–XVI XVI* XVII–XXXIII: 34 stipple-engraved plates, printed in colors and enhanced with hand-coloring, engraved by Perry, J. Strutt, W. Hinton, L. Sailliar, and Kirtland, after drawings by Sydenham Edwards, W. Darton, J. Walker, Boyne, W. Hinton, Strutt, Perry, Cruickshank, Kirtland, and "R.W."

GM 3985. *Heirs of Hippocrates* 1155. Norman 2241. Waller 10306.

Robert Willan, a Yorkshire-born physician who practiced at the Public Dispensary in London, is acknowledged as the founder of the specialty of dermatology. He developed and introduced a classification which brought a welcome measure of order to the chaos that characterized the study of skin diseases at the beginning of the nineteenth century. His classification was based on minute observation and precise description of the "elementary lesions," the primordial morphologic changes that make up all cutaneous eruptions. *On Cutaneous Diseases* influenced most of the significant works on its subject in the generations that followed, and it is in fact the earliest treatise on skin diseases that can be read by the modern physician with any degree of comfort or understanding.

Willan published the results of his studies in a series of four fascicles that appeared between 1798 and 1808, paper-bound in heavy red wrappers bearing the cover title *Description and Treatment of Cutaneous Diseases.* With the appearance of the last part, the first three were reprinted with some changes to text and plates, and the whole text was published under the title *On Cutaneous Diseases,* Volume I. At the same time the complete volume was published, copies of the fourth part, together with a title page, a list of the orders of skin diseases, and directions to the binder, were made available to complete sets consisting of the separate fascicles; copies bound from the original parts may be distin-

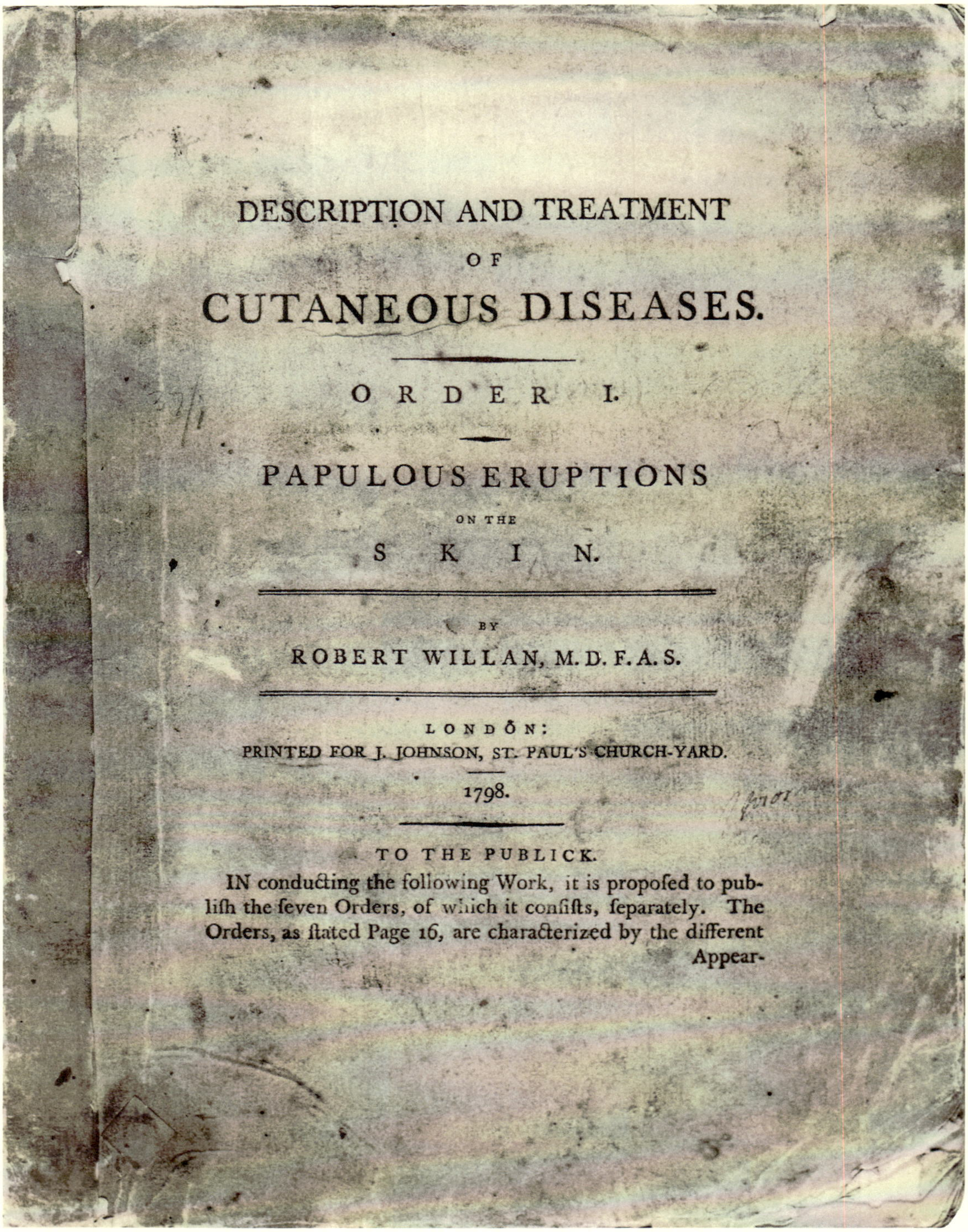

DESCRIPTION AND TREATMENT
OF
CUTANEOUS DISEASES.

ORDER I.

PAPULOUS ERUPTIONS
ON THE
SKIN.

BY
ROBERT WILLAN, M.D. F.A.S.

LONDON:
PRINTED FOR J. JOHNSON, ST. PAUL'S CHURCH-YARD.
1798.

TO THE PUBLICK.

IN conducting the following Work, it is propoſed to publiſh the ſeven Orders, of which it conſiſts, ſeparately. The Orders, as ſtated Page 16, are characterized by the different Appear-

Fig. 101. No. 55. Willan. Front wrapper of the first fascicle (1798).

guished by the variant collations of quires P and 2E, as well as by differences in the text.[1] In addition to the scientific contributions embodied in the text, the value of *On Cutaneous Diseases* was greatly enhanced by the systematic use of illustrations to supplement disease descriptions. Thirty-four plates were printed in color from stipple-engraved copperplates and were further colored by hand under the supervision of the author to assure clinical authenticity. The eruptions are well rendered and distinctive enough in most cases to allow diagnoses to be made with reasonable certainty even today. Plate I depicts the "elementary lesions," and because of the power and utility of the idea it represents, it can be considered one of the most important dermatological illustrations ever published.

Willan was at work on the second volume of his treatise when he began to suffer from symptoms attributable to heart disease. In October 1811 he journeyed to Madeira, where he hoped to regain his health, but his condition deteriorated, and he died on 7 April 1812 at the age of fifty-five.

A single fascicle of Volume II of *On Cutaneous Diseases* was edited and published in 1814 by Ashby Smith as *A Practical Treatise on Porrigo, or Scalled Head, and on Impetigo, the Humid or Running Tetter.* The authentic completion of Willan's grand scheme, however, is to be found in the works of his pupil, Thomas Bateman, who completed the text intended for Volume II in his own *Practical Synopsis of Cutaneous Diseases* (1813), and the plates in his *Delineations of Cutaneous Diseases* (1817).[2]

On Cutaneous Diseases, Volume I, was also published in German (1799–1816) in a translation made from the parts, and an American edition was published in Philadelphia in 1809.

JTC

1. T.S.L. Beswick, "Robert Willan: The Solution of a Ninety-Year-Old Mystery," *Journal of the History of Medicine and Allied Sciences* 12 (1957): 349–65; F. M. Sutherland, "Willan's *Cutaneous Diseases*," ibid. 13 (1958): 92–94. Beswick summarizes the textual differences between fasc. 1 and 2 and the corresponding sections as reprinted in 1808.

2. The full titles of these works express Bateman's indebtedness to Willan: *A Practical Synopsis of Cutaneous Diseases According to the Arrangement of Dr. Willan, Exhibiting a Concise View of the Diagnostic Symptoms and the Methods of Treatment* (London, 1813), and *Delineations of Cutaneous Diseases: Exhibiting the Characteristic Appearances of the Principal Genera and Species Comprised in the Classification of the Late Dr. Willan; and Completing the Series of Engravings Begun by that Author* (London, 1817).

See color plate XXVI.

MÉMOIRES

DE

CHIRURGIE MILITAIRE,

ET

CAMPAGNES

DE D. J. LARREY,

Premier Chirurgien de la Garde et de l'Hôpital de la Garde de S. M. I. et R., Baron de l'Empire, Commandant de la Légion-d'Honneur, Chevalier de l'Ordre de la Couronne de Fer; Inspecteur général du service de santé des Armées; ex-Professeur au ci-devant Hôpital militaire d'instruction du Val-de-Grâce; Docteur en Chirurgie et en Médecine; Membre de l'Institut d'Égypte, des Sociétés de la Faculté de Médecine de Paris, d'Émulation, Philomatique; Associé correspondant de celles de Montpellier, de Toulouse, de Bruxelles, etc.; de l'Académie Joséphine impériale de Vienne; de celles de Turin, de Madrid, de Naples, de Munich et d'Jéna.

Eò adductus sum ut multis meorum æqualium hinc indè errantibus viam monstrarem et aliquantulùm munirem. BAGL. PRAX. MED., *lib. 1, cap. 1.*

TOME I.

PARIS,

Chez J. SMITH, Imprimeur-Libraire, rue de Montmorency.

1812.

Fig. 102. No. 56. Larrey. Title page of Volume I.

56

DOMINIQUE JEAN LARREY
(1766–1842)

Mémoires de chirurgie militaire, et campagnes.

Paris: Chez J. Smith, 1812–17.

[Vol. I] 8º: $[a]^8$ b^6 $1–23^8$ 24^4 25^4 $(–25_4)$. 205 leaves, pp. *i–v* vi–xxviii *1* 2–382. Pl. I–VIII: 8 engraved plates.

[Vol. II] 8º: π^2 $1–32^8$. 258 leaves, pp. [4] *1* 2–512. Pl. IX–X: 2 engraved plates. Cancels noted in some copies: 15_4, 22_7, 27_5.

[Vol. III] 8º: π^2 $1–30^8$ 31^6 $[32]^4$ $(–32_4)$. 251 leaves, pp. [4] *1* 2–272 275–499 [i.e., 497] [1]. Pl. XI: 1 engraved plate. Cancels noted in some copies: 3_1, 3_3, 3_4.

[Vol. IV] 8º: π^2 $1–29^8$ 30^8 $(–30_8)$ 31^2 32^8. 251 leaves, pp. [4] *1* 2–478 *481* 482–500 [i.e. 498]. 5 engraved plates (1 folding), one signed "Dr. Sarlandière del.; Plée sc."; 1 folding engraved map after a drawing by J. B. Sarlandière. Some copies collate: π^4 $1–30^8$ 32^8. 252 leaves, pp. *i–v* vi–viii *1* 2–480 *485* 486–500 [i.e., 496]. Cancel noted in some copies: 1_2.

Relation médicale de campagnes et voyages, de 1815 à 1840.

Paris: J.-B. Ballière, 1841.

8º: π^2 $1–25^8$ 26^6. 208 leaves, pp. [4] *1* 2–412. 2 folding engraved plates.

GM 2160. *Heirs of Hippocrates* 1212. Norman 1280. Osler 3162. Waller 5610, 5613. Wellcome III, p. 451.

Early in his medical career, Dominique Jean Larrey accompanied the French fishing fleet to the Grand Banks of North America, but with the rise of Napoleon he became a military surgeon of great renown, serving as chief surgeon to Napoleon's *Grande Armée.* His devotion to his patients made him extremely popular with the troops as well as with Napoleon, who characterized him as "the most virtuous man I have known." As early as 1790 Larrey had devised the *ambulance volante* or flying ambulance for the French republican army, modeled after the highly mobile French field artillery. With the flying ambulance, the wounded from battle were not left on the field but were picked up and promptly delivered to field hospitals for treatment, and the high morale for which the French army was known was due in no little way to Larrey's invention. Larrey was one of the first to amputate successfully at the hip joint; his doctrine of early amputation in the case of compound fracture led to the saving of many soldiers' lives and remained the standard of practice until Lister developed antiseptic surgery some seventy-five years later. Larrey also recognized the importance of wound debridement and primary wound clo-

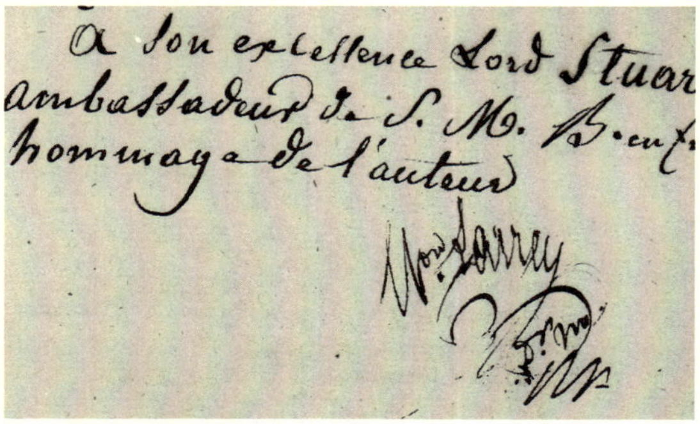

Fig. 103. No. 56. Larrey. Presentation inscription to the British ambassador to France, Lord Charles Stuart. The inscription has been cropped in the original.

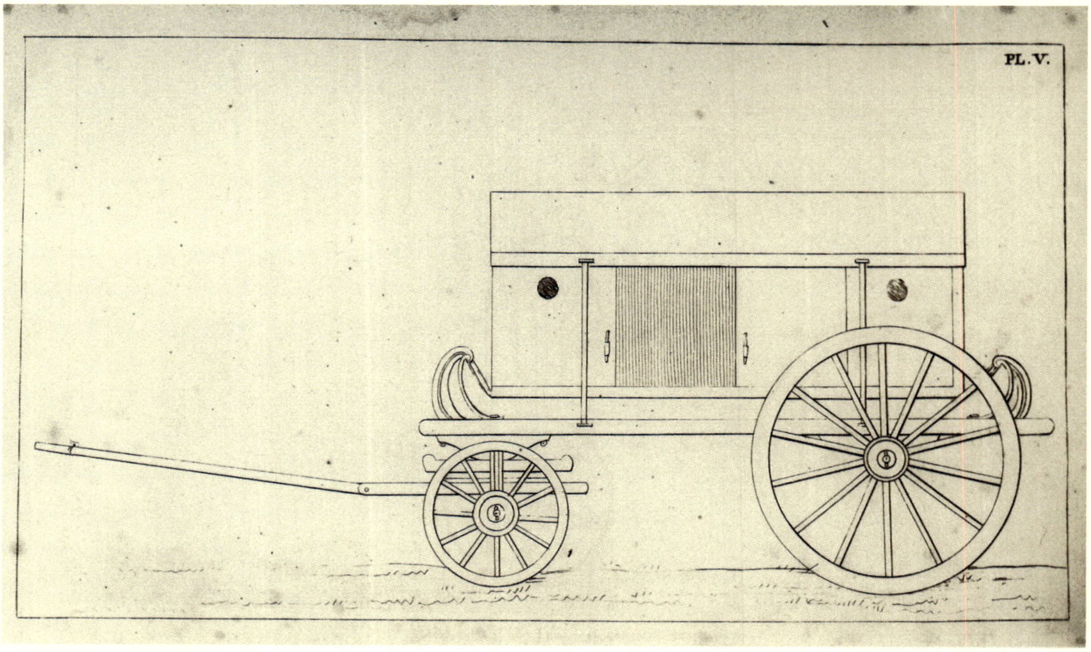

Fig. 104. No. 56. Larry's *ambulance volante*, used to transport wounded soldiers from the battlefield to the field hospital.

sure. During Napoleon's Egyptian campaign, he published a classic description of trachoma (infectious conjunctivitis), a major cause of blindness. He was present at most of the famous battles fought by Napoleon's army and survived the disastrous Russian campaign. After Waterloo Larrey took up civilian practice and teaching in Paris. Among his American students was Oliver Wendell Holmes.

Larrey wrote several books describing his experiences with the French army, the most important of which was his *Mémoires de chirurgie militaire, et campagnes.* His writings are very readable, and in addition to their accounts of military surgery, they include much information of general historical interest. Larrey was proud of his reputation and he frequently annotated his books for presentation, inking in his most recent honors and decorations on the title page after his name.

AEL

There are two issues of the *Mémoires.* Volumes I–III, describing Larrey's career through 1811, were published in 1812 with the imprint "Paris: Chez J. Smith . . . Et chez F. Buisson . . . De l'imprimerie de J. H. Stône." Volume IV, containing accounts of the campaigns of 1812–14 and a general index, appeared in 1817 with the imprint "Paris: Chez J. Smith"; it was presumably at that time that Volumes I and II were reissued with the first quire of each reset to give a revised imprint matching that of Volume IV, but retaining the publication date 1812. Volume III appears to be recorded only with the original imprint, and there is no clear correlation between the variant imprints and the pattern of cancels observed in individual copies. There are also two issues of Volume IV. In one, signed "De l'imprimerie de J. Smith" on the verso of the title page, the index to the volume is printed in quire 31 (pp. 481–84); the main text ends on leaf 30_7 verso (p. 478), and leaf 30_8 (presumably blank, corresponding to pp. 479–80) is cancelled. In the other issue, signed "Imprimerie de Demonville" at the foot of p. 500, the index to Volume IV is printed in the preliminary quire, which consists of four leaves; the main text ends on leaf 30_8 verso (p. 480); and quire 31 is omitted, with a resulting gap in pagination. In both issues, the general index to the four volumes fills quire 32.

Relation médicale de campagnes et voyages, de 1815 à 1840, an account of Larrey's later career, was published by Ballière in 1841 and may be regarded as the fifth volume of the author's memoirs. Volumes I–III were translated into English by Richard Willmott Hall and published in two volumes in Baltimore in 1814.

[ED.]

DE

L'AUSCULTATION

MÉDIATE

OU

TRAITÉ DU DIAGNOSTIC DES MALADIES

DES POUMONS ET DU COEUR,

FONDÉ PRINCIPALEMENT SUR CE NOUVEAU
MOYEN D'EXPLORATION.

PAR R. T. H. LAENNEC,

D. M. P., Médecin de l'Hôpital Necker, Médecin honoraire des Dispensaires, Membre de la Société de la Faculté de Médecine de Paris et de plusieurs autres sociétés nationales et étrangères.

Optimo patruo
altero patri
Théo Laennec

Μέγα δὲ μέρος ἡγεῦμαι τῆς τέχνης εἶναι τὸ δύνασθαι σκοπεῖν.
Pouvoir explorer est, à mon avis, une grande partie de l'art. HIPP., *Epid. III.*

TOME PREMIER.

A PARIS,

CHEZ J.-A. BROSSON et J.-S. CHAUDÉ, Libraires,
rue Pierre-Sarrazin, nº 9.

1819.

Fig. 105. No. 57. Laennec. Title page.

57

RENÉ THÉOPHILE HYACINTHE LAENNEC
(1781–1826)

De l'auscultation médiate ou traité du diagnostic des maladies des poumons et du coeur, fondé principalement sur ce nouveau moyen d'exploration.

Paris: Chez J.-A. Brosson & J.-S. Chaudé, 1819.

[Vol. I] 8°: π^2 a^{*4} χ1 b–c^8 1–28^8 29^4 ^{*4}. 255 leaves, pp. [5] viii–xlviii [i.e., xlvi] *1* 2–456 [8]. Pl. I–IV: 4 folding engraved plates. Printed wrappers

[Vol. II] 8°: π^8 1–29^8 30^4. 244 leaves, pp. *i–v* vi–xvi *1* 2–472. Printed wrappers.

EFDT 226. GM 2673. *Heirs of Hippocrates* 1364. Norman 1253. Osler 1318. PMM 280. Viets 1. Waller 5491. Wellcome III, p. 429.

The invention of the stethoscope by René Théophile Hyacinthe Laennec occurred within a French tradition of bedside observation and clinical empiricism that combined new methods of physical diagnosis with meticulous autopsy correlation. Percussion of the chest, as described by Leopold Auenbrugger (see no. 45) and practiced in Paris under Jean-Nicolas Corvisart, introduced the first useful clinical technique for diagnosis of thoracic diseases at the bedside. At the same time, distrust of theoretical systems of clinical philosophy during the turbulent political climate of the Revolutionary and post-Revolutionary eras in France focused attention on the empirical correlation of clinical histories with autopsy findings, as exemplified previously in the work of Giovanni Battista Morgagni (see no. 46). Integrated and expanded by Laennec, these concepts led to a revolution in the practice and teaching of medicine.

Laennec recognized that many respiratory disorders shared similar presenting symptoms, and he observed in the autopsy room how frequently pneumonia and pleurisy had been overlooked or misdiagnosed prior to the improved recognition afforded by percussion. He also realized the limitations of percussion alone for identifying specific chest disorders and for the early detection of heart disease. Clearly, physicians needed to be able to distinguish additional physical signs of disease. Direct, or immediate, auscultation by application of the ear to the chest had been described in a limited sense by Hippocrates, and while Corvisart taught that the beat of the heart could be appreciated by listening close to the chest wall, objections to this method reduced its applicability. As noted by Laennec, in a statement somewhat colorfully embellished in Forbes's translation, "It is always inconvenient both to the physician and patient; in the case of females it is not only indelicate but often impracticable; and in that class of persons found in hospitals it is disgusting."[1]

These inconveniences were overcome by Laennec's discovery and application of mediate auscultation. "In 1816," he reported, "I was consulted by a young woman laboring under general symptoms of diseased heart, and in whose case percussion and the application of the hand were of little avail on account of the great degree of fatness." Since immediate auscultation was indelicate, or at least impractical, in this situation, Laennec recalled the "augmented impression of sound when conveyed through certain solid bodies; as when we hear the scratch of a pin at one end of a piece of wood, on applying our ear to the other." Rolling a quire of paper into a cylinder and placing one end over the heart, he was able to "perceive the action of the heart in a manner much more clear and distinct than I had ever been able to do by the immediate application of the ear." It was quickly recognized that this new method "might furnish means for enabling us to ascertain the character, not only of the action of the heart, but of every species of sound produced by the motion of all the thoracic viscera." The rolled paper was replaced by a solid wood cylinder about one foot in length, through which the drilling of a central bore was soon discovered to improve transmission of the breath sounds. "This instrument," Laennec stated, "I commonly designate simply the *Cylinder*, sometimes the *Stethoscope*."[2]

Although the invention of the stethoscope introduced the first tool for physical diagnosis, even more remarkable was Laennec's energetic application of this new instrument. Within three years *De l'auscultation médiate* (On mediate auscultation) was published in Paris. The first edition of this epochal work, which appeared in 1819, offers a masterful correlation of stethoscopic signs of chest disease with corresponding autopsy findings that serves still as the foundation for bedside diagnosis of chest disorders. The early impact of Laennec's work was important and widespread, and four French editions were published in Paris and Brussels by 1837. Because the accurate use of the stethoscope could not be learned from the lecture method that had characterized eighteenth-century medical instruction, Paris in the 1820s became the center of clinical training in the use of the instrument. Hospital rounds were conducted with an increasingly international group of student observers, and when these early advocates of diagnostic auscultation and pathologic anatomy returned home, they also spread the French methods of bedside observation and instruction.

The first English translation of *De l'auscultation médiate*, by John Forbes, was published in London in 1821, and British enthusiasm for the use of the stethoscope followed the appearance of confirmatory treatises by Forbes, William Stokes, and Charles Scudamore. Important experimental studies by Charles Williams and James Hope soon led to the accurate classification and description of heart sounds and murmurs. In America, Forbes's translation was published in Philadelphia in 1823; diagnostic use of the stethoscope was recommended by James Jackson in lectures to medical students at Harvard before 1827; and the utility of auscultation was emphasized by Oliver Wendell Holmes in the Boylston prize essay for 1836. In Germany, a translation of Laennec's work was published in 1832, and Josef Skoda's *Abhandlungen über Perkussion und Auskultation* (1839) signalled the acceptance of percussion and auscultation in bedside practice. An Italian edition of Laennec's book was published in 1836–38.

In *De l'auscultation médiate* there are two known states of the second leaf of a*. In the first, the original leaf a*2 is present and unsigned; in the second, this has been replaced by a cancel signed * and exhibiting some minor typographical changes:

	ORIGINAL LEAF	*CANCEL LEAF*
signature:	unsigned	signed "*"
recto, line 14:	comma after "Corvisarto"	comma after "erepta"
recto, line 17:	"quibus hanc"	"quos hanc"
recto, footnote:	"(b) AVENBRUGGER"	"(a) AVENBRUGGER"
verso, line 1:	"constat;"	"constat,"[3]

PK

1. René T. H. Laennec, *A Treatise on the Diseases of the Chest,* trans. John Forbes, 2d ed. (London, 1827), p. 4.
2. All quotations in this paragraph are taken from pp. 284–86 of the first edition of Forbes's translation (London, 1821).
3. The last point may not hold true for every copy.

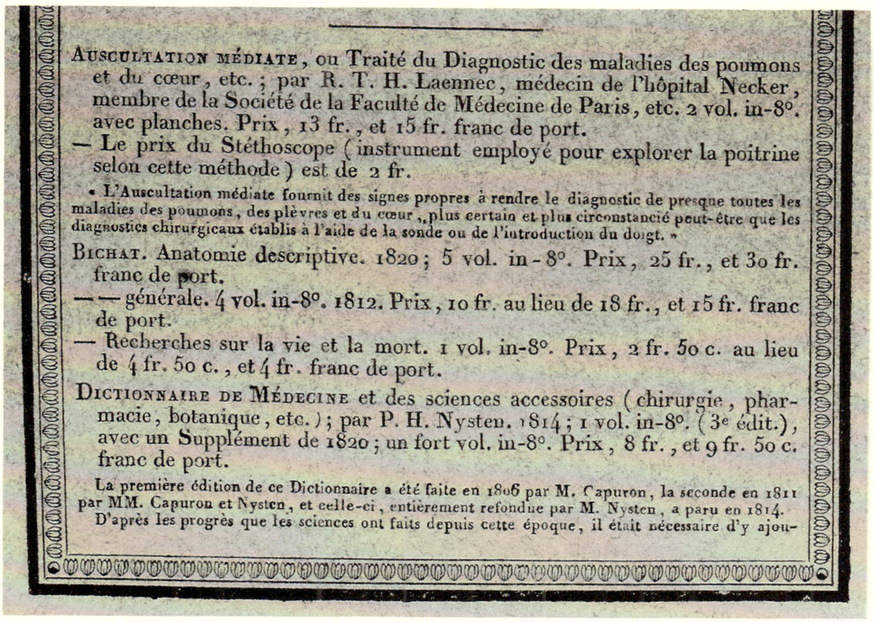
AUSCULTATION MÉDIATE, ou Traité du Diagnostic des maladies des poumons et du cœur, etc.; par R. T. H. Laennec, médecin de l'hôpital Necker, membre de la Société de la Faculté de Médecine de Paris, etc. 2 vol. in-8°. avec planches. Prix, 13 fr., et 15 fr. franc de port.
— Le prix du Stéthoscope (instrument employé pour explorer la poitrine selon cette méthode) est de 2 fr.

« L'Auscultation médiate fournit des signes propres à rendre le diagnostic de presque toutes les maladies des poumons, des plèvres et du cœur, plus certain et plus circonstancié peut-être que les diagnostics chirurgicaux établis à l'aide de la sonde ou de l'introduction du doigt. »

BICHAT. Anatomie descriptive. 1820; 5 vol. in-8°. Prix, 25 fr., et 30 fr. franc de port.
— — générale. 4 vol. in-8°. 1812. Prix, 10 fr. au lieu de 18 fr., et 15 fr. franc de port.
— Recherches sur la vie et la mort. 1 vol. in-8°. Prix, 2 fr. 50 c. au lieu de 4 fr. 50 c., et 4 fr. franc de port.

DICTIONNAIRE DE MÉDECINE et des sciences accessoires (chirurgie, pharmacie, botanique, etc.); par P. H. Nysten. 1814; 1 vol. in-8°. (3e édit.), avec un Supplément de 1820; un fort vol. in-8°. Prix, 8 fr., et 9 fr. 50 c. franc de port.

La première édition de ce Dictionnaire a été faite en 1806 par M. Capuron, la seconde en 1811 par MM. Capuron et Nysten, et celle-ci, entièrement refondue par M. Nysten, a paru en 1814.
D'après les progrès que les sciences ont faits depuis cette époque, il était nécessaire d'y ajou-

Fig. 106. No. 57. Laennec. The back wrapper, advertising both Laennec's treatise and his stethoscope.

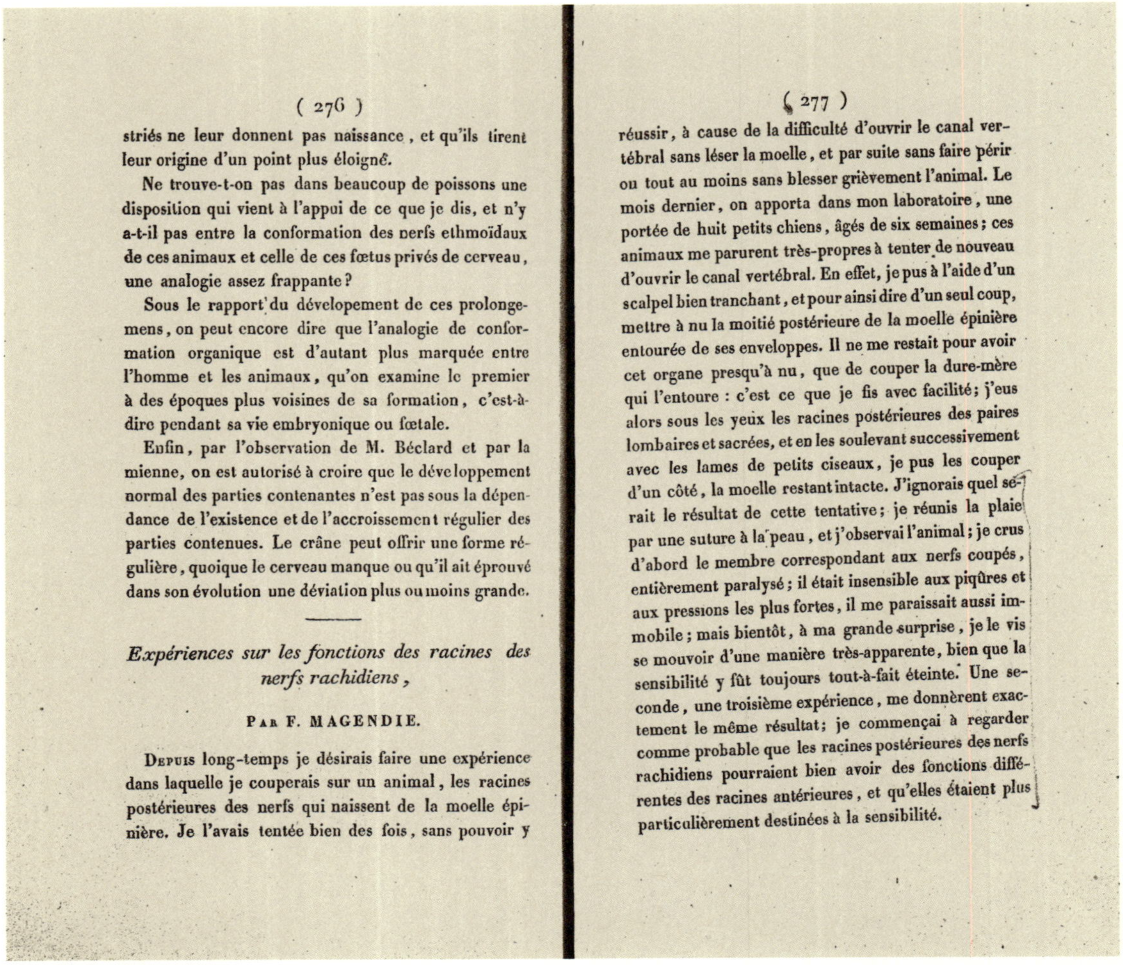

(276)

striés ne leur donnent pas naissance, et qu'ils tirent leur origine d'un point plus éloigné.

Ne trouve-t-on pas dans beaucoup de poissons une disposition qui vient à l'appui de ce que je dis, et n'y a-t-il pas entre la conformation des nerfs ethmoïdaux de ces animaux et celle de ces fœtus privés de cerveau, une analogie assez frappante?

Sous le rapport du dévelopement de ces prolongemens, on peut encore dire que l'analogie de conformation organique est d'autant plus marquée entre l'homme et les animaux, qu'on examine le premier à des époques plus voisines de sa formation, c'est-à-dire pendant sa vie embryonique ou fœtale.

Enfin, par l'observation de M. Béclard et par la mienne, on est autorisé à croire que le développement normal des parties contenantes n'est pas sous la dépendance de l'existence et de l'accroissement régulier des parties contenues. Le crâne peut offrir une forme régulière, quoique le cerveau manque ou qu'il ait éprouvé dans son évolution une déviation plus ou moins grande.

Expériences sur les fonctions des racines des nerfs rachidiens,

PAR F. MAGENDIE.

DEPUIS long-temps je désirais faire une expérience dans laquelle je couperais sur un animal, les racines postérieures des nerfs qui naissent de la moelle épinière. Je l'avais tentée bien des fois, sans pouvoir y

(277)

réussir, à cause de la difficulté d'ouvrir le canal vertébral sans léser la moelle, et par suite sans faire périr ou tout au moins sans blesser grièvement l'animal. Le mois dernier, on apporta dans mon laboratoire, une portée de huit petits chiens, âgés de six semaines; ces animaux me parurent très-propres à tenter de nouveau d'ouvrir le canal vertébral. En effet, je pus à l'aide d'un scalpel bien tranchant, et pour ainsi dire d'un seul coup, mettre à nu la moitié postérieure de la moelle épinière entourée de ses enveloppes. Il ne me restait pour avoir cet organe presqu'à nu, que de couper la dure-mère qui l'entoure : c'est ce que je fis avec facilité; j'eus alors sous les yeux les racines postérieures des paires lombaires et sacrées, et en les soulevant successivement avec les lames de petits ciseaux, je pus les couper d'un côté, la moelle restant intacte. J'ignorais quel serait le résultat de cette tentative; je réunis la plaie par une suture à la peau, et j'observai l'animal; je crus d'abord le membre correspondant aux nerfs coupés, entièrement paralysé; il était insensible aux piqûres et aux pressions les plus fortes, il me paraissait aussi immobile; mais bientôt, à ma grande surprise, je le vis se mouvoir d'une manière très-apparente, bien que la sensibilité y fût toujours tout-à-fait éteinte. Une seconde, une troisième expérience, me donnèrent exactement le même résultat; je commençai à regarder comme probable que les racines postérieures des nerfs rachidiens pourraient bien avoir des fonctions différentes des racines antérieures, et qu'elles étaient plus particulièrement destinées à la sensibilité.

Fig. 107. No. 58. Magendie. Opening pages of text.

58

FRANÇOIS MAGENDIE
(1783–1855)

Expériences sur les fonctions des racines des nerfs rachidiens.

In: *Journal de physiologie expérimentale et pathologique* 2 (1822): 276–79.

[journal number] Vol. 2, No. 3: 8°: π^{2} 14–18^{8} 19^{6}. 48 leaves, pp. [4] 191–282. Dark green printed wrappers.

[article] 19_{3}^{v}–19_{5}^{r}, pp. 276–279.

GM 1256. Norman 1418.

François Magendie, a native of Bordeaux, was a child of revolutionary France, the son of a surgeon steeped in republican philosophy. A brilliant student, Magendie was one of the first required to defend a medical thesis, an innovation instituted under the Napoleonic educational reforms. He received his degree in medicine in 1808 and became demonstrator in anatomy at the new Faculté de Médecine in Paris. After 1813 he abandoned plans for a surgical career and devoted his professional life to experimental physiology, the field that he originated.

Magendie had become convinced that one could begin to understand the physiology of the body only through experimentation on live laboratory animals, and it was on the basis of such experiments that the French school of experimental physiology became preeminent in the nineteenth century. In contrast, English scientists, who were generally opposed to vivisection, were hostile to Magendie's methods, and this difficulty in dealing with experimentation on live animals retarded British physiological research for years.

In 1821 Magendie founded the *Journal de physiologie expérimentale,* which was published quarterly until April 1831. Starting with Volume II the words *et pathologique* were added to the title, reflecting Magendie's belief that pathology was the physiology of the sick organism. This was the first journal devoted to its subject, and Magendie became its main contributor. His research interests were varied, and he made original contributions in many areas of physiology: the action of drugs, the functions of the stomach, the nature of the spinal fluid, and the activity of the peripheral nervous system. He also helped introduce such alkaloids as strychnine, morphine, codeine, and quinine into medical practice.

Magendie is most famous for identifying and proving by experiment the distinct functions of the dorsal and ventral nerve roots of the spinal cord (the "Bell-Magendie" law). His findings were in some part anticipated by the work of the Scottish anatomist Charles

Bell (1774–1842), who had experimented with separately cutting the spinal roots and had published a pamphlet proposing his idea of the separation of sensory and motor function.[1] Bell, however, did not establish experimentally the distinct properties of the two types of root. Magendie may have learned of Bell's work from Bell's nephew John Shaw, who visited Magendie's laboratory in 1821 and alluded to Bell's research in an article on partial paralysis published in 1822.[2] Magendie repeated Bell's work, using unanesthetized puppies, and not only validated Bell's findings but went much further. He showed the dorsal roots to be purely sensory and the ventral roots unequivocally motor, thus proving experimentally that the nervous system has a rational and understandable arrangement. This discovery was as significant for the study of the nervous system as Harvey's discovery of the circulation of the blood had been for the understanding of the cardiovascular system.

Disputes over priority erupted between Bell and Magendie, exacerbated by the long-standing political antipathy between the French and the English. The famous Bell-Magendie controversy outlasted the principals and continued to be argued, with remarkable passion, for many years. Recently, however, Paul F. Cranefield has exhaustively surveyed the evidence and awarded full credit to Magendie.[3]

AEL

1. Charles Bell, *Idea of a New Anatomy of the Brain* (London, 1811).

2. John Shaw, "On Partial Paralysis," *Medico-Chirurgical Transactions* 12 (1822): 105–51.

3. Paul F. Cranefield, *The Way In and the Way Out: François Magendie, Charles Bell and the Roots of the Spinal Nerves* (Mt. Kisco, N.Y., 1974). This work includes facsimile reprints of the sources relating to the controversy.

59

KARL ERNST VON BAER
(1792–1876)

De ovi mammalium et hominis genesi epistolam ad Academiam Imperialem Scientiarum Petropolitanam.

Leipzig: Sumptibus Leopoldi Vossii, 1827.

π^4 1–5[4] [6]$_1$. 25 leaves, pp. [8] *1* 2–40 [2]. 1 hand-colored folding engraved plate after drawings by the author. Cream printed wrappers.

GM 477. *Heirs of Hippocrates* 1493. Horblit 9b. Waller 594.

Karl Ernst von Baer's discovery of the mammalian ovum, announced in *De ovi mammalium,* ended a search that had begun over one hundred and fifty years earlier when William Harvey, in his *Exercitationes de generatione animalium* (1651), first proposed the idea that all animals come from eggs. Baer first discovered the mammalian ovum in a dog, and later in other mammals, while he was professor of zoology at Königsberg, a position he held from 1826 to 1834. He published his findings in the form of a letter to the Academy of Sciences at St. Petersburg, of which he was then a corresponding member. The major significance of his work is summarized in the first of the conclusions to *De ovi mammalium: Omne animal, quod coitu maris et feminae gignitur, ex ovo evolvitur, nullum ex mero liquore formativo* (Every animal that springs from the coition of male and female is developed from an ovum, and none from a simple formative liquid).[1]

In the same year, 1827, that *De ovi mammalium* appeared, Baer also published the first volume of his *Ueber Entwicklungsgeschichte der Thiere,* a work that was not completed until twelve years after his death. In contrast to *De ovi mammalium,* the *Entwicklungsgeschichte* is a large work, offering a careful examination and interpretation of the whole course of vertebrate embryonic development. Continuing the work of his friend and collaborator Christian Heinrich Pander (1794–1865), Baer observed the formation of the germ layers and established the germ layer theory. He described the way in which the layers formed various organs by tubulation, and he emphasized that the development of the embryo is from the apparently homogeneous to the obviously heterogeneous. In this he finally refuted the long held and much discussed theory that embryonic parts might be preformed in the egg. The publication of this book provided a solid basis for the further systematic study of mammalian development. In response to demands by subscribers, the

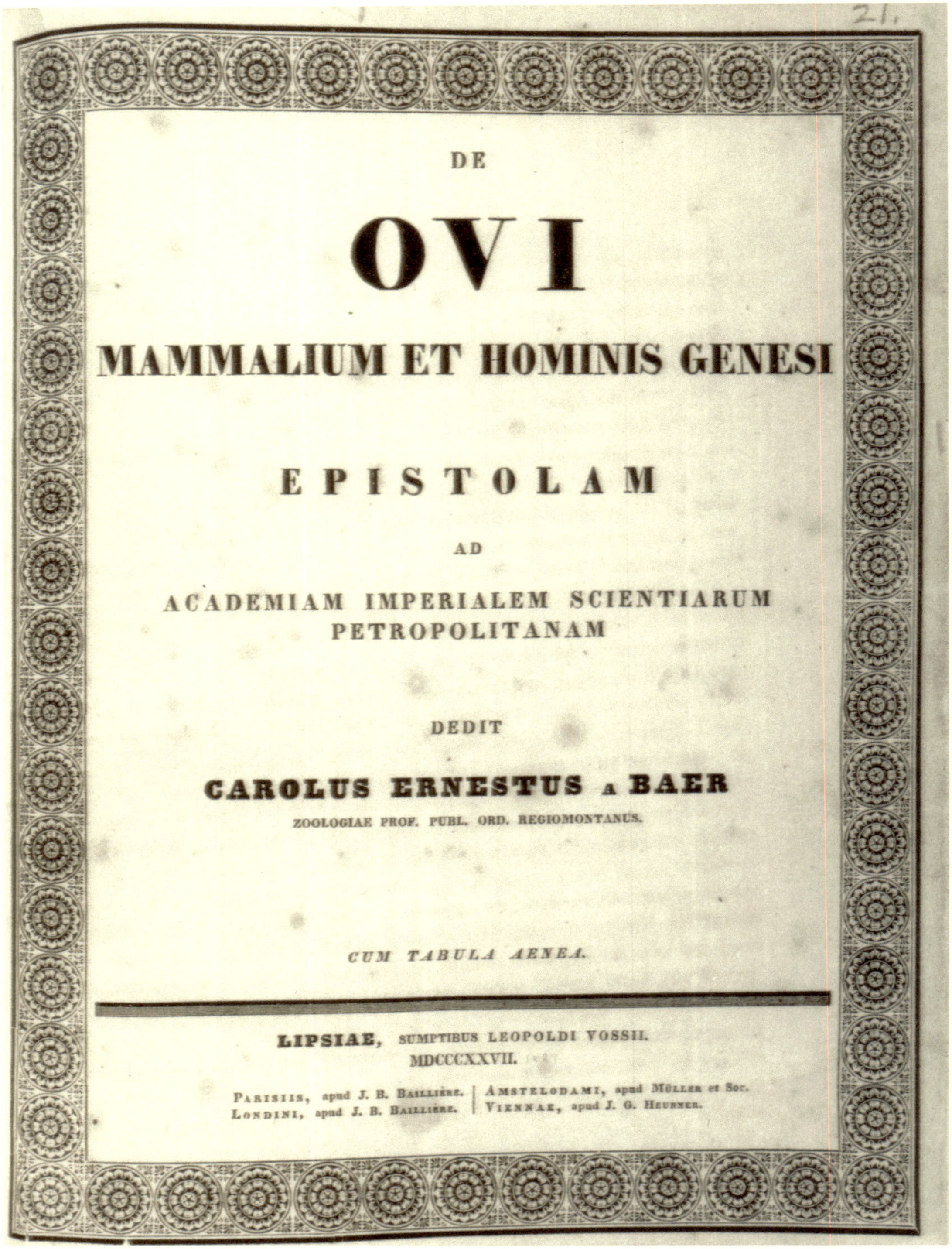

DE

OVI

MAMMALIUM ET HOMINIS GENESI

EPISTOLAM

AD

ACADEMIAM IMPERIALEM SCIENTIARUM
PETROPOLITANAM

DEDIT

CAROLUS ERNESTUS A BAER

ZOOLOGIAE PROF. PUBL. ORD. REGIOMONTANUS.

CUM TABULA AENEA.

LIPSIAE, SUMPTIBUS LEOPOLDI VOSSII.
MDCCCXXVII.

PARISIIS, apud J. B. BAILLIÈRE. | AMSTELODAMI, apud MÜLLER et Soc.
LONDINI, apud J. B. BAILLIÈRE. | VIENNAE, apud J. G. HEUBNER.

Fig. 108. No. 59. Baer. Front wrapper.

publishers released the second volume in incomplete form in 1837, but the conclusion to that volume, which is of great rarity, was not published until 1888.

From 1834 to 1867 Baer resided in St. Petersburg, where he pursued a variety of interests. As academician for comparative anatomy and physiology at the Academy of Sciences, he took charge of the academy's anatomical museum and established a craniological collection there. Long interested in anthropology and ethnology, he sought to classify man based on degrees of primitiveness and attempted to standardize systems for measuring skulls. He made a number of scientific expeditions, leading to discoveries in natural history and geology, and he contributed to the founding of the Russian Geographical Society, the Russian Entomological Society, and the German Anthropological Society. Although he had objections to the theory of evolution as expounded by Darwin (see no. 70), his discoveries in embryology provided a foundation for further developments in this area.

NP

1. Karl Ernst von Baer, "On the Genesis of the Ovum of Mammals and of Man," trans. Charles D. O'Malley, *Isis* 47 (1956): 117–53, at p. 149.

See color plate XXVII.

REPORTS

OF

MEDICAL CASES,

SELECTED

WITH A VIEW OF ILLUSTRATING

THE SYMPTOMS AND CURE OF DISEASES

BY A REFERENCE TO

MORBID ANATOMY.

By RICHARD BRIGHT, M.D. F.R.S. &c.

LECTURER ON THE PRACTICE OF MEDICINE,

AND ONE OF THE PHYSICIANS TO

GUY'S HOSPITAL.

LONDON:

PRINTED BY RICHARD TAYLOR, RED LION COURT, FLEET STREET.

PUBLISHED BY LONGMAN, REES, ORME, BROWN, AND GREEN.

1827.

Fig. 109. No. 60A. Bright. Title page.

60

RICHARD BRIGHT
(1789–1858)

A] *Reports of Medical Cases, Selected with a View of Illustrating the Symptoms and Cure of Diseases by a Reference to Morbid Anatomy.*

London: Printed by Richard Taylor; Published by Longman, Rees, Orme, Brown, and Green, 1827–31.

[Vol. I] 4°: [a]^4 b^4 B–Z^4 2A–2G^4 χ1–16χ1. 140 leaves, pp. *i–vii* viii–xvi *1* 2–231 [1] [32]. Pl. I–VI VI* VII–XV: 16 hand-colored engraved plates by William Say after Frederick Richard Say. Leaves χ1–16χ1 represent the plate captions, each bound as a separate leaf opposite the plate it describes.

[Vol. II, part 1] 4°: [a]^4 b–e^4 χ1 B–Z^4 2A–2Z^4 3A–3L^4 3M^4 (–3M2.3, 4). 246 leaves, pp. *i–vii* viii–xl [2] *1* 2–450.

[Vol. II, part 2] 4°: π^4 (–π4) 3M^4 (–3M1) 3N–3Z^4 4A–4Y^4 4Z^2 χ1–38χ1. 178 leaves, pp. [6] *451–452* 453–724 [76]. Pl. I–III V–VII IX–XL: 31 hand-colored engraved plates (1 folding) by William Say, C. J. Canton, and William Thomas Fry after drawings by F. R. Say, C. J. Canton, and F. F. Giraud; and 7 uncolored lithographed plates (4 folding) by Thomas and William Fairland after drawings by C. J. Canton and George Scharfe. Plates IV and VIII, as explained in the captions, were never engraved. Leaves χ1–38χ1 represent the plate captions, each bound as a separate leaf opposite the plate it describes. Plates I–XVI and their captions are sometimes bound with Vol. II, part 1.

GM 2285. *Heirs of Hippocrates* 1451. Hill 6. Norman 341. Osler 1340. Waller 1460. Wellcome II, p. 239.

B] THOMAS HODGKIN (1798–1866). On Some Morbid Appearances of the Absorbent Glands and Spleen.

In: *Medico-Chirurgical Transactions* 17 (1832): 68–114.

[journal volume] Vol. 17: [a]^8 b^4 B–Z^8 AA–LL^8. 276 leaves, pp. *i–vi* vii–xxiii [1] *1* 2–527 [1]. Pl. 1–4: 4 folding lithographed plates.

[article] F2^v–I1^v, pp. *68* 69–114.

[offprint] *On Some Morbid Appearances of the Absorbent Glands and Spleen.* From the Seventeenth Volume of the Medico-Chirurgical Transactions published by the Medical and Chirurgical Society of London. London: Printed by G. Woodfall, 1832.

[A]1 B–D^8. 25 leaves, pp. [2] *1* 2–47 [1].

GM 3762.

c] Thomas Addison (1793–1860). *On the Constitutional and Local Effects of Disease of the Supra-Renal Capsules.*

London: Samuel Highley, 1855.

[A]4 B–F4 G2. 26 leaves, pp. *i–vii* viii *1* 2–43 [1]. Pl. I–XI: 11 hand-colored lithographed plates by W. Hurst and M. and N. Hanhart after drawings by W. Hurst and John Tupper. Green gilt-blocked cloth.

GM 3864. *Heirs of Hippocrates* 1502. Norman 8. Osler 1744. Waller 225.

Richard Bright graduated from the medical school at the University of Edinburgh in 1813. In 1820 he was appointed assistant physician at Guy's Hospital in London, where he began to devote himself to teaching and research, emphasizing the importance of the study of pathology in the understanding of disease. In 1827 he published the first volume of his *Reports of Medical Cases, Selected with a View of Illustrating the Symptoms and Cure of Diseases*; this volume contains ninety case histories, of which twenty-three, studied during the years 1811–27, comprise the classic section on kidney disease. Bright was the first to establish the relationship between edema (dropsy), albuminuria (coagulable urine), and kidney pathology, and he was also the first to distinguish between cardiac and renal edema. He recognized three basic types of diseased kidney: (1) the large red kidney of acute glomerulonephritis; (2) the large white kidney associated with the nephrotic syndrome; and (3) the small contracted kidney of chronic glomerulonephritis and chronic renal failure. Ten years after the publication of Bright's observations, the French authority on renal diseases, Pierre François Olive Rayer, referred to the complex of kidney disorders that Bright described as "maladie de Bright" or "Bright's disease." The second volume of Bright's *Reports*, published in two parts in 1831, is devoted entirely to neuropathology and contains three hundred detailed case histories describing such conditions as brain tumor, acute and chronic hydrocephalus, tuberculous meningitis, subarachnoid hemorrhage, epilepsy, Jacksonian epilepsy, and hysteria.

The plates in Bright's *Reports* are among the most beautiful of medical illustrations. Bright himself was an artist, and he supervised the drawings done for him by Frederick Richard Say (whose portrait of Bright hangs in the Royal College of Physicians in London) and the engravings made from them by the artist's father, William Say, and others. According to publisher's records, 242 copies of Volume I and 171 copies of Volume II were printed, which explains why Volume I is more common than a complete set.

Bright was the most charismatic of the great triumvirate at Guy's Hospital which consisted of himself, Thomas Hodgkin, and Thomas Addison, each of whom also had a disease named after him. Thomas Hodgkin, the second member of the triumvirate, studied medicine at Guy's Hospital and on the Continent before receiving his doctorate from the University of Edinburgh. In Paris he studied under René Théophile Laennec (see no. 57), and on his return to London he introduced the stethoscope in the examination of pa-

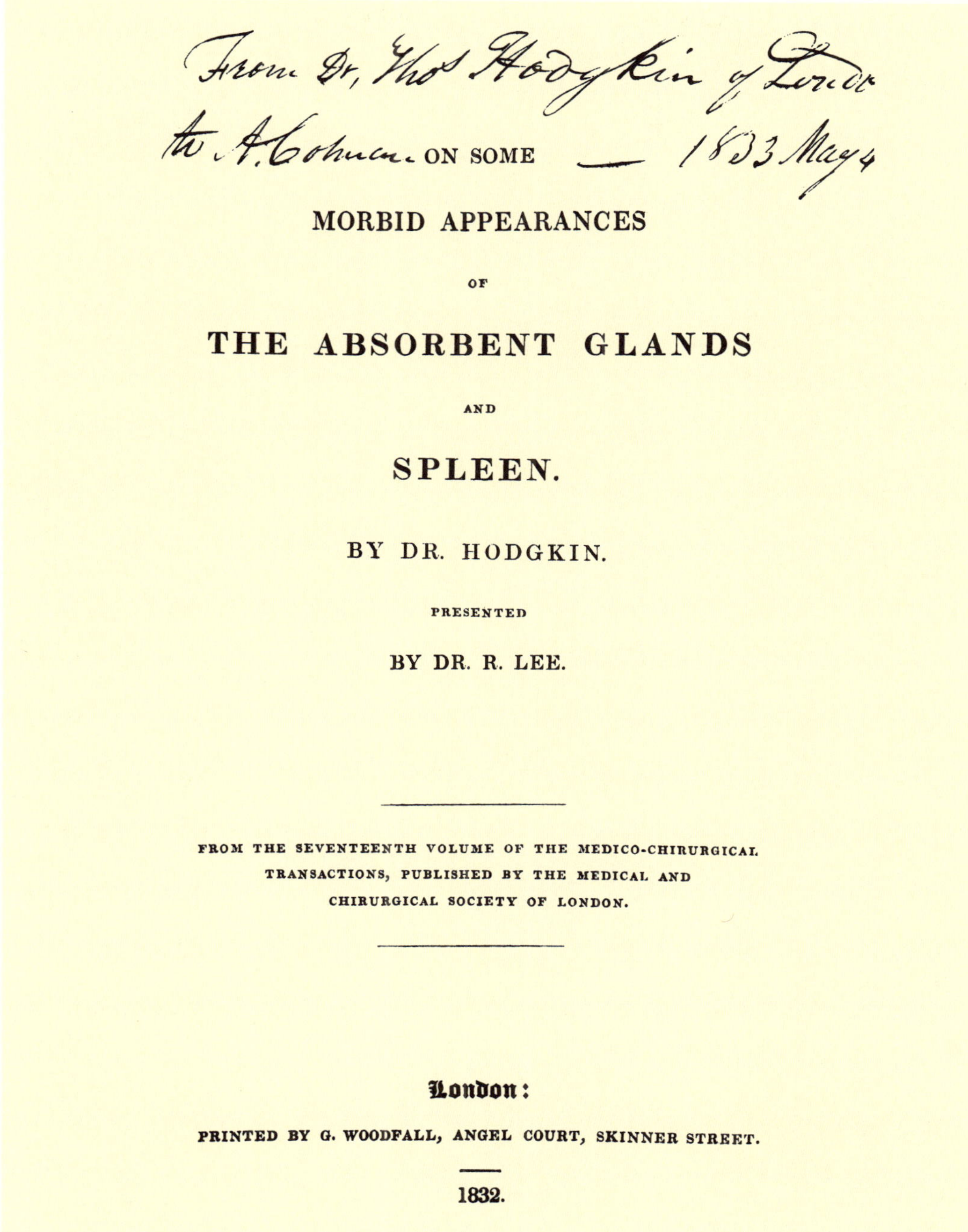

From Dr. Thos Hodgkin of London
to A. Colman — 1833 May 4

ON SOME

MORBID APPEARANCES

OF

THE ABSORBENT GLANDS

AND

SPLEEN.

BY DR. HODGKIN.

PRESENTED

BY DR. R. LEE.

FROM THE SEVENTEENTH VOLUME OF THE MEDICO-CHIRURGICAL TRANSACTIONS, PUBLISHED BY THE MEDICAL AND CHIRURGICAL SOCIETY OF LONDON.

London:

PRINTED BY G. WOODFALL, ANGEL COURT, SKINNER STREET.

1832.

Fig. 110. No. 60B. Hodgkin. Title page of the offprint.

ON THE

CONSTITUTIONAL AND LOCAL EFFECTS

OF

DISEASE

OF THE

SUPRA-RENAL CAPSULES.

BY

THOMAS ADDISON, M.D.,

SENIOR PHYSICIAN TO GUY'S HOSPITAL.

LONDON:

SAMUEL HIGHLEY, 32 FLEET STREET.

1855.

Fig. III. No. 60C. Addison. Title page.

tients. He became a member of the Royal College of Surgeons and in 1825 was appointed lecturer on morbid anatomy and curator of the museum at Guy's. In 1832 he published "On Some Morbid Appearances of the Absorbent Glands and Spleen," which included the first full description of lymphadenoma. In 1865 Sir Samuel Wilkes was the first to call this disorder by the eponym "Hodgkin's disease."

Thomas Addison was elected assistant physician at Guy's Hospital in 1824 and full physician in 1837. In his work *On the Constitutional and Local Effects of Disease of the Supra-Renal Capsules*, an expansion of an address published in 1849,[1] Addison gave a full description of two new diseases: pernicious anemia (Addison's anemia), and adrenal insufficiency (Addison's disease). J. S. Combe had previously published an account of pernicious anemia,[2] but it attracted little attention, and it was Addison who made the disease known to the medical profession. His identification of chronic disease with the adrenals and his recognition that the adrenals are necessary to human life contributed to the beginning of modern endocrinology. The importance of Addison's work was first recognized in Paris, particularly through the efforts of Charles Édouard Brown-Séquard. Brown-Séquard based his work on Addison's research, confirming Addison's findings in a series of experiments in which he excised the adrenals of a large number of animals, all of which contracted and died of Addison's disease.[3]

RDG

1. Thomas Addison, "Anaemia; Disease of the Supra-Renal Capsules," *London Medical Gazette* 43 (1849): 517–18.
2. James Scarth Combe, "History of a Case of Anaemia," *Transactions of the Medico-Chirurgical Society of Edinburgh* 1 (1824): 194–204. The paper was read on 1 May 1822.
3. Charles Édouard Brown-Séquard, "Recherches expérimentales sur la physiologie et la pathologie des capsules surrénals," *Comptes rendus hebdomadaires des séances de l'Académie des Sciences* 43 (1856): 422–25, 542–46.

See color plates XXVIII *and* XXIX.

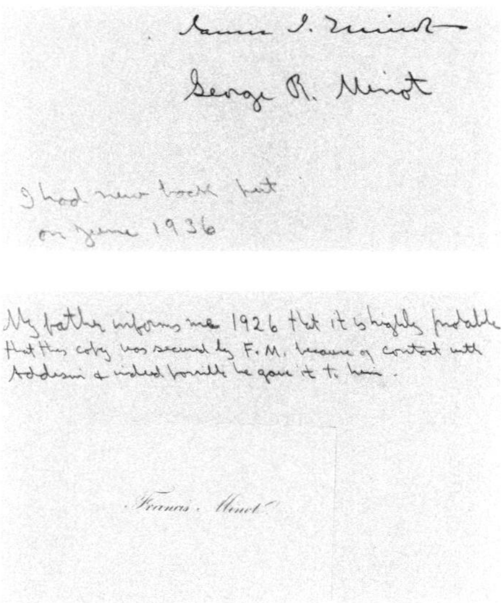

Fig. 112. No. 60c. George R. Minot's notes on the provenance of the Minot family copy of Addison's work. Minot's signature and that of his father, James Jackson Minot, are seen above. Francis Minot, whose bookplate appears below, was George R. Minot's great uncle and a teacher at Harvard Medical School. George R. Minot discovered the cure for pernicious anemia, one of the diseases discussed in Addison's monograph.

To Wm Dunlap Esqr
with the respects of the Author

EXPERIMENTS

AND

OBSERVATIONS

ON THE

GASTRIC JUICE,

AND THE

PHYSIOLOGY OF DIGESTION.

BY WILLIAM BEAUMONT, M. D.

Surgeon in the U. S. Army.

PLATTSBURGH,

PRINTED BY F. P. ALLEN.

1833.

Fig. 113. No. 61. Beaumont. Title page.

61

WILLIAM BEAUMONT
(1785–1853)

Experiments and Observations on the Gastric Juice, and the Physiology of Digestion.

Plattsburgh: Printed by F. P. Allen, 1833.

8º: [A]4 B–Z4 2A–2M4. 140 leaves, pp. *1–5* 6–280. 3 wood-engraved figures in text. Cloth-backed boards, or sheep.

GM 989. Grolier *American* 38. *Heirs of Hippocrates* 1411. Horblit 10. Norman 152. Osler 1972. Peters & Fulton 1. Waller 805. Wellcome II, p. 123.

William Beaumont's contribution to medical history resulted from the opportunity created in 1822 when, as the army surgeon at Fort Mackinac, Michigan, he attended a French-Canadian voyageur, Alexis St. Martin, who had had a hole blown into his stomach by the accidental discharge of a musket loaded with duck shot. The permanent gastric fistula or "window" that this wound left in St. Martin's abdomen enabled Beaumont to make the first accurate scientific study of the physiological processes of gastric digestion. Beaumont conducted his experiments and observations over a period of eight years, the major investigative phase taking place at the primitive log hospital at Fort Crawford on the upper Mississippi River during the winter of 1830–31.[1] His researches established the presence and role of hydrochloric acid in the stomach, the temperature of the stomach during digestion, the movement of the stomach walls, and the relative digestibility of certain foods, all findings that revolutionized current theories of the physiology of digestion.

Although he made the first significant American contribution to physiology, the sum of Beaumont's life work in science is disappointing. "Truth, like beauty, 'when unadorned is adorned the most,' and in prosecuting experiments and inquiries I believe I have been guided by its light," is how Beaumont described his own gift for objective observation.[2] After 1833, however, St. Martin refused further cooperation, and Beaumont never again engaged in research on gastric physiology. He went on to a successful career in private practice and died in St. Louis in 1853 from the effects of a fall suffered while making a house call.

William Beaumont's immortality is assured by what Sir William Osler called a "brown backed, poorly printed octavo volume of 280 pages with the imprint 'Plattsburgh, printed by F. P. Allen 1833'."[3] The first edition, which included three wood-engraved illustrations of St. Martin's wound and stomach after drawings by a Mr. King, was originally offered for sale at three dollars a copy. Later, Senator Edward Everett, a cousin of Beaumont, observed that ". . . if the price were lower" the book would have had a larger sale.[4] It was printed in Plattsburgh, where Beaumont had previously practiced medicine, because the work could be done more quickly and cheaply there than in New York or Philadelphia and because Beaumont did not find New York a congenial place to work. A rare second issue has a cancel title page with the imprint "Boston: Lilly, Wait, and Company, 1834." Andrew Combe reprinted the book in Edinburgh in 1838, with added notes of his own, and Beaumont's cousin Samuel Beaumont edited a slightly "corrected" second edition of 1500 copies published in Burlington, Vermont, in 1847. A German translation was published in Leipzig in 1834. John Fulton's copy of the original edition served as the source for a facsimile that was published in three issues in 1929, and other reproductions have appeared since then.

The size of the first edition has long been a point of controversy. A reasonable interpretation, first suggested by John Fulton, is that only a thousand copies were printed in 1833 in Plattsburgh, as stated in Beaumont's letter to Surgeon General Joseph Lovell, dated 3 December 1833. The same month Beaumont asked Mr. E. Smith (the binder) to send "400 or 500" copies to New York to Carvill's, a Broadway bookseller. An autograph memorandum by Beaumont, also from 1833, lists "agents and subscribers" and contains the entry "Lilly, Wait." Still other memoranda by Beaumont suggest that he personally sold and distributed a hundred or so copies, including fifty sent to Daniel Drake. All this leads to a tentative conclusion that the first edition consisted of only a thousand copies: five hundred (plus an additional fifty presentation copies bound in sheep) with the Plattsburgh imprint, and a smaller number issued by Lilly, Wait, and Company. Probably it was hoped that the Boston imprint would enhance marketability. Samuel Beaumont later claimed, when he wrote the preface to the second edition, that first edition consisted of three thousand copies, but this seems exaggerated, especially since correspondence between Beaumont and his New Haven bookseller, Hezekiah Howe, suggests that sales of the first edition were slow.[5]

RBN

1. Beaumont's preliminary reports on St. Martin were published as "A Case of Wounded Stomach," *Medical Recorder* 8 (1825): 14–19, 840; and "Further Experiments on the Case of Alexis St. Martin, Who Was Wounded in the Stomach by a Load of Buckshot," *Medical Recorder* 9 (1826): 94–97. The first article was published under the name of Joseph Lovell.

2. Quoted in Jesse S. Myer, *William Beaumont: A Pioneer American Physiologist*, 3d ed. (St. Louis, 1981), p. 21.

3. William Osler, in his introduction to Jesse S. Myer, *Life and Letters of Dr. William Beaumont* (St. Louis, 1912), p. xxiii; quoted in *Bibliotheca Osleriana* (Oxford, 1929), no. 1972.

4. Quoted in R. B. Nelson, *Beaumont: America's First Physiologist* (Geneva, Ill., 1990), p. 221.

5. Charlotte H. Peters and John F. Fulton, "William Beaumont's Letter to His New Haven Bookseller, Hezekiah Howe, with a Bibliographical Description of the Editions of Beaumont's Book," *Yale Journal of Biology and Medicine* 6 (1933): 9–17.

62

THEODOR SCHWANN
(1810–1882)

Mikroskopische Untersuchungen über die Uebereinstimmung in der Struktur und dem Wachsthum der Thiere und Pflanzen.

Berlin: Verlag der Sander'schen Buchhandlung (G. E. Reimer), 1839.

8°: π^8 $2\pi 1$ $1–9^8$ 10^8 $(\pm 10_2)$ $11–16^8$ $17^8(–17_8)$. 144 leaves, pp. *I–III* IV–XVIII *1* 2–270. Tab. I–IV: 4 folding engraved plates by C. E. Weber after drawings by the author.

GM 113. cf. *Heirs of Hippocrates* 1754. Horblit 93a. Norman 1914. PMM 307b. Waller 11002.

In 1665 Robert Hooke, in his *Micrographia*, observed the cellular nature of plant construction and coined the word "cell." Nehemiah Grew and Marcello Malpighi (see no. 30) in the following decade also observed the cellular construction of parts of plants and formulated a rough hypothesis of a cellular theory of plant life. In 1831 Robert Brown described the nucleus as the essential characteristic of the plant cell,[1] and in 1838 Matthias Schleiden, in his own study of vegetable cells, became the first to construct a theory of cell formation and to present the concept that a living body—in this case a plant—was made up of an aggregate of cells and cell products.[2] After Schleiden pointed out to Theodor Schwann the importance of the nucleus in the development of plant cells, Schwann demonstrated the existence of cellular structures in animal tissue. At this point Schwann discarded Schleiden's erroneous *Uhrglastheorie* of cell formation, which had postulated that cells crystallize in a formative liquid, and formulated a cell theory that insisted on the cellular origin of all living tissue. His theory of the actual formation of cells was erroneous and was later corrected by Rudolf Virchow (see no. 69), but he had succeeded in establishing that the cell was the universal unit of life throughout the animal and vegetable kingdoms, thus ending the search for a common structural principle of live organisms.

Mikroskopische Untersuchungen is divided into three parts. The first is devoted to a microscopic study of the *chorda dorsalis* of frog larvae, in which Schwann developed his theory of cell formation. In the second part he applied the notion he had just promulgated to the individual animal tissue, be it muscle or bone, feather or fat. He found that all these are the product of cellular differentiation, and that although quite different physiologically, they are in their most elementary state only developments of cells. Schwann also coined the term "metabolism" in the course of his attempt to define the physicochemical processes of cellular differentiation. The third part of *Mikroskopische Unter-*

Mikroskopische

Untersuchungen

über

die Uebereinstimmung in der Struktur und dem Wachsthum

der

Thiere und Pflanzen

von

Dr. *Th. Schwann.*

Mit vier Kupfertafeln.

Berlin 1839.

Verlag der Sander'schen Buchhandlung.

(G. E. Reimer.)

Fig. 114. No. 62. Schwann. Title page.

suchungen is a philosophical discussion of Schwann's cell theory as expounded in the first two parts. The book was published in English translation in 1847.[3]

NP

1. Robert Brown, "On the Organs and Mode of Fecundation in Orchideae and Asclepiadeae," *Transactions of the Linnean Society* 16 (1833): 685–742. Printed for private distribution in 1831.
2. Matthias Schleiden, "Beiträge zur Phytogenesis," *Archiv für Anatomie, Physiologie und wissenschaftlicher Medicin* 5 (1838): 137–76.
3. Theodor Schwann, *Microscopical Researches into the Accordance in the Structure and Growth of Animals and Plants*, trans. Henry Smith (London, 1847).

Fig. 115. No. 62. Schwann. Schwann's presentation inscription to Gilbert Breschet. This copy was also owned by August Weismann, formulator of the first modern cell-based theory of inheritance, and Clifford Dobell, biographer of pioneer microbiologist Antoni van Leeuwenhoek.

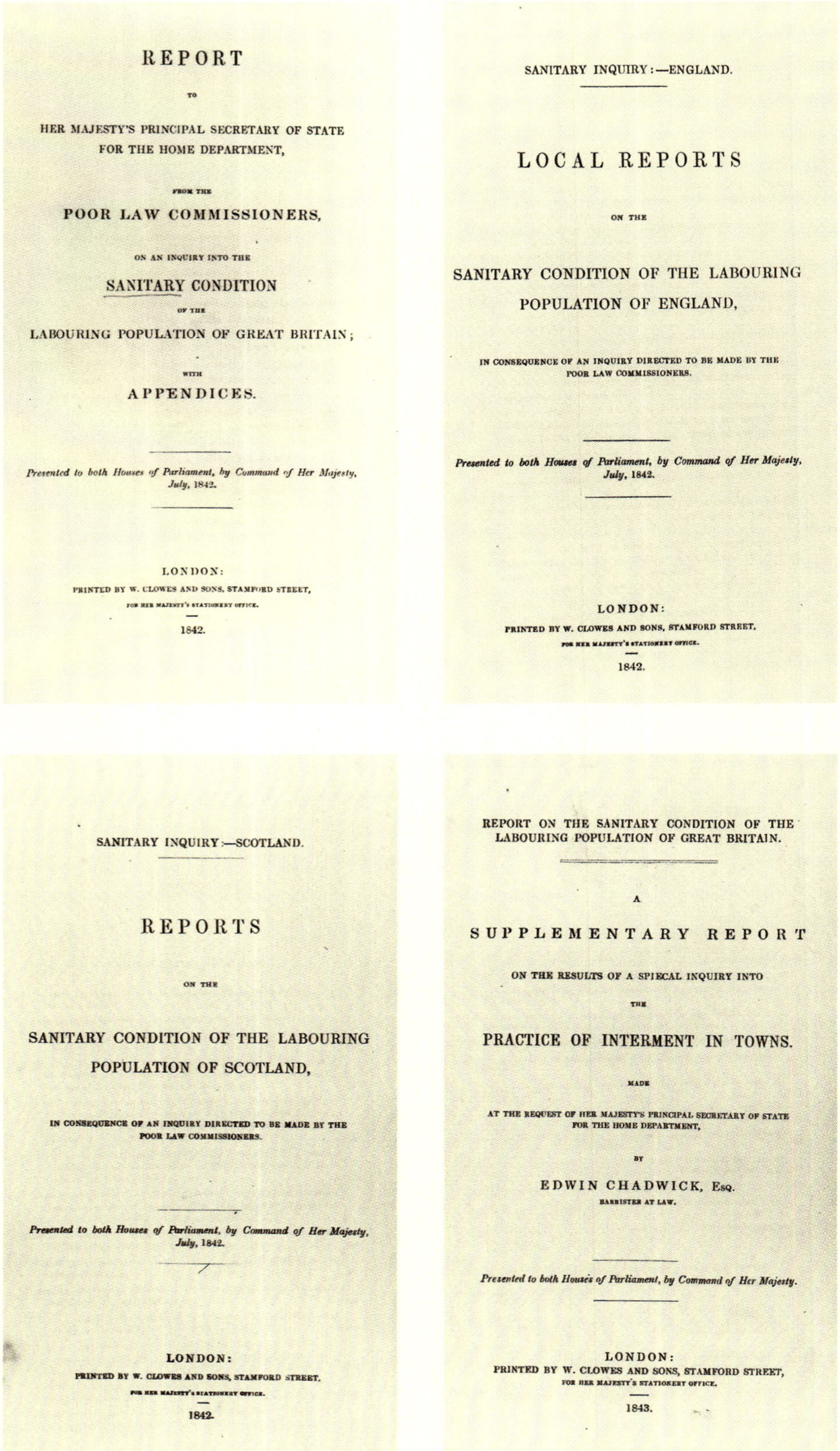

REPORT

TO

HER MAJESTY'S PRINCIPAL SECRETARY OF STATE
FOR THE HOME DEPARTMENT,

FROM THE

POOR LAW COMMISSIONERS,

ON AN INQUIRY INTO THE

SANITARY CONDITION

OF THE

LABOURING POPULATION OF GREAT BRITAIN;

WITH

APPENDICES.

Presented to both Houses of Parliament, by Command of Her Majesty,
July, 1842.

LONDON:
PRINTED BY W. CLOWES AND SONS, STAMFORD STREET,
FOR HER MAJESTY'S STATIONERY OFFICE.
1842.

SANITARY INQUIRY:—ENGLAND.

LOCAL REPORTS

ON THE

SANITARY CONDITION OF THE LABOURING
POPULATION OF ENGLAND,

IN CONSEQUENCE OF AN INQUIRY DIRECTED TO BE MADE BY THE
POOR LAW COMMISSIONERS.

Presented to both Houses of Parliament, by Command of Her Majesty,
July, 1842.

LONDON:
PRINTED BY W. CLOWES AND SONS, STAMFORD STREET,
FOR HER MAJESTY'S STATIONERY OFFICE.
1842.

SANITARY INQUIRY:—SCOTLAND.

REPORTS

ON THE

SANITARY CONDITION OF THE LABOURING
POPULATION OF SCOTLAND,

IN CONSEQUENCE OF AN INQUIRY DIRECTED TO BE MADE BY THE
POOR LAW COMMISSIONERS.

Presented to both Houses of Parliament, by Command of Her Majesty,
July, 1842.

LONDON:
PRINTED BY W. CLOWES AND SONS, STAMFORD STREET,
FOR HER MAJESTY'S STATIONERY OFFICE.
1842.

REPORT ON THE SANITARY CONDITION OF THE
LABOURING POPULATION OF GREAT BRITAIN.

A

SUPPLEMENTARY REPORT

ON THE RESULTS OF A SPIECAL INQUIRY INTO

THE

PRACTICE OF INTERMENT IN TOWNS.

MADE

AT THE REQUEST OF HER MAJESTY'S PRINCIPAL SECRETARY OF STATE
FOR THE HOME DEPARTMENT,

BY

EDWIN CHADWICK, Esq.
BARRISTER AT LAW.

Presented to both Houses of Parliament, by Command of Her Majesty.

LONDON:
PRINTED BY W. CLOWES AND SONS, STAMFORD STREET,
FOR HER MAJESTY'S STATIONERY OFFICE.
1843.

Fig. 116. No. 63. Chadwick. Title pages.

63

SIR EDWIN CHADWICK
(1800–1890)

Report to Her Majesty's Principal Secretary of State for the Home Department, from the Poor Law Commissioners, on an Inquiry into the Sanitary Condition of the Labouring Population of Great Britain.

London: Printed by W. Clowes and Sons, for Her Majesty's Stationery Office, 1842.

a–b^8 B–Q^8 R^2 S–Z^8 2A–2G^8 2H^4 (–2H4). 245 leaves, pp. *i–iii* iv–xxx [2] *1* 2–457 [1]. 1 folding engraved map, with brown aquatint shading, overprinted in red and blue; 1 folding lithographed map, printed in black and brown; 1 folding lithographed table; 16 lithographed plates (5 in two parts); 6 wood-engraved figures and 2 wood-engraved maps in text. Purple cloth.

Local Reports on the Sanitary Condition of the Labouring Population of England, in Consequence of an Inquiry Directed to Be Made by the Poor Law Commissioners.

London: Printed by W. Clowes and Sons, for Her Majesty's Stationery Office, 1842.

[A]^2 B–Z^8 2A–2E^8 2F^6. 224 leaves, pp. *i–iii* iv *1* 2–444. 8 lithographed plates (2 in two parts); 1 wood-engraved figure in text. Purple cloth.

Reports on the Sanitary Condition of the Labouring Population of Scotland, in Consequence of an Inquiry Directed to Be Made by the Poor Law Commissioners.

London: Printed by W. Clowes and Sons, for Her Majesty's Stationery Office, 1842.

[A]^2 B–Y^8. 170 leaves, pp. *i–iii* iv *1* 2–334 [2]. Purple cloth.

Report on the Sanitary Condition of the Labouring Population of Great Britain. A Supplementary Report on the Results of a Special Inquiry into the Practice of Interment in Towns.

London: Printed by W. Clowes and Sons, for Her Majesty's Stationery Office, 1843.

[A]^4 B–S^8 T^4. 144 leaves, pp. *i–iii* iv–vii [1] 1–279 [1]. 3 wood-engraved figures in text; 1 wood-engraved diagram in text. Purple cloth.

GM 1608. *Heirs of Hippocrates* 1626, 1627. Norman 434. PMM 313. Wellcome II, p. 322.

As a sanitary reformer Edwin Chadwick was responsible for three great achievements. His first was the series of reports written, edited, or commissioned by him, in which he was able to prove beyond doubt the connection between environment and disease. His second achievement was his suggestion of what was in effect a blueprint for a public health department, a revolutionary proposal for the time. His third achievement was his practical proposal for a new system of drainage, based on the work of a new generation of engineers.

A barrister and journalist, and an associate of Jeremy Bentham, Chadwick was appointed in 1832 to England's Poor Law Commission. In 1838 after an outbreak of disease in the East End of London, he charged a group of three doctors to report on its causes. Their findings called forth similar investigations of living conditions in other parts of the country and led to the publication of the present reports. Based on the eye-witness accounts of medical men, sent in from towns of all sizes located all over Britain, these reports revealed appalling conditions. For example, in medium-sized towns such as Truro and Tiverton, adjoining streets with quite different standards of hygiene and sanitation housed people with quite different standards of health, and in Windsor a street with open drains and foul cesspits went right up to the Long Walk adjoining Windsor Park and the castle.

In the principal volume of the 1842 report Chadwick forcefully summed up his conclusions as to the relationship between living conditions and disease:

> . . . the various forms of epidemic, endemic, and other disease caused, or aggravated, or propagated chiefly amongst the labouring classes by atmospheric impurities produced by decomposing animal and vegetable substances, by damp and filth, and close and overcrowded dwellings prevail amongst the population in every part of the kingdom, whether dwelling in separate houses, in rural villages, in small towns, in the larger towns—as they have been found to prevail in the lowest districts of the metropolis.
>
> . . . such disease, wherever its attacks are frequent, is always found in connexion with the physical circumstances above specified, and . . . where those circumstances are removed by drainage, proper cleansing, better ventilation, and other means of diminishing atmospheric impurity, the frequency and intensity of such disease is abated; and where the removal of the noxious agencies appears to be complete, such disease almost entirely disappears.
>
> . . . the annual loss of life from filth and bad ventilation are greater than the loss from death or wounds in any wars in which the country has been engaged in modern times.

Realizing that "the formation of all habits of cleanliness is obstructed by defective supplies of water," Chadwick saw that any effective system of drainage was dependent on the universal availability of water at high pressure. To protestations that his proposals would be very expensive, he replied, ". . . the expense of public drainage, of supplies of water laid on in houses, and of means of improved cleansing would be a pecuniary gain, by diminishing the existing charges attendant on sickness and premature mortality." Although Chadwick's sanitary reforms were not accomplished until long after his retirement, he made two crucial innovations: he adapted the arterial system of town drainage invented by John Roe, and he introduced glazed earthenware pipes.

The Poor Law Commissioners' report was issued in three volumes, two containing local reports for England and Scotland, and the third, by Chadwick, summing up the results of the inquiry and proposing steps for remedial action. Chadwick also wrote a supplementary report on the subject of interment in towns. In this he determined that the long retention of unburied bodies in the homes of the poor, as was then customary, contributed to the spread of disease and that burials in urban church cemeteries often led to the contamination of the air from shallow burials or of ground water from deeper ones; as solutions to these problems, he recommended a system of town cemeteries and crematoria.

From his position as secretary to the Poor Law Commissioners and from his experiences as a commissioner, Chadwick realized that any effective remedy to the problems caused by bad sanitation required a considerable extension of government power. It was the strength of the 1842 report that it not only exposed abuses in such a way as to create a force for reform, but it also suggested ways in which this might be achieved. From Chadwick's administrative reforms came the Public Health Act of 1848, in which for the first time a British government assumed responsibility for the health of its subjects. Chadwick also introduced the system of centrally controlled inspectors, on which all subsequent public health administration has depended.

RDG

THE

BOSTON MEDICAL AND SURGICAL JOURNAL.

EDITED BY

J. V. C. SMITH, M.D.

Whole No. 979. WEDNESDAY, NOVEMBER 18, 1846. Vol. XXXV. No. 16.

CONTENTS.

Published every Wednesday—each Number containing one sheet, subject to newspaper postage only.—Price $3 a year, in advance.

BOSTON:

DAVID CLAPP, PRINTER AND PUBLISHER,

184 Washington St., corner of Franklin St.

Fig. 117. No. 64A. Bigelow. Wrapper of the *Boston Medical and Surgical Journal* for 18 November 1846. Bigelow's article on surgical anesthesia appeared in this number.

64

HENRY JACOB BIGELOW
(1818–1890)

A] Insensibility during Surgical Operations Produced by Inhalation.

In: *Boston Medical and Surgical Journal* 35 (1846–47): 309–17, 379–82.

[journal numbers] Vol. 35, no. 16, 18 November 1846: 16^{12}. 12 leaves, pp. [2] *309* 310–328 [2]. Vol. 35, no. 19, 9 December 1846: 19^{12}. 12 leaves, pp. [2] *369* 370–388 [2]. Self wrappers, printed integrally with the text of each journal number.

[article] 16_2^r–16_6^r, pp. *309* 310–317. 19_7^r–19_8^v, pp. 379–382.

GM 5651. *Heirs of Hippocrates* 1859. Norman 232. Osler 1355. Wellcome II, p. 166.

[separate] *Insensibility during Surgical Operations Produced by Inhalation* [head title]. Reprinted from the Boston Medical and Surgical Journal. Vol. XXXV. Wednesday, November 18, 1846. No. 16.

$[1]^4$. 4 leaves, pp. *309* 310–316.

Completely reset, omitting the last seven paragraphs of the original article.

Norman 233.

B] William Thomas Green Morton (1819–1868). *To Surgeons and Physicians* [advertising circular].

Boston, [1846].

1 leaf, folded.

C] William Thomas Green Morton. *Remarks on the Proper Mode of Administering Sulphuric Ether by Inhalation.*

Boston: Dutton and Wentworth, Printers, 1847.

$[1]^6$ 2–3^6 4^4. 22 leaves, pp. *1–7* 8–44. Solid dark blue, or patterned black and white printed wrappers.

GM 5653. Norman 1556. Osler 1354.

Probably no other event has had such an immediate and profound effect on medical practice as the discovery of surgical anesthesia. Surgery has been practiced since Antiquity, but before anesthetics were known it had always been associated with intense, unrelievable pain, frequently and understandably unbearable. Thus surgery was most often restricted to emergency situations and only seldom carried out in other circumstances, as it was a

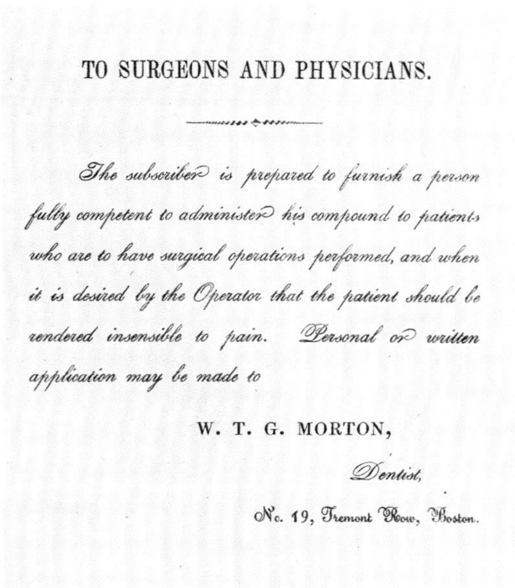

TO SURGEONS AND PHYSICIANS.

The subscriber is prepared to furnish a person fully competent to administer his compound to patients who are to have surgical operations performed, and when it is desired by the Operator that the patient should be rendered insensible to pain. Personal or written application may be made to

W. T. G. MORTON,

Dentist,

No. 19, Tremont Row, Boston.

Fig. 118. No. 64B. Morton. His advertising circular, "To Surgeons and Physicians," was his first reference in print to surgical anesthesia.

rare individual who would deliberately subject himself to the surgeon's knife with only the doubtful mitigation of opium or alcohol. It is not surprising that in the year prior to the first successful public demonstration of the effectiveness of ether anesthesia, no more than nine major operations were carried out at the Massachusetts General Hospital. With the discovery of anesthesia, however, this number soon increased to nine per week.

The anesthetic effect of inhaled substances had first been noticed by Sir Humphry Davy, the discoverer of nitrous oxide ("laughing gas"). Davy's *Researches, Chemical and Philosophical, Chiefly concerning Nitrous Oxide, or Dephlogisticated Nitrous Air, and Its Respiration* (1800) described his discovery of the anesthetic properties of the gas; however, his suggestion that it might have a use in surgery was ignored. In 1818 the physicist Michael Faraday reported similar results from the use of sulfuric ether, but this too made no impression on the medical community. Ether vapor was not used successfully as an anesthetic until 1842, when it was employed by the American dentist Dr. Crawford Long of Georgia; Long, however, failed to publish his results until 1849, three years after the first announcement of ether's anesthetic properties. Horace Wells, another American dentist, attempted in 1845 to demonstrate the anesthetic effects of nitrous oxide but failed and was denounced as a charlatan. Painless surgery remained an impossible dream until 16 October 1846, when W.T.G. Morton, a former associate of Wells, demonstrated the effectiveness of ether anesthesia during an operation performed at the Massachusetts General Hospital. Morton originally intended to keep the identity of his anesthetic substance a secret so that he could patent it; however, Henry Jacob Bigelow, a Boston surgeon who witnessed the demonstration, revealed the substance's identity in his epoch-making paper, "Insensibility during Surgical Operations Produced by Inhalation." After being presented

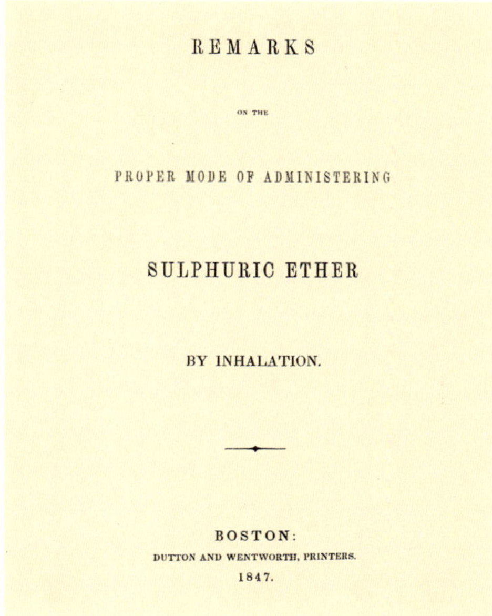
REMARKS

ON THE

PROPER MODE OF ADMINISTERING

SULPHURIC ETHER

BY INHALATION.

BOSTON:
DUTTON AND WENTWORTH, PRINTERS.
1847.

Fig. 119. No. 64c. Morton. Title page of his *Remarks on the Proper Mode of Administering Sulphuric Ether by Inhalation* (1847).

in abstract to the American Academy of Arts and Sciences on 3 November 1846, this was read before the Boston Society for Medical Improvement on 9 November and was published in the 18 November 1846 number of the *Boston Medical and Surgical Journal.* Morton subsequently advertised his ability to produce painless surgical operations, sought compensation for his discovery from Congress (without success), and spent the next few years contending priority of discovery with a Boston physician, Charles Jackson, who engaged him in a series of ruinous lawsuits.

Following the appearance of Bigelow's article, papers on anesthesia were published in the United States and in Europe. Both the medical profession and the general public immediately embraced surgical anesthesia: surgeons could now plan and carry out surgical operations in an unhurried and careful manner, and patients could agree to operations knowing that they would suffer no pain during the procedure. Within a year, textbooks of surgical anesthesia had been published, including Morton's *Remarks on the Proper Mode of Administering Sulfuric Ether by Inhalation*, and the use of anesthesia was extended to obstetrics, as first reported by the Edinburgh physician James Young Simpson in September 1847. The term "anesthesia" itself was coined by the physician, poet, and essayist Oliver Wendell Holmes, who suggested the name to Morton in a letter written on 21 November 1846.

Surgery as it is practiced today exists in large part because of anesthesia: anesthesia, discovered in 1846, and surgical antisepsis, discovered in 1868, are the nineteenth-century cornerstones of modern surgical practice. History has more than confirmed Bigelow's prediction: "[Anesthesia] now promises to be one of the important discoveries of the age."

AEL

See color plate XXX.

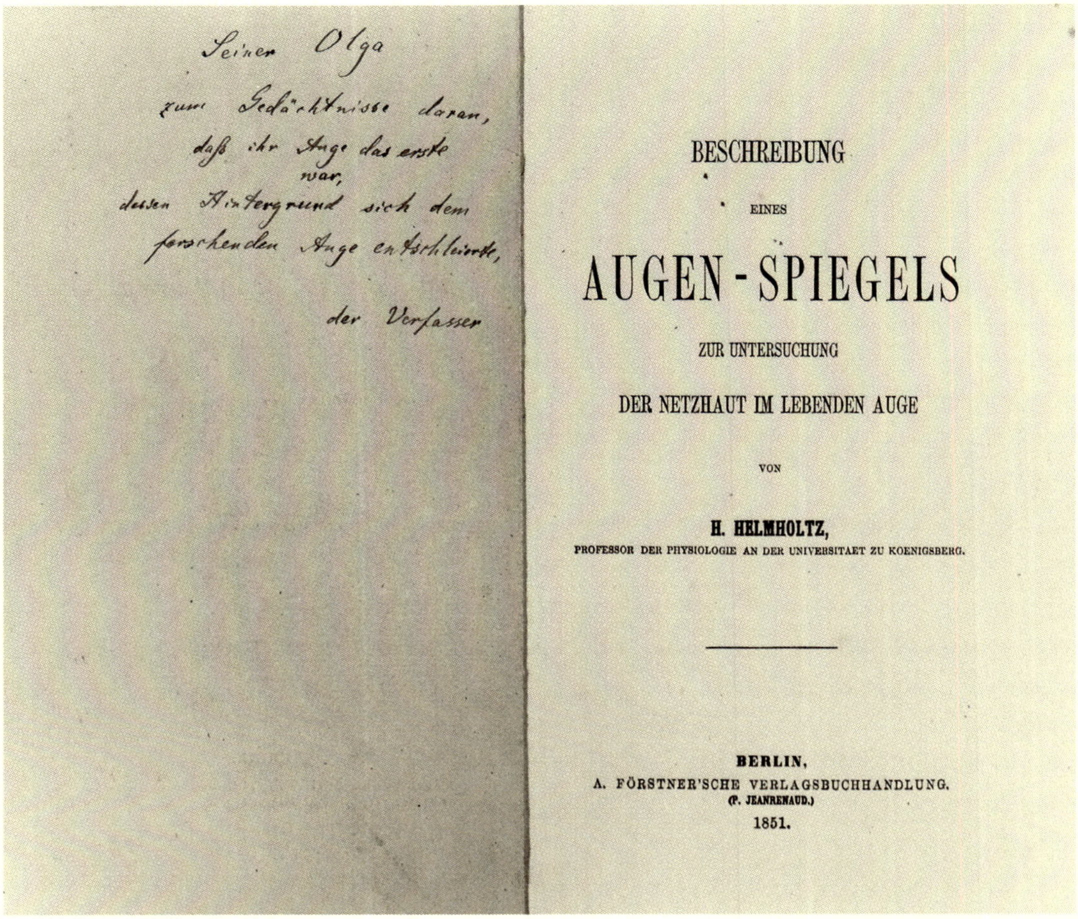

Fig. 120. No. 65. Helmholtz. Title page, with the author's presentation inscription to his wife Olga on the wrapper opposite.

65

HERMANN VON HELMHOLTZ
(1821–1894)

Beschreibung eines Augen-Spiegels zur Untersuchung der Netzhaut im lebenden Auge.

Berlin: A. Förstner'sche Verlagsbuchhandlung (P. Jeanrenaud), 1851.

1–3^8. 24 leaves, pp. *1–3* 4–43 [5]. 1 engraved plate by Afinger after drawings by Helmholtz. Yellow printed wrappers.

GM 5866. *Heirs of Hippocrates* 1886. Norman 1041. cf. PMM 323. Waller 4294.

Hermann von Helmholtz described his invention of the ophthalmoscope in a monograph of 1851 entitled *Beschreibung eines Augen-Spiegels.* The ophthalmoscope was a by-product of Helmholtz's attempt to demonstrate to his students that when the human eye is made to glow with reflected light, the light emitted from the pupil follows the same course it took in entering the pupil. It occurred to Helmholtz that the light could be brought to a focus and the details of the retina made visible. Although visualization of the fundus had been accomplished prior to Helmholtz's publication, both by Johannes Evangelista Purkyně and by Charles Babbage, Helmholtz was the first to convince the world of the importance of the ophthalmoscope. The value of the instrument was immediately appreciated by ophthalmologists, including William Bowman, Frans Cornelis Donders, and Albrecht von Graefe, and it was through Graefe's efforts in particular that the ophthalmoscope became part of the armamentarium of ophthalmologists throughout Europe and America.

Helmholtz is known for his contributions both to physiology and to physics, the latter including a seminal statement of the first law of thermodynamics (*Über die Erhaltung der Kraft* [1847]). Trained in medicine, he spent his life as a professor and researcher. He never practiced ophthalmology, but his invention, which gave ophthalmologists the ability to examine what had previously been called "the black cataract," greatly improved the capacity for diagnosis of eye diseases and thus revolutionized visual science.

DMA

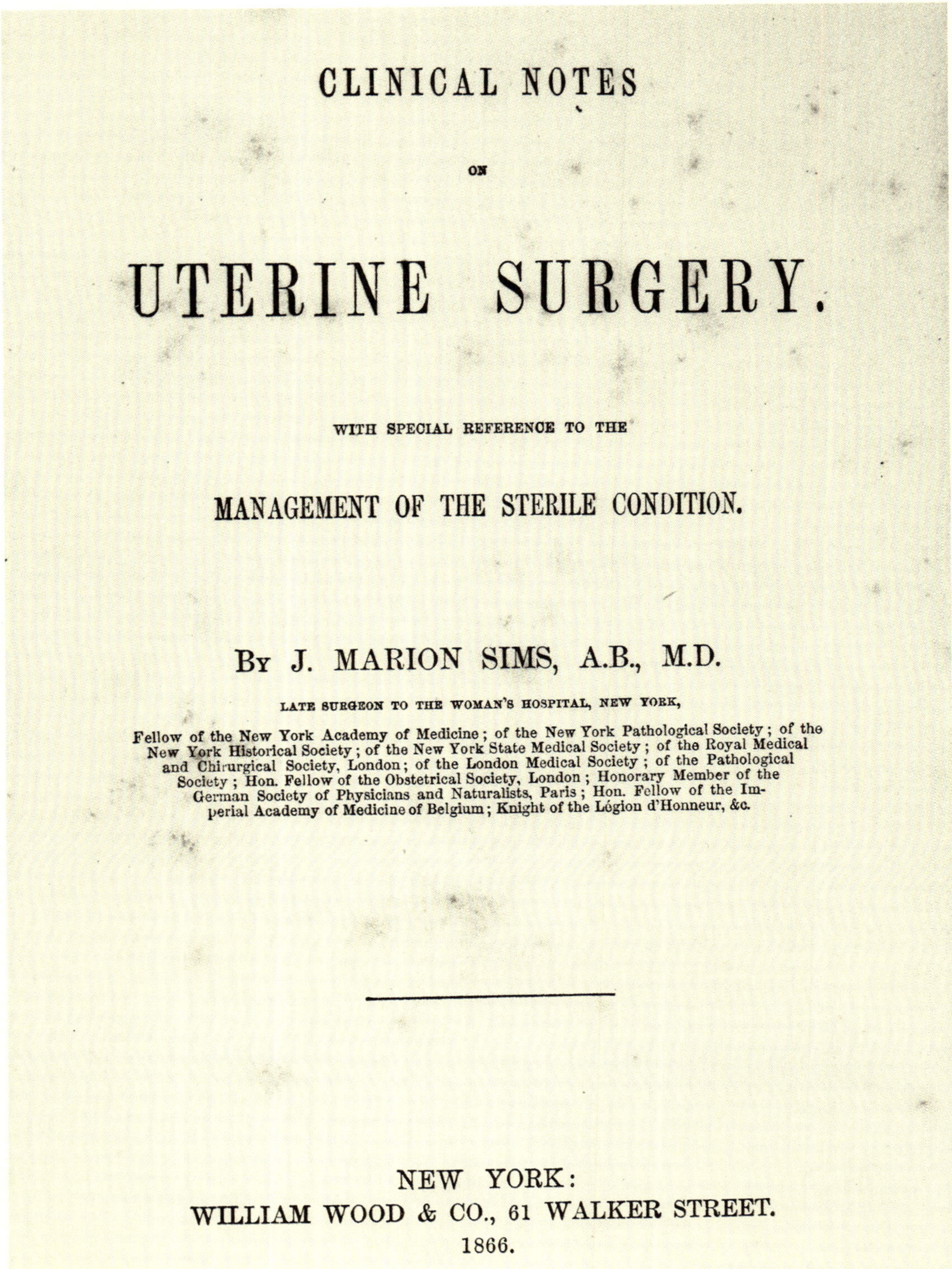

CLINICAL NOTES

ON

UTERINE SURGERY.

WITH SPECIAL REFERENCE TO THE

MANAGEMENT OF THE STERILE CONDITION.

BY J. MARION SIMS, A.B., M.D.

LATE SURGEON TO THE WOMAN'S HOSPITAL, NEW YORK,

Fellow of the New York Academy of Medicine; of the New York Pathological Society; of the New York Historical Society; of the New York State Medical Society; of the Royal Medical and Chirurgical Society, London; of the London Medical Society; of the Pathological Society; Hon. Fellow of the Obstetrical Society, London; Honorary Member of the German Society of Physicians and Naturalists, Paris; Hon. Fellow of the Imperial Academy of Medicine of Belgium; Knight of the Légion d'Honneur, &c.

NEW YORK:
WILLIAM WOOD & CO., 61 WALKER STREET.
1866.

Fig. 121. No. 66B. Sims. Title page.

66

JAMES MARION SIMS
(1813–1883)

A] On the Treatment of Vesico-Vaginal Fistula.

In: *American Journal of the Medical Sciences*, N.S. 23 (1852): 59–82.

[journal number] N.S. Vol. 23, No. 45, January 1852: $\pi 1$ $[1]^6$ $2–18^8$ 19^6. 149 leaves, pp. [2] *1* 2–60 51–286 [i.e., 296].

[article] $5_5^r–6_8^v$, pp. (second series) 59–82. Fig. 1–22: 22 wood-engraved figures in text.

GM 6037.

[offprint] *On the Treatment of Vesico-Vaginal Fistula* [wrapper title]. Philadelphia: Blanchard & Lea, 1853.

1_1 2^4 3^8. 13 leaves, pp. *3–5* 6–28 [i.e., 26]. Fig. 1–22: 22 wood-engraved figures in text. Pink printed wrappers.

With a preface dated 1 November 1853, announcing the opening of Sims's New York practice. Quire 2 reimposed with different page breaks.

B] *Clinical Notes on Uterine Surgery. With Special Reference to the Management of the Sterile Condition.*

[first English edition] London: Robert Hardwicke, 1866.

$[A]^6$ $B–Z^8$ $2A–2E^8$ $2F^2$. 224 leaves, pp. [2] *i–v* vi–viii [2] *1* 2–436. Fig. 1–142: 142 wood engravings in text, by Léveillé, Lackerbauer, Vien, and Orrin Smith after drawings by Sims. Purple publisher's cloth.

GM 6057.

[first American edition] New York: William Wood & Co., 1866.

π^6 $[1]^8$ $2–25^8$ 26^2. 208 leaves, pp. *i–v* vi–xi [1] *1* 2–401 [3]. Fig. 1–142: 142 wood engravings in text, by Léveillé, Lackerbauer, Vien, and Orrin Smith after drawings by Sims. Brown publisher's cloth.

A different setting of type.

Heirs of Hippocrates 1805. Norman 1949.

J. Marion Sims, a native of South Carolina who practiced medicine there and in Alabama, moved to New York City in 1853 for reasons of health. Two years later he founded the Women's Hospital in New York, which opened on 4 May 1855; this was the first American institution devoted exclusively to the treatment of gynecologic disorders. There Sims and his colleagues achieved a brilliant success record for their fistula repairs and vaginal

proximal ends of the wires, and to push it along them into the vagina, till it occupies a position in front of the fistula, corresponding exactly with the one behind it.

Fig. 15 shows the two clamps, one on each side of the fistula, and every-

Fig. 15.

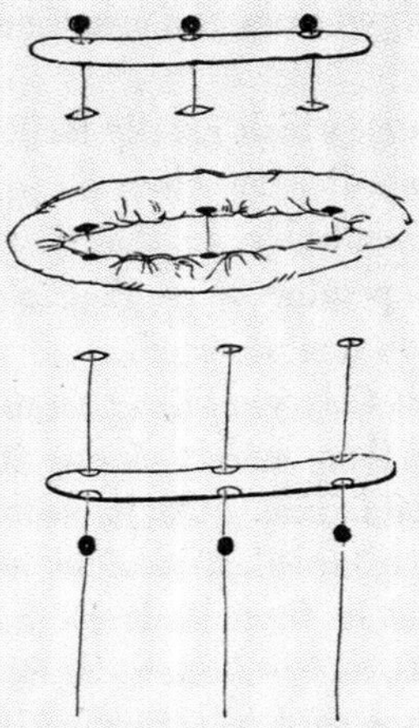

Fig. 16.

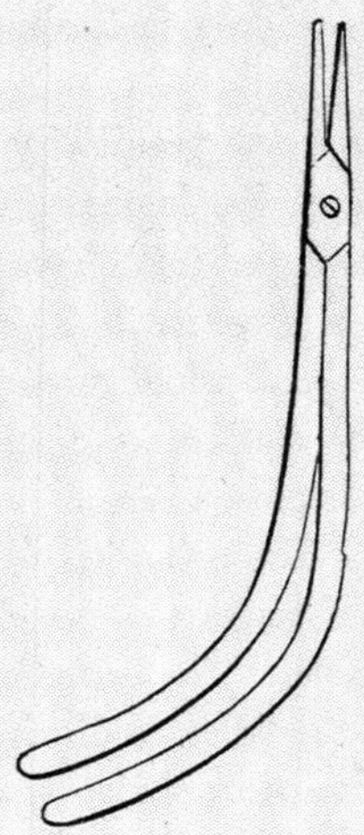

thing ready for closing it. The proximal clamp is pushed up by the crescent-shaped fork, while the wires are held firmly. This brings the denuded edges of the fistula into such close contact that it would be difficult to enter a common sized probe between them. The force necessary for tightening the clamps will depend upon the judgment of the operator; not enough will allow the parts to gape, while too much, which is the most frequent fault, will produce the bad effects formerly alluded to.

Fig. 17.

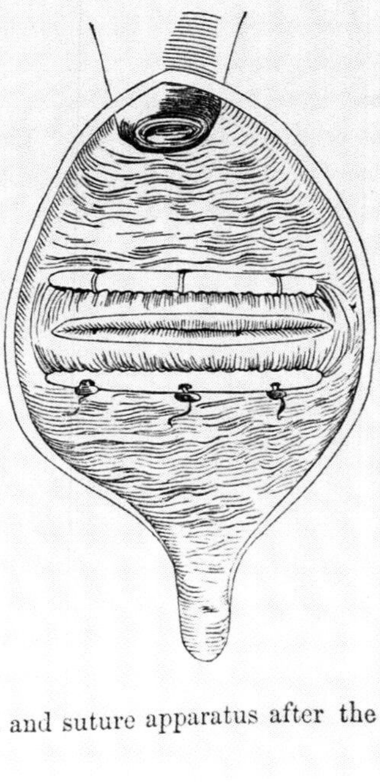

A simple and perfect contrivance now serves to hold the clamps in their proper places. A small bird shot, perforated, is passed along each wire close against the proximal clamp; when, the wires being held securely, they are gently but firmly compressed by means of a long strong pair of forceps (Fig. 16), whereby they are made to perform the office of a knot in preventing the clamp from slipping off the wire. The wires are cut off about a fourth or eighth of an inch from the shot, and then bent over, which effectually prevents their slipping off.

Fig. 17 shows the appearance of the fistula and suture apparatus after the

Fig. 122. No. 66A. Sims's method of repairing vesico-vaginal fistula.

plastic operations and established modern gynecologic surgery in the United States. Sims attained international renown as one of the world's foremost gynecologists.

Sims's 1852 paper contains the original description of his operation for the surgical cure of vesico-vaginal fistula. After repeated fruitless attempts (about forty in number) to cure several women suffering from this malady, Sims ultimately succeeded with the aid of silver sutures, the improved exposure provided by the knee-chest position, and a vaginal speculum now named for him. Sims's technique initiated a new era in the history of gynecology. In his *Silver Sutures in Surgery* (1858), his anniversary discourse before the New York Academy of Medicine, he reviewed the trials and tribulations leading to his eventual success and presented his experience with the use of silver sutures for other operative procedures.

Clinical Notes on Uterine Surgery, written while Sims was in Europe during the American Civil War, was printed in part in the *Lancet* in 1864 and 1865;[1] then in 1866 it was published as a book both in London and in New York. It includes the description of Sims's duck-bill speculum and discusses his controversial research on artificial and instrumental impregnation. Sims's method of uterine investigation made it possible to determine pathologic conditions with unprecedented ease and precision. His examination of cervical mucus soon after intercourse led to important insights into the role of the cervix in infertility but also exposed him to bitter criticism from his more conservative colleagues.

LDL

1. *Lancet*, 1864, 2: 413–16, 457–58, 542–44, 627–28; 1865, 1: 224–25, 253–54, 338–39, 587–88.

Nº D'ORDRE
167.

THÈSE

PRESENTEE

A LA FACULTÉ DES SCIENCES DE PARIS

POUR OBTENIR

LE GRADE DE DOCTEUR ÈS SCIENCES NATURELLES,

PAR M. CLAUDE BERNARD.

THESE DE ZOOLOGIE. RECHERCHES SUR UNE NOUVELLE FONCTION DU FOIE, CONSIDÉRÉ COMME ORGANE PRODUCTEUR DE MATIÈRE SUCRÉE CHEZ L'HOMME ET LES ANIMAUX.

— — PROPOSITIONS DE BOTANIQUE, DE GÉOLOGIE, D'ANATOMIE ET DE PHYSIOLOGIE, DONNÉES PAR LA FACULTÉ.

Soutenue le 17 mars 1853 devant la Commission d'examen.

MM. MILNE EDWARDS, *Président.*

DUMAS, }
A. DE JUSSIEU, } *Examinateurs.*

PARIS,
IMPRIMERIE DE L. MARTINET,
RUE MIGNON, 2.
1853.

Fig. 123. No. 67A. Bernard. Title page of the thesis publication of his treatise on a new function of the liver.

67

CLAUDE BERNARD
(1813–1878)

A] *Recherches sur une nouvelle fonction du foie, considéré comme organe producteur de matière sucrée chez l'homme et les animaux.*

[thesis publication] Paris: Imprimerie de L. Martinet, 1853.

[1]^4 2–12^4 13^2. 50 leaves, pp. *1–7* 8–97 [3]. 1 wood-engraved figure in text. Blue printed wrappers.

cf. EFDT 288. Grmek 9. Malloizel, p. 349. cf. PMM 353. Waller 969.

[monograph publication] *Nouvelle fonction du foie considéré comme organe producteur de matière sucrée chez l'homme et les animaux.* Paris: Chez J.-B. Ballière, 1853.

[1]^4 2–11^4 12^4. 48 leaves, pp. *1–7* 8–92 [4]. 1 wood-engraved figure in text. Gray-green printed wrappers.

cf. EFDT 288. Grmek 10. Horblit 11a. Norman 200. cf. PMM 353.

B] Mémoire sur le pancréas et sur le role du suc pancréatique dans les phénomènes digestifs particulièrement dans la digestion des matières grasses neutres.

In: *Comptes rendus hebdomadaires des séances de l'Académie des Sciences,* Supplement 1 (1856): 379–563.

[journal volume] π^4 1–56^4 57^4 ($\pm 57_{1.4}$) 58–70^4 71^2. 286 leaves, pp. [8] *1* 2–563 [1]. Pl. 1–23: 23 hand-colored engraved plates; Pl. 1–2, 3–4, 5–6, 7–8, 9: 5 folding engraved plates, 3 hand-colored (pl. 5–6, 7–8, 9).

[article] $48_2{}^r$–$71_2{}^r$, pp. 379–563. Pl. 1–2, 3–4, 5–6, 7–8, 9: 5 folding engraved plates by Borromée after Bernard, Lackerbauer, and Léveillé, 3 hand-colored (p. 5–6, 7–8, 9).

cf. EFDT 288. Grmek 163. Malloizel, p. 353. cf. PMM 353.

[monograph publication] Paris: Chez J.-B. Baillière, 1856.

π1 1–9^4 10^4 ($\pm 10_{1.4}$) 11–23^4 24^4 ($\pm 24_{2.3}$; -24_4). 96 leaves, pp. [2] *1–2* 3–190. Pl. 1–2, 3–4, 5–6, 7–8, 9: 5 folding engraved plates by Borromée after Bernard, Lackerbauer, and Léveillé, 3 hand-colored (pl. 5–6, 7–8, 9). Tan printed wrappers.

cf. EFDT 288. Grmek 22. Norman 202. cf. PMM 353. Waller 964.

Claude Bernard is regarded as the most important contributor to experimental physiology in the nineteenth century. Born in St. Julien, a village in the wine country of Beaujo-

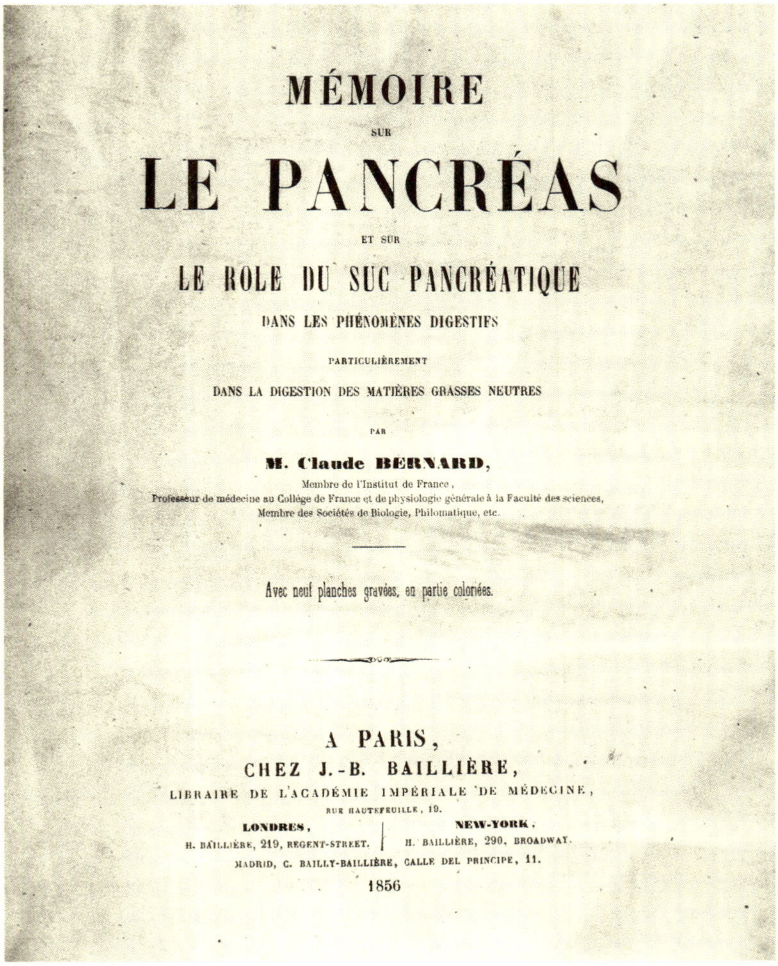
MÉMOIRE

SUR

LE PANCRÉAS

ET SUR

LE ROLE DU SUC PANCRÉATIQUE

DANS LES PHÉNOMÈNES DIGESTIFS

PARTICULIÈREMENT

DANS LA DIGESTION DES MATIÈRES GRASSES NEUTRES

PAR

M. Claude BERNARD,

Membre de l'Institut de France,
Professeur de médecine au Collège de France et de physiologie générale à la Faculté des sciences,
Membre des Sociétés de Biologie, Philomatique, etc.

Avec neuf planches gravées, en partie coloriées.

A PARIS,
CHEZ J.-B. BAILLIÈRE,
LIBRAIRE DE L'ACADÉMIE IMPÉRIALE DE MÉDECINE,
RUE HAUTEFEUILLE, 19.

LONDRES, H. BAILLIÈRE, 219, REGENT-STREET. | NEW-YORK, H. BAILLIÈRE, 290, BROADWAY.

MADRID, C. BAILLY-BAILLIÈRE, CALLE DEL PRINCIPE, 11.

1856

Fig. 124. No. 67B. Bernard. The front wrapper of the separate publication of his paper on the pancreas.

lais, Bernard's early education was humanistic rather than scientific. He at one time aspired to be a playwright, but when his efforts met with discouragement from the critic Saint Marc-Girardin, he entered the Faculté de Médecine in Paris in 1834. While still a student, Bernard came under the influence of the famous physiologist François Magendie (see no. 58), working as Magendie's assistant from 1841 to 1844 and learning from him the use of animal vivisection for physiological experimentation. It was under Magendie's influence that Bernard performed some of his most important researches into the physiology of digestion and nerves.

Bernard's contributions are so important and so numerous that it is difficult to select one work to represent them. His major physiological discoveries included the role of the pancreas in digestion, the glycogenic function of the liver, the vasomotor innovation, and the effects of curare on neuromuscular transmission. He also introduced seminal theoretical concepts, such as that of "internal secretion," and was the author of the landmark medico-philosophical work, *Introduction à l'étude de la médecine expérimentale* (1865), in which he analyzed the philosophical basis of the scientific method and its application to the study of living beings.

Bernard began investigating the glycogenic function of the liver in the 1840s, publishing his first communication on the subject in 1848. In order to determine whether glycemia (sugar in the blood) is a normal or abnormal physiological phenomenon, Bernard conducted experiments in which series of animals were fed either starchy or meat diets, or in some cases were not fed at all for several days. He found sugar in blood samples taken from all of these groups, from which he concluded that glycemia results from a normal and constant metabolic process independent of food intake and that blood sugar must be produced by a source within the animal body. Upon further investigation, Bernard identified this source as the liver, demonstrating that it produces sugar and discharges it into the bloodstream. He termed this the "glycogenic" function of the liver. A summary of his results was published in 1850.[1] In 1853, as his thesis for the doctorate in science, Bernard published his *Recherches sur une nouvelle fonction du foie consideré comme organe producteur de matière sucrée chez l'homme et les animaux*; this work was also issued in monograph form the same year, under a slightly modified title beginning *Nouvelle fonction du foie.*

In 1846 Bernard began studying the pancreatic juices and their role in digestion, and in 1849 he published a paper in which he described his discovery of the role of pancreatic juices in the first stage of metabolism, the emulsification of fats.[2] By observing the processes of digestion in dogs and rabbits, and by experimentation with pure pancreatic juices collected from temporary pancreatic fistulae, Bernard was able to show that pancreatic juices made fats absorbable by breaking them down into fatty acids and glycerine. In 1856 he published his most complete statement on the function of the pancreas, "Mémoire sur le pancréas et sur le role du suc pancréatique dans les phénomènes digestifs, particulièrement dans la digestion des matières grasses neutres." This appeared in Volume I of the supplement to the *Comptes rendus hebdomadaires de l'Académie des Sciences*, and it was also published as a separate edition in book form. The work has only recently been translated into English.[3]

HFN

1. Claude Bernard, "Sur une nouvelle fonction du foie chez l'homme et les animaux," *Comptes rendus hebdomadaires des séances de l'Académie des Sciences* 31 (1850): 571–74.
2. Claude Bernard, "Du suc pancréatique et de son role dans les phénomènes de la digestion," *Mémoires de la Société de Biologie* 1 (1849): 99–115.
3. Claude Bernard, *Memoir on the Pancreas and on the Role of Pancreatic Juice in Digestive Processes, Particularly in the Digestion of Neutral Fat*, trans. John Henderson (London, 1985).

See color plate XXXI.

ANATOMY

DESCRIPTIVE AND SURGICAL.

BY

HENRY GRAY, F.R.S.

LECTURER ON ANATOMY AT SAINT GEORGE'S HOSPITAL.

THE DRAWINGS

BY H. V. CARTER, M.D.

LATE DEMONSTRATOR OF ANATOMY AT ST. GEORGE'S HOSPITAL.

THE DISSECTIONS

JOINTLY BY THE AUTHOR AND DR. CARTER.

LONDON:

JOHN W. PARKER AND SON, WEST STRAND.

1858.

Fig. 125. No. 68. Gray. Title page.

68

HENRY GRAY
(1825/27–1861)

Anatomy, Descriptive and Surgical.

London: John W. Parker and Son, 1858.

[a]^4 b^8 c^4 B–Z^8 AA–ZZ^8 3A–3B^8. 392 leaves, pp. *i–vii* viii–xxxii *1* 2–750 [2]. Fig. 1–363: 363 wood engravings in text, after drawings by Henry Vandyke Carter. Brown publisher's cloth.

GM 418. *Heirs of Hippocrates* 1914. Norman 939.

[first American edition] Philadelphia: Blanchard and Lea, 1859.

[1]^8 2–49^8 50^2. 394 leaves, pp. *i–vii* viii–xxxii *1* 2–754 [2]. Fig. 1–363: 363 wood engravings in text, after drawings by Henry Vandyke Carter.

Reset, with corrections, from the English edition.

Heirs of Hippocrates 1915.

Henry Gray began the preface to the first edition of his *Anatomy* thus: "This work is intended to furnish the Student and Practitioner with an accurate view of the Anatomy of the Human Body, and more especially the application of this science to Practical Surgery." Such was the success of this enterprise that the first edition, seven hundred and fifty copies, was sold out within two years, and the book has continued to appear in revised editions up to the present—a thirty-seventh edition was published in 1989. The first American edition was published in June 1859 by Blanchard and Lea in Philadelphia, utilizing a complete set of wood blocks imported for the illustrations. The American editions of the work, with American editors, at first consisted of corrected reprints, but from the sixteenth edition on the text has been rewritten by American authors.

Little is known of Gray's life beyond his formal career and written work, yet his name is known to every English-speaking medical man and woman. He was evidently a very bright and hard-working young man—while still a student, he won the triennial prize of the Royal College of Surgeons for his paper on the comparative anatomy of the eye. This and subsequent original work on embryology and on the ductless glands led to his being elected a Fellow of the Royal Society in 1852, while still in his mid-twenties. His book, *The Structure and Use of the Spleen* (1854), was a pioneering work on that subject. As demonstrator of anatomy and lecturer at St. George's Hospital Medical School in London, Gray

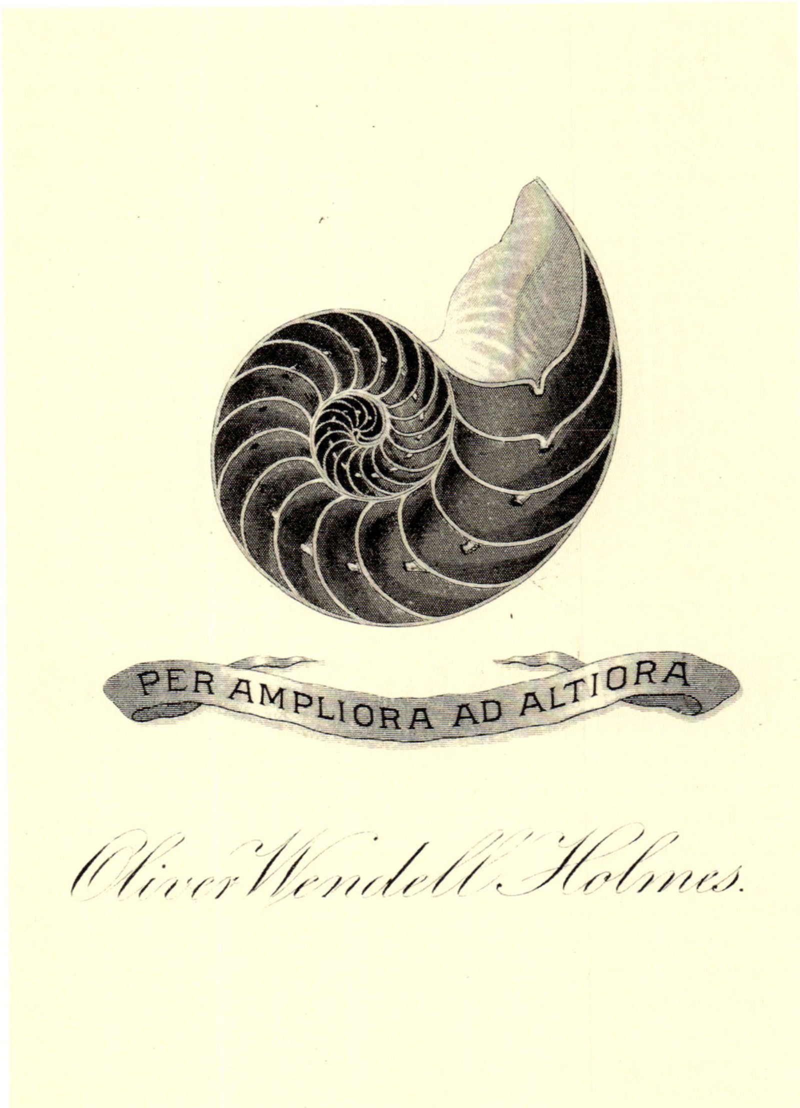

Fig. 126. No. 68. Oliver Wendell Holmes's bookplate in his copy of Gray's *Anatomy.*

obtained the necessary experience and background for his *Anatomy* and established the reputation that helped bring about its immediate success.

Gray's *Anatomy* was published at a time when there were already several rival anatomical textbooks, some by distinguished authors such as Jones Quain and Erasmus Wilson. The success of Gray's work may be due to the fact that he wrote clearly and arranged the contents of his book well, integrating surgical anatomy into the main text. The excellent illustrations may also have contributed—these were wood engravings after drawings by Henry Vandyke Carter, Gray's assistant at St. George's Medical School. The subjects were mainly fresh dissections by Gray and Carter, and explanatory text was included with the illustrations themselves, rather than in separate lists. Colored illustrations were introduced in the eleventh edition (1887). Dr. Charles Goss, who read the original reviews of Gray's work, commented in his *Brief Account of Henry Gray* that "one is struck . . . by the frequency of the comment that Gray has a new and skillful approach to giving students and practitioners what they need in an accessible form."[1] Whatever the reasons, Gray's *Anatomy* was and has remained a great success.

RDG

1. Charles Mayo Goss, *A Brief Account of Henry Gray F.R.S. and His Anatomy, Descriptive and Surgical During a Century of Its Publication in America* (Philadelphia, 1959). See also F.N.L. Poynter, "Gray's Anatomy: The First Hundred Years," *British Medical Journal*, 1958, 2: 610–11.

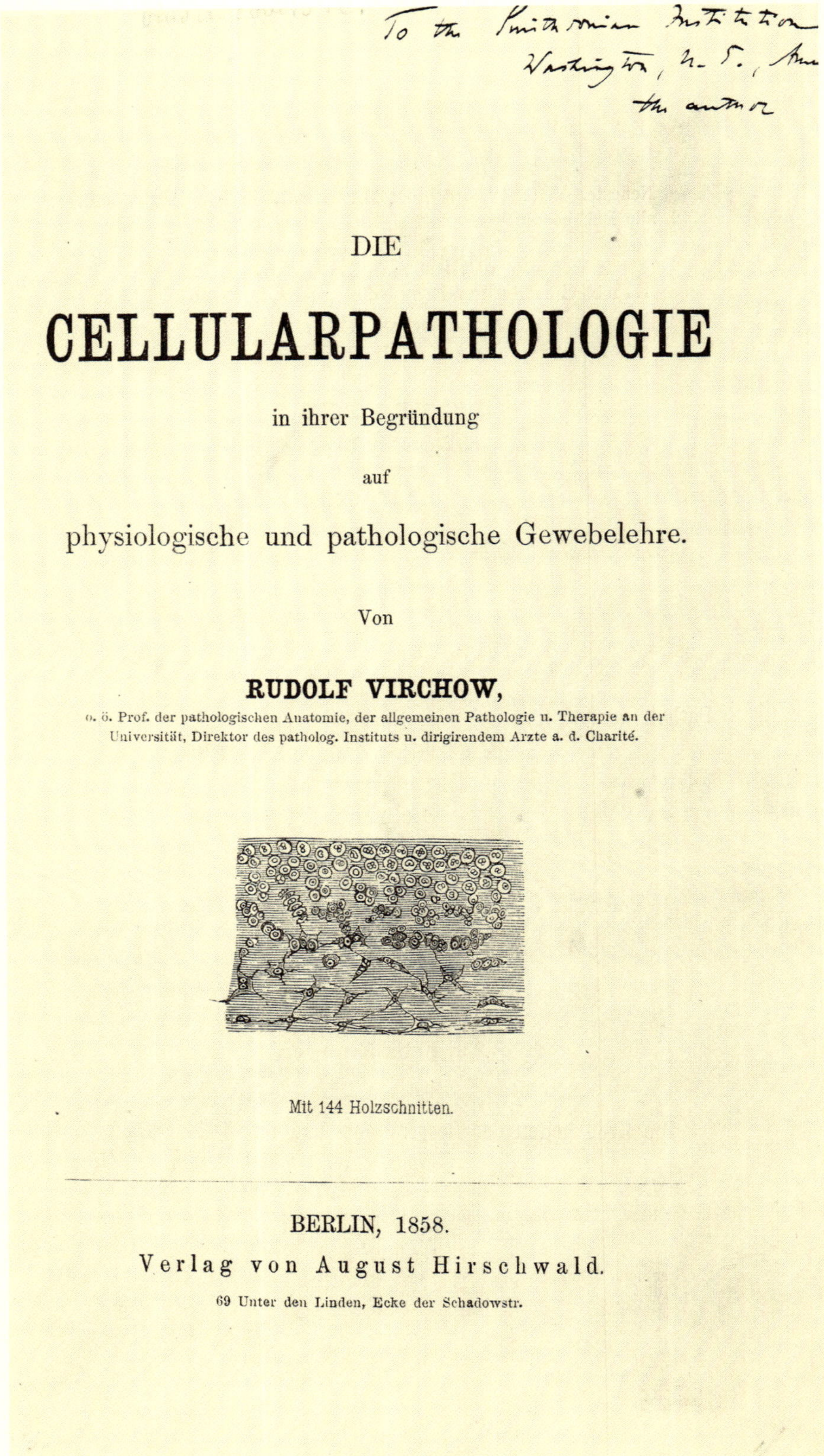

To the Smithsonian Institution
Washington, U. S., from
the author

DIE

CELLULARPATHOLOGIE

in ihrer Begründung

auf

physiologische und pathologische Gewebelehre.

Von

RUDOLF VIRCHOW,

o. ö. Prof. der pathologischen Anatomie, der allgemeinen Pathologie u. Therapie an der Universität, Direktor des patholog. Instituts u. dirigirendem Arzte a. d. Charité.

Mit 144 Holzschnitten.

BERLIN, 1858.

Verlag von August Hirschwald.

69 Unter den Linden, Ecke der Schadowstr.

Fig. 127. No. 69. Virchow. Front wrapper of the copy presented by Virchow to the Smithsonian Institution.

69

RUDOLF VIRCHOW
(1821–1902)

Die Cellularpathologie in ihrer Begründung auf physiologische und pathologische Gewebelehre.

Berlin: Verlag von August Hirschwald, 1858.

π^8 1–27^8 28^4. 228 leaves, pp. *I–V* VI–XVI *1* 2–440. Fig. 1–144: 144 wood engravings in text. Cloth-backed printed boards, or printed wrappers.

GM 2299. *Heirs of Hippocrates* 1892. Horblit 99. Norman 2156. Osler 1624. PMM 307c. Schwalbe, p. 22. Waller 9996.

Rudolf Virchow provided the final link in the chain of pathological investigation begun by Giovanni Battista Morgagni (see no. 46). Morgagni had located the seat of a disease in a specific organ, a concept that was further refined when Xavier Bichat showed that individual tissues could be individually affected by diseases. Virchow, enlightened by the researches of Matthias Schleiden and Theodor Schwann (see no. 62), who declared that the cell was the unit of life in both the vegetable and the animal kingdoms, traced the seat of disease to the cell.

Virchow was the first to state the axiom *Omnis cellula e cellula* (Every cell from a cell), or as he explained more fully: "Where a cell arises, there a cell must have previously existed, just as an animal can spring only from an animal, a plant only from a plant. . . . There is no discontinuity of development of such a kind that a new generation can of itself give rise to a new series of developmental forms. No developed tissues can be traced back either to any large or small simple element, unless it be unto a cell."[1] Every morbid structure therefore consists of cells, which, according to this axiom, themselves come from pre-existing cells. The seat of any disease must therefore be in the cell. On this basis, Virchow analysed disease and diseased tissue and proposed the idea that disease is a conflict between healthy and morbid cells. This was the beginning of modern pathology, and Virchow has been called the greatest figure in its history.[2] *Die Cellularpathologie* was the product of a course of lectures given while he occupied the first chair of pathology at Berlin, although many of the observations it includes had been made earlier in his career.

NP

1. Rudolf Virchow, *Cellular Pathology as Based upon Physiological and Pathological Histology*, trans. Frank Chance, from the second German edition (London, 1860).
2. Esmond R. Long, *A History of Pathology* (Baltimore, 1928), p. 191.

~~THE~~ On

THE ORIGIN OF SPECIES

BY MEANS OF NATURAL SELECTION,

OR THE

PRESERVATION OF FAVOURED RACES IN THE STRUGGLE FOR LIFE.

BY CHARLES DARWIN, M.A.,

FELLOW OF THE ROYAL, GEOLOGICAL, LINNÆAN, ETC., SOCIETIES;
AUTHOR OF 'JOURNAL OF RESEARCHES DURING H. M. S. BEAGLE'S VOYAGE ROUND THE WORLD.'

LONDON:
JOHN MURRAY, ALBEMARLE STREET.
1859.

The right of Translation is reserved.]

Fig. 128. No. 70B. Darwin. Title page of the proof copy of *On the Origin of Species*, showing a correction in Darwin's hand.

70

CHARLES ROBERT DARWIN
(1809–1882)

ALFRED RUSSEL WALLACE
(1823–1913)

A] On the Tendency of Species to Form Varieties; and on the Perpetuation of Varieties and Species by Natural Means of Selection.

In: *Journal of the Proceedings of the Linnean Society*, Zoology 3 (1858–59): 45–62.

[journal number] Vol. 3, No. 9, August 1858: 1–4^8. 32 leaves, pp. *1* 2–62 [2]. Pink printed wrappers. Also issued together with *Journal of the Proceedings of the Linnean Society*, Biology 3, no. 9 (August 1858), in blue printed wrappers.

[article] 3_7^r–4_7^v, pp. 45–62.

[offprint] *On the Tendency of Species to Form Varieties; and on the Perpetuation of Varieties and Species by Natural Means of Selection* [head title]. From the Journal of the Proceedings of the Linnean Society for August 1858.

π^2 4^8. 10 leaves, pp. *45* 46–62 [2]. Buff printed wrappers.

Freeman 346–48. GM 219. Horblit 23a. Norman 591. Osler 1565. PMM 344a.

B] Charles Darwin. *On the Origin of Species by Means of Natural Selection, or the Preservation of Favoured Races in the Struggle for Life.*

London: John Murray, 1859.

[a]^4 b1 B–X^{12} Y^{12} (–Y12). 256 leaves, pp. *i–v* vi–ix [1] *1* 2–502. 1 folding lithographed diagram. Green publisher's cloth.

Freeman 373. GM 220. *Heirs of Hippocrates* 1724. Horblit 23b. Norman 593. Osler 1566. PMM 344b. Waller 10786.

Charles Darwin's exposition of the theory of evolution by means of natural selection led eventually to the establishment of natural selection as a central organizing concept in biology. Previous writers on species had tended to think of species populations as defined by their correspondence to an ideal type, or as fixed rungs on a ladder made up of a progression of species from simple forms to the more complex. In contrast to this, Darwin, when studying a given species population, tended to see more deviation from the ideal type than correspondence to it, and he postulated that this deviation from the standard definition of a given species, called variation, could be understood if certain varieties were better adapted than others to survive and reproduce in a changing environment. The variety most successful in adapting to new environmental conditions would, in time (exactly how much time was unclear) become a new species.

As a result of the "Darwinian revolution," species came to be viewed as dynamic populations adapting over generations to environmental change by means of natural selection. Evolutionary theory stimulated thought about medically related subjects such as anatomy, embryology, physiology, and psychology by offering a framework and mechanism for understanding and interpreting evidence of development. With advances in microbiology and immunology, natural selection was eventually observed at the cellular level. Many disease entities came to be understood as microbial species populations (bacteria and viruses) rapidly evolving in response to sophisticated natural immunologic defenses which had, in turn, evolved by the perpetual struggle between these diverse, extremely mutable populations of microorganisms and their hosts. Through natural selection, populations of bacteria may become resistant to artificially introduced defenses such as antibiotics, making it necessary to develop new drugs to fight new disease entities. Some species of viruses may evolve so rapidly, it has been theorized, that it will be necessary to interfere with the mechanism of their replication before any effective vaccine for them can be developed.

Darwin and Wallace's paper "On the Tendency of Species to Form Varieties" represents the first published exposition of the Darwinian theory of evolution by natural selection. Darwin had developed the essential elements of his theory by 1838 and set them down on paper in 1844; however, he chose to keep his work on evolution unpublished for the time, instead concentrating his energies first on the preparation for publication of the geological work he had done on his voyage with the *Beagle*, and then on an exhaustive eight-year study of the barnacle genus *Cirripedia.* In 1856, at the urging of Charles Lyell, Darwin began writing an encyclopedic work on natural selection; however, it is possible that the extremely cautious Darwin might not have published his evolutionary theories during his lifetime had not Alfred Russel Wallace independently discovered the theory of natural selection. According to one of the most celebrated anecdotes in the history of science, Wallace conceived the theory in Febuary 1858, while delirious during an attack of malarial fever in Ternate in the Mollucas. Knowing that Darwin was working on the same problem, Wallace sent a manuscript summary to Darwin, who feared that his discovery would be pre-empted. However, Joseph Hooker and Charles Lyell suggested joint publication of Wallace's paper, "On the Tendency of Varieties to Depart Indefinitely from the

Original Type," prefaced by a section of a manuscript of a work on species written by Darwin in 1844, plus an abstract of a letter by Darwin to Asa Gray dated 1857, to show that Darwin's views on the subject had not changed between 1844 and 1857. The two papers were read by Lyell before the Linnean Society on 1 July 1858 and published on 20 August. In the following year, Darwin published *On the Origin of Species by Means of Natural Selection*, which he characterized as an abstract of his planned (but never published) larger work on the subject. The first edition consisted of 1,250 copies and, according to Darwin, sold out on the day of publication; by the time of his death the book had gone through six editions and thirty-seven printings.

JMN

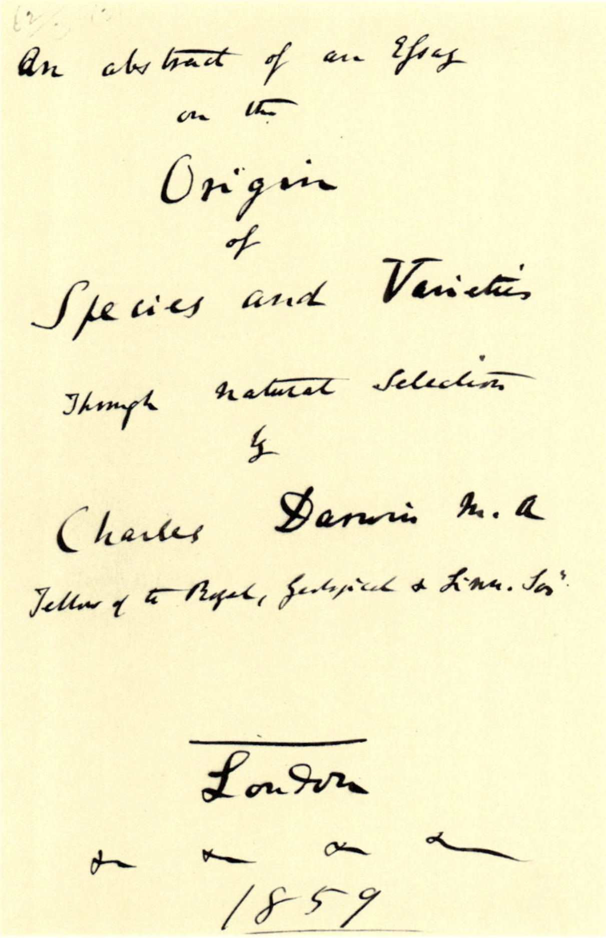

An abstract of an Essay
on the
Origin
of
Species and Varieties
Through natural Selection
by
Charles Darwin M.A.
Fellow of the Royal, Geological & Linn. Soc.

London

1859

Fig. 129. No. 70B. Darwin. The title page of Darwin's manuscript of *On the Origin of Species.* The manuscript itself was broken up by Darwin and now exists only in fragments like this one.

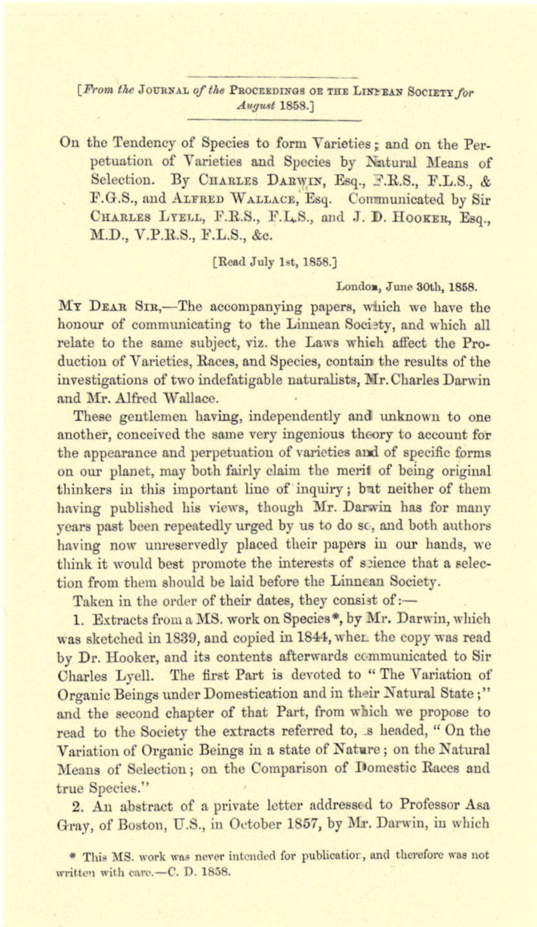

[*From the* Journal *of the* Proceedings of the Linnean Society *for August* 1858.]

On the Tendency of Species to form Varieties; and on the Perpetuation of Varieties and Species by Natural Means of Selection. By Charles Darwin, Esq., F.R.S., F.L.S., & F.G.S., and Alfred Wallace, Esq. Communicated by Sir Charles Lyell, F.R.S., F.L.S., and J. D. Hooker, Esq., M.D., V.P.R.S., F.L.S., &c.

[Read July 1st, 1858.]

London, June 30th, 1858.

My Dear Sir,—The accompanying papers, which we have the honour of communicating to the Linnean Society, and which all relate to the same subject, viz. the Laws which affect the Production of Varieties, Races, and Species, contain the results of the investigations of two indefatigable naturalists, Mr. Charles Darwin and Mr. Alfred Wallace.

These gentlemen having, independently and unknown to one another, conceived the same very ingenious theory to account for the appearance and perpetuation of varieties and of specific forms on our planet, may both fairly claim the merit of being original thinkers in this important line of inquiry; but neither of them having published his views, though Mr. Darwin has for many years past been repeatedly urged by us to do so, and both authors having now unreservedly placed their papers in our hands, we think it would best promote the interests of science that a selection from them should be laid before the Linnean Society.

Taken in the order of their dates, they consist of:—

1. Extracts from a MS. work on Species*, by Mr. Darwin, which was sketched in 1839, and copied in 1844, when the copy was read by Dr. Hooker, and its contents afterwards communicated to Sir Charles Lyell. The first Part is devoted to "The Variation of Organic Beings under Domestication and in their Natural State;" and the second chapter of that Part, from which we propose to read to the Society the extracts referred to, is headed, "On the Variation of Organic Beings in a state of Nature; on the Natural Means of Selection; on the Comparison of Domestic Races and true Species."

2. An abstract of a private letter addressed to Professor Asa Gray, of Boston, U.S., in October 1857, by Mr. Darwin, in which

* This MS. work was never intended for publication, and therefore was not written with care.—C. D. 1858.

Fig. 130. No. 70A. Darwin and Wallace. The opening page of their article on natural selection (1858), the first published discussion of the subject.

NOTES ON NURSING:

WHAT IT IS, AND WHAT IT IS NOT.

BY

FLORENCE NIGHTINGALE.

LONDON:
HARRISON, 59, PALL MALL,
BOOKSELLER TO THE QUEEN.

Fig. 131. No. 71. Nightingale. Title page.

71

FLORENCE NIGHTINGALE
(1820–1910)

Notes on Nursing: What It Is, and What It Is Not.

London: Harrison, [1860].

π^8 C–F^8. 40 leaves, pp. *1–5* 6–79 [1]. Charcoal cloth.

Bishop & Goldie 4(i). GM 1612. *Heirs of Hippocrates* 1884. Norman 1600–2. Osler 1667, 7737–38. cf. PMM 343. Waller 6872.

[New York edition] New York: D. Appleton and Company, 1860.

1–6^{12}. 72 leaves, pp. *1–3* 4–140 [4]. Brown cloth, or buff printed wrappers.

Reset from the London edition.

Bishop & Goldie 4(ii). *Heirs of Hippocrates* 1885.

[Boston edition] Boston: William Carter, 1860.

[1–3^6 4–6^{12} 7^6]. 60 leaves, pp. *i–ii* iii–iv, i–xii, 1–104. Frontispiece: 1 lithographed portrait (color-lithographed with cloth binding; black-and-white with wrappers); 1 wood-engraved figure in text. Red gold-blocked publisher's cloth, or yellow printed wrappers.

Reset from the London edition, with additional material pertaining to Nightingale's life. The type was originally set for imposition in a single preliminary quire of 8 and text quires of 6 leaves; printed signatures 1–9 appear on pp. 1, 13, 25, and every twelfth page thereafter.

The modern secular training of nurses in Britain can be dated from the opening of the Nightingale School at St. Thomas's Hospital in London in June 1860. Florence Nightingale had become a national heroine as the result of her work in the hospitals of the Crimean War (1853–56), where, by introducing sanitary measures and patient comforts, she had drastically reduced the mortality rate among British troops. Upon her return to England, a large sum of money was collected for her use by public subscription, and the new school of nursing, strongly influenced by her ideas, was financed out of the "Nightingale fund." The school was a success, and by the late 1870s it was turning out large numbers of trained nurses, many of whom went to teach Nightingale's methods in America and other countries.

Six months before the opening of the school, *Notes on Nursing: What It Is, and What It Is Not* was published. This was intended, not as a textbook, but as a book of hints for those nursing in the hospital ward and in the domestic sick room. The principles of

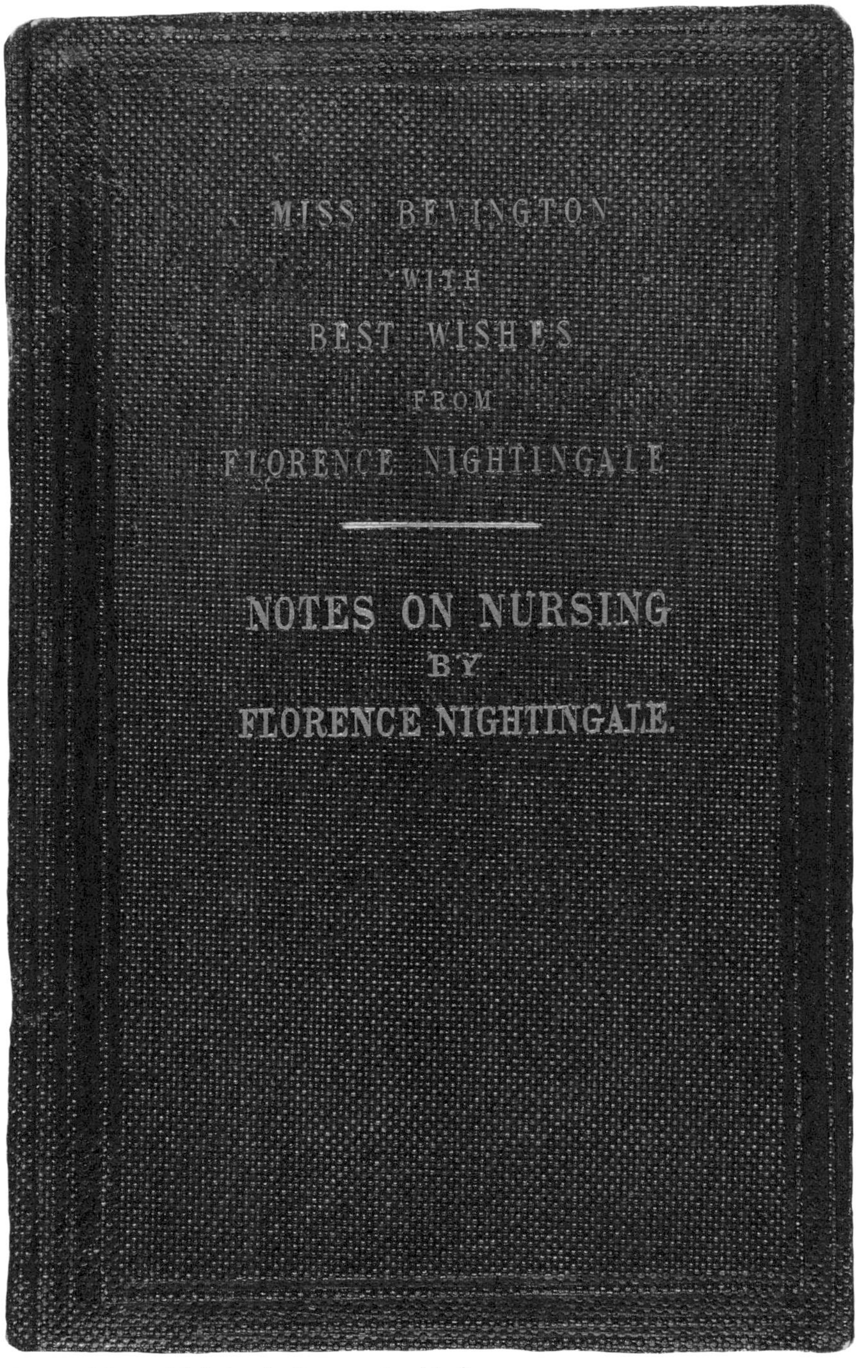

Fig. 132. No. 71. Nightingale. Presentation binding.

hygiene and sanitation which Nightingale had applied with such success in the military hospital at Scutari, in the Crimea, were fundamental. As she stated in the introductory paragraphs to *Notes on Nursing*:

> In watching disease, both in private houses and in public hospitals, the thing which strikes the experienced observer most forcibly is this, that the symptoms or the sufferings generally considered to be inevitable and incident to the disease are very often not symptoms of the disease at all, but of something quite different—of the want of fresh air, or of light, or of warmth, or of quiet, or of cleanliness, or of punctuality and care in the administration of diet, of each or of all of these.

Notes on Nursing described in great practical detail the nurse's duties in supplying her patient's needs, and it indicated a new and more responsible role for nurses, one that required proper training and medical knowledge. *Notes on Nursing* was the first major work on its subject and remained influential for many years.

The first edition of *Notes on Nursing* is undated. It was advertised in the *Publishers' Circular* for 14–31 December 1859, and a copy exists with a presentation inscription in Florence Nightingale's hand dated "New Years Day 1860." This copy has plain yellow endpapers and does not include a statement reserving translation rights. Endpapers with advertisements were soon substituted for the plain ones, and in February 1860 the book was reissued, without correction of textual errors but with "[*The right of Translation is reserved*]" printed on the title page below the imprint. Within a few months fifteen thousand copies had been sold, and an enlarged and corrected version was published in mid-1860. Two American editions were published in the same year, and translations soon appeared in a number of European languages. Nightingale herself prepared an abridged version, with some additional material, that was published as *Notes on Nursing for the Labouring Classes* (1861).[1]

Florence Nightingale's most lasting achievement was to upgrade the nursing profession so that it attracted able and intelligent women. Previously, apart from a few isolated groups, such as Roman Catholic religious orders and Elizabeth Fry's order of nursing sisters, nurses had been ignorant and often disreputable. Although Nightingale was no feminist, her example encouraged other women to follow careers beyond the very restricted choice until then thought suitable.

RDG

1. W. J. Bishop and Sue Goldie, *A Bio-Bibliography of Florence Nightingale* (London, 1962), pp. 15–20; Edward Cook, *The Life of Florence Nightingale* (2 vols., London, 1913), vol. 2, pp. 439–40. For recent discussions of the bibliographical complexity of *Notes on Nursing*, see Victor Skretkowicz, "Florence Nightingale's *Notes on Nursing*: The First Version and Edition," *The Library*, 6th series, 15 (1993): 24–46; idem, "The New York, Boston, and London Editions of Nightingale's *Notes on Nursing*," *Notes on Nursing Science: The Newsletter of the Nightingale Society* 4 (1991): 2–8; and *Florence Nightingale's Notes on Nursing*, ed. with an introduction, notes, and guide to identification by Victor Skretkowicz (rev. ed., London, 1992).

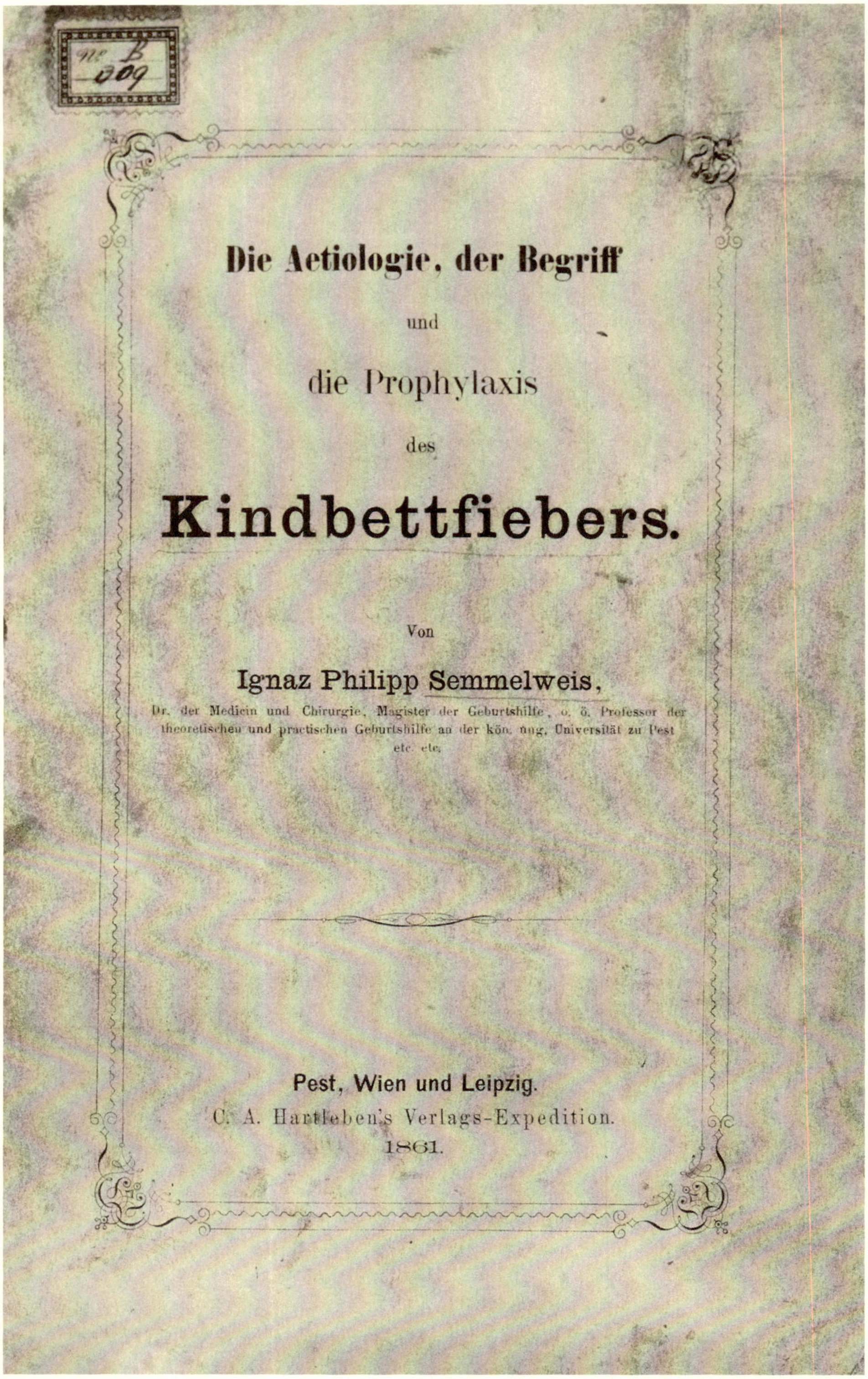

Die Aetiologie, der Begriff

und

die Prophylaxis

des

Kindbettfiebers.

Von

Ignaz Philipp Semmelweis,

Dr. der Medicin und Chirurgie, Magister der Geburtshilfe, o. ö. Professor der theoretischen und practischen Geburtshilfe an der kön. ung. Universität zu Pest etc. etc.

Pest, Wien und Leipzig.

C. A. Hartleben's Verlags-Expedition.

1861.

Fig. 133. No. 72A. Semmelweis. Front wrapper.

72

IGNAZ PHILIPP SEMMELWEIS
(1818–1865)

A] *Die Aetiologie, der Begriff und die Prophylaxis des Kindbettfiebers.*

Pest, Vienna & Leipzig: C. A. Hartleben's Verlags-Expedition, 1861.

π^4 (π4 signed "1") 1^8 (-1_1; $\pm 1_{4,7}$) 2–33^8 34^6 35^2. 275 leaves, pp. *I–III* IV–VI *1* 2–543 [1]. Pink printed wrappers.

GM 6277. *Heirs of Hippocrates* 1851. Norman 1926. PMM 316b2. Waller 8830.

B] Oliver Wendell Holmes (1809–1894). The Contagiousness of Puerperal Fever.

In: *The New England Quarterly Journal of Medicine and Surgery* 1 (1842–43): 503–30.

[journal number] Vol. 1, No. 4, April 1843: π^2 40–51^6 52^2. 76 leaves, pp. *i* ii–iii [1] *449* 450–595 [1].

[article] $44_4{}^r$–$46_5{}^v$, pp. 503–530.

[offprint] *The Contagiousness of Puerperal Fever* [wrapper title].

1–3^4 4^2. 14 leaves, pp. *1* 2–28. Buff printed wrappers.

Reimposed, with different page breaks.

BAL 8738. GM 6274. Grolier *American* 50. *Heirs of Hippocrates* 1744. Norman 1088. Osler 2989. PMM 316a. Waller 6847.

C] Oliver Wendell Holmes. *Puerperal Fever, As a Private Pestilence.*

Boston: Ticknor and Fields, 1855.

1–5^6. 30 leaves, pp. *1–5* 6–60. Printed wrappers, and publisher's cloth.

BAL 8768. GM 6276. Norman 1089. Osler 2989A. Waller 4852.

Ignaz Philipp Semmelweis's discovery of the etiology and prevention of childbed fever was an epochal event in the history of medicine for its importance in saving the lives and preventing the suffering of women in childbirth. In 1844 Semmelweis, a native of Hungary, was appointed assistant lecturer in the First Obstetrical Clinic of the Allgemeines Krankenhaus, Vienna, under Johann Klein. At the time, mortality from puerperal sepsis was very high, particularly in maternity hospitals. In Klein's clinic the rate was rarely under five percent and during one two-year period, between 1841 and 1843, 829 of 5,139 parturi-

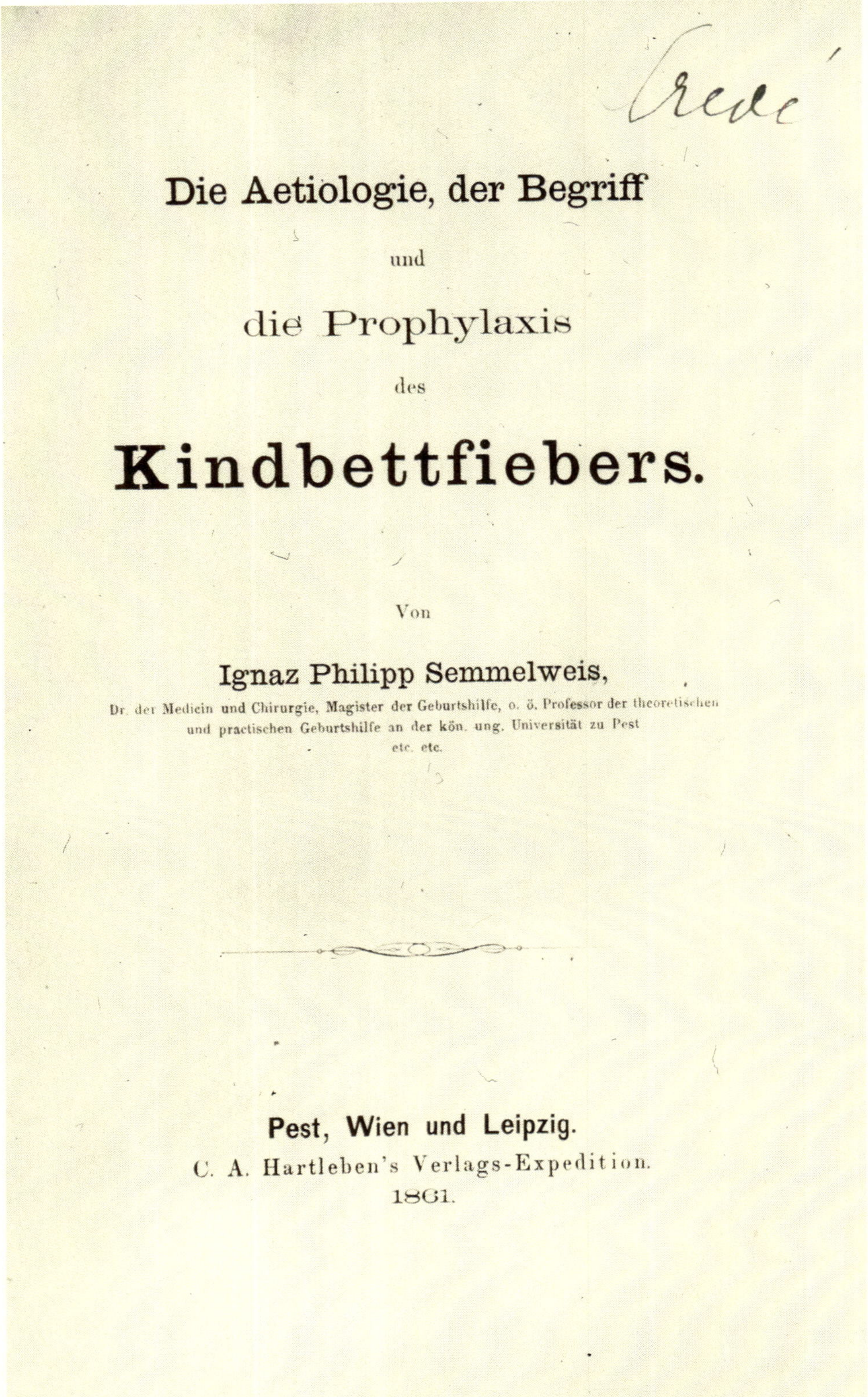

Credé

Die Aetiologie, der Begriff

und

die Prophylaxis

des

Kindbettfiebers.

Von

Ignaz Philipp Semmelweis,

Dr. der Medicin und Chirurgie, Magister der Geburtshilfe, o. ö. Professor der theoretischen und practischen Geburtshilfe an der kön. ung. Universität zu Pest etc. etc.

Pest, Wien und Leipzig.

C. A. Hartleben's Verlags-Expedition.

1861.

Fig. 134. No. 72A. Semmelweis. Title page, with the signature of Carl Sigmund Franz Credé, an early reviewer of the work.

ent women died, a mortality rate of sixteen percent. Semmelweis noticed that this high rate prevailed only in the wards attended by medical students and not in the wards managed by midwives, in which the death rate averaged about two percent. Later he was to write that the identity between sepsis and fatal puerperal cases was suggested to him by the death of his friend Jakob Kolletschka, who contracted blood poisoning from a wound accidentally sustained during a postmortem examination. This tragic event caused him to think about the pathology of septicemia, and led him to reason correctly that the medical students carried infective material directly from the autopsy dissecting rooms to the delivery room, whereas the midwives, who did not attend autopsies, were not exposed to this source of infection. In 1847 Semmelweis instituted a policy in the maternity division that required hand-washing with chlorinated limewater; within one month the mortality from puerperal fever plummeted from 12.4 to 2.4 percent, and it continued that year at a rate of about 3 percent. The following year, the mortality fell further to 1.3 percent, surpassing even the rate of the midwives. Semmelweis's superiors, however, remained unconvinced, and Klein, acting largely from vanity and jealousy, finally succeeded in driving him from Vienna in 1849. Semmelweis returned to Pest where he was later appointed obstetric physician in the maternity department of St. Rochus Hospital. In six years he reduced the mortality there to 0.85 percent.

Although Semmelweis's important discoveries were made in the 1840s, he did not publish them immediately. The first printed reports of his findings were written by his colleagues and were published or abstracted in various German, French, or English journals. Semmelweis himself gave three lectures before the Imperial and Royal Medical Society of Vienna in 1850 but did not publish his complete discussion of "The etiology, concept, and prophylaxis of childbed fever" until 1861, having previously contributed several shorter accounts to Hungarian medical journals.[1]

Semmelweis's conclusions met with considerable opposition, and the controversy inaugurated in medical circles by his doctrine was exceptionally bitter. As the conflict progressed, Semmelweis became more and more unbalanced, and in 1865 he was committed to an asylum, suffering from extreme mental disturbance. He died there within a few weeks of his admission, ironically, from sepsis contracted via an infected wound to his finger.

Independently of Semmelweis, in one of the greatest American contributions to medicine, Oliver Wendell Holmes established that puerperal (childbed) fever was contagious and that it was carried by the unwashed hands of the physician from bed to bed. Although not an obstetrician, Holmes, who later taught at the Harvard Medical School, amassed considerable evidence for his thesis and wrote with clear argument, drawing both on his own knowledge of the disease and on the observations and writings of others. His advice to accouchers was to wash their hands in calcium chloride and to change their clothes after treating cases of puerperal fever or performing postmortems. This recommendation was received favorably in some circles, but it aroused the scorn and animosity of many of

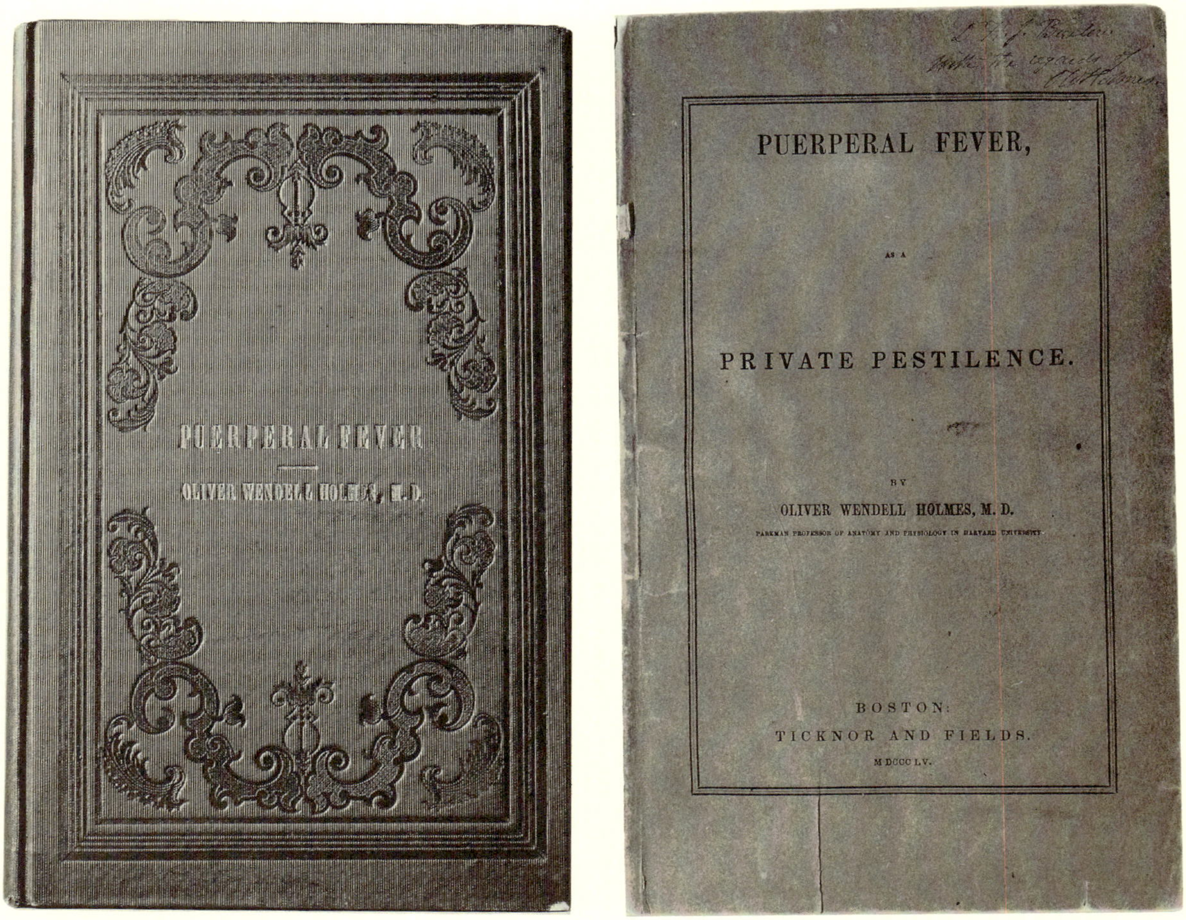

Fig. 135. No. 72C. Holmes. Two copies of *Puerperal Fever as a Private Pestilence* (1855), one in wrappers and one bound in publisher's cloth. Holmes inscribed the copy in wrappers to Dr. Henry J. Bigelow, author of the first paper on surgical anesthesia.

Holmes's fellow physicians, whose outspoken opposition to his ideas prevented their more widespread acceptance.

The New England Quarterly Journal of Medicine and Surgery, in which Holmes's paper first appeared, was published for only one year, producing a single volume. In 1855, recognizing that his essay had never received the wide circulation enjoyed by the views of his opponents, Holmes had it reprinted in pamphlet form, under a different title. He added a twenty-page introduction answering his opposition and mentioning the steps already taken by Semmelweis, and at the end he included a two-page list of "Additional References and Cases." The publisher's records show that only 500 copies of the pamphlet were printed and that by 1865 a remainder of 159 copies had been put in storage.

LDL

1. Frank P. Murphy, "Ignaz Philipp Semmelweis (1818–1865): An Annotated Bibliography," *Bulletin of the History of Medicine* 20 (1946): 653–707.

Fig. 136. No. 72B. Holmes inscribed this offprint of his 1843 paper on "The Contagiousness of Puerperal Fever" to Dr. Abel Lawrence Peirson.

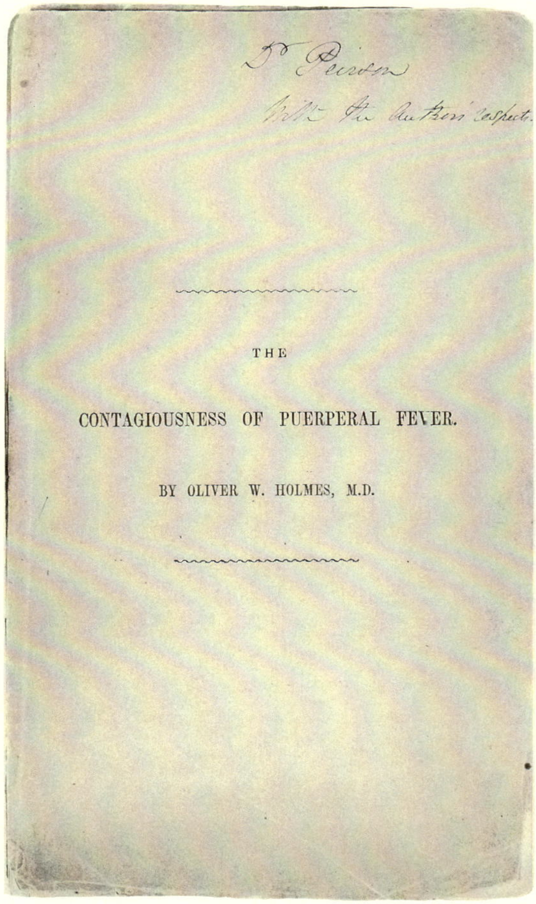

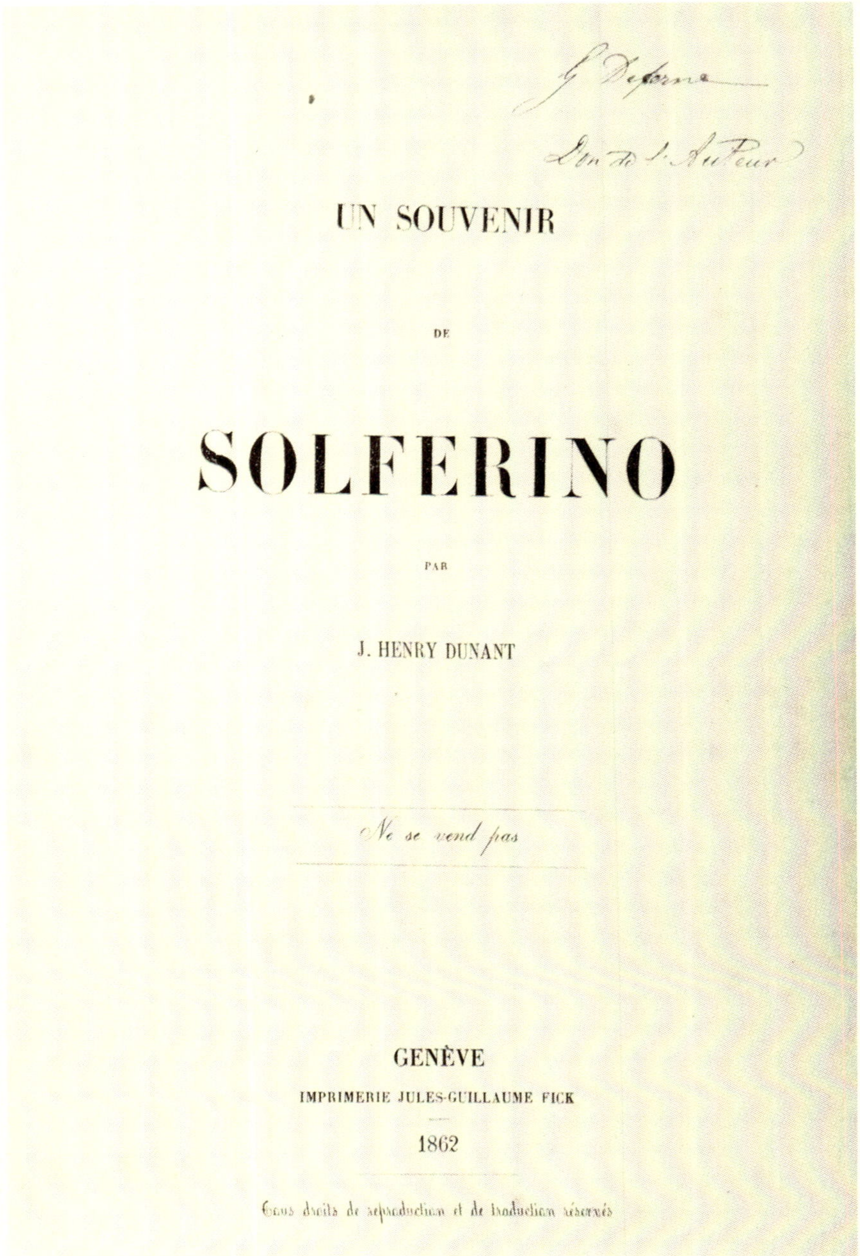

Don de l'Auteur

UN SOUVENIR

DE

SOLFERINO

PAR

J. HENRY DUNANT

Ne se vend pas

GENÈVE

IMPRIMERIE JULES-GUILLAUME FICK

1862

Tous droits de reproduction et de traduction réservés

Fig. 137. No. 73A. Dunant. Title page.

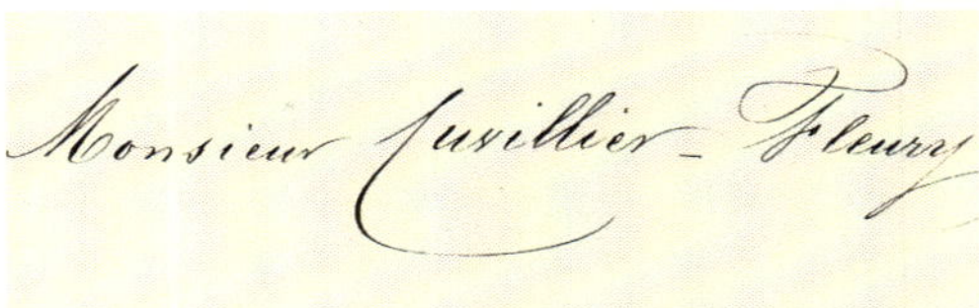

Monsieur Cuvillier-Fleury

Hommage respectueux.

J. Henry Dunant.

Fig. 138. No. 73A. Dunant. The author's presentation inscription to Monsieur Cuvillier-Fleury.

73

J. HENRY DUNANT
(1828–1910)

A] *Un souvenir de Solferino.*

Geneva: Imprimerie Jules-Guillaume Fick, 1862.

π^2 [1]^4 2–14^4 [15]^2. 60 leaves, pp. [4] *1* 2–115 [1]. 1 double-page lithographed map, overprinted with blocks of color. Brown printed wrappers.

EFDT 284. GM 2166. *Heirs of Hippocrates* 1945. Norman 670. PMM 350. Waller 2639.

B] SIR JOHN PRINGLE (1707–1782). *Observations on the Diseases of the Army, in Camp and Garrison.*

London: Printed for A. Millar and D. Wilson; and T. Payne, 1752.

8°: A^8 a^4 B–Z^8 Aa–Ee^8. 228 leaves, pp. *i–iii* iv–xxiii [1] *1* 2–431 [1].

GM 2150. *Heirs of Hippocrates* 879. Norman 1755.

J. Henry Dunant, a Swiss businessman inspired by the example of Florence Nightingale, made it his life's work to alleviate suffering in war. Such were the force of his convictions and the brilliance of his advocacy that he was able, within the space of a few years, to persuade most of the governments of the world to collaborate in creating an organization, the International Red Cross, based on his ideas.

With the support of Napoleon III, Dunant was present as an observer during the Italian war of 1859, in which France supported Piedmont against the occupying power, Austria. The culminating battle, at Solferino, was one of the bloodiest engagements of the nineteenth century. After witnessing it, Dunant, with a handful of local volunteers, struggled to improvise ambulance services and field hospitals for the nearly forty thousand casualties left to die on the battlefield.

Un souvenir de Solferino begins with a straightforward account of the battle. This, although graphic, is tactful, all honor being paid to military valor on all sides. Nevertheless, the inadequacy of the medical arrangements is not concealed, and the full horror of the aftermath is graphically described. In the second part of the book, Dunant outlined his suggestions for the formation of an international organization, consisting of a central committee in Switzerland and committees in all countries, run by eminent citizens. This organization would form bodies of volunteers ready in peace and war to tend the wounded. Central to the plan was an international agreement that the wounded, those places where they are housed, and those working among them should be regarded as neutral. Later Dunant extended this concept to prisoners of war and to civilians directly affected by war.

Dunant's work had such an impact that within a year of its publication an unofficial international conference had met in Geneva and had formulated proposals that were submitted to an official international conference called by the Swiss government. At this conference, in August 1864, the Geneva Convention was signed, creating the International Red Cross. Dunant continued to work for the Red Cross for several years, but in 1867 his business failed and he lost his money. Afterwards he faded into obscurity but enjoyed a brief revival of fame at the end of his life, when, together with Frédéric Passy, he was awarded the first Nobel Peace Prize in 1901.

The first edition of *Un souvenir de Solferino* consisted of sixteen hundred copies printed in November 1862 for private distribution. Only four hundred of these were actually distributed; these copies, constituting the original issue, have a title page stating "Ne se vend pas" above the imprint. A month later, in December 1862, Dunant had another thousand copies bound with a title page indicating "deuxième édition." The third edition, in which Dunant suggested the extension of Red Cross services to victims of natural disasters, appeared in 1863. An English translation was published by the American Red Cross in 1939.

A century before the publication of Dunant's work, Sir John Pringle was the first prominent physician to concern himself with hygiene and sanitation in the army. Pringle recognized the dangers to health from poor diet, poor ventilation, overcrowding, and inadequate sanitation, particularly in hospitals, barracks, and military encampments. He made a special study of the epidemic diseases current in his day, and recognizing the similarity of jail fever to hospital fever, now identified as typhus, he treated it successfully through cleanliness and fresh air. In his practicality and in his emphasis on prevention, Pringle anticipated the movement for medical reform in the nineteenth century.

In 1742 Pringle became physician to the Earl of Stair, the allied commander-in-chief on the Continent, and he was also named physician to the military hospital in Flanders. In 1745 he was appointed physician-general to the British army. From his experiences he wrote *Observations on the Diseases of the Army*, which is essentially a year-by-year account of the epidemics occuring during the War of the Austrian Succession (1742–48). In Pringle's words: "Upon my first being employed in the army . . . I began to note down such observations as occurred, in hopes of finding them afterwards useful in practice . . . and continued this method to the end of the war." From these notes came his suggestions for improving the lot of the ordinary soldier.

On the Diseases of the Army was published in a number of editions during its author's lifetime; it was also translated into German (1754), French (1755), Italian (1757), Dutch (1763), and Spanish (1775), and most of these versions were reprinted several times in the eighteenth century.

Pringle made a remarkable proposal in the introduction to this work, which was that in war, hospitals holding the wounded should be regarded as sanctuaries. Pringle described how this was proposed by Lord Stair and accepted by the French commander-in-chief, the Duc de Noailles. It is thought that this idea, formalized in the Geneva Convention of 1864, came from Pringle.

RDG

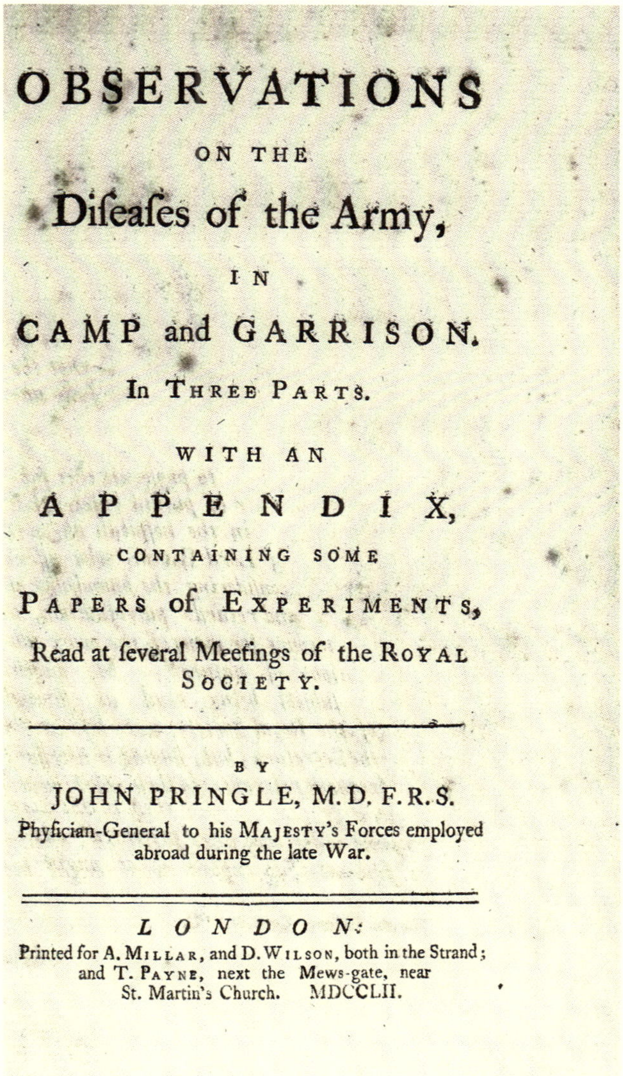

OBSERVATIONS
ON THE
Diſeaſes of the Army,
IN
CAMP and GARRISON.
In THREE PARTS.
WITH AN
APPENDIX,
CONTAINING SOME
PAPERS of EXPERIMENTS,
Read at ſeveral Meetings of the ROYAL SOCIETY.

BY
JOHN PRINGLE, M.D. F.R.S.
Phyſician-General to his MAJESTY's Forces employed abroad during the late War.

LONDON:
Printed for A. MILLAR, and D. WILSON, both in the Strand; and T. PAYNE, next the Mews-gate, near St. Martin's Church. MDCCLII.

Fig. 139. No. 73B. Pringle. Title page.

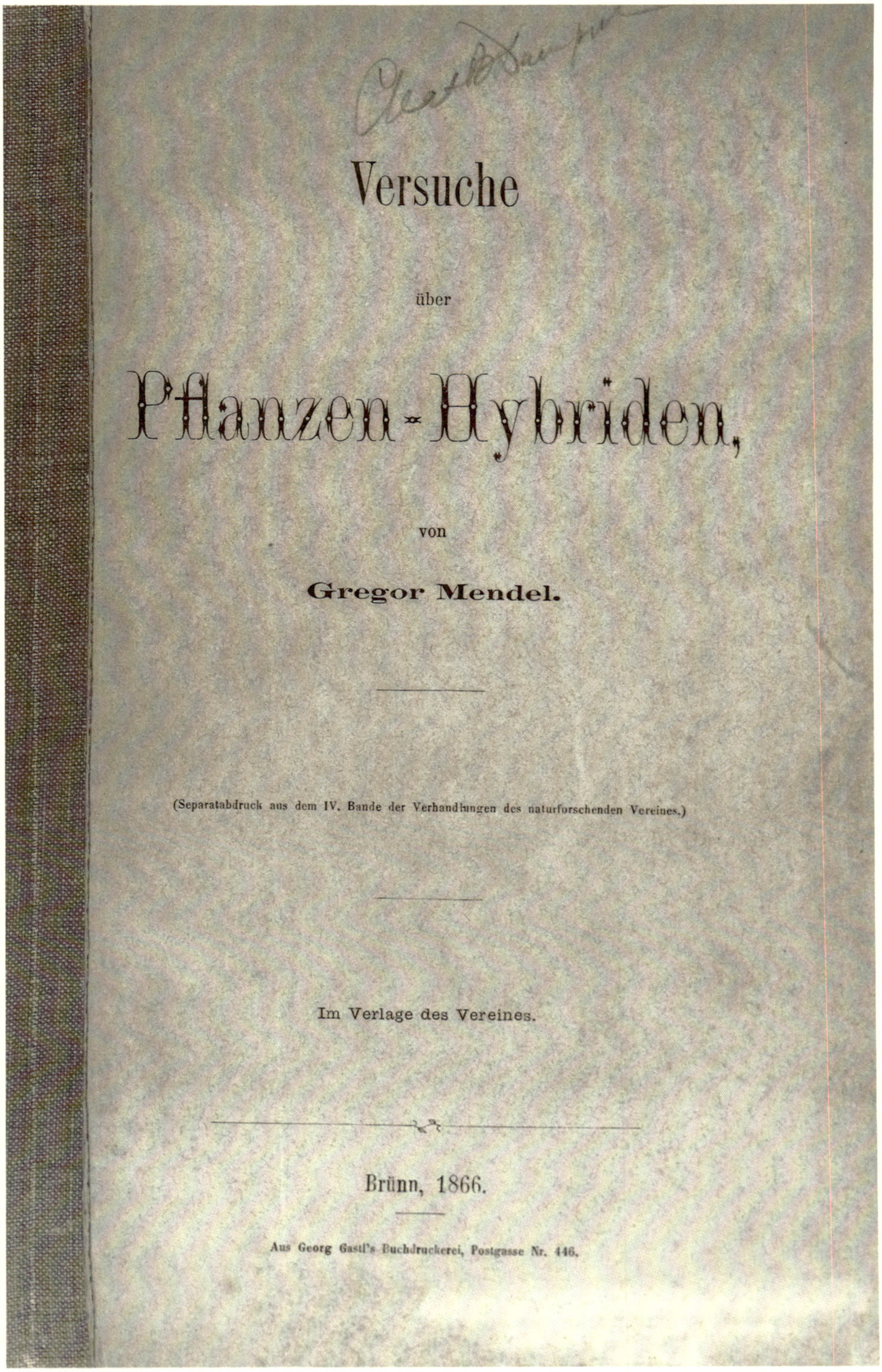

Versuche

über

Pflanzen-Hybriden,

von

Gregor Mendel.

(Separatabdruck aus dem IV. Bande der Verhandlungen des naturforschenden Vereines.)

Im Verlage des Vereines.

Brünn, 1866.

Aus Georg Gastl's Buchdruckerei, Postgasse Nr. 446.

Fig. 140. No. 74. Mendel. Title page of the offprint.

74

[JOHANN] GREGOR MENDEL
(1822–1884)

Versuche über Pflanzen-Hybriden.

In: *Verhandlungen des naturforschenden Vereines in Brünn* 4 (1865): 3–47.

[journal volume] $*^8$ $**4(-**1)$ $1\text{–}6^8$ 7^4, $1\text{–}20^8$ 21^4 $[22]_1$. 228 leaves, pp. *I–III* IV–XXI [1] *1–3* 4–104, *1–3* 4–330. Gray printed wrappers.

[article] (second series) $1_2^r\text{–}3_8^r$, pp. *3* 4–47.

[offprint] *Versuche über Pflanzen-Hybriden.* Separatabdruck aus dem IV. Bande der Verhandlungen des naturforschenden Vereines. Brünn: Im Verlage des Vereines; Aus Georg Gastl's Buchdruckerei, 1866.

$1\text{–}3^8$. 24 leaves, pp. *1–3* 4–47 [1].

The title page, which has the appearance of a wrapper, is printed on f. 1_1^r.

GM 222. Horblit 73a. Norman 1489. PMM 356a.

The discovery of the Mendelian ratios, set forth in the present paper, has been called the most significant event in the history of genetics. This paper reports the results of Mendel's ten years of experimental work on artificial plant hybridization, during which he followed a program designed to test his working hypothesis that hereditary matter is discrete and particulate. Mendel bred and cultivated nearly thirty thousand pea plants, performing careful statistical analyses of the distribution of seven pairs of mutually exclusive seed and plant characteristics—a manageable number that allowed him to observe all possible combinations of traits. He found that crossing plants that differed in only one characteristic—smooth seed versus wrinkled seed, for instance—produced offspring that all exhibited one of the parental characteristics in unchanged form; he called such a characteristic "dominant" and its latent partner "recessive." Crossing two of these first-generation hybrids resulted in offspring exhibiting the following distribution of characteristics, where *A* represents the dominant trait and *a* the recessive one:

$$\tfrac{1}{4}\,AA + \tfrac{1}{4}\,Aa + \tfrac{1}{4}\,aA + \tfrac{1}{4}\,aa$$

Thus in hybrid offspring, the parental forms *AA* and *aa* reappear along with the hybrid ones. This principle, which Mendel extended to cover any number of traits, is now referred to as Mendel's law of segregation. Mendel also found, in contradiction to theories of "blended inheritance," generally accepted at the time, that the behavior of each set of traits in a hybrid is independent of all other differences in the two parental plants, a principle later named Mendel's law of independent assortment.

A monk in the Augustinian monastery in Brünn, Austria (now Brno in the Czech Republic), Mendel read his paper before the local natural history society, an organization made up of about three hundred members. The paper was published in the society's journal, which was distributed to 134 scientific institutions in various countries as well as to the society's membership. Mendel also commissioned forty copies of an offprint, of which about ten are now known.

Although Mendel's work was cited in several publications during the second half of the nineteenth century, his achievement failed to gain the recognition of his contemporaries. This was no doubt due both to the originality of the work—Mendel's use of statistical analysis and numerical ratios to answer basic biological questions was then entirely new—and to the obscurity of the journal in which it was published. About 1900 Mendel's findings were replicated by Hugo de Vries, Carl Correns, and Erich von Tschermak, each of whom referred to Mendel's work. The English biologist William Bateson had "Experiments in Plant-Hybridisation" translated into English and defended Mendel's principles of heredity in several publications of his own.[1] Following this rediscovery of Mendel's work, genetics progressed rapidly, and with it, the study of inherited diseases.[2]

JMN

1. The translation, which first appeared in the *Journal of the Royal Horticultural Society* 26 (1901): 1–32, was reprinted in William Bateson, *Mendel's Principles of Heredity* (Cambridge, 1909).
2. Vítezslav Orel, *Mendel*, trans. Stephen Finn (Oxford, 1984), pp. 94–103.

75

JOSEPH LISTER
(1827–1912)

On a New Method of Treating Compound Fracture, Abscess, etc. With Observations on the Conditions of Suppuration.

In: *Lancet*, 1867, 1: 326–29, 357–59, 387–89, 507–9; 2: 95–96.

[journal numbers] No. 2272, 16 March 1867: L^{16}. 16 leaves, pp. *323* 324–354. No. 2273, 23 March 1867: M^{14} χ1. 15 leaves, pp. *355* 356–384. No. 2274, 30 March 1867: N^{14}. 14 leaves, pp. *385* 386–412. No. 2278, 27 April 1867: R^{14}. 14 leaves, pp. *505* 506–532. No. 2291, 27 July 1867: D^{14} χ1. 15 leaves, pp. *91* 92–120.

[article] $L2^v$–$L4^r$, pp. 326–329. $M2^r$–$M3^r$, pp. 357–359. $N2^r$–$N3^r$, pp. 387–389. $R2^r$–$R3^r$, pp. 507–509. $D3^r$–$D3^v$, pp. 95–96.

GM 5634. Le Fanu *Lister* 27. Norman 1366. PMM 316c.

Joseph Lister was born and educated in London but took his surgical instruction in Edinburgh under James Syme, the foremost British surgeon of the period. In 1860 he was appointed Regius Professor of Surgery in Glasgow, and it was there that he carried out his greatest work. At that time, the mortality rate in his hospital for amputations and compound fractures was over fifty percent, the result of uncontrolled infection. Lister, an experienced microscopist, identified surgical infection with decomposition. Decomposition, as he knew from the work of Louis Pasteur (see no. 78), was due to the action of bacteria, so to prevent bacterial infection Lister began using dressings saturated with carbolic acid, a chemical then used routinely by the city of Carlisle to disinfect sewage. In the series of surgical cases described in this landmark article in *Lancet*, he succeeded in completely eliminating infection. Although Lister was in error in assuming that the primary sources of infection were airborne, he had established the principle that the control of infection depended on the control of microorganisms. With the further work of Ernst von Bergmann in Berlin, antisepsis and clouds of irritating carbolic acid mist gave way in the 1880s to aseptic surgery and the aseptic routines which characterize the modern operating room.

Antisepsis soon gained acceptance on the Continent, where German surgeons in particular rapidly adopted Lister's ideas: Karl Thiersch in Leipzig and Richard von Volkmann in Halle were among the early enthusiastic supporters of Listerism. In contrast, older surgeons in England and America resisted the innovation. The American surgeon William Stewart Halsted had to resort to carrying out antiseptic surgery in a tent on the grounds of Bellvue Hospital as a result of both professional and institutional opposition.

intercostal spaces. Under such circumstances, there are several characters of considerable importance in diagnosis—viz.:

a. The bulging of the side of the chest is more uniform in pleurisy, and not abruptly limited to the lower part, as in diseases of the liver.

b. In pleuritic effusion, the upper margin of the dull space is horizontal (Fig. 6), instead of arched as in enlargements of the liver.

c. In pleuritic effusion, the upper level of the dull space will often be found to vary with the position of the patient. In enlargement of the liver, it is the same in all positions.

d. In pleuritic effusion, the lower margin of the liver is not depressed upon deep inspiration, which is the case in enlargements of the liver, unless there be firm adhesions to the diaphragm.

e. Eversion of the lower right costal cartilages would indicate hepatic enlargement, and not pleuritic effusion.

f. When there is sufficient effusion into the pleura to cause downward bulging of the diaphragm, a depression may be sometimes observed between the lower margin of the ribs and the lowest upper surface of the liver, which is not met with in hypertrophy of the liver.

Effusion into the pericardium will be recognised by the outline of the area of dulness on percussion. It is the left lobe of the liver that is mainly displaced by it.

In arriving at a diagnosis, it must not be forgotten that inflammation of the pleura or of the base of the right lung may coexist with enlargement of the liver. This is a not uncommon occurrence in hydatid tumours or abscesses of the liver, and often precedes their bursting upwards through the diaphragm. So also after an hydatid tumour of the liver has burst into the pleura, extensive emphysema may coexist with great enlargement of the liver. I shall hereafter have an opportunity of bringing under your notice the particulars of a case in which this occurred.

VI. *A tumour or collection of fluid between the upper surface of the liver and the diaphragm* may also cause great depression of the liver, and apparent enlargement of the organ. The upper margin of hepatic dulness will be arched, and it will probably be impossible during life to distinguish the case from one of real enlargement of the liver. You will find a case recorded by the late Dr. Bright, where a large abscess situated between the diaphragm and the liver produced apparent enlargement of the liver.* Such cases, however, are rare.

VII. *Various abnormal conditions of the abdominal viscera* may displace the liver upwards, so that it encroaches upon the cavity of the chest, and appears enlarged. This happens not unfrequently in cases of ascites, and in ovarian and uterine tumours, in aneurism of the abdominal aorta, &c.; and hence elevation of the liver above its usual height must not, under such circumstances, be regarded as a sign of enlargement. Greater difficulty, however, in diagnosis may result from tumours in the omentum or in the right kidney, being in the immediate proximity of the liver, and appearing to be tumours of the liver itself. The difficulty will be increased if such tumours compress the common bile-duct, so as to occasion jaundice. The diagnosis of an omental tumour under such circumstances must mainly depend on the want of all uniformity in the apparent hepatic enlargement, the dimensions of the liver in every other direction being normal; while in tumours of the kidney the urine usually presents important changes, and at the same time, when the patient lies on his back, the finger can usually be inserted between the ribs and the upper part of the tumour.

Accumulations of fæces in the transverse colon also constitute a condition which it is often most difficult to distinguish from enlargement of the liver. Such cases are constantly occurring in practice, and it is important to bear in mind that, if you are to rely on the patient's statements, these accumulations are far from being necessarily associated with constipation. The resemblance to hepatic disease in these cases may be further increased by the hardened scybala imparting to the tumour a nodulated character like that of cancer, and by the development of such symptoms as jaundice, vomiting, and hiccup. The diagnosis of these cases from true enlargement of the liver must rest mainly on—

1. The occurrence of spasmodic pains like those resulting from obstructed bowels, &c.

2. The disappearance of the tumour, and the amelioration of the symptoms under such treatment as poultices and fomentations, purgatives, enemata, and belladonna.

* Clinical Memoirs on Abdominal Tumours. Syd. Soc. ed., p. 257.

Lastly.

VIII. *Abnormal conditions of the abdominal parietes* may simulate enlargements of the liver.

Firm contraction of the bellies of the recti muscles, owing either to inflammation of the subjacent peritoneum or stomach, or, in cases of increased muscular irritability, to the mere application of the hand, is frequently mistaken by inexperienced observers for hepatic enlargement. It is distinguished by—

1. The situation, size, and form of the apparent tumour corresponding to those of the recti.

2. The sound on percussion being usually clear and tympanitic.

The diagnosis may also be considerably embarrassed by an inflammatory swelling in the abdominal parietes over the liver. This has often been mistaken for an abscess of the liver itself. Not long since a remarkable instance of this sort came under my notice in a patient recovering from typhus fever with parotid buboes. For some days the diagnosis was very doubtful. The following characters usually suffice to distinguish this condition from hepatic disease:—

1. The margin of inflammation and of dulness on percussion is ill-defined, and does not correspond to the boundary of an enlarged liver.

2. There is a greater amount of hardness and tightness of the superimposed integuments.

3. The constitutional symptoms are comparatively slight, and there are no indications of hepatic derangement.

Keeping in view these sources of fallacy, we may now proceed to consider the various causes of true enlargement of the liver.

(To be continued.)

ON A

NEW METHOD OF TREATING COMPOUND FRACTURE, ABSCESS, ETC.

WITH OBSERVATIONS ON THE CONDITIONS OF SUPPURATION.

By JOSEPH LISTER, Esq., F.R.S.,

PROFESSOR OF SURGERY IN THE UNIVERSITY OF GLASGOW.

PART I.

ON COMPOUND FRACTURE.

The frequency of disastrous consequences in compound fracture, contrasted with the complete immunity from danger to life or limb in simple fracture, is one of the most striking as well as melancholy facts in surgical practice.

If we inquire how it is that an external wound communicating with the seat of fracture leads to such grave results, we cannot but conclude that it is by inducing, through access of the atmosphere, decomposition of the blood which is effused in greater or less amount around the fragments and among the interstices of the tissues, and, losing by putrefaction its natural bland character, and assuming the properties of an acrid irritant, occasions both local and general disturbance.

We know that blood kept exposed to the air at the temperature of the body, in a vessel of glass or other material chemically inert, soon decomposes; and there is no reason to suppose that the living tissues surrounding a mass of extravasated blood could preserve it from being affected in a similar manner by the atmosphere. On the contrary, it may be ascertained as a matter of observation that, in a compound fracture, twenty-four hours after the accident the coloured serum which oozes from the wound is already distinctly tainted with the odour of decomposition, and during the next two or three days, before suppuration has set in, the smell of the effused fluids becomes more and more offensive.

This state of things is enough to account for all the bad consequences of the injury.

The pernicious influence of decomposing animal matter upon the tissues has probably been underrated, in consequence of the healthy state in which granulating sores remain in spite of a very offensive condition of their discharges. To argue from this, however, that fetid material would be innocuous in a recent wound would be to make a great mistake. The granulations being composed of an imperfect form of tissue, insen-

Fig. 141. No. 75. Lister. Opening page.

Lister received many honors for his pioneering work. He returned to London in 1877 when invited to fill the chair of Surgery at King's College Hospital, and Queen Victoria elevated him to the peerage in 1897. At the 1881 International Medical Congress in London, when Richard von Volkmann honored Lister as "indissolubly bound up with the greatest advance that surgery had ever made," Lister, whose work was to lead to the saving of millions of lives, modestly gave the greater credit to Pasteur, whom he personally escorted to the dais.

AEL

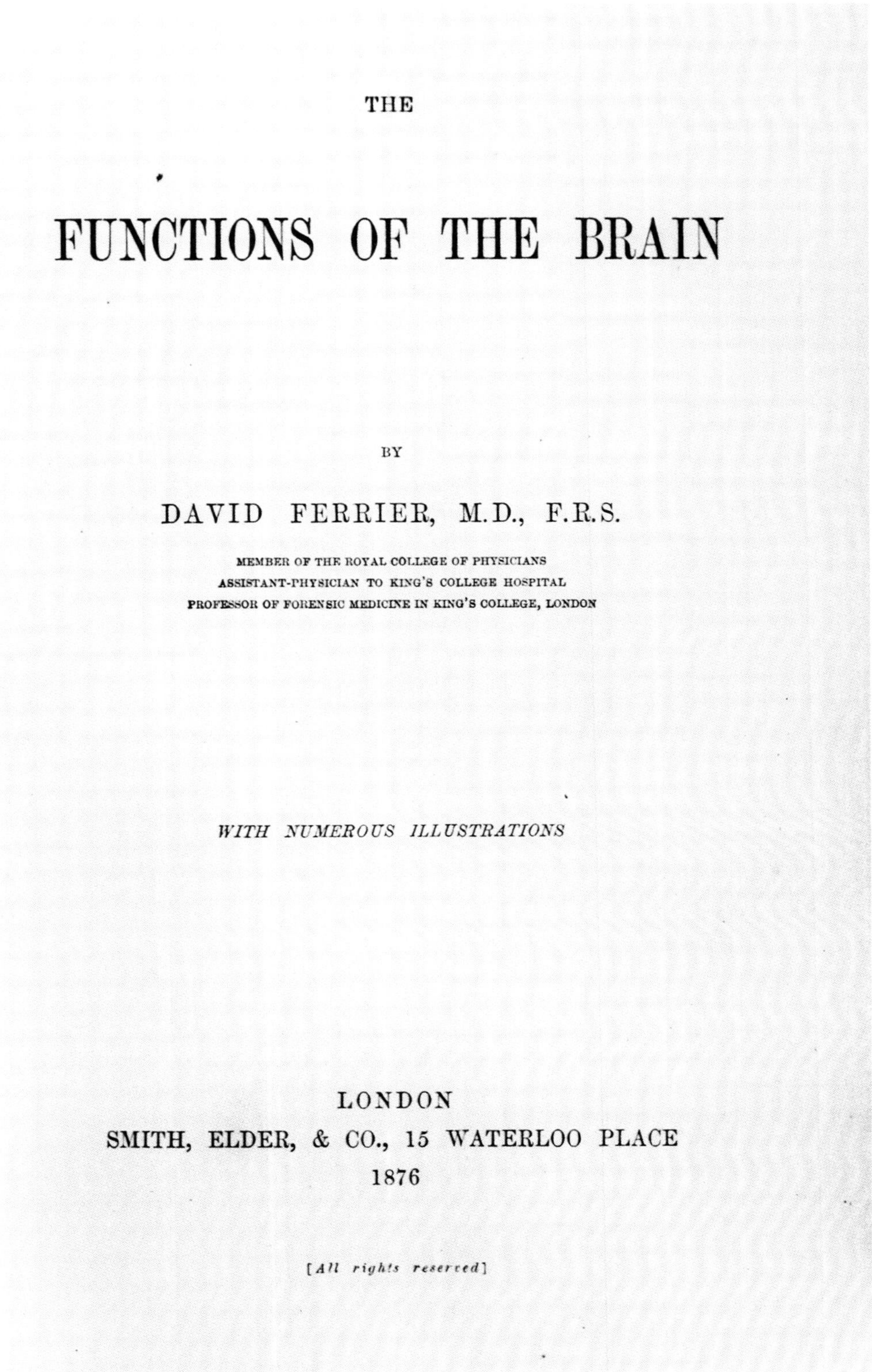

THE

FUNCTIONS OF THE BRAIN

BY

DAVID FERRIER, M.D., F.R.S.

MEMBER OF THE ROYAL COLLEGE OF PHYSICIANS
ASSISTANT-PHYSICIAN TO KING'S COLLEGE HOSPITAL
PROFESSOR OF FORENSIC MEDICINE IN KING'S COLLEGE, LONDON

WITH NUMEROUS ILLUSTRATIONS

LONDON
SMITH, ELDER, & CO., 15 WATERLOO PLACE
1876

[All rights reserved]

Fig. 142. No. 76. Ferrier. Title page.

76

SIR DAVID FERRIER
(1843–1928)

The Functions of the Brain.

[English issue] London: Smith, Elder, & Co., 1876.

[A]^8 B–X^8 Y^4. 172 leaves, pp. *i–ix* x–xv [1] *1* 2–323 [1] *1* 2–4. Fig. 1–68: 68 wood engravings in text. Green publisher's cloth.

GM 1409. *Heirs of Hippocrates* 2059. Norman 791.

[American issue] New York: G. P. Putnam's Sons, 1876.

[A]^8 B–X^8 Y^2. 170 leaves, pp. *i–ix* x–xv [1] *1* 2–323 [1]. Fig. 1–68: 68 wood engravings in text. Dark brown publisher's cloth.

The same setting of type, with the title page reset.

Ferrier was born in Aberdeen, Scotland, and was educated there and in Edinburgh. He spent a year studying psychology in Heidelberg and then attended medical school. After graduating he served briefly as an assistant to Thomas Laycock, his professor of medicine at Edinburgh; Laycock, a deeply intellectual and speculative thinker, influenced both Ferrier and Hughlings Jackson, with whom Ferrier later worked. Ferrier entered private practice in Bury St. Edmunds and obtained his M.D. degree at Edinburgh after submitting his thesis on the anatomy of the mid-brain. Then he moved to London, where he was appointed demonstrator in anatomy at King's College Hospital.

Ferrier's pioneering experimental work in neurophysiology established the basis for modern neurology and neurosurgery. In 1870, Gustav Theodor Fritsch and Eduard Hitzig published the results of their research on experimental stimulation of the brain, in which they showed that movement in discrete parts of the body on the opposite side could be consistently reproduced in the experimental animal. Ferrier realized the significance of this discovery and brought his keen mind and extraordinary technical skill to the task of expanding their work and confirming or refuting Jackson's theoretical suggestions as to localized areas of function in the cortex. During a period of ten years or more Ferrier made important experiments on the brain, publishing his results in a series of papers beginning in 1873. His book summarizing this research, *The Functions of the Brain*, was published in 1876, with a second edition in 1886.

Ferrier and his associates established that cerebral localization of neurologic function was a reality. Using electrical stimulation and cortical ablation, Ferrier showed conclusively that various neurologic functions were controlled by separate parts of the cerebrum and that damage or loss of that part created an irrevocable and particular deficit. He showed that these areas were much more discrete as one ascended the phylogenetic scale and that, accordingly, the effects of brain damage in rabbits, dogs, and cats could not be compared to the effects in monkeys, apes, and human beings. Using minute electrical currents and small electrodes, Ferrier was able to map the entire cortex in monkeys. For example, he showed that there existed a definite strip of cortex in the mid-parietal lobe which subserved motor function in the opposite limbs and that stimulation of the superior temporal lobe induced the animal to turn his head and eyes to the other side. He also demonstrated that the occipital lobe, when ablated, resulted in blindness in the opposite field of vision. In general, Ferrier's work confirmed the idea that there existed in the nervous system a rational and understandable organization. This had immense clinical significance in both the diagnosis and the treatment of diseases of the brain.

Ferrier was a slight man with tireless energy. While carrying out his experimental research he maintained an active medical practice in London and also held staff appointments at the West London Hospital and the National Hospital in Queens Square. At the latter, he is said to have been one of the last physicians to make his hospital ward rounds wearing the traditional top hat and long-tailed coat. With several others, he was a founder of the journal *Brain,* the foremost neurological periodical in the English language. He received many honors during his lifetime, including election to the Royal Society in 1876 and a knighthood in 1911.

Modern neurologists consider that Ferrier provides the connection between Hughlings Jackson, with whom he worked in the 1870s, and Charles Sherrington (see no. 90), who worked with him in the 1890s. Through him the theoretical and clinical neurology of the former was linked with the experimental neurophysiology of the latter.

AEL

77

PAUL BERT
(1833–1886)

La pression barométrique. Recherches de physiologie expérimentale.

Paris: G. Masson, Éditeur, 1878.

π^4 a^4 1–73^8. 592 leaves, pp. [8] *I* II–VIII *1–3* 4–1168. Fig. 1–9, 9, 10–89: 90 wood engravings in text, signed J. Blanadet, J. Fouché, Chauvet, O.F., E.C., A. Tissandier, Smeeton Tilly, and Belhatte. Maroon publisher's cloth.

EFDT 305. GM 944. Norman 218.

Paul Bert had degrees in both law and medicine and devoted his life at different times to each profession, as well as being active in French politics and in the implementation of national educational reforms following France's defeat in the Franco-Prussian War (1870–71). He obtained the M.D. degree in 1863 at age thirty, and from 1863 to 1866 he served as laboratory assistant to Claude Bernard (see no. 67), learning from him the methods of experimental physiology. In 1864 Bert became interested in the question of whether the amount of gases dissolved in the blood depended on atmospheric pressure. This question had also interested Dr. Denis Jourdanet, a wealthy patron of the arts and sciences who had experienced mountain sickness while traveling in Mexico. Jourdanet constructed pressure chambers for therapeutic use and formulated the hypothesis that the blood contained less oxygen under the low atmospheric pressure of high altitudes, a condition that he termed "barometric anoxemia." The two men met in 1869 and divided the field of altitude physiology between them, Jourdanet taking the observational fieldwork and Bert the laboratory research. Jourdanet subsequently published his own book, *Influence de la pression de l'air sur la vie de l'homme: climats d'altitude et climats de montagne* (1875).

Jourdanet subsidized Paul Bert's experiments, enabling Bert to build several low-pressure chambers with which to study the effects of varying atmospheric pressures on animals and man. In an experiment using himself as the subject, Bert found that when oxygen pressure was lowered to 406 millimeters of mercury, he experienced acceleration of his heart and pulse, slowing of digestive processes, nausea, expansion of intestinal gases, lowering of body temperature, and a state of atrophy or torpor. However, when the oxygen pressure was kept constant, no ill effects were noted, even when total barometric pressure was lowered. Bert arranged for balloon ascents in order to determine the constituents of the upper atmosphere, and these experiments demonstrated that the cause of high

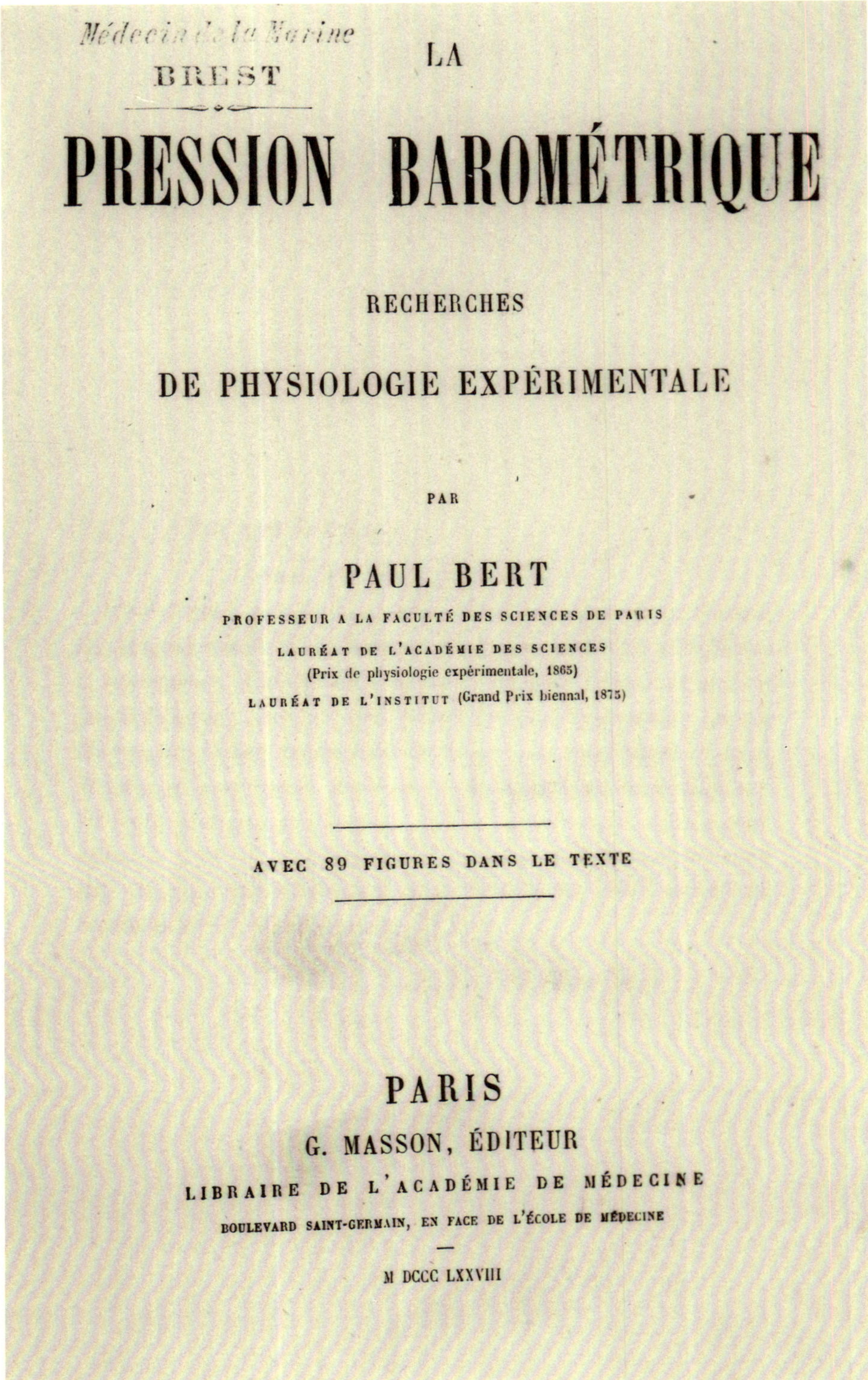

LA

PRESSION BAROMÉTRIQUE

RECHERCHES

DE PHYSIOLOGIE EXPÉRIMENTALE

PAR

PAUL BERT

PROFESSEUR A LA FACULTÉ DES SCIENCES DE PARIS
LAURÉAT DE L'ACADÉMIE DES SCIENCES
(Prix de physiologie expérimentale, 1865)
LAURÉAT DE L'INSTITUT (Grand Prix biennal, 1875)

AVEC 89 FIGURES DANS LE TEXTE

PARIS
G. MASSON, ÉDITEUR
LIBRAIRE DE L'ACADÉMIE DE MÉDECINE
BOULEVARD SAINT-GERMAIN, EN FACE DE L'ÉCOLE DE MÉDECINE

M DCCC LXXVIII

Fig. 143. No. 77. Bert. Title page.

altitude sickness was a decrease in oxygen pressure rather than the reduction of barometric pressure per se. This was the first application to human respiration of Dalton's Law of Partial Pressure, which states that in a mixture of gases, every gas acts as an independent entity.

Bert's book, considered to be the classic work in altitude physiology, describes his 670 experiments, which he had previously published in scientific journals between 1871 and 1875. It is organized in three parts: (1) review of the history of altitude physiology; (2) experimental protocols; and (3) summary and conclusions. The book was dedicated to Jourdanet with the following statement, "I have been very happy to see physiological experimentation on one of the most important points of my study confirm entirely the theory which your intelligence had deduced from numerous pathological observations collected on the high Mexican plateaux." Bert's book was translated into English in 1943 during World War II, the translators stating in their preface that "we know nothing would please Paul Bert more than the knowledge that his work had been of use to the Allied nations in their struggle to free his beloved country from the shackles of its traditional enemy."[1]

HFN

1. Paul Bert, *Barometric Pressure: Researches in Experimental Physiology*, trans. Mary Alice Hitchcock and Fred A. Hitchcock (Columbus, Ohio, 1943).

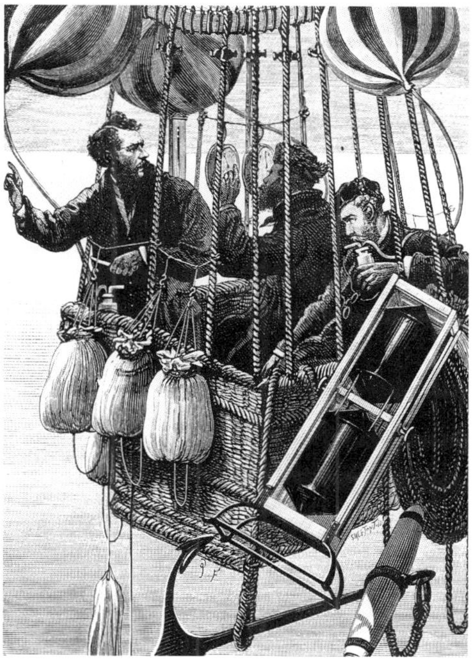

Fig. 144. No. 77. Bert. High altitude observations, made in the balloon *Zénith.* The man on the right holds an oxygen inhaler.

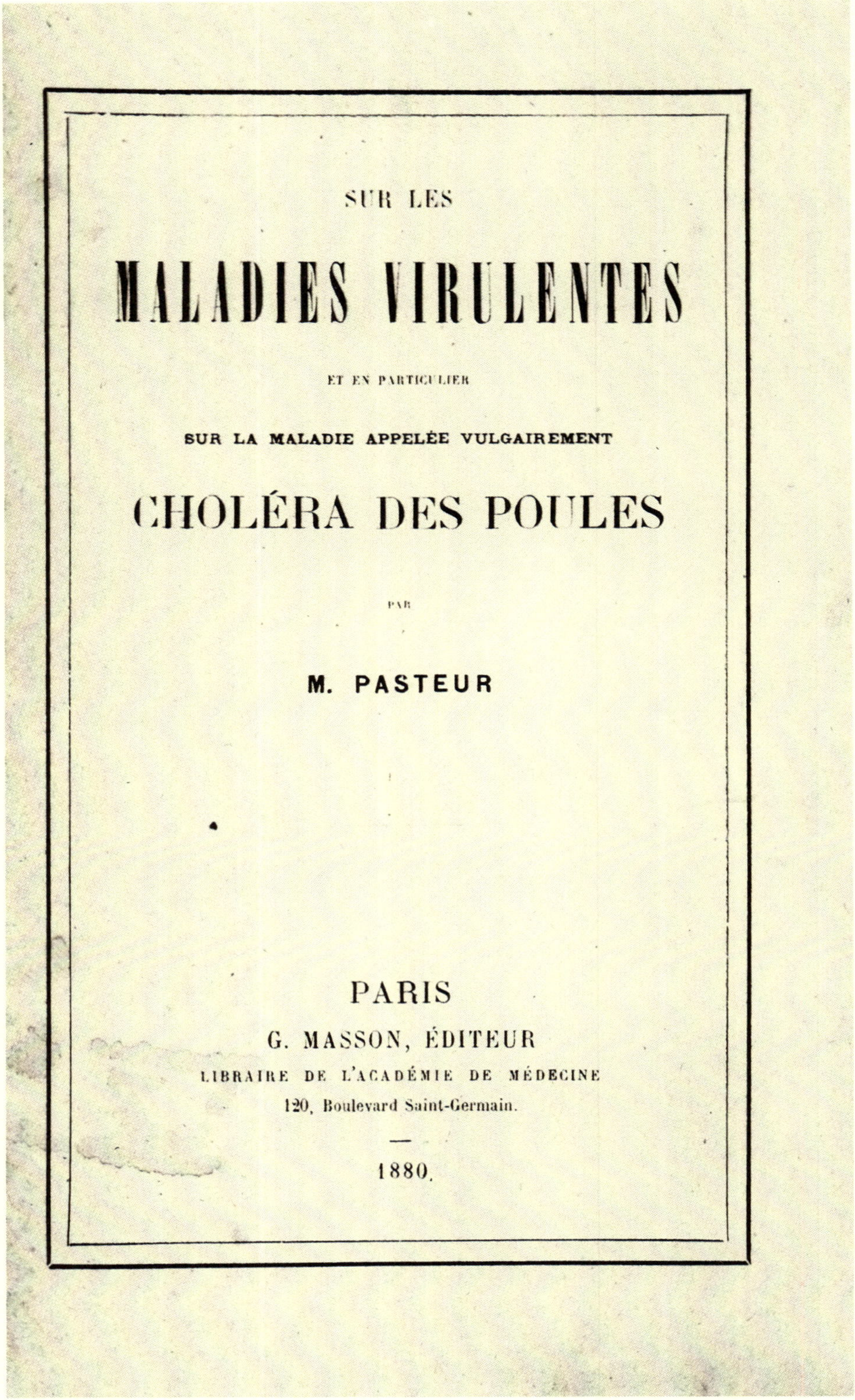

SUR LES

MALADIES VIRULENTES

ET EN PARTICULIER

SUR LA MALADIE APPELÉE VULGAIREMENT

CHOLÉRA DES POULES

PAR

M. PASTEUR

PARIS

G. MASSON, ÉDITEUR

LIBRAIRE DE L'ACADÉMIE DE MÉDECINE

120, Boulevard Saint-Germain.

—

1880.

Fig. 145. No. 78. Pasteur. Front wrapper of the offprint.

78

LOUIS PASTEUR
(1822–1895)

Sur les maladies virulentes et en particulier sur la maladie appelée vulgairement choléra des poules.

In: *Comptes rendus hebdomadaires des séances de l'Académie des Sciences* 90 (1880): 239–48.

[journal number] Vol. 90, No. 6, Séance du lundi 9 février 1880: $31–33^4$ 34^2. 14 leaves, pp. *233* 234–260.

[article] $31_4^r–32_4^v$, pp. 239–248.

EFDT 272. GM 2537. PMM 336e.

Also published in: *Bulletin de l'Académie de Médecine* 44, 2me série 9 (1880): 121–34.

[journal number] Vol. 44, No. 6, Séance du 10 février 1880: 10^8 11^4. 12 leaves, pp. *113* 114–136. Blue-green printed wrappers.

[article] $10_5^r–11_3^v$, pp. 121–134.

[offprint] *Sur les maladies virulentes et en particulier sur la maladie appelée vulgairement choléra des poules.* Paris: G. Masson, Éditeur, 1880.

$[1]^8$. 8 leaves, pp. *1–3* 4–16. Blue-green printed wrappers.

Reimposed, with different page breaks.

Norman 1661.

It had been known since Antiquity that recovery from certain diseases, such as smallpox, conferred lifelong immunity to the disease in question. Variolation, the practice of inoculating with infected material from smallpox cases, had been proven to accomplish similar results, and Edward Jenner (see no. 53) demonstrated at the end of the eighteenth century that cowpox vaccination provided a safer and more efficacious approach to smallpox immunity. However, the mechanism responsible for this protection and the means of extending it to other infectious diseases remained a mystery until Louis Pasteur published the present paper. This established the field of immunology as an experimental science, just as his earlier work had contributed to bacteriology by showing that each infectious disease (of wine, of beer, of silkworms, or of man) is due to a specific living microorganism that may be isolated, characterized morphologically, and cultured *in vitro* in a pure state.

After an opening discussion of the complicated nature of infectious diseases, Pasteur stated, "I dare to think that the Academy will see, in the facts that I have the honor to communicate, some unexpected explanations of the problems raised by the study of virulent diseases." Then, describing the first well-planned and controlled immunological experiment, he showed how, in the case of fowl cholera organisms, the virulence of the pathogen may be attenuated by altering the conditions of culture so as to render it non-lethal for rabbits and fowl. He also showed that animals immunized with the attenuated strain were subsequently protected from the deadly effects of inoculation with the virulent wild strain. Pasteur predicted the general applicability of this approach, which he later demonstrated brilliantly in his famous experiments on anthrax, rabies, and other infectious diseases.

AMS

79

CHARLES LOUIS ALPHONSE LAVERAN
(1845–1922)

Un nouveau parasite trouvé dans le sang de plusieurs malades atteints de fièvre palustre.

In: *Bulletins et mémoires de la Société médicale des hôpitaux de Paris,* Mémoires, 2me série 17 (1880): 158–64.

[journal volume] π^4 [1]^8 2–24^8 25^2, [1]^8 2–11^8 12^2. 288 leaves, pp. [8] *1–3* 4–387 [1], *1–3* 4–180. 1 lithographed chart; 3 black-and-white lithographed plates; 3 color-lithographed plates; 1 colored photo-lithograph.

[article] (second series) 10_7^v–11_2^v, pp. *158* 159–164. 1 wood-engraved figure in text.

GM 5236. *Heirs of Hippocrates* 2086.

This brief note contained Alphonse Laveran's first announcement, made from his laboratory in Constantine, Algeria, of the discovery of the malaria parasite. On 20 October 1880, while studying the characteristic pigmentation of the blood found in the brains and livers of malaria sufferers, Laveran noted other bodies, which he suspected might be parasites, in a sample of fresh blood. Later he wrote, "I had proceeded thus far with my researches, and was still hesitating whether these elements were parasites, when on November 6th, 1880, on examining the pigmented bodies mentioned above, I observed on the edge of several of these elements movable filaments of flagella, whose extremely rapid and varied movements left no doubt as to their nature."[1]

His paper on this subject was read at a meeting of the Académie de Médecine in Paris on 24 December 1880. It ended with an uncompromising declaration: "Parasitic elements are found in the blood of patients who are ill with malaria. Up to now these elements were thought to be pigmented leucocytes. The presence of these parasites in the blood is the principal cause of malaria." Laveran was not the first to see these parasites in the microscope, but he was the first to realize what they were and to recognize the enormous importance of this knowledge.

Although his discovery met with widespread skepticism, Laveran was to prove a determined and effective publicist for his views. In his first book on the subject, he was able to produce compelling additional evidence in support of his theory: he found the parasite in 148 out of 192 specimens of blood examined, and showed how they disappeared after

UN NOUVEAU PARASITE

TROUVÉ DANS LE SANG DES MALADES ATTEINTS DE FIÈVRE PALUSTRE

ORIGINE PARASITAIRE DES ACCIDENTS DE L'IMPALUDISME

Communication faite à la Société médicale des hôpitaux

DANS LA SÉANCE DU 24 DÉCEMBRE 1880

Par A. LAVERAN

Médecin-major, professeur agrégé au Val-de-Grâce

Le 20 octobre dernier, en examinant au microscope le sang d'un malade atteint de fièvre palustre, j'ai constaté la présence, au milieu des globules rouges du sang, d'éléments qui m'ont paru être d'origine parasitaire; depuis ce moment j'ai examiné le sang de 44 malades atteints de fièvre palustre et j'ai retrouvé 26 fois ces mêmes éléments, dont la nature parasitaire me paraît aujourd'hui démontrée. J'ai recherché en vain ces éléments dans le sang des malades atteints d'affections étrangères à l'impaludisme. Je décrirai ces éléments sous les noms de : corps n° 1, n° 2 et n° 3; la suite de ce travail montrera l'utilité de ces dénominations, qui ne préjugent en rien la nature du parasite.

I. *Description des éléments parasitaires trouvés dans le sang.* — Corps n° 1. Ce sont des éléments allongés, plus ou moins effilés à leurs extrémités, souvent incurvés en croissant (fig. 3 et fig. 4), quelquefois de forme ovalaire (fig. 5).

La longueur de ces corps est de 8 à 9 millièmes de millimètre; leur largeur de 3 millièmes de millimètre en moyenne. Les contours sont indiqués par une ligne très fine; le corps est transparent, incolore, sauf vers la partie moyenne où il existe une tache noirâtre constituée par une série de granulations arrondies, qui paraissent être des granulations pigmentaires. Par exception, cette tache peut être située près d'une des extrémités du corps n° 1. Les granulations affectent assez souvent

Fig. 146. No. 79. Laveran. Opening page.

treatment with quinine.[2] Later books continued to present his views, and by the late 1880s, these were generally accepted. Laveran did further original work in parasitology and was awarded the Nobel Prize for Medicine in 1907 in recognition of his work on the role played by protozoa in causing disease.

RDG

1. Alphonse Laveran, *Paludism,* trans. J. W. Martin (London, 1893), p. 9.
2. Alphonse Laveran, *Nature parasitaire des accidents de l'impaludisme. Description d'un nouveau parasite trouvé dans le sang* (Paris, 1881).

Die Aetiologie der Tuberkulose

von Dr. **R. Koch**, Geh. Regierungsrath.

Eine Reihe von Untersuchungen, welche ich in den letzten Jahren über die Aetiologie der Tuberkulose anstellte, haben mich zu Resultaten geführt, über welche zuerst gelegentlich eines Vortrages in der physiologischen Gesellschaft zu Berlin am 24. März 1882 berichtet wurde (Berliner klin. Wochenschr., 1882, No. 15.). Meine damaligen Mittheilungen konnten sich indessen nur auf die wichtigsten Punkte beschränken, während die eingehende Beschreibung der Versuche für einen ausführlichen Bericht vorbehalten bleiben musste. Seitdem ist durch fortgesetzte Untersuchungen noch manche Lücke ergänzt, auch Einzelnes neu hinzugekommen. Der hierdurch vervollständigte und erweiterte Bericht über meine Arbeiten zur Erforschung der Tuberkulose-Aetiologie soll im Nachstehenden gegeben werden.

Die Frage, ob die Tuberkulose eine durch übertragbare Krankheitsstoffe bedingte Krankheit sei, kann auf verschiedene Weise in Angriff genommen werden und es ist dies auch thatsächlich geschehen. Man hat theils mit Hülfe der klinischen Beobachtung, theils durch anatomische und schliesslich durch experimentelle Untersuchungen Gewissheit über das Wesen dieser Krankheit zu gewinnen gesucht.

Am unsichersten sind die Resultate gewesen, welche die am Krankenbett gesammelten Erfahrungen geliefert haben. Es begegnen zwar jedem einigermassen beschäftigten Arzte hin und wieder Fälle, in denen er nicht umhin kann, eine Uebertragung der Tuberkulose von einem Menschen auf andere anzunehmen. Dann aber folgen wieder zahlreiche Fälle, in denen jede Infection ausgeschlossen zu sein scheint. Es ist wiederholt der Versuch gemacht, mit Hülfe des gesammelten klinischen Materials die Ansteckungsfähigkeit der Phthisis zu beweisen, doch müssen diese Versuche als gescheitert angesehen werden, da es nicht gelungen ist, jener Anschauung Eingang in die Wissenschaft zu verschaffen. Manche Kliniker haben allerdings die Möglichkeit einer Ansteckung nicht aus dem Auge gelassen, aber im Grossen und Ganzen gilt die Phthisis bei den Aerzten als eine von constitutionellen Anomalien ausgehende, nicht infectiöse Krankheit.

Einen nicht zu verkennenden Hinweis auf den infectiösen Charakter der Tuberkulose lieferte dagegen die pathologische Anatomie, als Buhl auf den Zusammenhang der Miliartuberkulose mit primären käsigen Herden aufmerksam machte und den Satz aufstellte, dass die allgemeine Tuberkulose als eine Krankheit aufzufassen sei, welche durch die Resorption eines im primären Käseherd vorhandenen Virus, also gewissermassen durch Selbstinfection zu Stande kommt. Ueber den Weg, auf welchem das tuberkulöse Virus sich durch den Körper verbreitet, haben dann ferner die Entdeckungen von Ponfick über die Tuberkulose des Ductus thoracicus

Mittheilungen des Kaiserl. Gesundheitsamtes. II. Bd. 1

Fig. 147. No. 80. Koch. Opening page.

80

ROBERT KOCH
(1843–1910)

Die Aetiologie der Tuberkulose.

In: *Mittheilungen aus dem kaiserlichen Gesundheitsamte* 2 (1884): 1–88.

[journal volume] Vol. 2: π^4 1–31^8 32^2. 254 leaves, pp. [8] *1* 2–499 [1]. Taf. I–XIII: 13 color-lithographed plates (3 double). Gray-green printed wrappers, or cloth-backed gray-green printed boards.

[article] 1_1^r–6_4^v, pp. *1* 2–88. Taf. I–X: 10 color-lithographed plates.

cf. GM 2331. cf. PMM 366c.

Robert Koch was born and raised in Clausthal, a mining town in the Harz Mountains of northern Germany. He received his university and medical training at Göttingen, where among his early teachers were Friedrich Wöhler, Friedrich Gauss, Rudolf Hermann Lotze, and Jakob Henle. After completing his medical education in 1866 he spent some time in Berlin, where he attended the lectures of Rudolf Virchow (see no. 69). He then practiced medicine in small towns in northern Germany, served briefly in the military during the Franco-Prussian War (1870–71), and became a District Medical Officer in Wollstein, a German city in the otherwise Polish countryside of Silesia. It was there that he did the research on anthrax that first brought his name to the attention of the medical world.

Koch initially studied anthrax using microscopic techniques he had perfected as a naturalist. Through patient work with slide cultures and experimental animals, he was able to demonstrate the complete life cycle of the anthrax bacillus. Koch's work on anthrax provided the first firm evidence for the germ theory of disease and gave important insights into the control of anthrax in livestock and in people. Koch traveled to Breslau (now Wrocław, Poland) to demonstrate his work to the botantist Ferdinand Cohn and the pathologist Julius Cohnheim, and his paper on the etiology of anthrax was published in a botanical journal edited by Cohn.[1] This paper is universally recognized as a classic of experimental medicine. Both Cohn and Cohnheim became champions of Koch and his work and were responsible for his eventual move to Berlin, where he became the director of a laboratory of hygiene in the Imperial Health Office.

Koch was a pioneer in the use of the microscope in bacteriological research. He was among the first to employ the new optical devices that had been developed at the Carl

Zeiss company by Ernst Abbe, and he was the first to publish photomicrographs of bacteria.[2] In his final years at Wollstein, Koch set up extensive experiments on the nature of wound infections, culminating in his first book, *Untersuchungen über die Aetiologie der Wundinfectionskrankheiten* (Investigations into the etiology of traumatic infective diseases [1878]). In this work, Koch first developed procedures for staining bacteria in diseased tissues with aniline dyes, procedures that were to become critical in his research on tuberculosis a few years later.

After moving to Berlin, Koch carried out the studies that were to make him most famous. Many of these were published in the *Mittheilungen aus dem kaiserlichen Gesundheitsamte*, a "house organ" of the Imperial Health Office. In 1881 he described his development of the plate technique for cultivating bacteria, which provided the first consistent method for obtaining pure cultures of virtually any species of bacteria.[3] Using this plate culture technique, and applying his skill in the use of the microscope and experimental animals, Koch was able to show that tuberculosis was caused by a specific bacterium. His famous lecture of 24 March 1882 on the discovery of the tubercle bacillus was attended by the most noteworthy representatives of the Berlin medical profession and was quickly published.[4] Two years later, in an expanded version of "Die Aetiologie der Tuberculose" (The etiology of tuberculosis), he presented his detailed studies of the tubercle bacillus and announced what became known as "Koch's postulates" for isolating a disease-causing organism and testing its role in the transmission of the disease.

Not resting on his laurels, Koch led a German scientific expedition to Egypt and India in 1883. The purpose was to investigate outbreaks of cholera, and Koch succeeded in discovering and characterizing the comma bacillus, the causal organism of this epidemic disease.[5] He returned from India a hero and was soon appointed a professor of hygiene at the University of Berlin. During this period he trained many of the most important figures in German medicine and hygiene, including Friedrich Loeffler, Georg Gaffky, Paul Ehrlich (see no. 92), Emil von Behring (see no. 81), and Shibasaburo Kitasato (see no. 81). Continuing his own medical research, Koch discovered the delayed hypersensitivity reaction, which led to the development of the tuberculin test, and initiated field studies on typhoid fever in Germany. The latter led to the first recognition of the carrier state, a major discovery in public health. Koch spent his later years travelling the world, carrying out complex and important field studies in tropical medicine, including work on malaria, rinderpest, sleeping sickness, and Rhodesian redwater.

Koch was awarded the Nobel Prize in 1905, primarily for his work on tuberculosis and cholera. More generally, his application of bacteriology to medicine can be said to have provided the first scientific approach to the control of infectious diseases. Without Koch's work, the elaborate public health controls that were established about the turn of the century in urban areas throughout the world would not have become possible.

TDB

1. Robert Koch, "Die Aetiologie der Milzbrand-Krankheit, begründet auf die Entwicklungsgeschichte des Bacillus Anthracis," *Beiträge zur Biologie der Pflanzen* 2 (1876): 277–310.
2. Robert Koch, "Verfahren zur Untersuchung, zum Conservieren und Photographieren der Bakterien," *Beiträge zur Biologie der Pflanzen* 2 (1876): 399–434.
3. Robert Koch, "Zur Untersuchung von pathogenen Organismen," *Mittheilungen aus dem kaiserlichen Gesundheitsamte* 1 (1881): 1–48.
4. Robert Koch, "Die Aetiologie der Tuberculose," *Berliner klinische Wochenschrift* 19 (1882): 221–30.
5. Robert Koch, *Bericht über die Tätigkeit der zur Erforschung der Cholera im Jahre 1883 nach Ägypten und Indien entsandten Kommission* (Arbeiten aus dem kaiserlichen Gesundheitsamte, 3; Berlin, 1887).

See color plate XXXII.

Donnerstag — № 49. — 4. December 1890.

DEUTSCHE

MEDICINISCHE WOCHENSCHRIFT.

Mit Berücksichtigung des deutschen Medicinalwesens nach amtlichen Mittheilungen, der öffentlichen Gesundheitspflege und der Interessen des ärztlichen Standes.

Begründet von Dr. Paul Börner.

Sechszehnter Jahrgang.

Redacteur Sanitäts-Rath **Dr. S. Guttmann** in Berlin W. — Verlag von **Georg Thieme**, Leipzig-Berlin.

I. Aus dem hygienischen Institut des Herrn Geheimerath Koch in Berlin.

Ueber das Zustandekommen der Diphtherie-Immunität und der Tetanus-Immunität bei Thieren.

Von Stabsarzt Dr. **Behring**, Assistenten am Institut, und Dr. **Kitasato** aus Tokio.

Bei unseren seit längerer Zeit fortgesetzten Studien über Diphtherie (Behring) und Tetanus (Kitasato) sind wir auch der therapeutischen und der Immunisirungsfrage nähergetreten, und bei beiden Infectionskrankheiten ist es uns gelungen, sowohl inficirte Thiere zu heilen, wie die gesunden derartig vorzubehandeln, dass sie später nicht mehr an Diphtherie bezw. am Tetanus erkranken.

Auf welche Weise die Heilung und die Immunisirung zu erreichen ist, darauf soll an dieser Stelle nur soweit eingegangen werden,[1]) als nothwendig ist, um die Richtigkeit des folgenden Satzes zu beweisen.

„Die Immunität von Kaninchen und Mäusen, die gegen Tetanus immunisirt sind, beruht auf der Fähigkeit der zellenfreien Blutflüssigkeit, die toxischen Substanzen, welche die Tetanusbacillen produciren, unschädlich zu machen."

Die Erklärung für die Immunität, welche im vorstehenden Satz zum Ausdruck gebracht ist, wurde in denjenigen Arbeiten, die in neuerer Zeit sich mit der Immunitätsfrage beschäftigten, noch nicht in Erwägung gezogen.

Ausser mit der Phagocytosenlehre, die in der vitalen Thätigkeit der Zellen die Erklärung suchte, wurde noch mit der bacterienfeindlichen Wirkung des Blutes und mit der Giftgewöhnung des thierischen Organismus gerechnet.

Wenn eins dieser Erklärungsprincipien nicht ausreichte, oder von experimentell arbeitenden Autoren als unrichtig erkannt wurde, so glaubte man auf dem Wege der Ausschliessung die anderen in Anspruch nehmen zu dürfen. So sagte Bouchard in seiner Rede auf dem X. internationalen medicinischen Congress, die vielleicht am prägnantesten den bisherigen Stand der Immunitätsfrage wiedergiebt, Folgendes: „Ne parlons donc plus d'entrainement des leucocytes et d'accoutumance des cellules nerveuses aux poisons bactériens: c'est pure rhétorique" und: „C'est en effet cet état bactéricide qui constitue la vaccination ou l'immunité acquise."

Diese positive Erklärung kommt auf dasselbe hinaus, was Roger[2]) früher mit folgenden Worten ausdrückte: „La vaccination détermine dans l'organisme des modifications chimiques qui rendent les humeurs et les tissus peu favorables à la végétation du microbe, contre lequel on a prémuni l'animal."

Nun konnte der eine von uns (Behring) bei seinen Studien an diphtherieimmunen Ratten und an immunisirten Meerschweinchen feststellen, dass keine der oben erwähnten Theorieen uns die Immunität dieser Thiere zu erklären vermag, und er sah sich genöthigt, nach einem anderen Erklärungsprincip zu suchen. Nach mannichfachen vergeblichen Bemühungen zeigte sich in der diphtheriegift-zerstörenden Wirkung des Blutes von diphtherieimmunen Thieren die Richtung, in welcher die Unempfänglichkeit für Diphtherie zu suchen ist. Aber erst bei der Anwendung der bei der Diphtherie gemachten Erfahrungen auf den Tetanus sind wir zu Ergebnissen gelangt, die, soweit wir erkennen können, an Beweiskraft nichts zu wünschen übrig lassen.

Die im folgenden angeführten Experimente beweisen:

1. Das Blut des tetanusimmunen Kaninchens besitzt tetanusgiftzerstörende Eigenschaften.

2. Diese Eigenschaften sind auch im extravasculären Blut und in dem daraus gewonnenen zellenfreien Serum nachweisbar.

3. Diese Eigenschaften sind so dauerhafter Natur, dass sie auch im Organismus anderer Thiere wirksam bleiben, so dass man imstande ist, durch die Blut- bezw. Serumtransfusion hervorragende therapeutische Wirkungen zu erzielen.

4. Die tetanusgiftzerstörenden Eigenschaften fehlen im Blut solcher Thiere, die gegen Tetanus nicht immun sind, und wenn man das Tetanusgift nicht immunen Thieren einverleibt hat, so lässt sich dasselbe auch noch nach dem Tode der Thiere im Blut und in sonstigen Körperflüssigkeiten nachweisen.

Wir theilen zum Beweise für diese Behauptungen folgende grössere Versuchsreihe mit:

Auf eine Art, die an anderer Stelle genau beschrieben werden wird[1]), wurde ein Kaninchen gegen Tetanus immunisirt. Bei der Prüfung des Grades der Immunität erhielt dasselbe 10 ccm einer keimhaltigen virulenten Tetanusbacillen-Cultur, von der für normale Kaninchen 0,5 ccm genügten, um dieselben ganz sicher am Tetanus zu Grunde gehen zu lassen. Jenes Kaninchen blieb ganz gesund.

[1]) Genauere Mittheilungen hierüber werden in der Zeitschrift für Hygiene erfolgen.

[2]) „Contribution à l'étude de l'immunité acquise." 1890.

[1]) In einer demnächst in der Zeitschrift für Hygiene erscheinenden Arbeit: Ueber die Eigenschaften des Tetanusgiftes, von Kitasato.

Fig. 148. No. 81. Behring and Kitasato. Opening page.

81

EMIL ADOLPH VON BEHRING
(1854–1917)

SHIBASABURO KITASATO
(1852–1931)

Ueber das Zustandekommen der Diphtherie-Immunität und der Tetanus-Immunität bei Thieren.

In: *Deutsche medicinische Wochenschrift* 16 (1890): 1113–14.

[journal number] Vol. 16, No. 49, 4 December 1890: $[1–4]^4$. 16 leaves, pp. *1113* 1114–1144.

[article] $[1]_1^r$–$[1]_1^v$, pp. *1113* 1114.

GM 2544, 5060.

In the decade following Louis Pasteur's publication in 1880 of the rules governing preventive vaccination against infectious diseases (see no. 78), little was discovered about the mechanisms involved in this process. A major dispute developed between those who held that immunity was mediated by cellular (phagocytic) mechanisms, as proposed by Elie Metchnikoff, and those who favored humoral (blood-borne) factors. Then in 1888 Émile Roux and Alexandre Yersin in Paris discovered diphtheria toxin, and it quickly became apparent that the disease could be produced by the toxin itself, independent of the intact organism. At the Institute of Hygiene in Berlin, Robert Koch assigned army doctor Emil Behring to work on diphtheria and visiting Japanese scientist Shibasaburo Kitasato to work on tetanus. Because of their similar approaches, the two were finally advised to collaborate with one another.

In their joint paper the authors demonstrated for both diphtheria and tetanus that immunization of animals with sublethal doses of the toxins led to their protection against the ill effects of the administration of subsequent lethal doses of the disease-producing organisms. They showed further that a protective factor, which they described as a "toxin-destroying property," appeared in the blood of immunized animals. Thus the blood or cell-free serum of the immunized animal could be passively transferred to a naive recipient, even of another species, to provide protection against lethal doses of the organism or toxin. The authors also showed that this antitoxic effect may be accomplished in the test tube prior to inoculation of the poison and that it is specific for the disease in question. This was the first discovery of circulating, protective antibodies, and it had important implications for the cellular-humoral controversy. Indeed, the authors ended their paper with the famous saying of Goethe, "Blut ist ein ganz besonderer Saft" (Blood is quite a special juice).

In his later work, Behring demonstrated the cure of diphtheritic children using immune serum. This won him the ennobling *von* and the first Nobel Prize in Physiology or Medicine in 1901.

AMS

82

SIR WILLIAM OSLER
(1849–1919)

The Principles and Practice of Medicine. Designed for the Use of Practitioners and Students of Medicine.

[American issue] New York: D. Appleton and Company, 1892.

[A]^8 B^2 2^8 χ1 3^{10} 4–20^8 21^8 (21$_4$ + 1) 22–32^8 33^8 (33$_6$ + 1) 34–43^8 44^8 (44$_1$ + 1.2, 44$_3$ + 1, 44$_6$ + 1) 45–67^8 68^6. 553 leaves, pp. [2] *i–vii* viii–xvi [2] *1* 2–1079 [7]. Fig. 1–5: 5 line-block figures in text; Charts I–XIX: 19 line-block charts in text (XI in two parts), 2 printed in red and black, 7 printed in red, blue, and black. Brown publisher's cloth, sheep, or half-morocco.

GM 2231. Golden & Roland 1375. *Heirs of Hippocrates* 2121. Norman 1612. Osler 3543.

[British issue] Edinburgh & London: Young J. Pentland, 1892.

[A]^8 (–A1, 2 + A1.2) B^2 2^8 χ1 3^{10} 4–20^8 21^8 (21$_4$ + 1) 22–32^8 33^8 (33$_6$ + 1) 34–43^8 44^8 (44$_1$ + 1.2, 44$_3$ – 1, 44$_6$ + 1) 45–67^8 68^6 (–68$_{4,5,6}$). 550 leaves, pp. [2] *i–vii* viii–xvi [2] *1* 2–1079 [1]. Fig. 1–5: 5 line-block figures in text; Charts I–XIX: 19 line-block charts in text (XI in two parts), 2 printed in red and black, 7 printed in red, blue, and black. Dark blue-green publisher's cloth.

The American sheets, with cancel title and half-title, and the American advertisements cancelled at the end.

Golden & Roland 1439.

William Osler, the most renowned physician of recent times, was born and educated in Canada; his career spanned three nations and two continents. As Professor of the Institutes of Medicine at McGill University in Montreal, he was the "potent ferment" of the medical faculty. In 1884, an established medical leader, he came to Philadelphia to accept the chair of Clinical Professor of Medicine at the University of Pennsylvania. Five years later he relocated to Baltimore to join the newly established Johns Hopkins Hospital and Medical School as Physican-in-Chief and Professor of Medicine. In 1905, at the zenith of his career, he was called to Oxford when he was appointed Regius Professor of Medicine. In addition to being a superb clinician, teacher, historian, and humanist, Osler was also an ardent bibliophile and insatiable collector. At his death, he left his splendid library to McGill University; the contents of this collection are described and Osler's comments on many of the books are recorded in the monumental catalogue *Bibliotheca Osleriana*, which still serves as an inspiration to medical book collectors and as a guide to the historical bibliography of medicine.

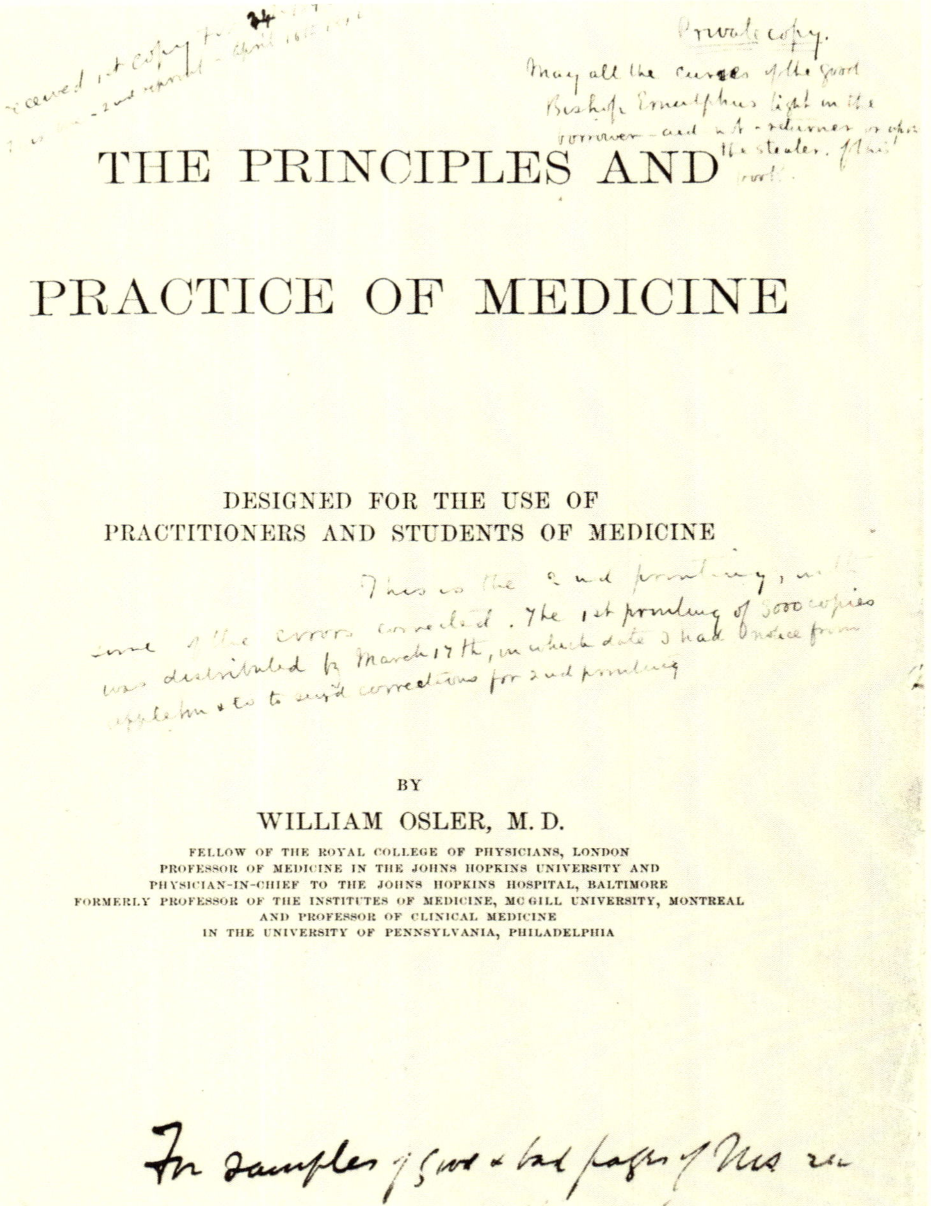

Private copy.
May all the curses of the good Bishop Ernulphus light on the borrower — and not-returner or else the stealer of this book!

THE PRINCIPLES AND

PRACTICE OF MEDICINE

DESIGNED FOR THE USE OF
PRACTITIONERS AND STUDENTS OF MEDICINE

This is the 2nd printing, with some of the errors corrected. The 1st printing of 5000 copies was distributed by March 17th, on which date I had notice from Appletons to send corrections for 2nd printing

BY

WILLIAM OSLER, M. D.

FELLOW OF THE ROYAL COLLEGE OF PHYSICIANS, LONDON
PROFESSOR OF MEDICINE IN THE JOHNS HOPKINS UNIVERSITY AND
PHYSICIAN-IN-CHIEF TO THE JOHNS HOPKINS HOSPITAL, BALTIMORE
FORMERLY PROFESSOR OF THE INSTITUTES OF MEDICINE, MCGILL UNIVERSITY, MONTREAL
AND PROFESSOR OF CLINICAL MEDICINE
IN THE UNIVERSITY OF PENNSYLVANIA, PHILADELPHIA

For samples of good & bad pages of Mss see
the end of this vol.

NEW YORK
D. APPLETON AND COMPANY
1892

Fig. 149. No. 82. Osler's own copy of the second issue of *The Principles and Practice of Medicine*, with his annotations.

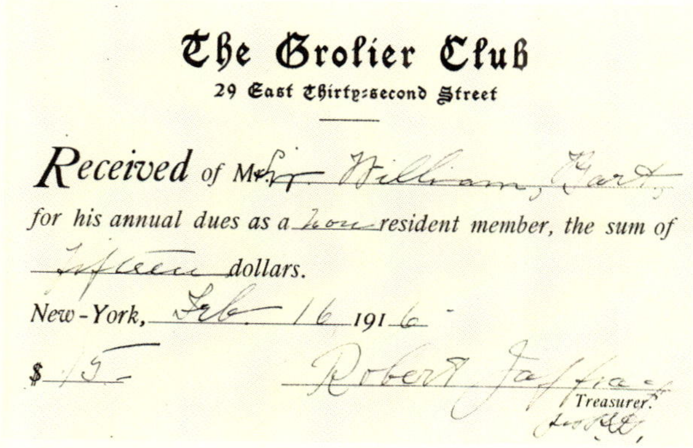
The Grolier Club
29 East Thirty-second Street

Received of Mr. William Osler
for his annual dues as a non-resident member, the sum of
Fifteen dollars.
New-York, Feb. 16 1916
$15 Robert Jaffray
Treasurer.

Fig. 150. No. 82. Receipt issued by the Grolier Club for Osler's 1916 membership dues.

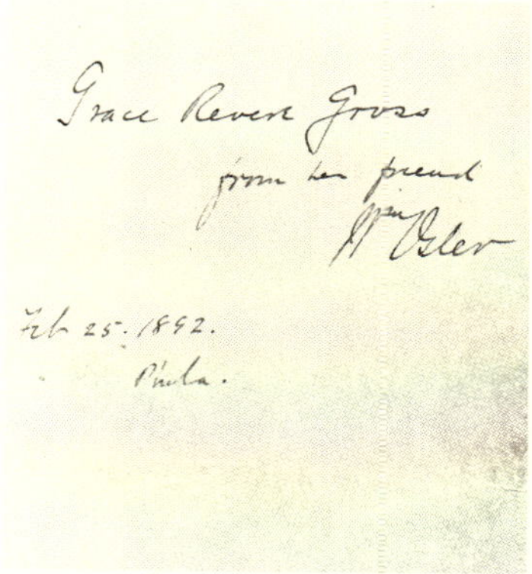
Grace Revere Gross
from her friend
Wm Osler
Feb 25. 1892.
Phila.

Fig. 151. No. 82. Osler inscribed this copy of *The Principles and Practice of Medicine* to Grace Revere Gross, who later became his wife.

While at Johns Hopkins, Osler wrote *The Principles and Practice of Medicine*, which continues to be an object of interest and admiration more than a century after its first publication in February 1892. Acclaimed as both a scientific and a literary masterpiece, it quickly became the standard textbook of medicine throughout much of the English-speaking world. The first issue of the first edition, consisting of the first three thousand copies, is distinguished by an error on the verso of the third leaf in which Plato's *Gorgias* is misspelled "*Georgias*" (in the second issue, this is spelled correctly). Osler's *Principles and Practice of Medicine* went through sixteen editions from 1892 to 1947, with new editions generally appearing at three- to five-year intervals. The first seven editions were prepared by Osler alone, but with the eighth edition (1912) and ninth edition (published posthumously in 1920) he was assisted by his former resident, Thomas McCrae, who continued the revisions through the twelfth edition (1935). Then the responsibility passed to Henry A. Christian of Harvard University, who, continuing the single-author tradition, carried *The Principles and Practice of Medicine* through the sixteenth edition (1947), the last edition published under Osler's name and depending substantially on his work. A medical textbook with the same title, published as the seventeenth edition in 1968 and most recently in a twenty-second edition (1988), is the work of many contributors under the direction of an editorial board. It has been estimated that almost 500,000 copies of Osler's work were sold. Translations of *The Principles and Practice of Medicine* appeared throughout the world, beginning with the Russian edition (1905–06), followed by the French (1908), German (1909), Chinese (1909–10), Spanish (1915), and Portuguese (1945) editions. The value of the book was ultimately in the impact it had on the education and practice of generations of students and physicians. The many translations attest to the global impact of Osler's teachings.

RLG

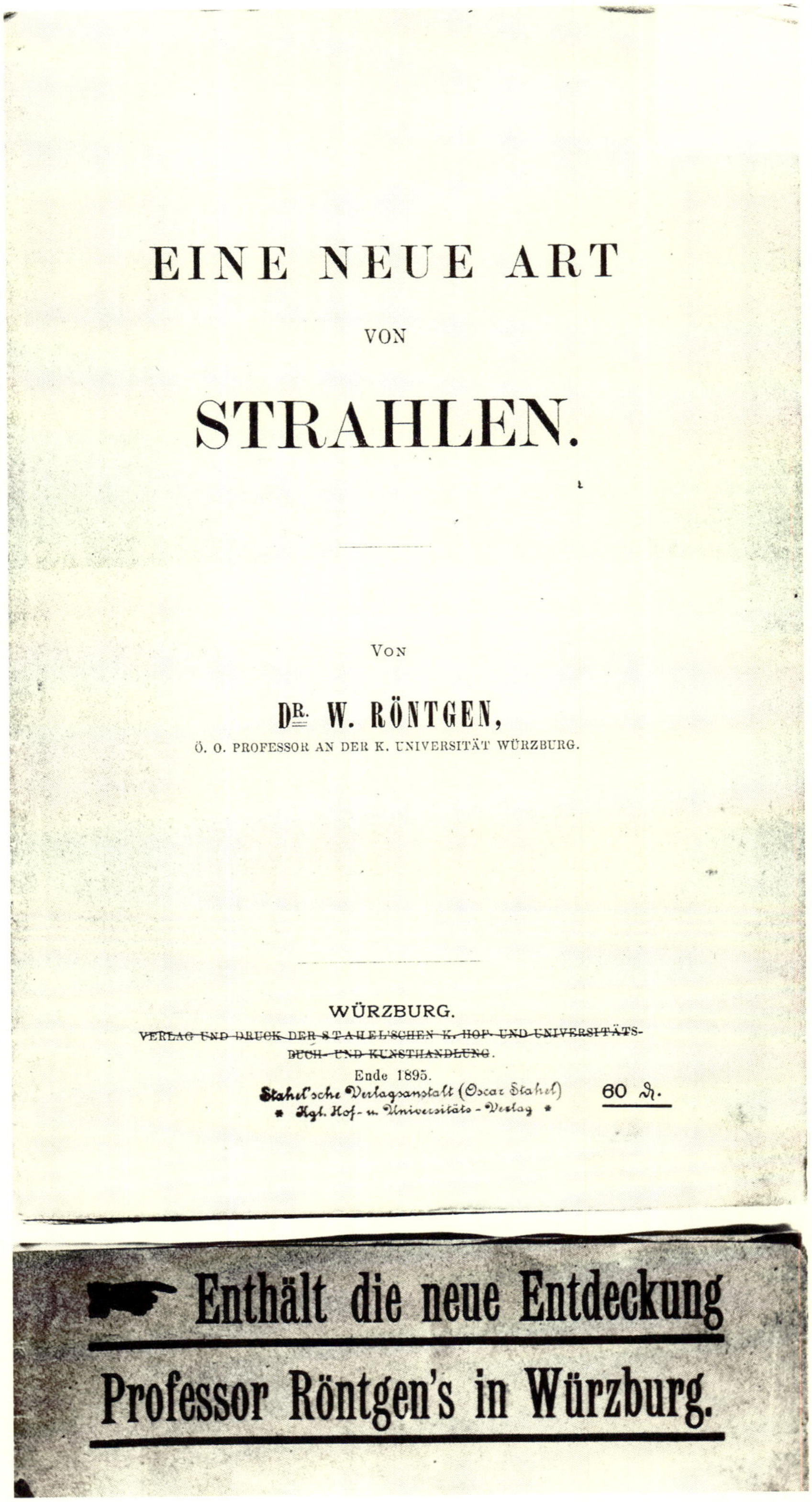

EINE NEUE ART

VON

STRAHLEN.

VON

DR. W. RÖNTGEN,

Ö. O. PROFESSOR AN DER K. UNIVERSITÄT WÜRZBURG.

WÜRZBURG.

~~VERLAG UND DRUCK DER STAHEL'SCHEN K. HOF- UND UNIVERSITÄTS-~~
~~BUCH- UND KUNSTHANDLUNG.~~

Ende 1895.

Stahel'sche Verlagsanstalt (Oscar Stahel) 60 ₰.
* Kgl. Hof- u. Universitäts-Verlag *

Enthält die neue Entdeckung
Professor Röntgen's in Würzburg.

Fig. 152. No. 83. Roentgen. Front wrapper of the 1895 offprint. Below is the printed paper band that the publishers wrapped around copies of the offprint; it reads: "Contains the new discovery of Professor Röntgen in Würzburg."

83

WILHELM CONRAD ROENTGEN
(1845–1923)

A] Ueber eine neue Art von Strahlen. (Vorläufige Mittheilung.).

In: *Sitzungs-Berichte der physikalisch-medicinischen Gesellschaft zu Würzburg,* 1895: 132–41.

[journal number] 1895, No. 9: 9^8 10^4. 12 leaves, pp. *129* 130–151 [1]. Yellow printed wrappers.

[article] 9_2^v–9_7^r, pp. 132–141.

[offprint] *Eine neue Art von Strahlen* [wrapper title]. Würzburg: Verlag und Druck der Stahel'schen K. Hof- und Universitäts- Buch- und Kunsthandlung, Ende 1895.

$[1]^6$. 6 leaves, pp. *1* 2–10 [2]. Yellow printed wrappers.

Reimposed, with different page breaks.

The first printing of the offprint has no title page and contains a blank leaf at the end. Four subsequent printings were printed from type pages reimposed so as to allow for a title leaf at the beginning rather than a final blank (these copies collate: $[1]^6$. 6 leaves, pp. *1–3* 4–12); all were dated 1896 and designated as 2., 3., 4., or 5. Auflage.

B] Ueber eine neue Art von Strahlen. II. Mittheilung.

In: *Sitzungs-Berichte der physikalisch-medicinischen Gesellschaft zu Würzburg,* 1896: 11–19.

[journal numbers] 1896, No. 1: 1^8. 8 leaves, pp. *1* 2–16. 1896, No. 2: 2^8. 8 leaves, pp. *17* 18–32.

[article] 1_6^r–2_2^r, pp. 11–19. 1 halftone illustration in text.

[offprint] *Eine neue Art von Strahlen. II. Mittheilung.* Würzburg: Verlag und Druck der Stahel'schen K. Hof- und Universitäts- Buch- und Kunsthandlung, 1896.

$[1]^6$. 6 leaves, pp. *1–3* 4–9 [3]. Orange printed wrappers.

Reimposed, with different page breaks.

GM 2683. Horblit 90. Norman 1841–42. Osler 1700. PMM 380. Waller 8078, 8083.

Wilhelm Conrad Roentgen, professor of physics, director of the Institute of Physics at the University of Würzburg, and rector of the university, was fifty years old when he discovered X-rays. Some have viewed Roentgen's discovery as accidental; however, "serendipitous" is a more appropriate term, since it was a product of experiment, and to quote Louis Pasteur, "Chance favors the prepared mind." In October 1895 Roentgen began to experiment with cathode rays, a field outside his usual area of study. On 8 November 1895, while he was experimenting with a Crookes tube or Lenard tube as a source of cathode rays, he noted that when he made the tube lightproof, something within the tube caused platinocyanide crystals to fluoresce. Further investigation revealed that the agent was not cathode rays but another unknown ray originating at the spot where the cathode rays hit the wall of the tube; Roentgen named this unknown ray the X-ray. These rays, he found, penetrated matter and had a photographic action.

> I have observed, and in part photographed, many shadow-pictures. . . . I possess, for instance, photographs of the shadow of the profile of a door. . . ; the shadow of the bones of the hand. . . ; the shadow of a covered wire wrapped on a wooden spool; of a set of weights enclosed in a box. . . ; of a compass in which the magnetic needle is entirely enclosed by metal. . . ; of a piece of metal whose lack of homogeneity . . . becomes noticeable by means of the X-rays, etc.[1]

In order to ensure immediate publication of his discovery, Roentgen sent his paper, "Eine neue Art von Strahlen (Vorlaufige Mittheilung)" (On a new kind of rays [preliminary communication]) to the Würzburg Physical-Medical Society for publication in its proceedings. The article appeared in the December 1895 number of the society's journal, although that number probably was not actually published until January 1896. There was also an offprint dated "Ende 1895" on the wrapper, and this went through four more printings in 1896.[2] Roentgen sent copies of the offprint, together with X-ray photographs, to a number of prominent scientists, and the news of his discovery quickly spread around the world. Within a year, over fifty books and pamphlets and about one thousand papers on X-rays had been published in the scientific and popular press, and within twenty years, the science of radiology was well established. Roentgen's discovery of X-rays marked the greatest advance in diagnostic medicine since the invention of the stethoscope by Laennec (see no. 57); it has also proved extremely useful to physicists, metallurgists, and photographers.

Roentgen published a second paper on X-rays in March of 1896 and a third in 1897, but he wrote no further papers on the subject, leaving the elucidation of the nature of X-rays and their application to others. For his discovery, he was awarded the first Nobel Prize for Physics in 1901.

HFN

1. Quoted in Otto Glasser, *Wilhelm Conrad Röntgen and the Early History of the Roentgen Rays* (Springfield, Ill., 1934; reprinted, San Francisco, 1993), p. 26.

2. E. Weil, "Some Bibliographical Notes on the First Publication on the Roentgen Rays," *Isis* 29 (1938): 362–65. See also Herbert S. Klickstein, *Wilhelm Conrad Röntgen On a New Kind of Rays: A Bibliographical Study.* Mallinckrodt Classics of Radiology, Vol. I, 1966.

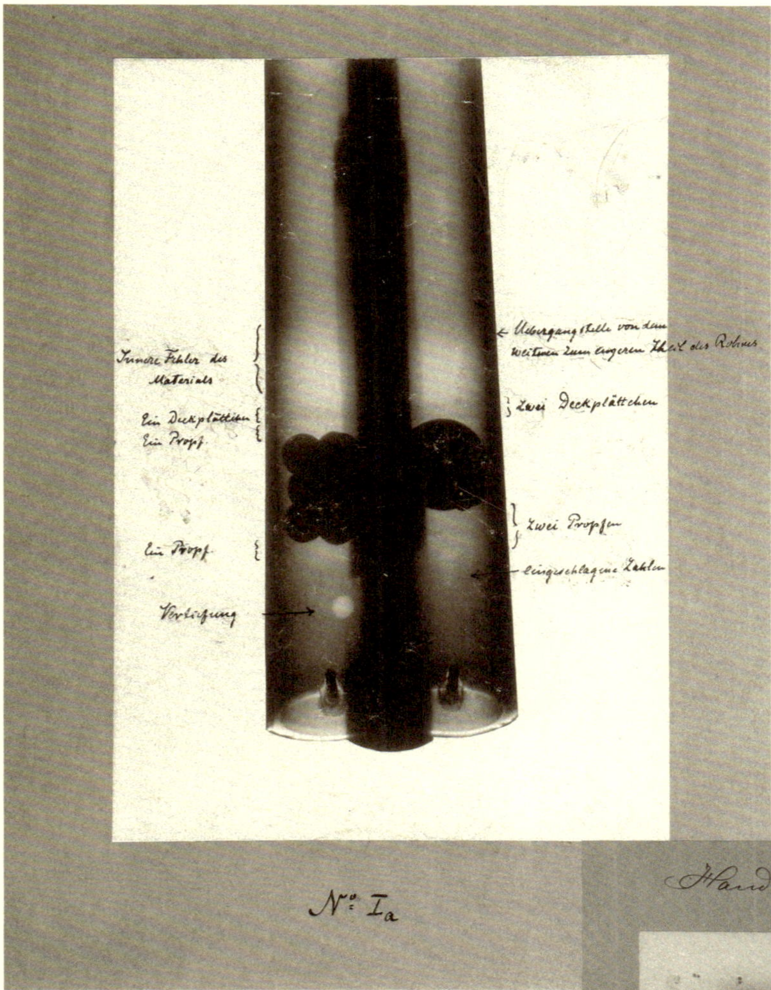

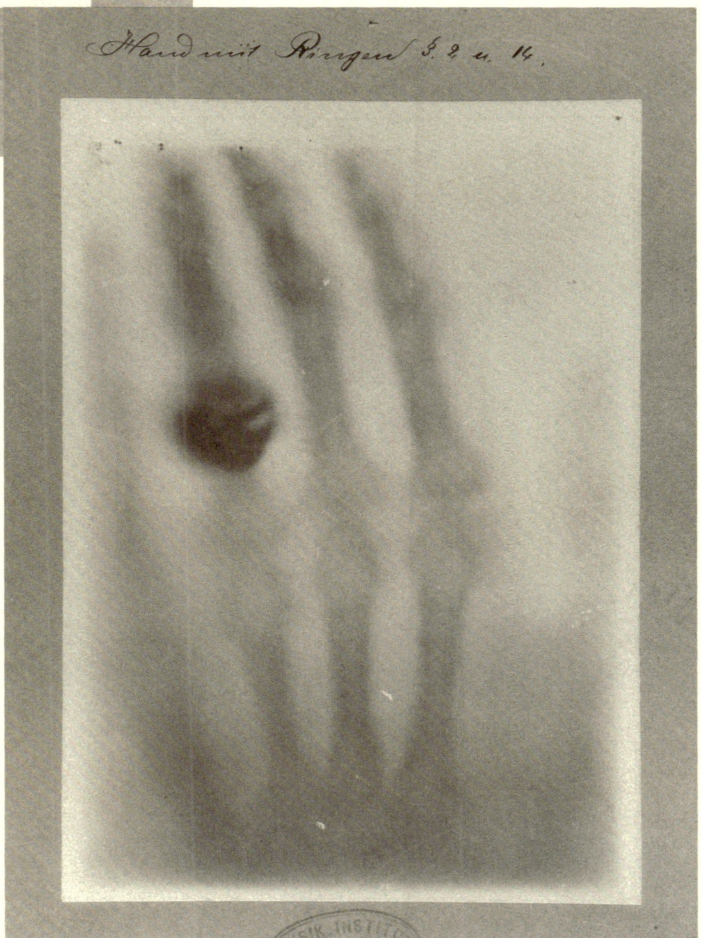

Fig. 153. No. 83. X-ray photographs taken by Roentgen of a rifle barrel and of his wife's hand.

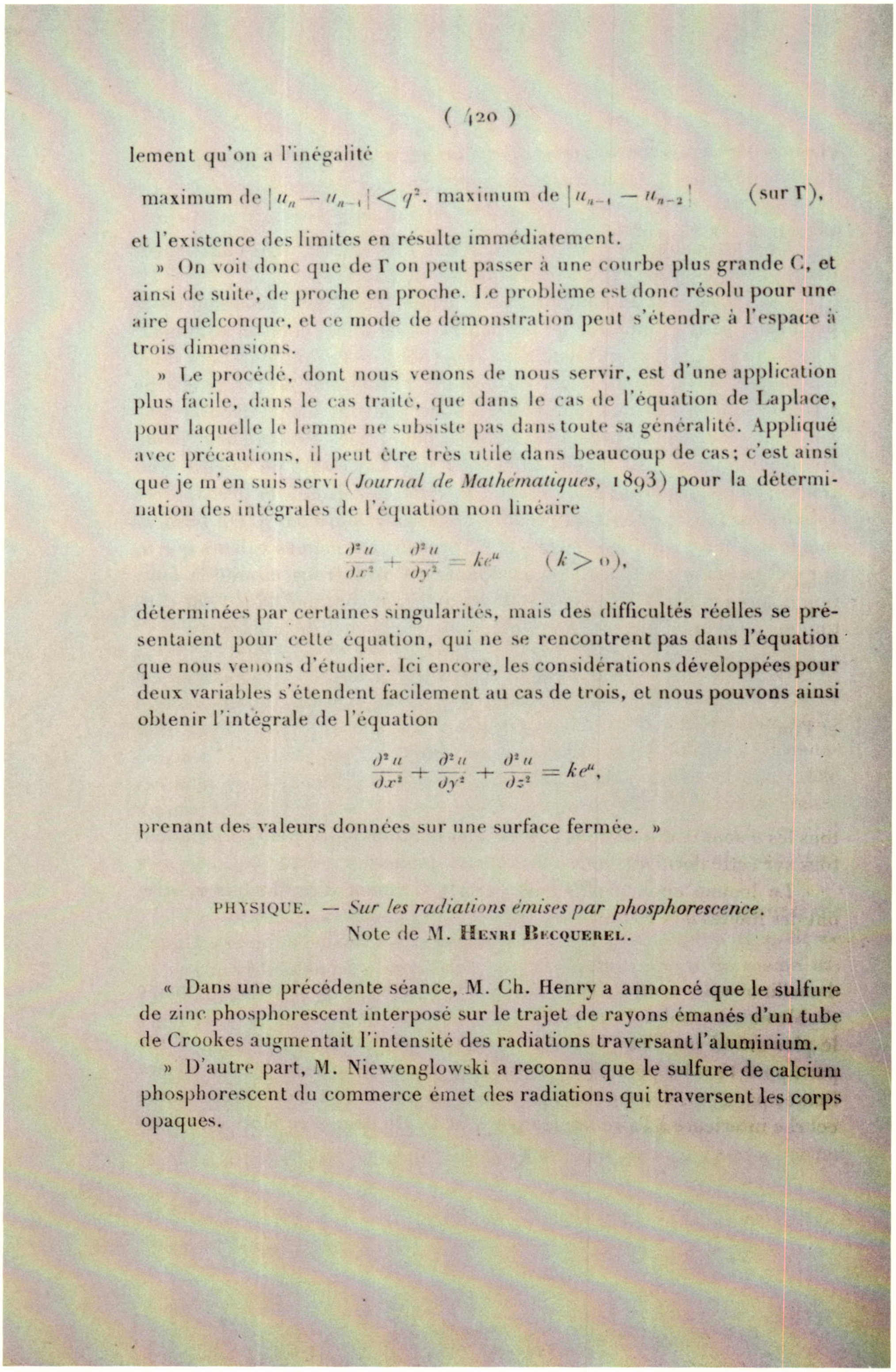

(420)

lement qu'on a l'inégalité

$$\text{maximum de } |u_n - u_{n-1}| < q^2 . \text{ maximum de } |u_{n-1} - u_{n-2}| \qquad (\text{sur } \Gamma),$$

et l'existence des limites en résulte immédiatement.

» On voit donc que de Γ on peut passer à une courbe plus grande C, et ainsi de suite, de proche en proche. Le problème est donc résolu pour une aire quelconque, et ce mode de démonstration peut s'étendre à l'espace à trois dimensions.

» Le procédé, dont nous venons de nous servir, est d'une application plus facile, dans le cas traité, que dans le cas de l'équation de Laplace, pour laquelle le lemme ne subsiste pas dans toute sa généralité. Appliqué avec précautions, il peut être très utile dans beaucoup de cas; c'est ainsi que je m'en suis servi (*Journal de Mathématiques*, 1893) pour la détermination des intégrales de l'équation non linéaire

$$\frac{\partial^2 u}{\partial x^2} + \frac{\partial^2 u}{\partial y^2} = ke^u \qquad (k > 0),$$

déterminées par certaines singularités, mais des difficultés réelles se présentaient pour cette équation, qui ne se rencontrent pas dans l'équation que nous venons d'étudier. Ici encore, les considérations développées pour deux variables s'étendent facilement au cas de trois, et nous pouvons ainsi obtenir l'intégrale de l'équation

$$\frac{\partial^2 u}{\partial x^2} + \frac{\partial^2 u}{\partial y^2} + \frac{\partial^2 u}{\partial z^2} = ke^u,$$

prenant des valeurs données sur une surface fermée. »

PHYSIQUE. — *Sur les radiations émises par phosphorescence.* Note de M. HENRI BECQUEREL.

« Dans une précédente séance, M. Ch. Henry a annoncé que le sulfure de zinc phosphorescent interposé sur le trajet de rayons émanés d'un tube de Crookes augmentait l'intensité des radiations traversant l'aluminium.

» D'autre part, M. Niewenglowski a reconnu que le sulfure de calcium phosphorescent du commerce émet des radiations qui traversent les corps opaques.

Fig. 154. No. 84A. Becquerel. Opening page.

84

HENRI BECQUEREL
(1852–1908)

A] Sur les radiations émises par phosphorescence.

In: *Comptes rendus hebdomadaires des séances de l'Académie des Sciences* 122 (1896): 420–21.

[journal number] Vol. 122, No. 8, Séance du lundi 24 février 1896: 55–64^4. 40 leaves, pp. *417* 418–496.

[article] 55_2^v–55_3^r, pp. 420–421.

cf. EFDT 332. GM 2001. Norman 157. cf. PMM 393.

B] MARIE CURIE (1867–1934), PIERRE CURIE (1859–1906), & Gustave Bémont. Sur une nouvelle substance fortement radio-active, contenue dans la pechblende.

In: *Comptes rendus hebdomadaires des séances de l'Académie des Sciences* 127 (1898): 1215–17.

[journal number] Vol. 127, No. 26, Séance du lundi 26 décembre 1898: 155–164^4. 40 leaves, pp. *1179* 1180–1257 [1]. Pink printed wrappers.

[article] 159_3^r–159_4^r, pp. 1215–1217.

cf. EFDT 333. GM 2003. Norman 545. cf. PMM 394.

Roentgen's discovery of X-rays initiated atomic physics and provided the first method for imaging the interior of the body without dissection. It also led to Henri Becquerel's discovery of radioactivity, which was soon followed by the discovery of radium and polonium by Marie and Pierre Curie. The destructive power of radioactivity from sources such as radium was later applied for medical purposes in nuclear medicine and radiation oncology. Further developments in nuclear physics led to the discovery in 1937 of the first artificial element, technitium (element 43), which was widely used as the first imaging agent for computed tomography.

At the beginning of 1896, inspired by Roentgen's discovery of X-rays, Becquerel began experimenting with luminescent crystals. On 24 February he announced to the Academy of Sciences in Paris that fluorescent crystals of potassium uranyl sulfate had exposed a photographic plate wrapped in black paper while both lay for several hours in direct sunlight; a week later, he reported similar exposures when both crystal and plate were placed in total darkness. In the following months Becquerel determined that only crystals con-

spectre et dispersion cathodiques, comme impliquant des analogies non justifiées avec la lumière ordinaire. Mais, dans son hypothèse, les rayons simples sont dus à des potentiels différents et donc ont des vitesses de propagation différentes; de plus ils sont successifs. Or les rayons simples de la lumière ordinaire, qui ont traversé un corps transparent, même gazeux, sont justement dans le même cas. Les analogies sont nettes au contraire (1). »

PHYSIQUE. — *Sur une nouvelle substance fortement radio-active, contenue dans la pechblende* (2). Note de M. **P. Curie**, de Mme **P. Curie** et de M. **G. Bémont**, présentée par M. Becquerel.

« Deux d'entre nous ont montré que, par des procédés purement chimiques, on pouvait extraire de la pechblende une substance fortement radio-active. Cette substance est voisine du bismuth par ses propriétés analytiques. Nous avons émis l'opinion que la pechblende contenait peut-être un élément nouveau, pour lequel nous avons proposé le nom de *polonium* (3).

» Les recherches que nous poursuivons actuellement sont en accord avec les premiers résultats obtenus; mais, au courant de ces recherches, nous avons rencontré une deuxième substance fortement radio-active et entièrement différente de la première par ses propriétés chimiques. En effet, le polonium est précipité en solution acide par l'hydrogène sulfuré; ses sels sont solubles dans les acides, et l'eau les précipite de ces dissolutions; le polonium est complètement précipité par l'ammoniaque.

» La nouvelle substance radio-active que nous venons de trouver a toutes les apparences chimiques du baryum presque pur : elle n'est précipitée ni par l'hydrogène sulfuré, ni par le sulfure d'ammonium, ni par

---

signalées entre les déviations des rayons simples dues à la déflexion et les déviations dues au champ magnétique (*Comptes rendus*, t. CXXV, p. 375) et, inversement, l'étude de ces différences peut permettre de remonter aux causes.

(1) M. Goldstein exagère donc lorsqu'il appelle la dispersion des rayons cathodiques une soi-disant dispersion, comparable à la dispersion par un miroir tournant.

(2) Ce Travail a été fait à l'École municipale de Physique et Chimie industrielles.

(3) M. P. Curie et Mme P. Curie, *Comptes rendus*, t. CXXVII, p. 175.

Fig. 155. No. 84B. Curie, Curie, and Bémont. Opening page.

taining uranium emitted the penetrating rays, that nonluminescent compounds of uranium also emitted the rays, and that the rays were capable of ionizing gases. On 18 May he reported that a disc of pure uranium produced penetrating radiation three to four times stronger than the rays emitted by the potassium uranyl sulfate crystals. With this last announcement, Becquerel's discovery was complete: he had demonstrated not only the occurrence and properties of radiation, but also—and more importantly—that the power of emitting radiation was a particular property of uranium.

Becquerel's discoveries prompted Marie Curie to investigate the phenomenon of radiation. Having found only two ray-emitters, thorium and uranium, among the then-known elements, Marie and her husband Pierre proceeded to search for unknown elements with radioactive properties. In 1898 they discovered two new radioactive elements, polonium and radium; both of these elements are present in pitchblende (uranium ore), but in such minute quantities that the Curies were unable to isolate either one, and had to rely on spectroscopic evidence to prove their existence. Marie Curie's work attracted the attention of Becquerel, who became the intermediary through whom the Curies' papers reached the Academy of Sciences.[1] In 1903 Becquerel and the Curies shared the Nobel Prize in Physics for their discoveries.

JMN

1. The discovery of polonium, named after Marie Curie's native Poland, was announced in Marie and Pierre Curie, "Sur une substance nouvelle radio-active, contenue dans la pechblende," *Comptes rendus hebdomadaires des séances de l'Académie des Sciences* 127 (1898): 175–78; the discovery of radium was presented in the paper cited above.

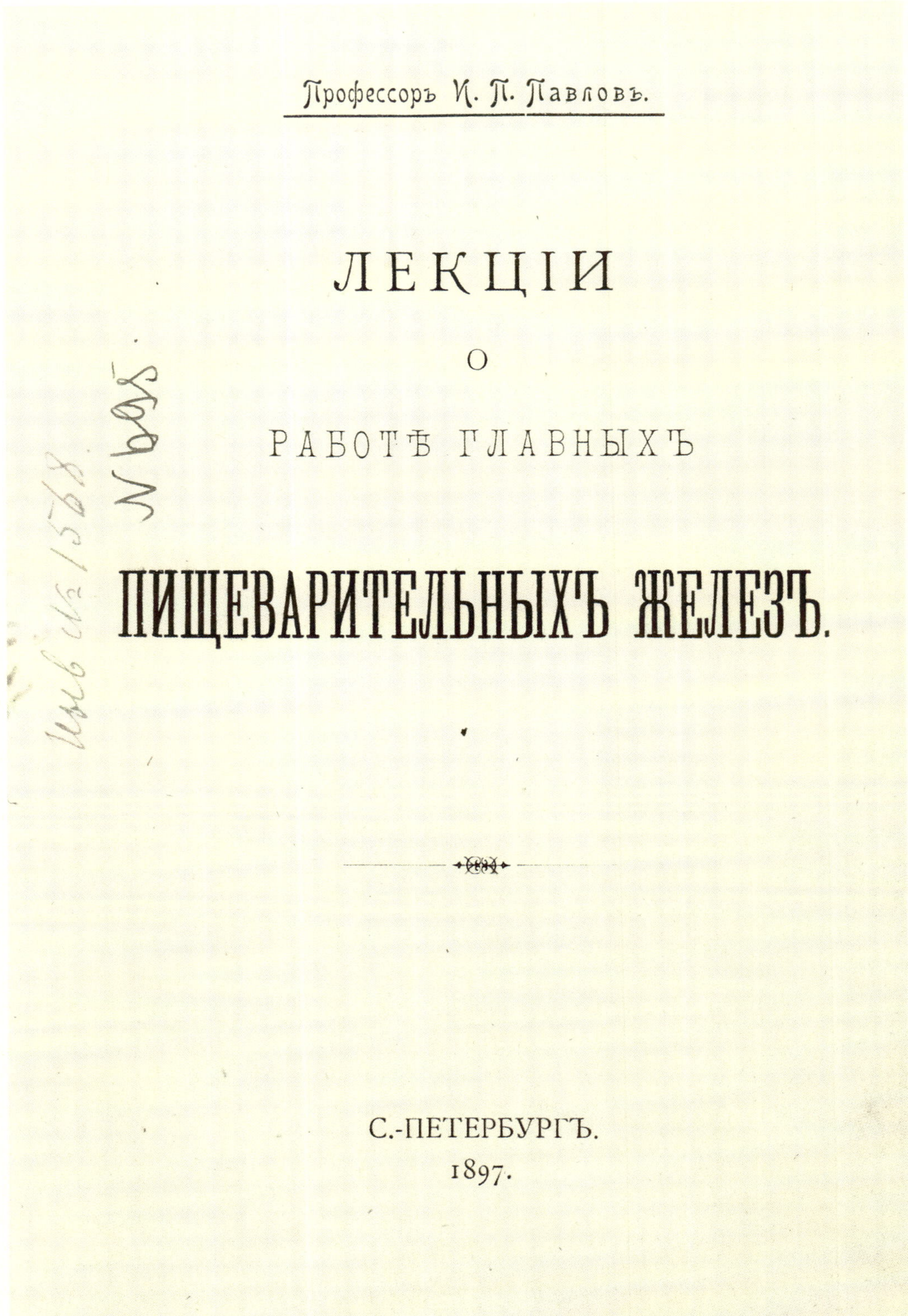

Профессоръ И. П. Павловъ.

ЛЕКЦІИ

О

РАБОТѢ ГЛАВНЫХЪ

ПИЩЕВАРИТЕЛЬНЫХЪ ЖЕЛЕЗЪ.

С.-ПЕТЕРБУРГЪ.

1897.

Fig. 156. No. 85. Pavlov. Title page.

85

IVAN PETROVICH PAVLOV
(1849–1936)

Лекціи о работѣ главныхъ пищеварительныхъ железъ. [Lectures on the work of the principal digestive glands.]

St. Petersburg: I. N. Kushnereff, 1897.

π4 1–14⁸. 116 leaves, pp. [6] *I* II *1* 2–223 [1]. 16 wood-engraved figures in text. Printed wrappers.

GM 1022. cf. *Heirs of Hippocrates* 2129. Horblit 83. cf. Norman 1664–65. PMM 385.

Ivan Petrovich Pavlov was born at Ryazan, Russia, in 1849, and died in Leningrad in 1936. In 1875 he earned a degree in natural sciences from the University of St. Petersburg, where he developed an interest in physiology, and he obtained his medical degree at the Medical Military Academy in 1879. During the summer of 1877 he visited Rudolf Heidenhain's laboratory in Breslau, Germany (now Wrocław, Poland), where he became interested in the physiology of digestion, one of the three major areas of research (the others being the physiology of the circulation and the physiology of the brain) to which he made significant contributions.

In 1852 Friedrich Bidder and Carl Schmidt had shown that the sight of food produced a copious flow of gastric juice in a gastrostomized dog, and in 1878 Charles Robert Richet observed a similar reaction in a man with a strictured esophagus who had to be fed through a gastric fistula. Heidenhain attempted to confirm these observations in 1880 by creating a gastric fistula in a dog; however, in doing so he damaged the nerve supply to the dog's stomach and was thus unable to complete the experiment. In his own researches on the physiology of digestion, Pavlov brought to the task great skill as a surgeon, as well as a method of long-term experiment that revolutionized the study of physiology. He was successful in producing gastric fistulas without damaging the nerve supply and was also able to create fistulas in the salivary glands, pancreas, and intestines. More importantly, he was able to restore his experimental animals postoperatively to a nearly normal state, and this enabled him to observe them over long periods, in keeping with his dictum that organs, and indeed the entire organism, must be studied under natural conditions. Through various experiments, Pavlov was able to demonstrate that the effects of feeding were transmitted to the gastric glands by nervous channels, so that gastric juice could be made to flow from the gastric glands even when food was prevented from entering the stomach. He called the flow of gastric juice that occurred without the actual ingestion of food in the stomach "psychic secretion," his name for glandular activity produced mentally rather than physiologically; this could be stopped either by severing both vagus nerves to the stomach or by removing the cerebral cortex of the animal.

Pavlov summarized his experiments in a series of lectures given in 1896 and published in Russian the following year. A German translation appeared in 1898 and an English one in 1902. For his work on the physiology of digestion Pavlov was awarded the Nobel Prize in 1904. In the interim, he had noted that his dogs ("Pavlov's dogs") learned the daily routine of the laboratory and would respond with secretion at the approach of the experimenter himself or in response to some other remote stimulus. This led him to formulate the concept of "conditioned reflex," which he announced for the first time in 1903 and discussed in his Nobel Prize lecture, "Physiology of Digestion," delivered on 12 December 1904.

HFN

86

SANTIAGO RAMÓN Y CAJAL
(1852–1934)

Textura del sistema nervioso del hombre y de los vertebrados.

Madrid: Imprenta y librería de Nicolás Moya, 1899–1904.

[Vol. I] π^6 1–35^8 36^4 (–36_4). 289 leaves, pp. *i–v* vi–xi [1] *1* 2–566. Fig. 1–206: 206 line-block or halftone illustrations in text (19 printed in blue; 5 in red and blue; 1 in red, blue, and black). Printed wrappers.

[Vol. II, part 1] π^2 1–38^8. 306 leaves, pp. [4] *1* 2–608. Fig. 207–532: 326 line-block or halftone illustrations in text (2 printed in blue; 1 in red and black). Printed wrappers.

[Vol. II, part 2] π^2 39–75^8 76^6. 304 leaves, pp. [4] *609* 610–1209 [3]. Fig. 533–887: 355 line-block or halftone illustrations in text (16 printed in blue; 2 in red; 1 in red and black; 1 in brown). Printed wrappers.

GM 1293.1.

The work of Santiago Ramón y Cajal provided the foundation for present concepts of the cellular composition of the nervous system. Improving and refining existing histological techniques and developing new ones of his own, he demonstrated the microscopic anatomy of the brain as it had never before been seen, and correlated the cellular structures of the brain, nerves, and spinal cord with their functions, giving neurophysiology for the first time a firm anatomic base. Utilizing his remarkable skill as an artist and draftsman, Cajal was able, through the illustrations in his books, to convey to the scientific world what was revealed of the nervous system through his microscope.

Cajal was born in Navarre in northeastern Spain, the son of a country doctor. In his autobiography he revealed that he was an unusually poor and inattentive student who preferred to draw rather than study.[1] He received his medical education in Saragossa, after which he served in the Spanish Army in Cuba. In 1877 he was appointed temporary professor of anatomy in Saragossa and later served as a full professor in Valencia, Barcelona, and Madrid successively. It was in Madrid that he carried out his major work.

Cajal was interested in histology from the first, beginning his work on the peripheral nervous system in 1880. At that time nerve cells and their processes were extremely difficult to observe because of their resistance to staining with conventional dyes. In 1887 Cajal learned of the precipitated silver chromate stain devised by the Italian anatomist Camillo Golgi, who had first reported its use in 1875; employing this stain, Golgi was able to observe minute details of nerve cells for the first time.[2] Although this was a major breakthrough, the stain had been largely ignored because it was very difficult to use. Cajal

Presented by the Author

TEXTURA DEL SISTEMA NERVIOSO

DEL

HOMBRE Y DE LOS VERTEBRADOS

ESTUDIOS SOBRE EL PLAN ESTRUCTURAL
Y COMPOSICIÓN HISTOLÓGICA DE LOS CENTROS NERVIOSOS
ADICIONADOS DE CONSIDERACIONES FISIOLÓGICAS
FUNDADAS EN LOS NUEVOS DESCUBRIMIENTOS

POR

S. RAMÓN CAJAL

Catedrático de Histología en la Universidad de Madrid.

Con numerosos grabados en negro y en color.

TOMO I

MADRID
IMPRENTA Y LIBRERÍA DE NICOLÁS MOYA
Carretas, 8, y Garcilaso, 6.
1899

Fig. 157. No. 86. Ramón y Cajal. Title page.

adopted Golgi's technique, refined it, made it more predictable, and thereafter based most of his work on this improved stain. He made other advances when he began concentrating on the more visible cells and fibers present in the less complicated embryologic and neonatal nervous system, and when he took advantage of the unique staining characteristics of degenerating neurons to reveal the separate paths that nerve cell processes follow through the brain. Cajal's work convinced him that each nerve or neuron was a distinct entity, touching but not being in continuity with other cells. In 1888 he published an important paper in which he affirmed this "neuron" doctrine—a controversial subject at the time, as it contradicted the widely accepted "reticular" theory that all nerves in the brain were in continuity.[3] In this controversy Cajal had no less an adversary than Golgi himself, an adherent of the reticular theory; however, subsequent research proved that the neuron doctrine was correct. Cajal and Golgi shared the Nobel Prize in Physiology or Medicine in 1906.

Cajal studied all parts of the nervous system in both humans and animals, sketching the microscopic appearance of the cells and their processes with the aid of a camera lucida attached to his microscope so that it projected images directly onto a sheet of paper. Cajal's articles and books are all magnificently illustrated, and his drawings of the microscopic appearance of the nervous system continue to be reprinted.

Cajal's most notable contribution is generally considered to be his *Textura del sistema nervioso del hombre y de los vertebrados.* Only eight hundred copies were printed of this work, which was originally published in fascicles (three for Volume I, four for Volume II) between 1897 and 1904. In it Cajal summarized his earlier research, consolidated his arguments, and presented his mature thinking on the organization of the nervous system. He proved many of the connections between one section of the brain and another, and he illustrated these, as well as the many connections one cell makes with others. He described many nerve cells for the first time and also pointed out the plasticity of nerve cells in the brain, a discovery that has only recently come to be appreciated in the course of modern work on nerve physiology. *Textura del sistema nervioso* is a model of beauty and clarity, and it earned Cajal world-wide recognition. A revised and enlarged French translation was published in 1909 and republished in 1952 on the anniversary of the author's birth.[4] This version was recently translated into English.[5]

AEL

1. Santiago Ramón y Cajal, *Recuerdos de mi vida*, 3d ed. (Madrid, 1923).

2. Camillo Golgi, "Sulla sostanza grigia del cervello," *Gazzetta medica italiana lombarda* 6 (1875): 244–46.

3. Santiago Ramón y Cajal, "Estructura de los centros nerviosos de los aves," *Revista trimestral de histología normal y patológica* 1 (1888): 305–15.

4. Santiago Ramón y Cajal, *Histologie du système nerveux de l'homme et des vertébrés*, trans. L. Azoulay (Paris, 1909–11; reprinted, Madrid, 1952).

5. Santiago Ramón y Cajal, *Cajal's Histology of the Nervous System*, trans. Neely and Larry W. Swanson (2 vols., Oxford, 1994).

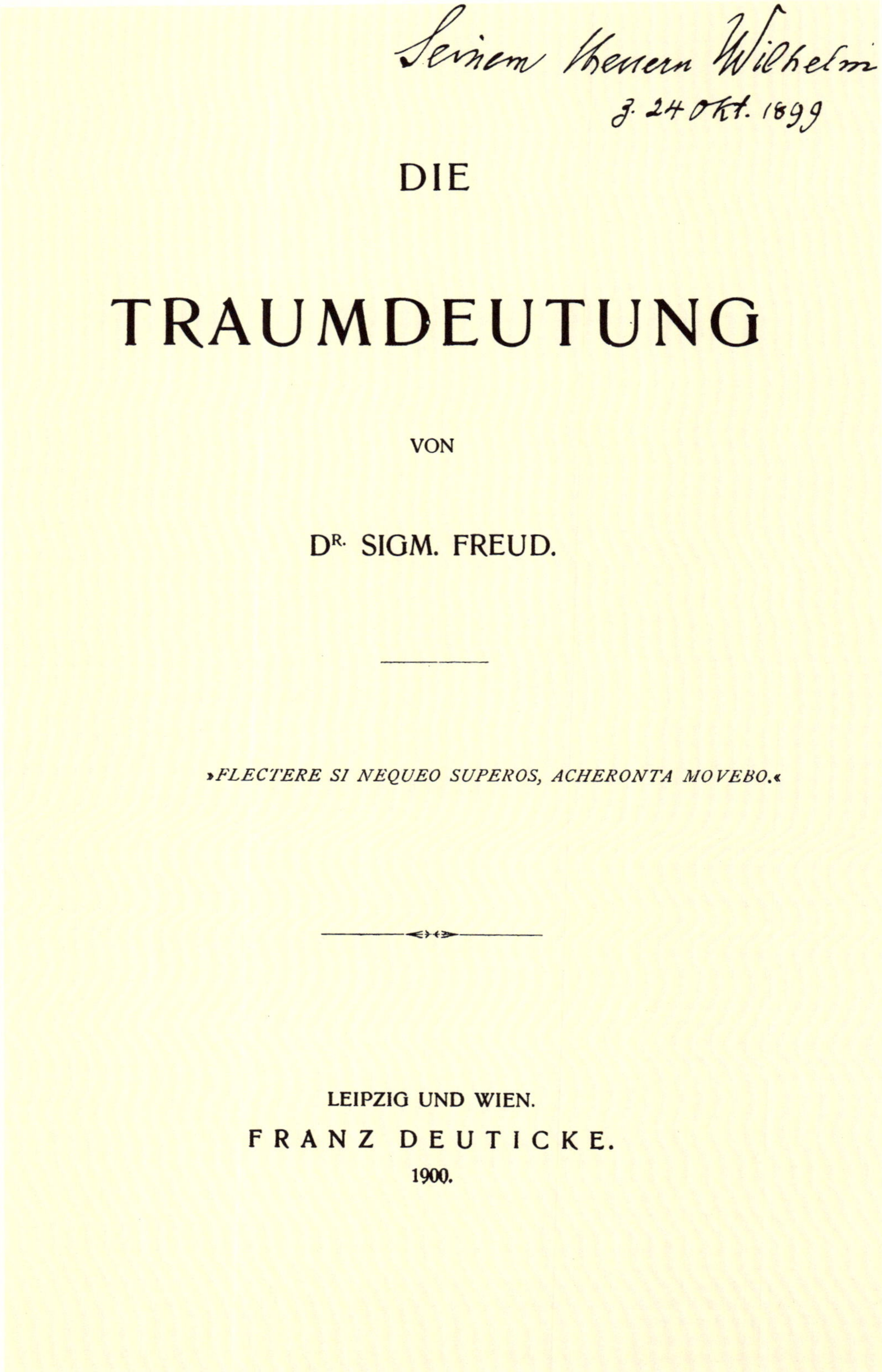

Seinem theuern Wilhelm
z. 24 Okt. 1899

DIE

TRAUMDEUTUNG

VON

DR. SIGM. FREUD.

»*FLECTERE SI NEQUEO SUPEROS, ACHERONTA MOVEBO.*«

LEIPZIG UND WIEN.
FRANZ DEUTICKE.
1900.

Fig. 158. No. 87. Freud. Presentation copy to Dr. Wilhelm Fliess, inscribed by Freud "To his dear Wilhelm."

87

SIGMUND FREUD
(1856–1939)

Die Traumdeutung.

Leipzig & Vienna: Franz Deuticke, 1900.

π^2 $1–23^8$ 24^4. 190 leaves, pp. [4] *1* 2–371 [5].

GM 4980. Grinstein 10614. *Heirs of Hippocrates* 2176. Horblit 32. Norman F33. PMM 389.

I. Bernard Cohen, in his *Revolution in Science*, ranked Freud with Charles Darwin and Karl Marx as one of the three great revolutionary thinkers of the nineteenth century and identified *Die Traumdeutung* as the manifesto of Freud's revolutionary thought.[1] This book remained for Freud his greatest achievement; as he wrote in 1932 in the introduction to the revised edition of the English translation, "It contains, even according to my present-day judgment, the most valuable of all the discoveries it has been my good fortune to make. Insight such as this falls to one's lot but once in a lifetime."[2]

Sigmund Freud began his medical career as a neurologist and made several important contributions in this field, including a method of gold chloride staining of nerve cells, researches on the pharmacological uses and effects of cocaine, studies of aphasia, and work on infantile cerebral palsy. His fame today, however, derives wholly from his discovery of psychoanalysis and his theory of the structure of the mind. In Freud's day, what are now called psychoneuroses (a term he introduced) were classed as neurological diseases, and as a neurologist Freud was called upon to treat a number of "neurotic" patients. After struggling unsatisfactorily with traditional modes of therapy, Freud began to use his colleague Joseph Breuer's technique of hypnotizing patients to stimulate them to talk about the traumatic events that led to the onset of their symptoms; Breuer had discovered that this treatment caused the symptoms to disappear. Freud collaborated with Breuer on the book *Studien über Hysterie* (Studies on hysteria [1895]), generally considered the first work on psychoanalysis, but the two men parted ways shortly thereafter when Breuer refused to accept some of Freud's more radical innovations, particularly his emphasis on sex.

When he discovered that not all patients were hypnotizable, Freud devised the technique of free association, requiring his patients to say everything that was on their minds regardless of how nonsensical or irrelevant it seemed; he named this new technique "psychoanalysis." Observing that patients often mentioned their dreams during free association, he was prompted to study his own dreams, and this led to his discovery in 1895 of the hidden meaning of dreams. During these years Freud psychoanalyzed himself using his own dreams, and in late 1899 he published *Die Traumdeutung* (The interpretation of dreams), in which he announced not only his understanding of the meaning of dreams but also the mechanism of their formation and their wish-fulfilling erotic nature. He described what was later to be called the Oedipus complex, the sexual attraction a child feels for the parent of the opposite sex and the corresponding rivalrous hatred for the parent of the same sex. He presented his theory of the mind as composed topographically of a conscious, a pre-conscious, and an unconscious, and showed how unconscious processes influence conscious thought in normal behavior. He also established the fact that the difference between the normal and the abnormal mind was one of degree. These once-revolutionary ideas have become an accepted part of psychological theory, and *Die Traumdeutung* is still studied as a text by psychiatrists, psychologists, social workers, sociologists, anthropologists, philosophers, historians, writers, and artists.

Freud's publisher dated *Die Traumdeutung* 1900, which inspired Freud to state that "Psychoanalysis may have been said to have been born with the twentieth century."[3] The book, however, was actually published on 4 November 1899, Freud having previously received two author's copies during the month of October. One of these he sent as a birthday present to Wilhelm Fliess, the Berlin otolaryngologist whom he regarded as the "godfather" of *Die Traumdeutung*.[4] The first edition of the work consisted of six hundred copies which took eight years to sell: 123 copies were sold in the first six weeks after publication and 228 in the next two years. A second edition was published in 1909 and a third in 1911; the latter was the source of the English translation, first published in 1913. A total of eight German editions, many of them revised and enlarged, appeared during Freud's lifetime. Translations, in addition to the English, include Russian (1913), Spanish (1922), French (1926), Swedish (1927), Japanese (1930), Hungarian (1934), and Czech (1938).

HFN

1. I. Bernard Cohen, *Revolution in Science* (Cambridge, Mass., 1985), p. 352. Cohen also called the Freudian revolution "the last revolution in science to be made public in a printed book rather than a paper in a scientific journal or in a series monograph" (pp. 356–57).

2. Reprinted in Sigmund Freud, *The Standard Edition of the Complete Psychological Works*, ed. and trans. James Strachey et al., vol. 4 (London & New York, 1953), p. xxxii.

3. Sigmund Freud, "A Short Account of Psycho-Analysis," in *The Standard Edition*, vol. 19 (London, 1961), p. 191. This essay was originally published in English translation as "Psychoanalysis: Exploring the Hidden Recesses of the Mind," in *These Eventful Years: The Twentieth Century in the Making, as Told by Many of Its Makers* (London & New York, 1924), pp. 511–23. Regarding Freud's claim about the birthdate of psychoanalysis, Cohen states that "Freud shared a common error in believing that the year 1900 began the twentieth century. Since the first year of our era is the year 1, the hundredth year (completing a century) is the year 100 and not the year 99. Thus the final or hundredth year of the nineteenth group of hundred years (the nineteenth century) is 1900 and not 1899, and the first year of the twentieth century must properly be 1901" (*Revolution in Science*, p. 359).

4. *The Complete Letters of Sigmund Freud to Wilhelm Fliess, 1887–1904*, ed. and trans. Jeffrey Masson (Cambridge, Mass., 1986), pp. 380–81. On 27 October 1899 Freud wrote to Fliess: "Thanks for the kind words in response to my sending you the dream book . . . Incidentally, it has not yet been issued; only our two copies so far have seen the light of day."

88

KARL LANDSTEINER
(1868–1943)

A] Ueber Agglutinationserscheinungen normalen menschlichen Blutes.

In: *Wiener klinische Wochenschrift* 14 (1901): 1132–34.

[journal number] Vol. 14, No. 46, 14 November 1901: $[1]^{12}$. 12 leaves, pp. *1121* 1122–1144. Green printed wrappers.

[article] $[1]_6^v$–$[1]_7^v$, pp. 1132–1134.

[offprint] *Ueber Agglutinationserscheinungen normalen menschlichen Blutes* [head title]. Abdruck aus der Wiener klinische Wochenschrift, 1901, Nr. 46.

$[1]^2$ $[2]_1$. 3 leaves, pp. *1* 2–5 [1].

Reimposed in single-column pages, with different page breaks.

Chase 17.

B] Zur Kenntnis der antifermentativen, lytischen und agglutinierenden Wirkungen des Blutserums und der Lymphe.

In: *Centralblatt für Bakteriologie, Parasitenkunde und Infektionskrankheiten.* Erste Abteilung: *Medicinisch-hygienische Bakteriologie und tierische Parasitenkunde* 27 (1900): 357–62.

[journal number] Vol. 27, No. 10/11, 23 March 1900: 23–26^8. 32 leaves, pp. *353* 354–416. Gray-green printed wrappers.

[article] 23_3^r–23_5^v, pp. 357–362.

[offprint] *Zur Kenntnis der antifermentativen, lytischen und agglutinierenden Wirkungen des Blutserums und der Lymphe* [head title]. Abdruck aus dem Centralblatt für Bakteriologie, Parasitenkunde und Infektionskrankheiten. I. Abteilung. XXVII. Bd. 1900. No. 10/11.

$[1]^2$ $[2]_1$. 3 leaves, pp. *357* 358–362. Cream printed wrappers.

Chase 13. GM 889. *Heirs of Hippocrates* 2265.

Karl Landsteiner, who was born and trained in Vienna and who spent the latter part of his career at the Rockefeller Institute in New York, made a number of important contributions to immunology during the first half of the twentieth century. He described the first autoimmune disease to be recognized (paroxysmal cold hemoglobinuria), was the

K. Landsteiner

henschrift, 1901, Nr. 46.
'1, Wickenburggasse 13.

Aus dem pathologisch-anatomischen Institute in Wien.

Ueber Agglutinationserscheinungen normalen menschlichen Blutes.

Von Dr. **Karl Landsteiner**, Assistenten am pathologisch-anatomischen Institute.

Vor einiger Zeit habe ich beobachtet und mitgetheilt[1]), dass öfters Blutserum von normalen Menschen rothe Blutkörperchen anderer gesunder Individuen zu verklumpen im Stande ist. Ich hatte damals den Eindruck, dass in manchen Krankheitsfällen diese verklumpende Eigenschaft des Blutserums fremden Blutkörperchen gegenüber besonders deutlich wäre und meinte, dass sie mit dem von Maragliano[2]) viel früher beobachteten starken Lösungsvermögen pathologischer Sera für normale Körperchen in Zusammenhang sein könne, da ja Agglutinations- und Lösungsvermögen häufig, wenn auch nicht immer, parallel sich ändern. Gegen die Gleichsetzung der Reactionen von Maragliano mit den jetzt so häufig untersuchten hämolytischen Reactionen der Blutsera spricht der Umstand, dass zwar nicht Erwärmen, wohl aber Zusatz von Kochsalz bis zu einem Gehalt, der dem normalen gleichkommt, das Lösungsvermögen der Sera aufhebt. Maragliano selbst unterscheidet seine Beobachtung von der Erscheinung von Landois — der Hämolyse durch artfremdes Serum, dadurch — dass in seinem Fall das Hämoglobin nicht nur gelöst, sondern auch zerstört wird. Ein wesentlicher Unterschied meiner Beobachtung und der von Maragliano besteht darin, dass im Falle von Maragliano das Serum auch auf die Körperchen, die vom selben Individuum stammen, wirkt und dass seine Reaction nur mit krankhaftem Blut gelingt. Meine Beobachtung zeigte aber gerade Unterschiede recht sinnfälliger Art zwischen Blutserum und Körperchen verschiedener anscheinend völlig gesunder Menschen.

Die Beobachtung von Shattock[3]) gehört dagegen nach der Beschreibung und Abbildung des Autors zweifellos hieher, wenn er auch die Reaction nur bei fieberhaften Krankheiten nachweist und sie bei normalem Blut vermisst. Shattock bringt

---

[1]) Centralblatt für Bacteriologie. XXVII, S. 361, v. 10. Februar 1900.
[2]) XI. Congress für innere Medicin. Leipzig 1892.
[3]) Journ. of Pathol. and Bacteriology. Februar 1900.

1

Fig. 159. No. 88A. Landsteiner. The opening page of his 1901 offprint on blood groups. A slip with Landsteiner's signature partially obscures the type in the upper left and center; the bottom part of a postmark is also visible.

first to produce experimental syphilis in monkeys, contributed significantly to studies of poliomyelitis, and was the chief founder of the field of immunochemistry, among many other accomplishments.

In a study, published in 1900, of the antibody properties of blood and lymph, Landsteiner recorded in a footnote the chance observation that human serum might agglutinate the erythrocytes, or red blood cells, of other humans. In 1901 he returned to this phenomenon, proving that it was not the result of a disease process but that it was demonstrable in the serum of healthy individuals. Further, he was able to show that each serum can agglutinate the red cells only of certain other individuals. He found that the sera could be divided into three distinct groups: group A agglutinates the red cells of group B, but not those of group A; group B agglutinates the red cells of group A, but not those of group B; and group C agglutinates both A and B red cells, but is not agglutinated by the sera of either group A or group B.

Landsteiner correctly concluded that among humans there exist at least two different blood types, represented on the erythrocytes as distinct agglutinogens and in the serum as distinct isoagglutinins. His notation is currently used for blood groups A and B, and his group C was later renamed blood type O; his initial series was not large enough for him to have identified the rarer blood type AB, which was discovered in his laboratory in 1902. Landsteiner correctly predicted that these findings would have important implications for forensic pathology as well as for blood transfusions. Blood grouping has also been employed extensively in epidemiological studies and by anthropologists in the study of racial interrelationships and mass population migrations.

Landsteiner maintained his interest in blood groups throughout his long career. In 1927 he and Philip Levine discovered the M, N, and P blood groups, and in 1940 he and Alexander Wiener discovered the Rh (Rhesus) system. For his discovery of human blood groups, Landsteiner received the Nobel Prize in Physiology or Medicine in 1930.

AMS

Galvanometrische registratie van het menschelijk electrocardiogram.

Tot nog toe kon het door AUG. D. WALLER ontdekte menschelijk electrocardiogram alleen met behulp van den capillair-electromer worden verkregen. De kromme,. die door dit werktuig geschreven wordt, geeft bij het gewone bekijken een geheel onjuiste voorstelling van de wisselingen in potentiaalverschil, die zich tijdens het registreeren werkelijk hebben voorgedaan. Om deze te leeren kennen, moet men ze berekenen uit den vorm der geregistreerde kromme en de eigenschappen van het gebruikte werktuig. Zoo komt men tot de constructie van een nieuwe kromme, welker vorm de juiste uitdrukking is van de werkelijk geheerscht hebbende potentiaalschommelingen.

Ter toelichting moge een voorbeeld dienen [1]).

Fig. 1 der hierbijgevoegde uitslaande plaat stelt de geschreven kromme voor van den Heer v. D. W. bij stroomafleiding van rechter- en linkerhand, terwijl fig. 2 de geconstrueerde kromme weergeeft. De verschillen springen in het oog. Men vergelijke vooral de toppen *C* en *D* in de geregistreerde kromme met de overeenkomstige toppen *R* en *T* in de geconstrueerde figuur. Alleen deze laatste geeft de verhouding der tophoogten juist weer.

Ik heb naar een middel gezocht, om de berekening en de constructie zooveel mogelijk te ontgaan en ten slotte een werktuig gevonden, dat het menschelijk electrocardiogram direct in

[1]) Zie „Onderzoekingen" Physiol. laborat. Leiden, 2e Reeks, Dl. 2.

Fig. 160. No. 89. Einthoven. Opening page.

89

WILLEM EINTHOVEN

(1860–1927)

Galvanometrische registratie van het menschelijk electrocardiogram.

In: *Herinneringsbundel Professor S. S. Rosenstein* (Leiden: Edouard Ijdo, 1902), pp. 101–6.

[book] π^4 $2\pi^6$ $[1]^8$ 2^8 $[3]^4$ $4–6^8$ 7^4 7^{*8} 8^8 9^4 $10–19^8$ $20–21^4$ 22^8 23^4 $24–27^8$ 28^6 $29–30^8$ 31^4 32^8 33^4 $34–35^8$ 36^4 $37–49^8$ 50^4 51^6 $(–51_6)$ 52^4. 385 leaves, pp. *i–v* vi–viii, *i–v* vi–xi [1], *1–3* 4–750. Frontispiece: 1 collotype plate; Pl. I–XV: 1 line-block plate; 4 halftone plates, and 10 collotype plates (1 colored). Gray-green publisher's cloth.

[article] $7^*{}_3{}^r–7^*{}_5{}^v$, pp. *101–103* 104–106. Pl. V: 1 line-block plate.

Willem Einthoven was born in 1860 in Semarang, Java. His family moved to Utrecht, Holland, following the death of his father. After Einthoven received his medical degree from the University of Utrecht, he became increasingly interested in physiology. His first publications dealt with the physiology of vision and the neural control of respiration; by 1894, however, his research was focused on electrophysiology, especially the electrical activity of the heart.

Einthoven was convinced that records of the electrical activity of the heart in humans would have clinical value, and his major contribution to medicine was the development of instrumentation leading to the introduction of clinical electrocardiography. In 1877 British physiologist Augustus D. Waller had recorded the first human electrocardiogram using a capillary electrometer, but this instrument was cumbersome, and the electrical signals it recorded were markedly damped by the poor high-frequency response of its mercury column. Einthoven was able to correct these curves mathematically to produce useful tracings, but he sought to develop an instrument that would make electrocardiography more practical. Although he tried first to improve upon the capillary electrometer, he then abandoned this approach in favor of using a galvanometer. Initially Einthoven employed a D'Arsonval moving coil galvanometer, but eventually he discovered that a string galvanometer was better suited to record graphically the electrical activity of the heart.

In 1902 Einthoven published an article in Dutch that included the first description of a human electrocardiogram recorded with a string galvanometer. This was followed by a series of papers in German, French, and English that brought the new technique to the attention of physiologists and clinicians throughout Europe and America. Soon thereafter,

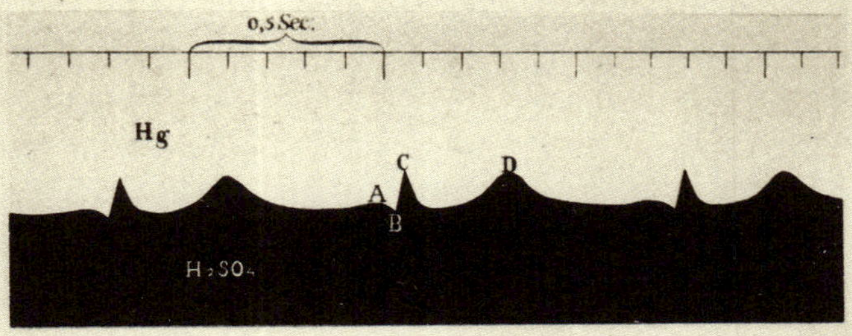

Fig. 1.

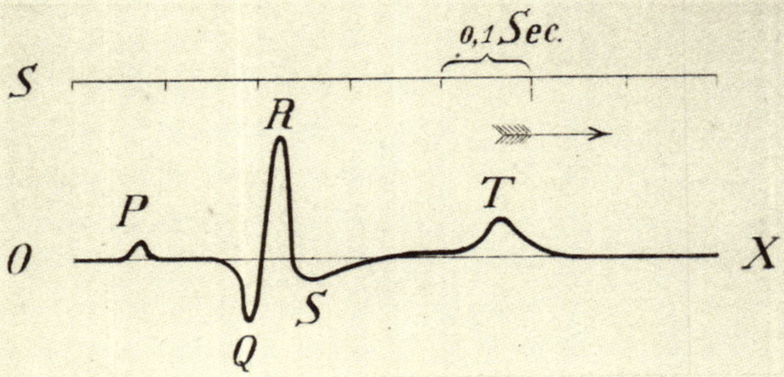

Fig. 2.

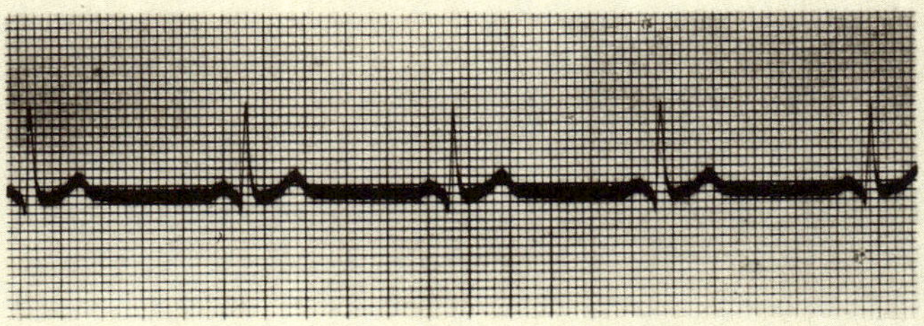

Fig. 3.

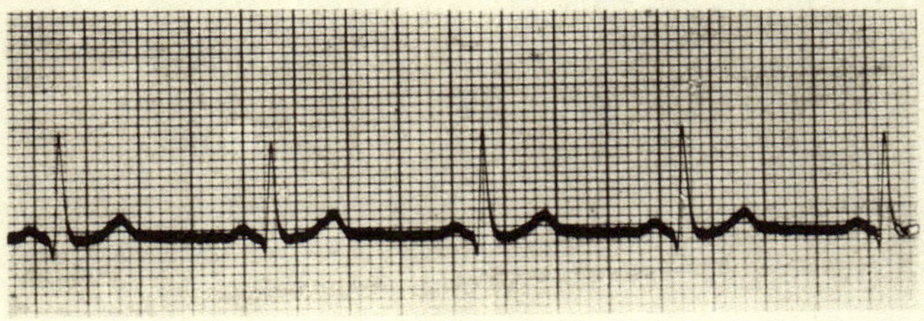

Fig. 4.

Prof. W. EINTHOVEN. — Galvanometrische registratie van het menschelijk electrocardiogram.

Fig. 161. No. 89. Einthoven. Figure 1 in this illustration represents the severely damped registered capillary electrometer recording of patient v.d.W. Figure 2 shows the mathematically corrected electrometer curve, labeled according to what is now standard electrocardiographic terminology. Figures 3 and 4 show accurate tracings derived directly from the new string galvanometer recording of the same patient.

papers and monographs from many laboratories reported the characteristic electrocardiographic findings in a wide variety of cardiac disorders.

Einthoven's string galvanometer and the instruments derived from it allowed scientists and physicians to study disorders of cardiac impulse formation and conduction in humans. The galvanometer was soon used to characterize the electrical manifestations of acute myocardial infarction, an important development that provided physicians with a reliable method of diagnosing this serious medical condition. The introduction of the electrocardiogram, together with the discovery of X-rays in 1896, revolutionized the practice of medicine, signalling the advent of the modern era of diagnosis.

WBF/PK

THE

INTEGRATIVE ACTION

OF THE

NERVOUS SYSTEM

BY

CHARLES S. SHERRINGTON

D.Sc., M.D., Hon. LL.D. Tor., F.R.S.

Holt Professor of Physiology in the University of Liverpool,
Honorary Member of the American Physiological Society,
&c.

WITH ILLUSTRATIONS

NEW YORK
CHARLES SCRIBNER'S SONS
1906

Fig. 162. No. 90. Sherrington. Title page.

90

SIR CHARLES SCOTT SHERRINGTON
(1857–1952)

The Integrative Action of the Nervous System.

[American issue] New York: Charles Scribner's Sons, 1906.

π^8 1–25^8 26^6. 214 leaves, pp. *i–xi* xii–xvi *1* 2–411 [1]. Fig. 1–29, 30A–B, 31A–B, 32–85: 87 line-block figures in text. Dark blue publisher's cloth.

[English issue] London: Archibald Constable & Co., Lt'd., 1906.

π^8 1–25^8 26^6. 214 leaves, pp. *i–xi* xii–xvi *1* 2–411 [1]. Fig. 1–29, 30A–B, 31A–B, 32–85: 87 line-block figures in text.

The American sheets, with the title page reset.

Fulton *Sherrington*, p. 182. GM 1432. *Great Names in Neurology*, p. 53. *Heirs of Hippocrates* 2198. Norman 1939. PMM 397.

Charles Scott Sherrington was born in London in 1857, the son of a country doctor. He matriculated at Cambridge and received his clinical medical training at St. Thomas's Hospital in London. While at Cambridge he became interested in physiology, and after hearing a paper presented by Friedrich Goltz at the Seventh International Medical Congress in London in 1881, he was inspired to continue his studies in the field of neurophysiology. Sherrington travelled to Germany to study with Goltz in Strassburg and later with Rudolf Virchow (see no. 69) and Robert Koch (see no. 80) in their laboratories in Berlin. On returning to England, Sherrington became director of the Brown Institution of the University of London, where he was able to engage in experimental work on the nervous system in animals. In 1895 he went to the University of Liverpool, where he remained as professor of physiology for eighteen years. It was during his tenure at Liverpool that Sherrington was invited to give the Silliman Lectures at Yale University in 1904; these later became his book on neurophysiology, *The Integrative Action of the Nervous System*, dedicated to David Ferrier (see no. 76). In 1913 Sherrington was appointed to the Waynfleet Chair of Physiology at Oxford, and he remained at Oxford until his retirement in 1935. He established what became in effect the English school of neurophysiology, training and inspiring dozens of men who later became famous in their own right; among these were A.S.F. Leyton, E.G.T. Liddell, Derrick Denny-Brown, John Fulton, John C. Eccles, and Wilder Penfield.

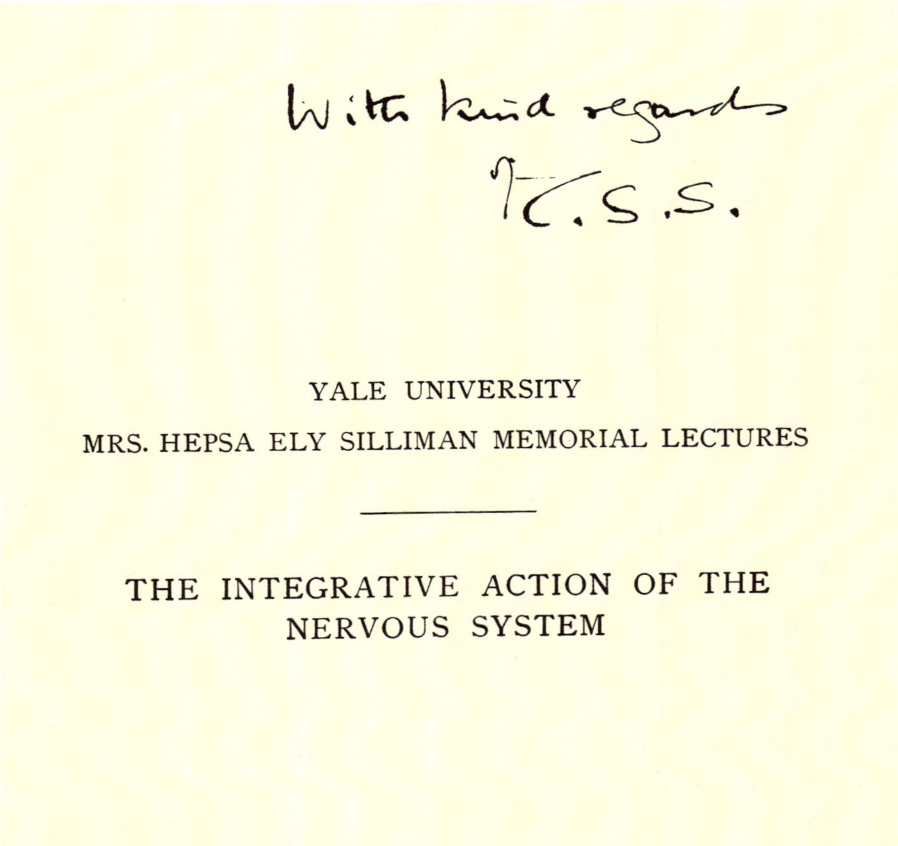

With kind regards
C. S. S.

YALE UNIVERSITY

MRS. HEPSA ELY SILLIMAN MEMORIAL LECTURES

THE INTEGRATIVE ACTION OF THE NERVOUS SYSTEM

Fig. 163. No. 90. Sherrington. Half-title, inscribed by the author.

Sherrington was the most important neurophysiologist Britain has produced, and perhaps the most remarkable neuroscientist ever to have lived. His work bridged the gap between the theoretical and speculative neurology of the nineteenth century and the empirical science of the twentieth. He carried out an extensive program of experimentation, and the results of these investigations placed clinical neurology on a sound scientific footing. His *Integrative Action of the Nervous System*, which summarized twenty years of intensive investigation, has been compared to William Harvey's *De motu cordis* (see no. 27A) for its significance as a turning point in the history of physiology.

In studying the nervous system, Sherrington began with the most primitive and simple nervous function, the reflex, which he spent years investigating and analyzing; he understood that as the atom was considered to be the most elemental particle of all material things, so the reflex was the most basic form of all nervous activity. At the heart of the reflex is the connection between nerve cells, which he was the first to call the synapse, and he hypothesized, long before it could be demonstrated, that secreted chemical mediators carried impulses from one neuron to another. Sherrington considered the most primitive animal reflexes to be protective, as when the iris of the eye closes in response to bright light; other reflexes are more elaborate and less easily understood. Reflexes and their arcs can be localized in the brain and spinal cord. They are all independent of voluntary control. Muscular responses depend on sensory organs (stretch receptors) present within them, which Sherrington first fully described. He also demonstrated that when one muscle contracts, its antagonist relaxes in an active process of reciprocal inhibition.

In Sherrington's view, the response of the living organism to its external environment is largely reflexive in nature. But the animal deprived of his cerebral cortex—i.e., the reflex animal—though he may stand, walk, scratch, eat, and blink, is not really alive without the higher functioning of the mind. Where is the mind? Sherrington, a dualist like Descartes three hundred years earlier, assumed that it is in the brain, but he had no explanation of how it works. He recognized that the separation of the mind from the brain was contrived for the convenience of investigation; however, no reflex activity could explain for Sherrington the psyche or the workings of the mind. The work of the past twenty years in the field of nerve transmitters and neurochemistry would have helped bridge that gap in Sherrington's understanding, but the mystery remains. Sherrington was not at all ambivalent as to whether a full understanding of the brain was desirable. Man's liberty depends on his free will, and "if anyone can fully understand how the brain does its thinking, then [mind control cannot be far off]. We need not be prophets to foresee that then will come the long-told speedy extinction of man."

Sherrington was knighted in 1924, and in 1932 he shared the Nobel Prize in Physiology or Medicine. After his retirement from Oxford, he published a number of books on historical or philosophical subjects, including *Man on His Nature* (1940), *Goethe on Nature and on Science* (1942), and *The Endeavour of Jean Fernel* (1946). At the age of ninety, in 1947, he reissued his *Integrative Action of the Nervous System* with a new preface.

AEL

The Integrative Action of the Nervous System originated in lectures given at Yale University in 1904. These were published in 1906 by Charles Scribner's Sons, New York, and Scribner's evidently provided copies of the American sheets to the English publisher, Archibald Constable of London. The 1906 edition was copyrighted in that year by Yale University, and the notice to that effect appears on the versos of both the American and the English title pages. In 1911 and subsequently the text was reissued over the imprint of the Yale University Press; these impressions were presumably made from plates, since they match the pagination of the original printing and the copyright date continued to be given as 1906. Although several bibliographies describe the first edition as having the imprint "New Haven: Yale University Press, 1906," this is an error that appears to originate in the substitution of the copyright date for the date of printing.

[ED.]

Reprinted from the Proceedings of the Society for Experimental Biology and Medicine, 1907, iv, pp. 140–143.

98 (241)

Observations on the living developing nerve fiber.

By **ROSS G. HARRISON.**

[*From the Anatomical Laboratory of the Johns Hopkins University.*]

The immediate object of the following experiments was to obtain a method by which the end of a growing nerve could be brought under direct observation while alive, in order that a correct conception might be had regarding what takes place as the fiber extends during embryonic development from the nerve center out to the periphery.

The method employed was to isolate pieces of embryonic tissue known to give rise to nerve fibers, as for example, the whole or fragments of the medullary tube, or ectoderm from the branchial region, and to observe their further development. The pieces were taken from frog embryos about 3 mm. long, at which stage, *i. e.*, shortly after the closure of the medullary folds, there is no visible differentiation of the nerve elements. After carefully dissecting it out the piece of tissue is removed by a fine pipette to a cover slip upon which is a drop of lymph freshly drawn from one of the lymph sacs of an adult frog. The lymph clots very quickly, holding the tissue in a fixed position. The cover slip is then inverted over a hollow slide and the rim sealed with paraffine. When reasonable aseptic precautions are taken, tissues will live under these conditions for a week and in some cases specimens have been kept alive for nearly four weeks. Such specimens may be readily observed from day to day under highly magnifying powers.

While the cell aggregates, which make up the different organs

(1)

Fig. 164. No. 91A. Harrison. Opening page of the 1907 offprint.

91

ROSS GRANVILLE HARRISON
(1870–1959)

A] Observations on the Living Developing Nerve Fiber.

In: *Anatomical Record* 1 (1906–08): 116–18.

[journal number] Vol. 1, No. 5, 1 June 1907: 13^{10}. 10 leaves, pp. *109* 110–128. Published as part of the *American Journal of Anatomy* 7, no. 1 (1 June 1907), in blue printed wrappers.

[article] $13_4{}^v$–$13_5{}^v$, pp. 116–118.

GM 521. Nicholas, p. 157.

Also published in: *Proceedings of the Society for Experimental Biology and Medicine* 4 (1906–07): 140–43.

[journal number] Vol. 4, No. 6, 15 June 1907: $[1]^{18}$. 18 leaves, pp. 111–146. Blue printed wrappers

[article] $[1]_{15}{}^v$–$[1]_{17}{}^r$, pp. 140–143.

[offprint] *Observations on the Living Developing Nerve Fiber* [head title]. Reprinted from the Proceedings of the Society for Experimental Biology and Medicine, 1907, iv, pp. 140–143.

$[1]^2$. 2 leaves, pp. 1–4.

Reimposed, with different page breaks.

B] The Outgrowth of the Nerve Fiber as a Mode of Protoplasmic Movement.

In: *Journal of Experimental Zoology* 9 (1910): 787–846.

[journal number] Vol. 9, No. 4, December 1910: $[1–13]^8$ $[14]^8$ (14_6 + 1). 113 leaves, pp. *657* 658–846 [4] *847–849* 850–870 [8]. Pl. 1–3: 3 collotype plates (2 folding). Green printed wrappers.

[article] $[9]_2{}^r$–$[13]_2{}^r$, pp. *787* 788–846 [6]. Pl. 1–3: 3 collotype plates (2 folding) after drawings by Harrison; Fig. 1–3: 1 line-block and 2 halftone illustrations in text.

[offprint] *The Outgrowth of the Nerve Fiber as a Mode of Protoplasmic Movement* [wrapper title] Reprinted from the Journal of Experimental Zoology. Volume 9, No. 4.

$[1]^8$ (-1_1) $[2–4]^8$ $[5]_1$ $[6]_1$, pp. *787* 788–846 [6]. Pl. 1–3: 3 collotype plates (2 folding) after drawings by Harrison; Fig. 1–3: 1 line-block and 2 halftone illustrations in text. Printed wrappers.

GM 558. Nicholas, p. 158.

Ross G. Harrison's greatest single accomplishment was the innovation of the technique of tissue culture, which he developed in order to demonstrate the origin and growth of nerve fiber. At the time when he began his work on nerve cells, there were three competing theories regarding the development of nerve fiber: the cell-chain theory, the plasmoderm theory, and the outgrowth theory. Harrison, an adherent of the outgrowth theory, saw that the theory could be proved experimentally by growing nerve cells outside the body. Between 1905 and 1907 he conducted a pioneering series of experiments in which he adapted the "hanging drop" technique to the study of embryonic tissues. Using this simple method, in which fragments of neural tissue from frog embryos were preserved in drops of frog lymph, Harrison was able to keep tissues alive for up to four weeks; he was thus able to demonstrate conclusively that nerve fibers are products (outgrowths) of the nerve cell itself.

This confirmation of the validity of the outgrowth theory, which also established the primary role of the cell in the development of multi-cellular organisms, was later characterized by Harrison himself as "the most important step ever taken in embryology."[1] Of broader significance, however, was the development of the method of tissue culture, one of the most important discoveries of Western medicine. Without tissue culture, much of what is now known about the growth and character of tumors, as well as normal cells of all sorts, could not have been learned. Moreover, since viruses can grow only in living cells, the development of a method of tissue culture made it easier to manufacture vaccines against viral diseases, for example, the vaccines now used to immunize against measles and poliomyelitis.

At the time, no one foresaw the indispensable role that tissue culture would play in immunology and tumor pathology, and so Harrison was not awarded the Nobel Prize, although he was considered by the Nobel Committee in both 1917 and 1933. In 1954 the Nobel Committee, aware of how important tissue culture had been in providing adequate amounts of poliomyelitis vaccine, awarded the prize in Physiology or Medicine to John F. Enders (see no. 98), whose modification of Harrison's tissue culture process supplied the procedure by which the poliomyelitis vaccine was made available for either the Salk or Sabin method of vaccination.

Harrison, who studied at Johns Hopkins and in Germany, held doctorates in both medicine and zoology. It was in 1907, while serving as associate professor of anatomy at the Johns Hopkins Medical School, that he first presented the results of his experiments in a paper read before the Society for Experimental Biology and Medicine on 22 May. It was published both in the 15 June 1907 number of the society's *Proceedings* and in the 1 June 1907 number of the *Anatomical Record.* Later in 1907 Harrison left Hopkins to head the department of zoology at Yale University, and it was from there that he published in 1910 his definitive paper on the outgrowth of the nerve fiber. He remained at Yale, teaching and engaging in research until his retirement in 1955.

JMN

1. Ross G. Harrison, "Embryology and Its Relations," *Science* 85 (1937): 372.

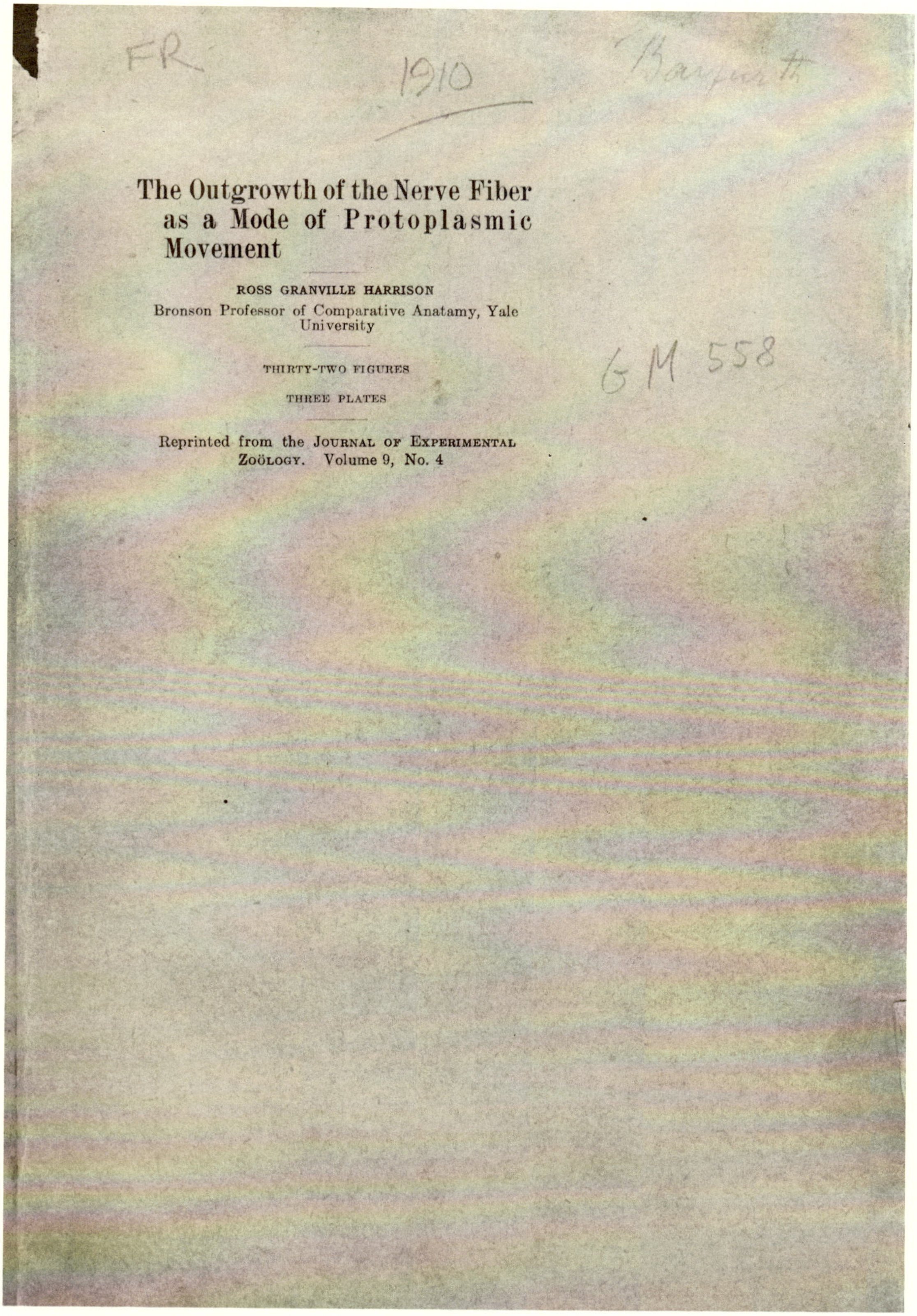

Fig. 165. No. 91B. Harrison. Front wrapper of the 1910 offprint.

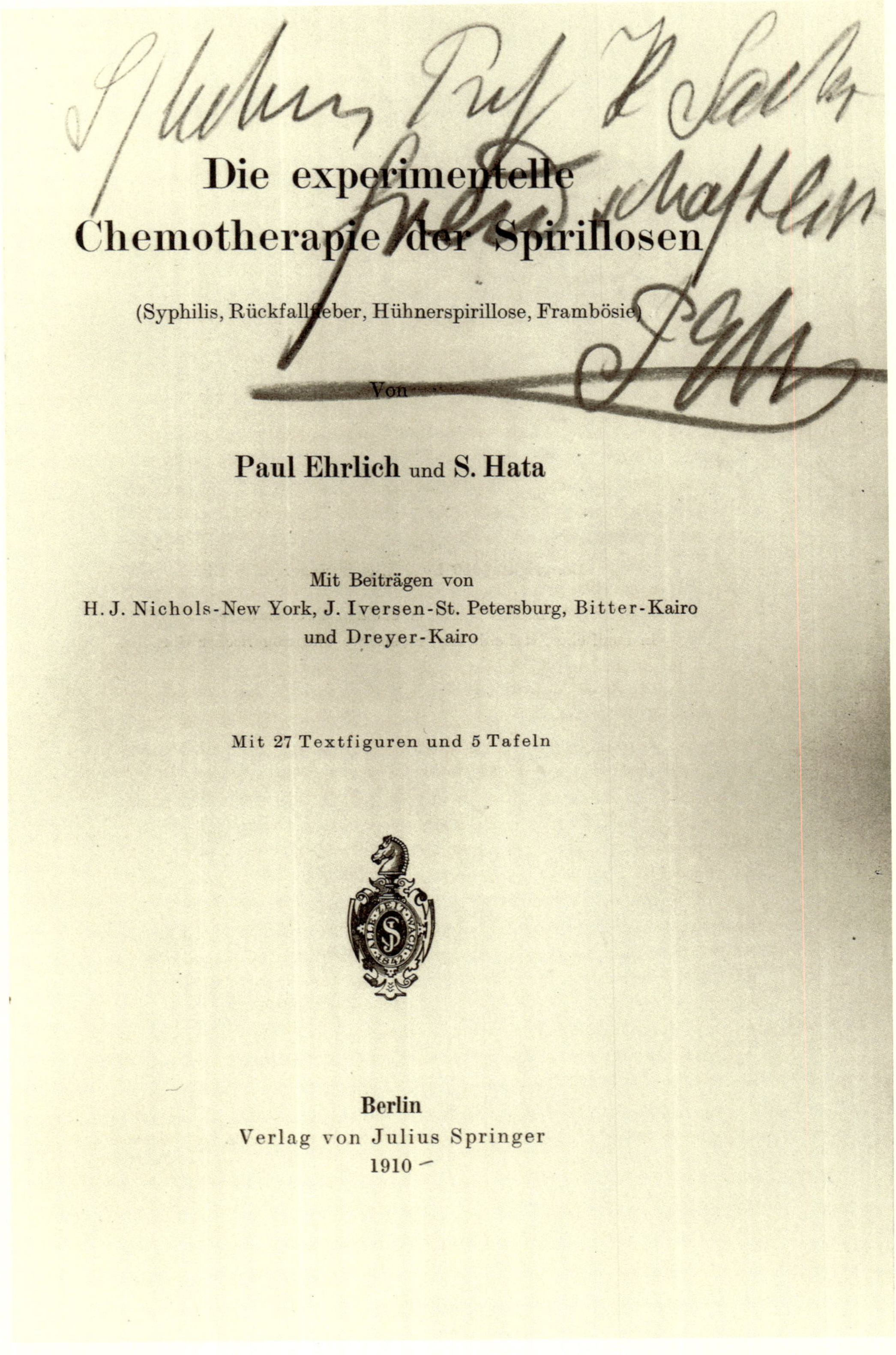
Die experimentelle
Chemotherapie der Spirillosen

(Syphilis, Rückfallfieber, Hühnerspirillose, Frambösie)

Von

Paul Ehrlich und S. Hata

Mit Beiträgen von
H. J. Nichols-New York, J. Iversen-St. Petersburg, Bitter-Kairo
und Dreyer-Kairo

Mit 27 Textfiguren und 5 Tafeln

Berlin
Verlag von Julius Springer
1910

Fig. 166. No. 92. Ehrlich and Hata. Title page, with Ehrlich's inscription in laboratory grease pencil to Hans Sachs, his pupil, co-worker, and bibliographer.

92

PAUL EHRLICH
(1854–1915)

SAHACHIRO HATA
(1873–1938)

Die experimentelle Chemotherapie der Spirillosen (Syphilis, Rückfallfieber, Hühnerspirillose, Frambösie).

Berlin: Verlag von Julius Springer, 1910.

π^4 1–10^8 11^4. 88 leaves, pp. *I–III* IV–VIII *1* 2–164 [4]. Taf. I–V: 5 halftone plates; Tab. I–XXXIII: 3 inserted, folding letterpress tables (Tab. XIV, XV, XVII) and 30 letterpress tables in text; Kurve 1–15, 1–12: 27 line-block graphs in text. Blue publisher's cloth, or printed wrappers.

GM 2403. *Heirs of Hippocrates* 2159. Norman 686. Osler 1697. PMM 402. Sachs, p. 628, and p. 635, no. 125. Waller 2707.

Paul Ehrlich made outstanding contributions to bacteriology, immunology, hematology, and chemotherapy. His researches in hematology led to the introduction of the differential white cell count as a diagnostic tool and to the establishment of methods for detecting leukemias and anemias, while his investigations into immunological processes resulted in his "side-chain" theory that postulated the production of immunologically specific antibodies against invading organisms. Much honored during his lifetime, he shared the Nobel Prize for Physiology or Medicine with Elie Metchnikoff in 1908 for his work in immunology, and he was renominated in 1912 and 1913 for his contributions to chemotherapy.

As a medical student at his cousin Carl Weigert's laboratory, Ehrlich began researches on the selective staining action of aniline dyes on cells and tissues. Experiments on differential staining of bacteria, which took up aniline dyes that left surrounding tissues unaffected, enabled him to demonstrate the presence of the tubercle bacillus in sputum and in tissues, thereby enhancing the importance of Robert Koch's discovery of the tubercle bacillus (see no. 80). His work on dyes impressed him with the selective affinity of chemicals for different tissues, a concept that had implications for therapeutics. Nowhere was this selective affinity more evident than in immunology, and Ehrlich referred to antibodies as "magic bullets" which could seek out and neutralize pathogenic microorganisms. In the early twentieth century he began a research program to synthesize substances that might act as chemical "magic bullets," destroying microorganisms in the body without harming the human host. The discovery in 1905 by H. W. Thomas and A. Breinl that atoxyl, an organic arsenic compound, was effective against typanosome infections in rodents led Ehrlich to synthesize and test hundreds of arsenic compounds in an effort to find one that would destroy trypanosomes in humans without the toxic side effects of atoxyl (which caused blindness in higher animals). The erroneous belief that the spirochete that caused syphilis, isolated by Fritz Schaudinn in 1905, was very similar to the trypanosome inspired Ehrlich to try his synthetic drugs against syphilis as well. In 1909 Ehrlich and his assistant Sahachiro Hata tested their 606th experimental compound, arsphenamine (later patented under the name Salvarsan), which proved to be effective against syphilis. This was Ehrlich's chemical "magic bullet," the discovery of which heralded the development of chemotherapy.

In 1910 Ehrlich and Hata published *Die experimentelle Chemotherapie der Spirillosen*, in which they announced the discovery of Salvarsan. The book contains Ehrlich's fifty-page essay on the chemotherapy of syphilis, together with Hata's presentation of the experiments with the drug. It paved the way for Gerhard Domagk's discovery of the sulfonamides (1935) and for the successful demonstration of the therapeutic action of penicillin *in vivo* by Howard Florey and Ernst Chain (1940).

HFN

93

HARVEY WILLIAMS CUSHING
(1869–1939)

The Pituitary Body and Its Disorders. Clinical States Produced by Disorders of the Hypophysis Cerebri.

Philadelphia & London: J. B. Lippincott Company, 1912.

π^6 1–21^8 22^4. 178 leaves, pp. [2] *i–v* vi–x *1* 2–341 [3]. Frontispiece: 1 five-color halftone plate; Fig. 1–114, 114a, 115–319: 1 inserted halftone plate (Fig. 225) and 319 halftone or line-block illustrations in text. Red publisher's cloth.

Cushing Society 1. GM 3896. *Heirs of Hippocrates* 2269. Norman 549. Waller 2252.

Harvey Cushing, the father of neurological surgery, was the first to devote himself entirely to the field of surgery of the nervous system. He obtained his undergraduate education at Yale University (1887–91) and his medical training at Harvard Medical School (1891–95). After his internship at Massachusetts General Hospital (1895–96), he began his training in surgery at Johns Hopkins Hospital as assistant resident under William Stewart Halsted, and he remained at Hopkins for sixteen years. It was there that he also worked with William Osler, who became a very important influence in his life. After graduation he spent a year in Europe, where he visited laboratories and clinics and worked with Theodor Kocher in Bern investigating problems of increased intracranial pressure. He returned to the United States in 1901, convinced that his future lay in the field of neurosurgery.

At the beginning of the twentieth century, neurosurgery was considered an interesting but generally discouraging field, marked by extraordinarily high rates of failure and mortality. Within a few years, Cushing changed this by refining old techniques and developing new ones. Applying lessons he had learned under Halsted, he combined meticulous technique with unusual attention to pre- and postoperative care, with the result that surgical cures became the rule rather than the exception. Cushing was convinced that the successful neurosurgeon must be an accomplished neurologist as well as a skilled technician, and this led to neurosurgery becoming a discrete specialty. This remains perhaps his most enduring legacy.

Cushing was a disciplined and prodigious writer. The corpus of his work is immense, comprising more than 330 books and articles. His first major monograph was devoted to the pituitary, the small pea-sized gland at the base of the brain. This work, which established the field of clinical endocrinology, is his most famous publication; it contains the

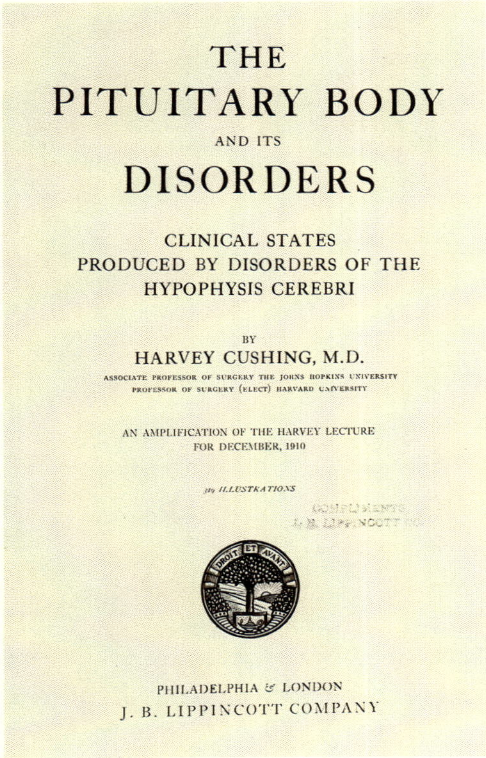
THE
PITUITARY BODY
AND ITS
DISORDERS

CLINICAL STATES
PRODUCED BY DISORDERS OF THE
HYPOPHYSIS CEREBRI

BY
HARVEY CUSHING, M.D.
ASSOCIATE PROFESSOR OF SURGERY THE JOHNS HOPKINS UNIVERSITY
PROFESSOR OF SURGERY (ELECT) HARVARD UNIVERSITY

AN AMPLIFICATION OF THE HARVEY LECTURE
FOR DECEMBER, 1910

319 ILLUSTRATIONS

COMPLIMENTS
J. B. LIPPINCOTT CO.

PHILADELPHIA & LONDON
J. B. LIPPINCOTT COMPANY

Fig. 167. No. 93. Cushing. Title page of the first issue.

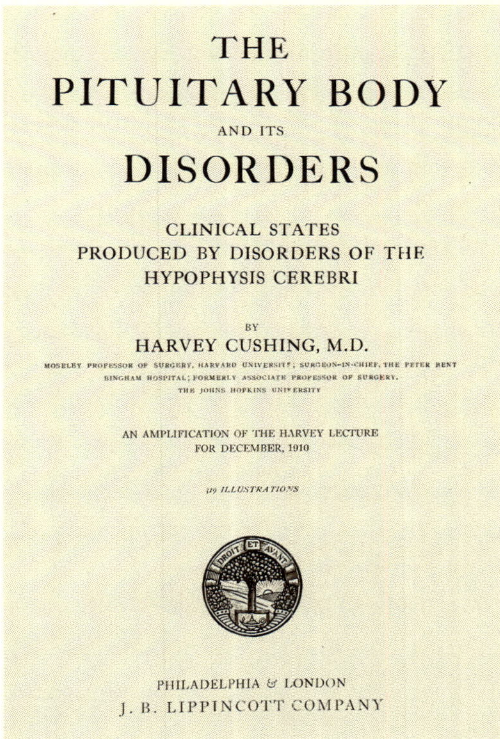
THE
PITUITARY BODY
AND ITS
DISORDERS

CLINICAL STATES
PRODUCED BY DISORDERS OF THE
HYPOPHYSIS CEREBRI

BY
HARVEY CUSHING, M.D.
MOSELEY PROFESSOR OF SURGERY, HARVARD UNIVERSITY; SURGEON-IN-CHIEF, THE PETER BENT
BRIGHAM HOSPITAL; FORMERLY ASSOCIATE PROFESSOR OF SURGERY,
THE JOHNS HOPKINS UNIVERSITY

AN AMPLIFICATION OF THE HARVEY LECTURE
FOR DECEMBER, 1910

319 ILLUSTRATIONS

PHILADELPHIA & LONDON
J. B. LIPPINCOTT COMPANY

Fig. 168. No. 93. Cushing. Title page of the second issue.

first description of his method of operating on the pituitary and the first account of hyperadrenalism (at that time erroneously attributed to pituitary basophilism), now known as Cushing's syndrome. As an author, Cushing did not limit himself strictly to medical subjects: in addition to works on all phases of neurosurgery, he published many books on bibliographical, biographical, and historical topics, including a bio-bibliography of the sixteenth-century anatomist Andreas Vesalius and a biography of his mentor William Osler.[1] The latter was awarded the Pulitzer Prize in 1925. He also amassed a large collection of rare medical and scientific books.

Harvey Cushing recognized the importance of training young men in the field of neurological surgery. He sought trainees from all over the world, and most of his students went on to become prominent neurosurgeons in their own right. During the first half of the twentieth century, virtually all chairs of neurosurgery were held by Cushing's students, and they invariably acknowledged their debt to their master.

After spending his early career at Johns Hopkins, Cushing in 1912 accepted an appointment as professor of surgery at the Harvard Medical School. Following his reluctant retirement from that position at age 63, he left Boston and ended his career as professor of the history of medicine at Yale, where his library and clinical records remain. He left a bequest to enable his friend, John Fulton, to write his biography following his death; this is also a history of American neurosurgery in the first half of the twentieth century.[2]

There are two issues of *The Pituitary Body and Its Disorders.* In the first, consisting of 2000 copies, the title leaf is integral and describes Cushing as "Associate Professor of Surgery the Johns Hopkins University Professor of Surgery (elect) Harvard University." In the second, of 1000 copies, the title leaf is a cancel, and Cushing is described as "Moseley Professor of Surgery, Harvard University; Surgeon-in-Chief, the Peter Bent Bingham [*sic*] Hospital; formerly Associate Professor of Surgery, The Johns Hopkins University."

AEL

1. Harvey Cushing, *A Bio-Bibliography of Andreas Vesalius* (New York, 1943; reprinted, Hamden, Conn., 1962); idem, *The Life of Sir William Osler* (2 vols., Oxford, 1925).
2. John F. Fulton, *Harvey Cushing: A Biography* (Springfield, Ill., 1946).

Die Vitamine

ihre Bedeutung für die Physiologie und Pathologie

mit besonderer Berücksichtigung der

Avitaminosen:

(Beriberi, Skorbut, Pellagra, Rachitis)

Anhang:

Die Wachstumsubstanz und das Krebsproblem

Von

Casimir Funk,

Leiter des physiologisch-chemischen Laboratoriums,
Cancer Hospital Research Institute, London

Mit 38 Abbildungen im Text und 2 Tafeln.

Wiesbaden
Verlag von J. F. Bergmann
1914

Fig. 169. No. 94. Funk. Title page.

94

CASIMIR FUNK
(1884–1967)

Die Vitamine ihre Bedeutung für die Physiologie und Pathologie mit besonderer Berücksichtigung der Avitaminosen: (Beriberi, Skorbut, Pellagra, Rachitis).

Wiesbaden: Verlag von J. F. Bergmann, 1914.

π^4 1–12^8 13^4. 104 leaves, pp. *I–VII* VIII *1* 2–193 [7]. Taf. I–II: 2 color–lithographed plates; Fig. 1–38: 38 halftone and line-block illustrations in text. Blue printed wrappers.

GM 1051. cf. *Heirs of Hippocrates* 2322. Norman 849.

In this pioneering work on vitaminology, Casimir Funk explored the relationship between nutritional deficiency and disease, presenting research that paved the way for a deeper understanding of the role of vitamins in growth and development.

Born in Warsaw, Poland, Funk was the son of a renowned dermatologist. In 1904 he received a Ph.D. in organic chemistry from the University of Bern. From 1904 to 1906 he worked at the Pasteur Institute, where his research centered on the isolation of amino acids. While in Berlin from 1906 to 1910 he assisted the chemists Emil Fischer and Emil Abderhalden, and for one year he held the post of biochemist at the Municipal Hospital in Wiesbaden.

It was while he was at the Lister Institute in London that Funk worked out the physiological and pathological implications of the "accessory food factors" discovered by the British biochemist Frederick Gowland Hopkins between 1906 and 1912. Funk induced beriberi in pigeons by feeding them a diet of polished rice, then prepared a concentrate of rice polishings which cured them. The active ingredient in the polishings was isolated and identified as thiamine (the first vitamin to be isolated), and thiamine was later found to cure beriberi in humans as well. Funk published the results of this research in 1911, and in 1912 he coined the term "vitamine" (from "vital amine") to describe vital compounds responsible in trace amounts for the cure or prevention of beriberi, scurvy, and rickets.[1] Although Funk was not the first to espouse the "vitamin hypothesis," it was through his researches and publications that awareness of the necessity of vitamins in nutrition became firmly fixed in the consciousness of the educated public.

After holding several industrial and academic positions in New York City, Funk returned to Warsaw in 1923 where, with the support of the Rockefeller Foundation, he be-

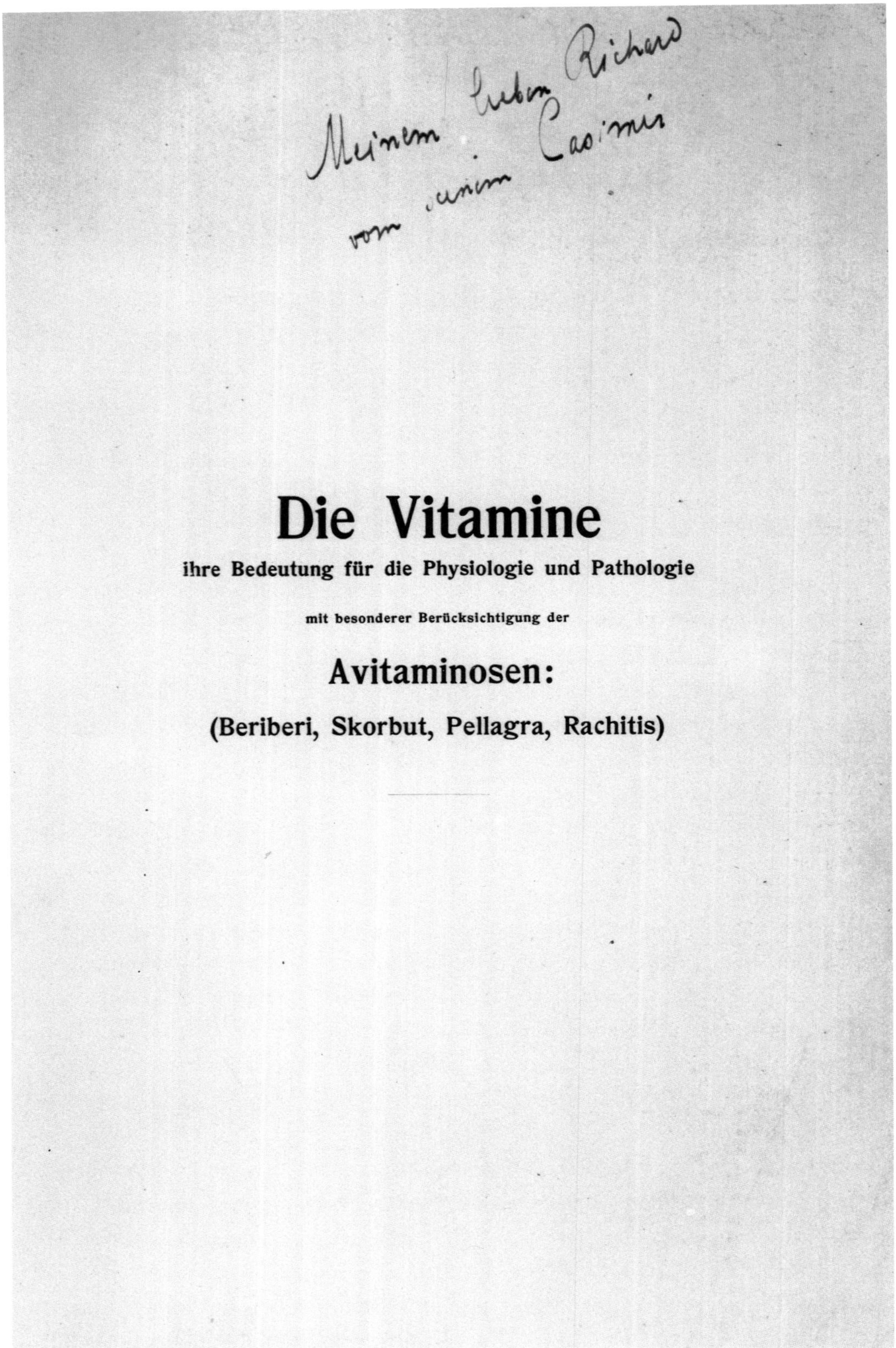

Meinem lieben Richard vom seinem Casimir

Die Vitamine

ihre Bedeutung für die Physiologie und Pathologie

mit besonderer Berücksichtigung der

Avitaminosen:

(Beriberi, Skorbut, Pellagra, Rachitis)

Fig. 170. No. 94. Funk. Half-title, inscribed by the author.

came chief of the biochemistry department in the State Institute of Hygiene; however, political unrest in Poland caused him to abandon this position in 1927. He then established a private research firm (Casa Biochemica) in Paris, but at the outbreak of World War II he returned to New York as consultant to the U.S. Vitamin Corporation.

Funk is well known for his extensive research on animal hormones, particularly the male sex hormone, and on the biochemistry of cancer and ulcers. He was among the first to link phosphoric acid to the action of insulin, and he studied the relationship between hormones and the production of insulin.

APH

1. Casimir Funk, "On the Chemical Nature of the Substance Which Cures Polyneuritis in Birds Induced by a Diet of Polished Rice," *Journal of Physiology* 43 (1911): 395–400; idem, "The Etiology of Deficiency Diseases," *Journal of State Medicine* 20 (1912): 341–68.

(1)

To Dr Harvey Cushing
Compliments
F. G. Banting.

THE INTERNAL SECRETION OF THE PANCREAS

By F. G. Banting and C. H. Best

(Read before the Academy of Medicine, February 7th, 1922)

Lantern slides to illustrate the following points: (by Best)—

1. Intravenous injections of dog's pancreas, removed from seven to ten weeks after ligation of the ducts, invariably exercises a reducing influence on the percentage sugar of the blood and the amount of sugar excreted in the urine.

2. Rectal injections are not effective.

3. The extent and duration of the reduction varies directly with the amount of extract injected.

4. Pancreatic juice destroys the active principle.

5. Extracts made 0.1% acid are effectual in lowering the blood sugar.

6. The presence of the extract enables a diabetic dog to retain a much larger percentage of injected sugar than it otherwise would.

7. Extracts prepared in neutral saline and kept in cold storage retain their potency for at least seven days.

8. Boiled extracts are ineffectual in reducing blood sugar.

9. That the reducing action is not a dilution phenomenon is indicated by the following facts: (1) Hemoglobin estimations before and after administration of the extract are identical; (2) Injections of large quantities of saline do not effect the blood sugar; (3) Similar quantities of extracts of other tissues do not cause a reduction of blood sugar.

The results so far reported occupied our time until the middle of November, 1921, when a new era was introduced by the discovery that the foetal calf pancreas of under five month's development did not contain pancreatic juice but did contain internal secretion.

Laguesse found that the Islets of Langerhans were comparatively more plentiful in the foetus and newborn than in the adult animal. On November 16th, the idea presented itself that by making an extract of the pancreas of foetal calves, we might be able to obtain large quantities of the internal secretion without the destroying influence of pancreatic juice. This was done and, to our great satisfaction, on the injection of such an extract, the blood sugar per cent. of a diabetic

Fig. 171. No. 95B. Banting and Best. The paper presented to the Academy of Medicine, Toronto, in 1922, and privately printed, inscribed by Banting to Harvey Cushing.

95

SIR FREDERICK GRANT BANTING
(1891–1941)

CHARLES HERBERT BEST
(1899–1978)

A] The Internal Secretion of the Pancreas.

In: *Journal of Laboratory and Clinical Medicine* 7 (1921–22): 251–66.

[journal number] Vol. 7, No. 5, February 1922: [1–3^{16} 4^{2}]. 50 leaves, pp. 1–16, 251–310, 17–40. Gray printed wrappers.

[article] $[1]_9^r$–$[1]_{16}^v$, pp. 251–266. Charts 1–6: 6 line-block charts in text (Chart 2 in two parts.)

[offprint] *The Internal Secretion of the Pancreas* [head title]. Reprint from the Journal of Laboratory and Clinical Medicine, St. Louis, Vol. VII, No. 5, February, 1922.

$[1]^8$. 8 leaves, pp. 1–16. Charts 1–6: 6 line-block charts in text (Chart 2 in two parts).

GM 3967. *Heirs of Hippocrates* 2333. Stevenson, p. 438.

B] The Internal Secretion of the Pancreas.

(Read before the Academy of Medicine, February 7th, 1922). N.p., n.d. [Toronto: Academy of Medicine, 1922.]

$[1]^2$. 2 leaves, pp. *1–4*.

Although the anti-diabetic function of the islets of Langerhans in the pancreas had been suspected for many years, it was Frederick Grant Banting (later Sir Frederick) who proved it by isolating the diabetes-preventing hormone insulin and demonstrating its function. Banting, demonstrator in anatomy and physiology at the University of Western Ontario, was preparing a lecture on the physiology of the pancreas when, on 30 October 1920, he came across an article by Moses Barron entitled "The Relation of the Islets of Langerhans to Diabetes with Special Reference to Cases of Pancreatic Lithiasis."[1] There Barron cited evidence that blockage of the pancreatic duct either by gallstones or by ligature produced atrophy and sclerosis of the pancreas but left the islets of Langerhans intact; in such cases, glycosuria did not develop. Inspired by this article, Banting conceived the idea of extracting the islet cells by ligating the pancreatic duct of experimental animals. Since his own

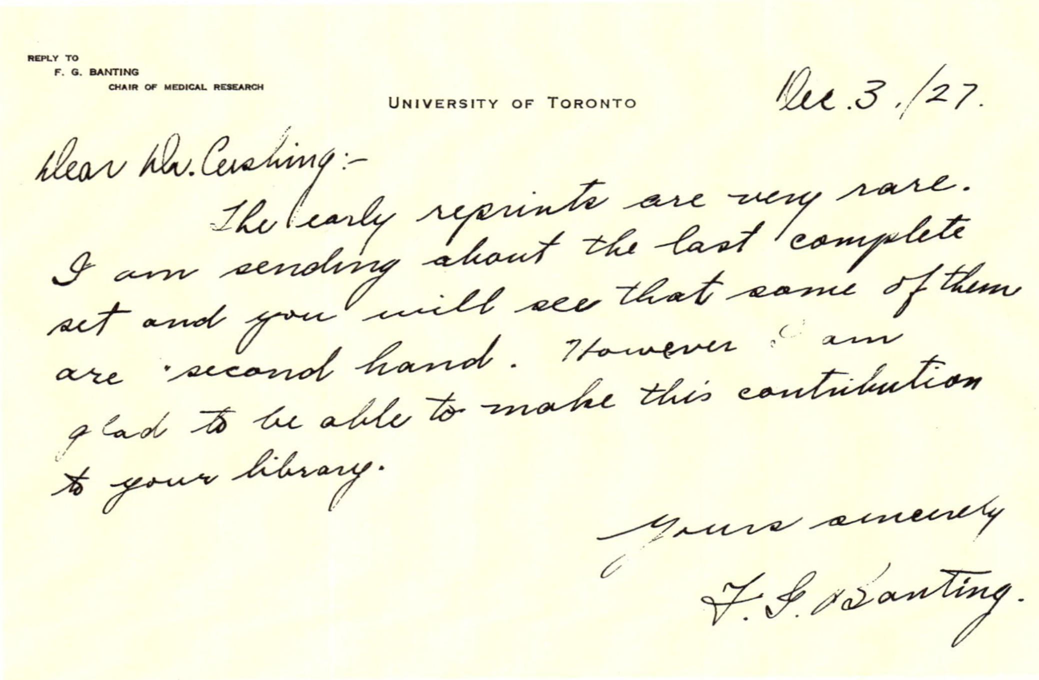
REPLY TO
F. G. BANTING
CHAIR OF MEDICAL RESEARCH

UNIVERSITY OF TORONTO

Dec. 3./27.

Dear Dr. Cushing:-

The early reprints are very rare. I am sending about the last complete set and you will see that some of them are 'second hand'. However I am glad to be able to make this contribution to your library.

Yours sincerely
F. G. Banting.

Fig. 172. No. 95. Note from Banting to Harvey Cushing regarding Banting's gift of offprints to Cushing's library.

institution was unable to provide him with the necessary laboratory space and animals, he appealed to Professor J.J.R. Macleod of the University of Toronto, who made the necessary facilities available and assigned to him as an assistant an undergraduate student, C. H. Best. Banting and Best set about ligating the pancreatic ducts of some dogs and depancreatizing others. By July 1921 they had successfully prepared both. They then made an extract from the degenerated gland of a ligated dog and injected it into a depancreatized animal; within two hours, the dog's condition had improved remarkably.

During the next few weeks, Banting and Best struggled to obtain a potent extract of the substance produced from the islets, which they had named "isletin." At this point, Professor Macleod, who had until then been skeptical about Banting's hypothesis, stepped in and enlisted the aid of a biochemist, J. B. Collip, to purify the extract. In January 1922 they had an extract pure enough to begin a clinical trial on a fourteen-year-old diabetic boy at the Toronto General Hospital. They found that when the boy received daily injections of the extract, he showed immediate clinical improvement, and the sugar and acetone bodies in his urine were much reduced. When the extract was withheld for ten days, however, the boy's symptoms and the chemistry of the urine were reversed. After this successful trial, the task became one of purifying and producing on a large scale the extract, which Macleod had now named "insulin." By November 1922 a pure, stable, and potent insulin was being produced commercially by the Eli Lilly Company.

On 14 November 1921 Banting and Best announced their findings at a meeting of the Physiological Journal Club of the University of Toronto, and on 28 December, joined by Macleod, they gave a report at a meeting of the American Physiological Society.[2] Their first paper on insulin research, "The Internal Secretion of the Pancreas," written in November 1921, was published the following February in the *Journal of Laboratory and Clinical Medicine.* Shortly afterwards, a four-page paper, also entitled "The Internal Secretion of the Pancreas," was privately printed by the Academy of Medicine in Toronto; it represents the paper that Banting and Best read before the Academy on 7 February 1922.[3]

In 1923, Banting and Macleod were awarded the Nobel Prize in Physiology or Medicine for their work; Banting shared his portion with Best and Macleod shared his with Collip. In 1930, the Banting Institute of the University of Toronto was established, and Banting spent the rest of his life there as director of the Banting-Best Department of Medical Research. During World War II he was involved in coordinating medical research with British colleagues and made frequent plane trips to England. On 21 February 1941 he died in a plane crash in Newfoundland while on such a mission.

HFN

1. *Surgery, Gynecology, and Obstetrics* 31 (1920): 437–48.
2. An abstract of the latter was published in *American Journal of Physiology* 59 (1922): 479.
3. Michael Bliss, *The Discovery of Insulin* (Chicago, 1982), pp. 90, 94, 123.

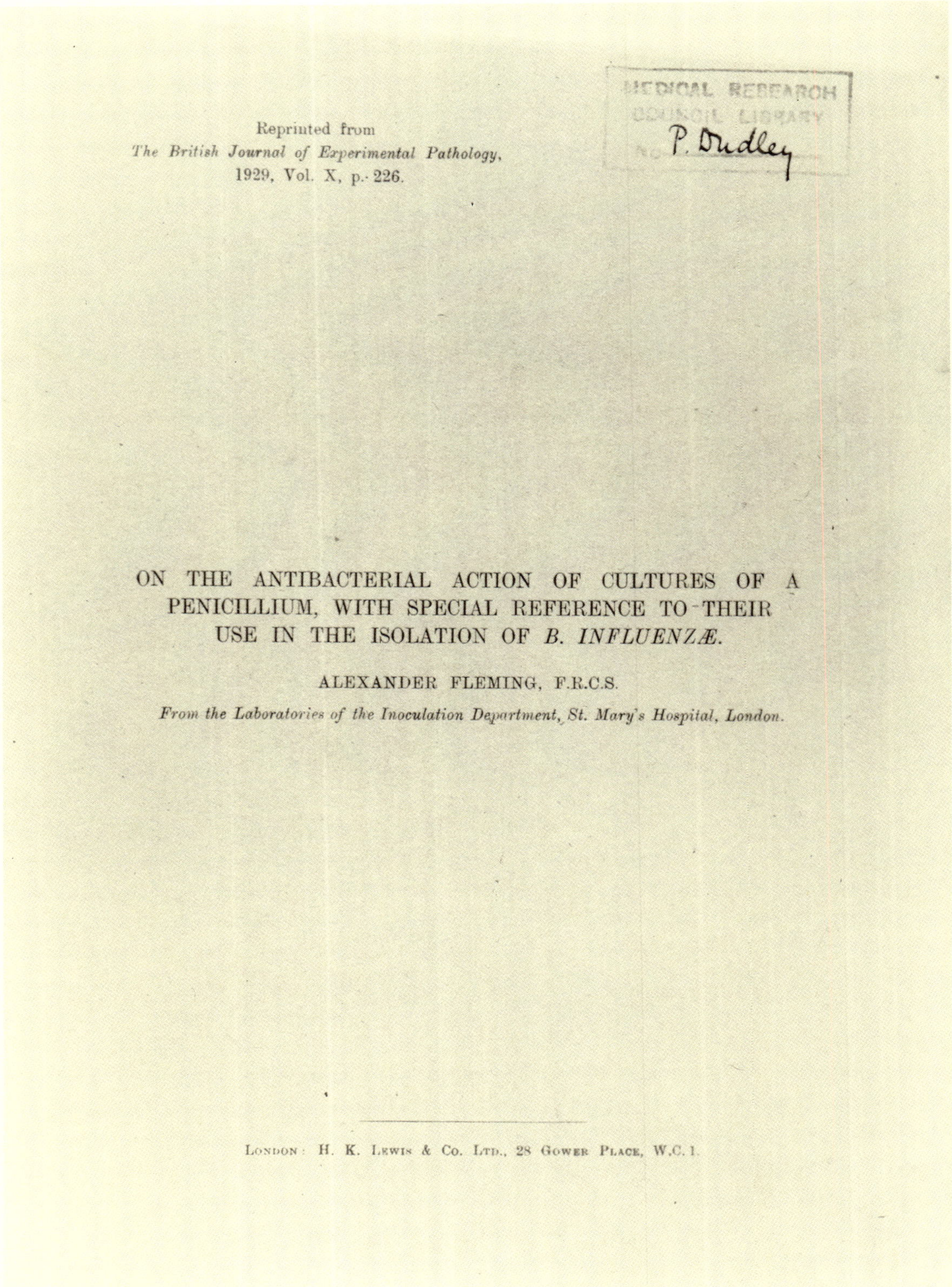

Reprinted from
The British Journal of Experimental Pathology,
1929, Vol. X, p. 226.

ON THE ANTIBACTERIAL ACTION OF CULTURES OF A PENICILLIUM, WITH SPECIAL REFERENCE TO THEIR USE IN THE ISOLATION OF *B. INFLUENZÆ.*

ALEXANDER FLEMING, F.R.C.S.

From the Laboratories of the Inoculation Department, St. Mary's Hospital, London.

London: H. K. Lewis & Co. Ltd., 28 Gower Place, W.C. 1.

Fig. 173. No. 96. Fleming. Front wrapper of the rare 1929 offprint from the *British Journal of Experimental Pathology.*

96

SIR ALEXANDER FLEMING
(1881–1955)

On the Antibacterial Action of Cultures of a Penicillium, with Special Reference to Their Use in the Isolation of *B. Influenzae.*

In: *British Journal of Experimental Pathology* 10 (1929): 226–36.

[journal number] Vol. 10, No. 3, June 1929: $15–17^8$ 18_1. 25 leaves, pp. *191* 192–194 [2] 195–228 [2] 229–236. Orange printed wrappers.

[article] 17_3^v–18_1^v, pp. 226–228 [2] 229–236. Fig. 1–4: 4 halftone illustrations in text.

[offprint] *On the Antibacterial Action of Cultures of a Penicillium, with Special Reference to Their Use in the Isolation of* B. Influenzae [wrapper title]. Reprinted from the British Journal of Experimental Pathology, 1929, Vol. X, p. 226.

$[1]^8$. 8 leaves, pp. 226–228 [2] 229–236 [3]. Fig. 1–4: 4 halftone illustrations in text. Orange printed wrappers.

The journal pages have been reimposed so that even-numbered pages are printed on the recto, odd-numbered pages on the verso.

Colebrook, p. 125. GM 1933. *Heirs of Hippocrates* 2320. Maurois, p. 284. Norman 798. PMM 420a.

[new setting] *On the Antibacterial Action of Cultures of a Penicillium with Special Reference to Their Use in the Isolation of* B. Influenzae [head title]. Reprinted from the British Journal of Experimental Pathology, 1929, Vol. X, p. 226.

$[1]^6$. 6 leaves, pp. 1–12. Fig. 1–4: 4 halftone illustrations in text.

Completely reset.

Alexander Fleming was born into a farmer's family in Ayrshire, Scotland, in 1881, but at an early age he went to London to live with one of his brothers who was a physician. In 1901 he enrolled as a student at St. Mary's Hospital Medical School, where he won almost every class prize and scholarship. He graduated in 1908 from London University, with honors in five subjects and a university gold medal. Thereafter at St. Mary's Hospital he became associated with the distinguished bacteriologist Sir Almoth Wright. From 1928 to 1948 he was professor of bacteriology at the University of London. After his retirement from that position he continued as director of the newly renamed Wright-Fleming Institute of Bacteriology until shortly before his death in 1955.

In 1928 Fleming made his great discovery: while working with culture plates of staphylococcus bacteria, he observed that some of his plates had become contaminated with a mold and that the bacterial colonies in contact with the mold had become transparent or dissolved. He concluded that the mold (later identified as *Penicillium notatum*) secreted a substance which had a bacteriolytic or bactericidal effect. After growing the mold in pure culture, he was able to demonstrate that the mold broth filtrate was nontoxic to laboratory animals and that it inhibited the growth of gram-positive pathogenic organisms, including staphylococcus, streptococcus, and meningococcus, as well as the gram-negative gonococcus. Fleming named the bactericidal substance "penicillin" and tried for some time to prepare a reliable extract of it, suspecting that such an extract "may be an efficient antiseptic for application to, or injection into, areas infected with penicillin-sensitive microbes." He was unsuccessful, however, due to his limited knowledge of chemistry, and the "mold juice" remained of limited use until 1940–41, when Ernst Boris Chain and Howard W. Florey, using Fleming's original culture, successfully prepared a pure and stable penicillin extract and demonstrated its usefulness in treating human bacterial infection. Within three years the United States government, in collaboration with the pharmaceutical industry, was producing penicillin on a large scale, with the result that many thousands of lives were saved during World War II. Fleming was knighted in 1944, and in 1945 Fleming, Chain, and Florey received the Nobel Prize in Physiology or Medicine.

Fleming reported his discovery in 1929 in a paper published in the *British Journal of Experimental Pathology.* For bibliophiles, the offprint of this paper has posed a special challenge. The original, true offprint contains eleven pages of text and two of photographs corresponding to those in the journal but reimposed so that the even-numbered pages are printed on the recto and the odd-numbered pages on the verso; it has an orange printed wrapper, on which is printed the statement "Reprinted from *The British Journal of Experimental Pathology*, 1929, Vol. X, p. 226." The edition was supposedly limited to 150 copies, and it is now exceedingly rare. The late Dr. Ernst Weil, a renowned dealer of rare books in science and medicine, wrote of it as follows:

> Several years before the war, the late Professor Fleming asked me through his assistant to find him an offprint of his classic paper on Penicillium of 1929, since he had retained none for himself. I was not able to find one. When after his death, the late Dr. Gilpin offered me a copy of it, which he had received himself from Prof. Fleming, I was only too pleased to accept this offer. I offered this copy in 1960 in my catalogue 28. But the story does not end there. Nearly two years after I had sold it to a collector in France, suddenly several copies turned up there, and it was soon established, that, although this was the first separate printing of the great paper and dated 1929, it was a reprint Prof. Fleming had ordered himself in 1944 to satisfy the numerous requests from scientists and friends. My client had been given one too, after the purchase from me. I took my copy back, and it is again offered as item no. 278. The great surprise, however, was that after long and

> careful investigations, apparently only one copy of the original excerpt from the Brit. Journ. of Experim. Pathol. given to Prof. Fleming has survived.[1]

Others have estimated that there are possibly three copies in existence. The "reprint" Weil mentions, which Fleming had made in 1944, was limited to 250 copies. Although the text is the same as that of the original, it was printed from a new setting of type; the pagination was changed to 1–12; the statement of reprinting is found at the head of page 1; and it was apparently issued without wrappers. The Parisian bookseller Alain Brieux was allegedly the person who obtained twenty copies of this reprint from Lady Fleming in the early 1960s, thereby making them available to the book trade and to collectors.

HFN

1. Ernst Weil, *Catalogue 31: Science and Medicine in the XIXth and XXth Centuries* (London, n.d. [1963]), p. 2.

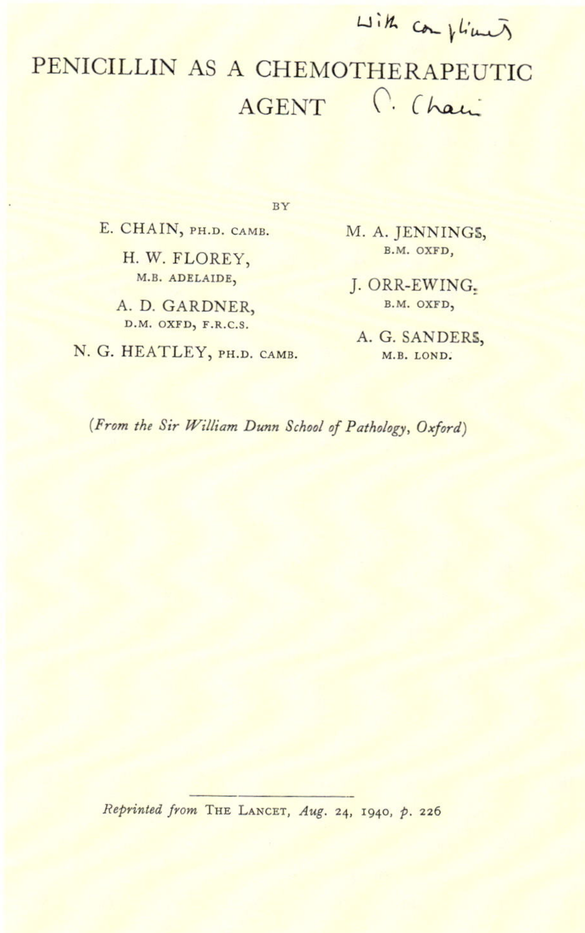

PENICILLIN AS A CHEMOTHERAPEUTIC AGENT

BY

E. CHAIN, PH.D. CAMB.
H. W. FLOREY, M.B. ADELAIDE,
A. D. GARDNER, D.M. OXFD, F.R.C.S.
N. G. HEATLEY, PH.D. CAMB.
M. A. JENNINGS, B.M. OXFD,
J. ORR-EWING, B.M. OXFD,
A. G. SANDERS, M.B. LOND.

(From the Sir William Dunn School of Pathology, Oxford)

Reprinted from THE LANCET, *Aug.* 24, 1940, *p.* 226

Fig. 174. Ernst Boris Chain, Howard Walter Florey, et al. "Penicillin as a Chemotherapeutic Agent," *Lancet*, 1940, 2: 226–28. Wrapper of the offprint. In this paper Chain and Florey announced their success in producing a stable penicillin drug suitable for therapeutic use. For this achievement they shared the Nobel Prize in Medicine with Fleming in 1945.

To Dr. W. Bruce Fye
from Helen B. Taussig

The Surgical Treatment of Malformations of the Heart

IN WHICH THERE IS PULMONARY STENOSIS
OR PULMONARY ATRESIA

ALFRED BLALOCK, M.D.
AND
HELEN B. TAUSSIG, M.D.
BALTIMORE

Reprinted from The Journal of the American Medical Association
May 19, 1945, Vol. 128, pp. 189-202

Printed and Published in the United States of America

Fig. 175. No. 97. Blalock and Taussig. Front wrapper of the offprint, with Taussig's presentation inscription.

97

ALFRED BLALOCK
(1899–1964)

HELEN BROOKE TAUSSIG
(1898–1986)

The Surgical Treatment of Malformations of the Heart in Which There Is Pulmonary Stenosis or Pulmonary Atresia.

In: *Journal of the American Medical Association* 128 (1945): 189–202.

[journal number] Vol. 128, No. 3, 19 May 1945: 74 leaves, pp. 1–32, 161–244, 33–62 [2]. Printed wrappers.

[article] pp. 189–202. Fig. 1–12: 7 halftone and 5 line-block illustrations in text.

[offprint] *The Surgical Treatment of Malformations of the Heart in Which There Is Pulmonary Stenosis or Pulmonary Atresia* [wrapper title]. Reprinted from the Journal of the American Medical Association, May 19, 1945, Vol. 128, pp. 189–202.

[1]^{22}. 22 leaves, pp. *1* 2–43 [1]. Fig. 1–12: 7 halftone and 5 line-block illustrations in text. Blue printed wrappers.

Reimposed in single-column pages, with different page breaks.

GM 3043. Ravitch 155.

Modern cardiac surgery emerged in response to many scientific and technical advances and through the bold innovations of surgeons around the world. It is impossible to identify one advance or operation as the pivotal development in this dynamic field. Nevertheless, cardiac surgery owes much to the team from Johns Hopkins that developed an operation for tetralogy of Fallot, a common form of cyanotic congenital heart disease. The "Blalock-Taussig" or "blue baby" operation, first performed by Alfred Blalock in 1944, was immediately recognized as a major advance. Surgeons from around the world came to Baltimore to observe and learn the new procedure, and the media attention was unprecedented.

The fundamental problem in patients with tetralogy of Fallot is that an inadequate blood supply reaches the lungs. Children born with tetralogy of Fallot are deeply cyanotic and have severely limited exercise tolerance; before the advent of the Blalock-Taussig operation they invariably died as a result of the condition and its complications. Helen Taussig, the pioneer pediatric cardiologist, was the first to suggest the creation of an anastomosis between the systemic and pulmonary circulations, and she urged Blalock to develop this innovative operation. Blalock, working with his African-American laboratory assistant Vivien Thomas, eventually succeeded in finding a means of connecting the left subclavian artery to the pulmonary artery, thus creating a shunt that dramatically increased the pulmonary blood flow.

Both Blalock and Taussig contributed greatly to the emergence of their disciplines. Blalock trained many individuals who made major contributions to the advance of cardiac surgery. The specialty of pediatric cardiology developed as a direct result of Taussig's active training program in Baltimore and her 1947 monograph on the subject.[1]

WBF

1. Helen B. Taussig, *Congenital Malformations of the Heart* (New York, 1947).

98

JOHN FRANKLIN ENDERS
(1897–1985)

THOMAS HUCKLE WELLER
(b. 1915)

FREDERICK CHAPMAN ROBBINS
(b. 1916)

A] Cultivation of the Lansing Strain of Poliomyelitis Virus in Cultures of Various Human Embryonic Tissues.

In: *Science* 109 (1949): 85–87.

[journal number] Vol. 109, No. 2822, 28 January 1949: 20 leaves, pp. 1–8, 77–102, 9–14. Printed wrappers.

[article] pp. 85–87.

[offprint] *Cultivation of the Lansing Strain of Poliomyelitis Virus in Cultures of Various Human Embryonic Tissues* [head title]. Reprinted from Science, January 28, 1949, Vol. 109, No. 2822, pages 85–87.

[1]^2. 2 leaves, pp. *1–2* [2].

Reimposed, with different page breaks.

GM 4671.1.

B] JONAS EDWARD SALK (1914–1995). Studies in Human Subjects on Active Immunization against Poliomyelitis. 1. A Preliminary Report of Experiments in Progress.

In: *Journal of the American Medical Association* 151 (1953): 1081–98.

[journal number] Vol. 151, No. 13, 28 March 1953: 86 leaves, pp. 1–34, 1055–1156, 35–68 [2].

[article] pp. 1081–1098. Fig. 1–16: 16 line-block charts in text.

[offprint] *Studies in Human Subjects on Active Immunization against Poliomyelitis. 1. A Preliminary Report of Experiments in Progress* [wrapper title]. Reprinted, with additions, from the Journal of the American Medical Association, March 28, 1953, Vol. 151, pp. 1081–1098.

[1]^{28}. 28 leaves, pp. *1* 2–56. Fig. 1–16: 16 line-block charts in text. Printed wrappers.

Reimposed in single-column pages, with different page breaks. The notes include acknowledgments and bibliographical references that did not appear in the journal.

GM 4672.2.

By the middle of the twentieth century polio epidemics in the industrialized western world had become a source of great alarm to the general public. The disease affected otherwise healthy children and adults, often causing death and inducing permanent paralysis in many of the survivors. Franklin Delano Roosevelt, polio's most famous victim, suffered permanent paralysis to his legs after being stricken in 1921; it was his experience that prompted him and his friends to establish in 1937 the National Foundation for Infantile Paralysis, the organization which, through its annual "March of Dimes" fundraising campaigns, provided the finances for the research that eventually helped reduce, if not eradicate, this disease.

Michael Underwood (see no. 48) provided the first accurate description of poliomyelitis in 1789, and in 1840 Jacob von Heine distinguished the paralysis caused by acute anterior poliomyelitis from other forms of paralysis; however, it was not until 1890 that the disease's epidemic character was first noted by Oscar Medin. In 1905 Otto Wickman produced the first evidence of the infectious nature of the disease, and in 1909 Karl Landsteiner and Erwin Popper transmitted poliomyelitis to monkeys by inoculating their brains with tissue taken from the spine of a human polio victim; since no bacteriological agent could be found, they concluded that the disease was caused by a virus. The polio virus was at first believed to be exclusively neurotropic, and early efforts to produce a vaccine were complicated by the impossiblity of completely separating the virus from the nervous tissue; the presence of this foreign material in the vaccine occasionally triggered a fatal allergic reaction. Although the polio virus had been found in human feces as early as 1911, it was not shown that it could grow in the alimentary canal until 1940, when Howard Howe and David Bodian produced polio in chimpanzees by feeding them the virus. In 1947 Joseph Melnick and Dorothy Horstmann demonstrated that animals who survived the infection were immune to reinfection thereafter. Between 1931 and 1947 three different strains of the virus were identified.

This was the stage at which Enders, Weller, and Robbins made their important discovery in 1949. John F. Enders, a bacteriologist, had become convinced as early as 1937 that viruses could be propagated by using tissue culture techniques (see no. 91), a procedure that would eliminate the difficult, time-consuming and costly process of cultivating viruses in live hosts. Thomas H. Weller, a specialist in tropical medicine, joined him in 1939, and after World War II Frederick C. Robbins, a specialist in the contagious diseases of children, became a member of the team. By the late 1940s and early 1950s, the team had succeeded in growing the polio virus in a variety of human tissues, including fetal intes-

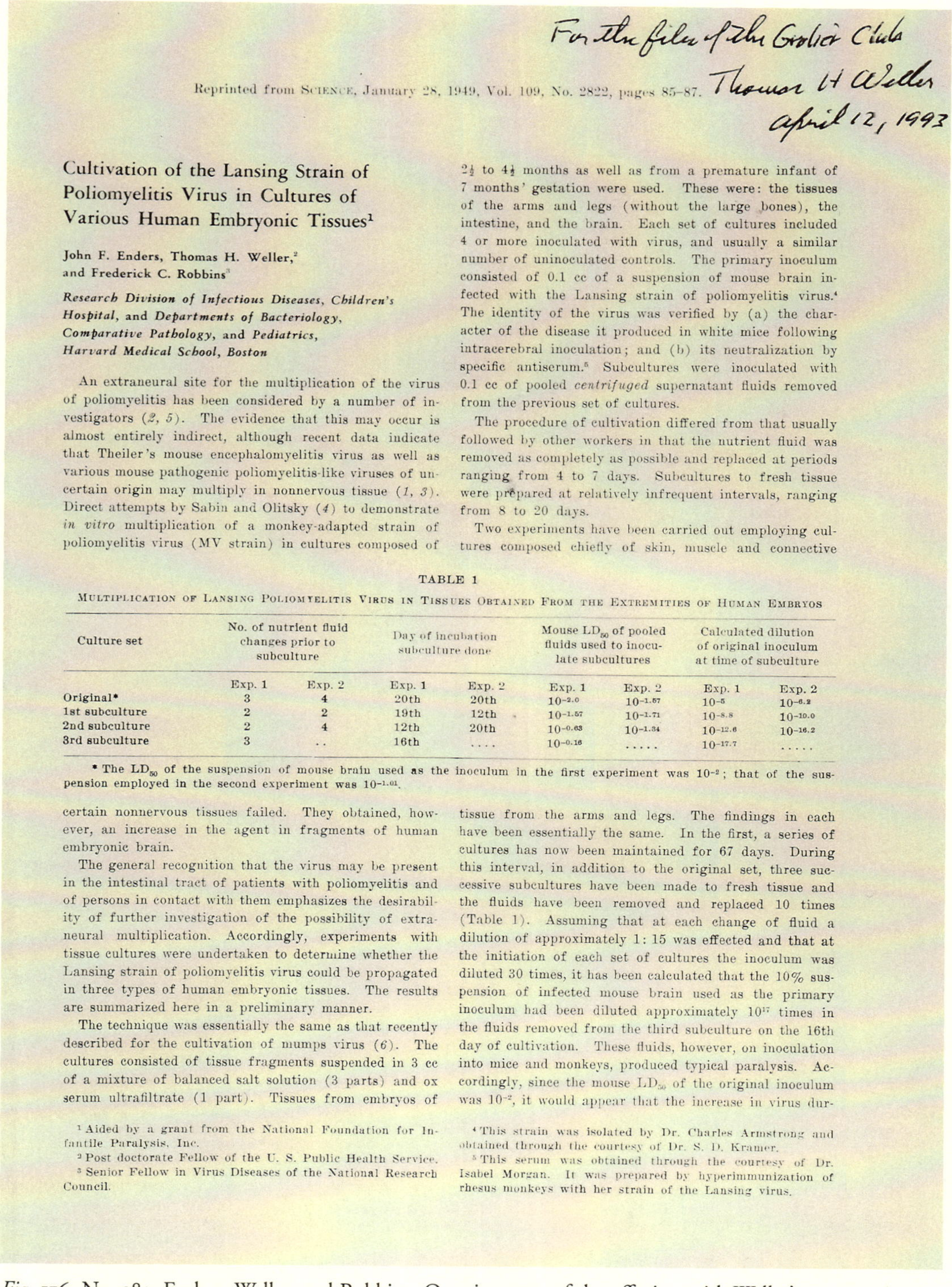

For the files of the Grolier Club
Thomas H Weller
April 12, 1993

Reprinted from SCIENCE, January 28, 1949, Vol. 109, No. 2822, pages 85-87.

Cultivation of the Lansing Strain of Poliomyelitis Virus in Cultures of Various Human Embryonic Tissues[1]

John F. Enders, Thomas H. Weller,[2] and Frederick C. Robbins[3]

Research Division of Infectious Diseases, Children's Hospital, and Departments of Bacteriology, Comparative Pathology, and Pediatrics, Harvard Medical School, Boston

An extraneural site for the multiplication of the virus of poliomyelitis has been considered by a number of investigators (*2, 5*). The evidence that this may occur is almost entirely indirect, although recent data indicate that Theiler's mouse encephalomyelitis virus as well as various mouse pathogenic poliomyelitis-like viruses of uncertain origin may multiply in nonnervous tissue (*1, 3*). Direct attempts by Sabin and Olitsky (*4*) to demonstrate *in vitro* multiplication of a monkey-adapted strain of poliomyelitis virus (MV strain) in cultures composed of certain nonnervous tissues failed. They obtained, however, an increase in the agent in fragments of human embryonic brain.

The general recognition that the virus may be present in the intestinal tract of patients with poliomyelitis and of persons in contact with them emphasizes the desirability of further investigation of the possibility of extraneural multiplication. Accordingly, experiments with tissue cultures were undertaken to determine whether the Lansing strain of poliomyelitis virus could be propagated in three types of human embryonic tissues. The results are summarized here in a preliminary manner.

The technique was essentially the same as that recently described for the cultivation of mumps virus (*6*). The cultures consisted of tissue fragments suspended in 3 cc of a mixture of balanced salt solution (3 parts) and ox serum ultrafiltrate (1 part). Tissues from embryos of $2\frac{1}{2}$ to $4\frac{1}{2}$ months as well as from a premature infant of 7 months' gestation were used. These were: the tissues of the arms and legs (without the large bones), the intestine, and the brain. Each set of cultures included 4 or more inoculated with virus, and usually a similar number of uninoculated controls. The primary inoculum consisted of 0.1 cc of a suspension of mouse brain infected with the Lansing strain of poliomyelitis virus.[4] The identity of the virus was verified by (a) the character of the disease it produced in white mice following intracerebral inoculation; and (b) its neutralization by specific antiserum.[5] Subcultures were inoculated with 0.1 cc of pooled *centrifuged* supernatant fluids removed from the previous set of cultures.

The procedure of cultivation differed from that usually followed by other workers in that the nutrient fluid was removed as completely as possible and replaced at periods ranging from 4 to 7 days. Subcultures to fresh tissue were prepared at relatively infrequent intervals, ranging from 8 to 20 days.

Two experiments have been carried out employing cultures composed chiefly of skin, muscle and connective tissue from the arms and legs. The findings in each have been essentially the same. In the first, a series of cultures has now been maintained for 67 days. During this interval, in addition to the original set, three successive subcultures have been made to fresh tissue and the fluids have been removed and replaced 10 times (Table 1). Assuming that at each change of fluid a dilution of approximately 1 : 15 was effected and that at the initiation of each set of cultures the inoculum was diluted 30 times, it has been calculated that the 10% suspension of infected mouse brain used as the primary inoculum had been diluted approximately 10^{17} times in the fluids removed from the third subculture on the 16th day of cultivation. These fluids, however, on inoculation into mice and monkeys, produced typical paralysis. Accordingly, since the mouse LD_{50} of the original inoculum was 10^{-2}, it would appear that the increase in virus dur-

TABLE 1

MULTIPLICATION OF LANSING POLIOMYELITIS VIRUS IN TISSUES OBTAINED FROM THE EXTREMITIES OF HUMAN EMBRYOS

Culture set	No. of nutrient fluid changes prior to subculture		Day of incubation subculture done		Mouse LD_{50} of pooled fluids used to inoculate subcultures		Calculated dilution of original inoculum at time of subculture	
	Exp. 1	Exp. 2	Exp. 1	Exp. 2	Exp. 1	Exp. 2	Exp. 1	Exp. 2
Original*	3	4	20th	20th	$10^{-2.0}$	$10^{-1.67}$	10^{-5}	$10^{-6.2}$
1st subculture	2	2	19th	12th	$10^{-1.57}$	$10^{-1.71}$	$10^{-8.8}$	$10^{-10.0}$
2nd subculture	2	4	12th	20th	$10^{-0.63}$	$10^{-1.34}$	$10^{-12.6}$	$10^{-16.2}$
3rd subculture	3	..	16th	....	$10^{-0.16}$	.....	$10^{-17.7}$	.....

* The LD_{50} of the suspension of mouse brain used as the inoculum in the first experiment was 10^{-2}; that of the suspension employed in the second experiment was $10^{-1.01}$.

[1] Aided by a grant from the National Foundation for Infantile Paralysis, Inc.

[2] Post doctorate Fellow of the U. S. Public Health Service.

[3] Senior Fellow in Virus Diseases of the National Research Council.

[4] This strain was isolated by Dr. Charles Armstrong and obtained through the courtesy of Dr. S. D. Kramer.

[5] This serum was obtained through the courtesy of Dr. Isabel Morgan. It was prepared by hyperimmunization of rhesus monkeys with her strain of the Lansing virus.

Fig. 176. No. 98A. Enders, Weller, and Robbins. Opening page of the offprint, with Weller's presentation inscription to the Grolier Club.

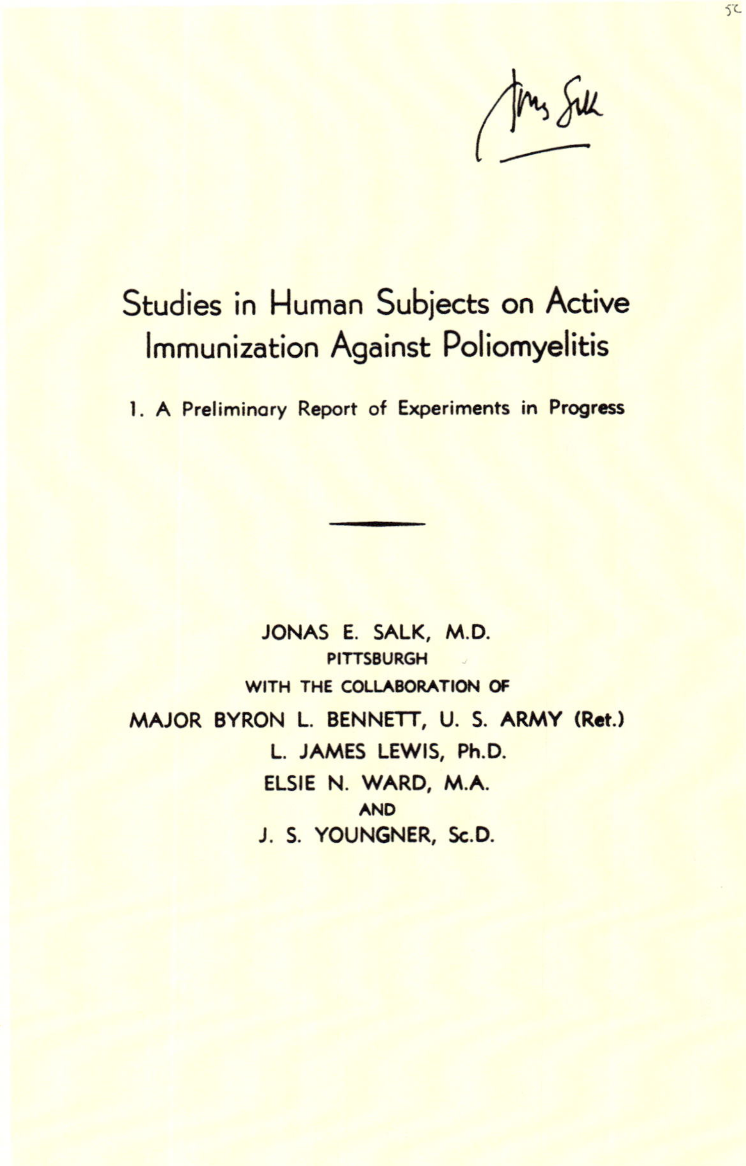
Studies in Human Subjects on Active Immunization Against Poliomyelitis

1. A Preliminary Report of Experiments in Progress

JONAS E. SALK, M.D.
PITTSBURGH
WITH THE COLLABORATION OF
MAJOR BYRON L. BENNETT, U. S. ARMY (Ret.)
L. JAMES LEWIS, Ph.D.
ELSIE N. WARD, M.A.
AND
J. S. YOUNGNER, Sc.D.

Fig. 177. No. 98B. Salk. Signed front wrapper of the offprint.

tine, embryonic skin, foreskin, kidney, and uterus. It was this development, which made possible the laboratory cultivation of large amounts of polio virus for experimental use, that led to great advances in research and enabled the preparation of a vaccine free of neural tissue. In 1954, Enders, Weller, and Robbins were awarded the Nobel Prize for their discovery.

The first important application of Enders's work to polio prevention was made at the

University of Pittsburgh by Jonas Salk and his colleagues, who appear to have been the first group of immunologists to master Enders's technique of tissue culture. By early 1950 Salk was ready to begin experiments in polio prevention by immunologic means. He hypothesized that the polio virus would multiply in non-neural tissue and only thereafter proceed from the portal of entry to the central nervous system, where it would either kill or cause paralysis in its host. He also assumed that if an antibody barrier could be created to intercept the virus before it invaded the central nervous system, the sequence of infection would be avoided. Salk and his team were able to show that poliomyelitis is not a single disease; rather, it is caused in man by any one of three immunologically different viruses, and the antibodies that protect against one virus do not guard against the rest. The team prepared a vaccine made of the three known polio viruses, which were killed by using a solution of formalin. When this was inoculated into monkeys, the vaccine produced antibody formation without evidence of infectivity. These experiments paved the way for human experimentation.

In 1952 Salk began to test his vaccine on human subjects, inoculating 161 children and young adults. He observed no signs of illness in the test subjects that could be attributed to the inoculations, and the level of antibody formation in the subjects compared favorably with the levels developed after natural infection. Salk reported this data in the *Journal of the American Medical Association* on 28 March 1953; although he called this paper a "preliminary communication" and concluded that his results "should not be interpreted to indicate that a practical vaccine is now at hand," the members of the National Foundation for Infantile Paralysis decided to conduct large-scale field trials of the Salk vaccine as soon as possible, on the ground that in 1952 more American children had died of polio than of any other communicable disease. The field trials occurred in the spring and summer of 1954, and on 12 April 1955 the results were announced to the general public: Salk's vaccine was successful in preventing paralytic poliomyelitis.

It is estimated that the Salk vaccine reduced poliomyelitis by ninety percent in the United States. After 1961 it was largely replaced in this country by the Sabin vaccine, which consists of a live attenuated virus administered orally, but the Salk vaccine is still used in some parts of the world, including Scandinavia and Holland.[1] Salk received numerous awards for his efforts, including a Congressional Medal, and a grateful public contributed to the establishment of the Salk Institute for Biological Studies.

HFN

1. For a discussion of the current state of the Salk vaccine, see H. V. Wyatt, "Poliomyelitis," in *The Cambridge World History of Human Disease*, ed. K. F. Kiple (Cambridge, 1993), pp. 942–50.

equipment, and to Dr. G. E. R. Deacon and the captain and officers of R.R.S. *Discovery II* for their part in making the observations.

[1] Young, F. B., Gerrard, H., and Jevons, W., *Phil. Mag.*, **40**, 149 (1920).
[2] Longuet-Higgins, M. S., *Mon. Not. Roy. Astro. Soc., Geophys. Supp.*, **5**, 285 (1949).
[3] Von Arx, W. S., Woods Hole Papers in Phys. Oceanog. Meteor., **11** (3) (1950).
[4] Ekman, V. W., *Arkiv. Mat. Astron. Fysik. (Stockholm)*, **2** (11) (1905).

MOLECULAR STRUCTURE OF NUCLEIC ACIDS

A Structure for Deoxyribose Nucleic Acid

WE wish to suggest a structure for the salt of deoxyribose nucleic acid (D.N.A.). This structure has novel features which are of considerable biological interest.

A structure for nucleic acid has already been proposed by Pauling and Corey[1]. They kindly made their manuscript available to us in advance of publication. Their model consists of three intertwined chains, with the phosphates near the fibre axis, and the bases on the outside. In our opinion, this structure is unsatisfactory for two reasons: (1) We believe that the material which gives the X-ray diagrams is the salt, not the free acid. Without the acidic hydrogen atoms it is not clear what forces would hold the structure together, especially as the negatively charged phosphates near the axis will repel each other. (2) Some of the van der Waals distances appear to be too small.

Another three-chain structure has also been suggested by Fraser (in the press). In his model the phosphates are on the outside and the bases on the inside, linked together by hydrogen bonds. This structure as described is rather ill-defined, and for this reason we shall not comment on it.

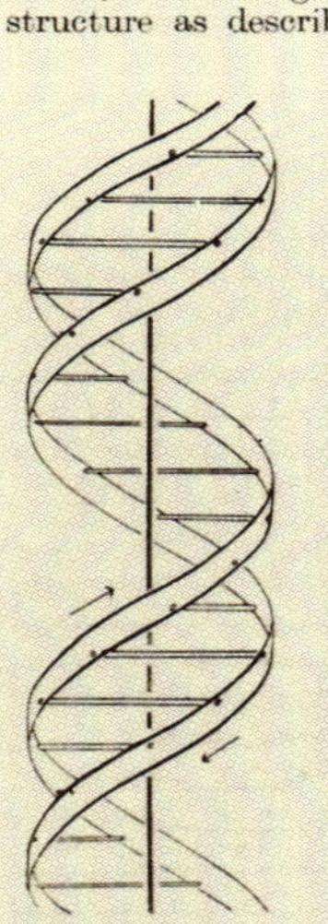

This figure is purely diagrammatic. The two ribbons symbolize the two phosphate—sugar chains, and the horizontal rods the pairs of bases holding the chains together. The vertical line marks the fibre axis

We wish to put forward a radically different structure for the salt of deoxyribose nucleic acid. This structure has two helical chains each coiled round the same axis (see diagram). We have made the usual chemical assumptions, namely, that each chain consists of phosphate diester groups joining β-D-deoxyribofuranose residues with 3′,5′ linkages. The two chains (but not their bases) are related by a dyad perpendicular to the fibre axis. Both chains follow right-handed helices, but owing to the dyad the sequences of the atoms in the two chains run in opposite directions. Each chain loosely resembles Furberg's[2] model No. 1; that is, the bases are on the inside of the helix and the phosphates on the outside. The configuration of the sugar and the atoms near it is close to Furberg's 'standard configuration', the sugar being roughly perpendicular to the attached base. There is a residue on each chain every 3·4 A. in the *z*-direction. We have assumed an angle of 36° between adjacent residues in the same chain, so that the structure repeats after 10 residues on each chain, that is, after 34 A. The distance of a phosphorus atom from the fibre axis is 10 A. As the phosphates are on the outside, cations have easy access to them.

The structure is an open one, and its water content is rather high. At lower water contents we would expect the bases to tilt so that the structure could become more compact.

The novel feature of the structure is the manner in which the two chains are held together by the purine and pyrimidine bases. The planes of the bases are perpendicular to the fibre axis. They are joined together in pairs, a single base from one chain being hydrogen-bonded to a single base from the other chain, so that the two lie side by side with identical *z*-co-ordinates. One of the pair must be a purine and the other a pyrimidine for bonding to occur. The hydrogen bonds are made as follows: purine position 1 to pyrimidine position 1; purine position 6 to pyrimidine position 6.

If it is assumed that the bases only occur in the structure in the most plausible tautomeric forms (that is, with the keto rather than the enol configurations) it is found that only specific pairs of bases can bond together. These pairs are: adenine (purine) with thymine (pyrimidine), and guanine (purine) with cytosine (pyrimidine).

In other words, if an adenine forms one member of a pair, on either chain, then on these assumptions the other member must be thymine; similarly for guanine and cytosine. The sequence of bases on a single chain does not appear to be restricted in any way. However, if only specific pairs of bases can be formed, it follows that if the sequence of bases on one chain is given, then the sequence on the other chain is automatically determined.

It has been found experimentally[3,4] that the ratio of the amounts of adenine to thymine, and the ratio of guanine to cytosine, are always very close to unity for deoxyribose nucleic acid.

It is probably impossible to build this structure with a ribose sugar in place of the deoxyribose, as the extra oxygen atom would make too close a van der Waals contact.

The previously published X-ray data[5,6] on deoxyribose nucleic acid are insufficient for a rigorous test of our structure. So far as we can tell, it is roughly compatible with the experimental data, but it must be regarded as unproved until it has been checked against more exact results. Some of these are given in the following communications. We were not aware of the details of the results presented there when we devised our structure, which rests mainly though not entirely on published experimental data and stereochemical arguments.

It has not escaped our notice that the specific pairing we have postulated immediately suggests a possible copying mechanism for the genetic material.

Full details of the structure, including the conditions assumed in building it, together with a set of co-ordinates for the atoms, will be published elsewhere.

We are much indebted to Dr. Jerry Donohue for constant advice and criticism, especially on interatomic distances. We have also been stimulated by a knowledge of the general nature of the unpublished experimental results and ideas of Dr. M. H. F. Wilkins, Dr. R. E. Franklin and their co-workers at

Fig. 178. No. 99. Watson and Crick. First page of the journal article.

99

JAMES DEWEY WATSON
(b. 1928)

FRANCIS HARRY COMPTON CRICK
(b. 1916)

A Structure for Deoxyribose Nucleic Acid.

In: *Nature* 171 (1953): 737–38.

[journal number] Vol. 171, No. 4356, 25 April 1953: $[1]^{40}$. 40 leaves, pp. *cclxix* cclxx–cclxxviii *709* 710–732 i–xii 733–758 cclxxix–cclxxxvi. Printed wrappers.

[article] $[1]_{26}{}^{r}$–$[1]_{26}{}^{v}$, pp. 737–738. 1 line-block illustration in text.

[offprint, 1-article version] *A Structure for Deoxyribose Nucleic Acid.* Reprinted from Nature, Vol. 171, p. 737, April 25, 1953.

1 leaf, pp. *1–2.* 1 line-block figure in text.

Reimposed, with different page breaks, and partially reset to accommodate the different placement of the figure.

[offprint, 3-article version] *Molecular Structure of Nucleic Acids.* Reprinted from Nature, Vol. 171, p. 737, April 25, 1953.

$[1]^{6}$ $[2]_{1}$. 7 leaves, pp. *1* 2–13 [1]. Fig. [1], 1–2, [1]: 2 line-block and 2 halftone illustrations in text.

Reimposed in single-column pages, with different page breaks and different placement of the illustrations; the paper by Watson and Crick partially reset (as in the 1-article offprint) to accommodate the different placement of the figure. Reprints three articles from *Nature* 171 (1953): Watson and Crick, "A Structure for Deoxyribose Nucleic Acid" (pp. 1–4); M.H.F. Wilkins, A. R. Stokes, and H. R. Wilson, "Molecular Structure of Deoxypentose Nucleic Acid" (pp. 4–9); and Rosalind E. Franklin and R. G. Gosling, "Molecular Configuration in Sodium Thymonucleate" (pp. 9–12).

GM 256.3. *Heirs of Hippocrates* 2342.

This paper by James D. Watson and Francis H.C. Crick records the discovery of the molecular structure of deoxyribonucleic acid (DNA), the main component of chromosomes and the material that transfers genetic characteristics in all life forms. Publication of this paper initiated the science of molecular biology. Forty years after Watson and Crick's discovery, so much of the basic understanding of medicine and disease has advanced to the

WATSON

(*Reprinted from Nature, Vol.* 171, *p.* 737, *April* 25, 1953)

A Structure for Deoxyribose Nucleic Acid

WE wish to suggest a structure for the salt of deoxyribose nucleic acid (D.N.A.). This structure has novel features which are of considerable biological interest.

A structure for nucleic acid has already been proposed by Pauling and Corey[1]. They kindly made their manuscript available to us in advance of publication. Their model consists of three intertwined chains, with the phosphates near the fibre axis, and the bases on the outside. In our opinion, this structure is unsatisfactory for two reasons: (1) We believe that the material which gives the X-ray diagrams is the salt, not the free acid. Without the acidic hydrogen atoms it is not clear what forces would hold the structure together, especially as the negatively charged phosphates near the axis will repel each other. (2) Some of the van der Waals distances appear to be too small.

Another three-chain structure has also been suggested by Fraser (in the press). In his model the phosphates are on the outside and the bases on the inside, linked together by hydrogen bonds. This structure as described is rather ill-defined, and for this reason we shall not comment on it.

We wish to put forward a radically different structure for the salt of deoxyribose nucleic acid. This structure has two helical chains each coiled round the same axis (see diagram). We have made the usual chemical assumptions, namely, that each chain consists of phosphate di-ester groups joining β-D-deoxyribofuranose residues with 3′,5′ linkages. The two chains (but not their bases) are related by a dyad perpendicular to the fibre axis. Both chains follow right-handed helices, but owing to the dyad the sequences of the atoms in the two chains run in opposite directions. Each chain loosely resembles Furberg's[2] model No. 1; that is, the bases are on the inside of the helix and the phosphates on the outside. The configuration of the sugar and the atoms near it is close to Furberg's 'standard configuration', the sugar being roughly perpendicular to the attached base. There is a residue on each chain every 3·4 A. in the z-direction. We have assumed an angle of 36° between adjacent residues in the same chain, so that the structure repeats after 10 residues on each chain, that is, after 34 A. The distance of a phosphorus atom from the fibre axis is 10 A. As the phosphates are on the outside, cations have easy access to them.

The structure is an open one, and its water content is rather high. At lower water contents we would expect the bases to tilt so that the structure could become more compact.

The novel feature of the structure is the manner in which the two chains are held together by the purine and pyrimidine bases. The planes of the bases are perpendicular to the fibre axis. They are joined together in pairs, a single base from one chain being

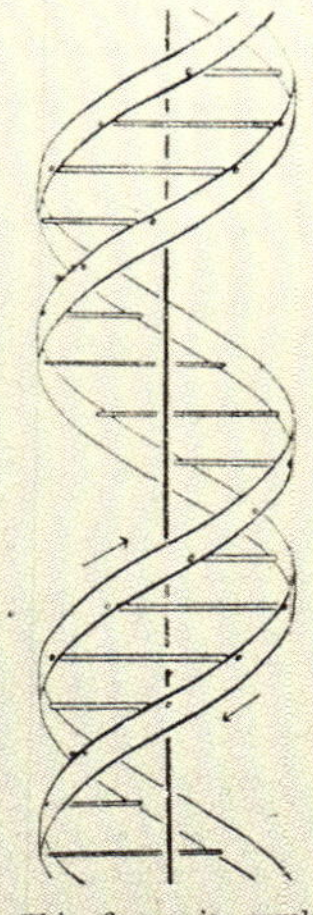

This figure is purely diagrammatic. The two ribbons symbolize the two phosphate—sugar chains, and the horizontal rods the pairs of bases holding the chains together. The vertical line marks the fibre axis

hydrogen-bonded to a single base from the other chain, so that the two lie side by side with identical z-co-ordinates. One of the pair must be a purine and the other a pyrimidine for bonding to occur. The hydrogen bonds are made as follows: purine position 1 to pyrimidine position 1; purine position 6 to pyrimidine position 6.

If it is assumed that the bases only occur in the structure in the most plausible tautomeric forms (that is, with the keto rather than the enol configurations) it is found that only specific pairs of bases can bond together. These pairs are: adenine (purine) with thymine (pyrimidine), and guanine (purine) with cytosine (pyrimidine).

In other words, if an adenine forms one member of a pair, on either chain, then on these assumptions the other member must be thymine; similarly for guanine and cytosine. The sequence of bases on a single chain does not appear to be restricted in any way. However, if only specific pairs of bases can be formed, it follows that if the sequence of bases on one chain is given, then the sequence on the other chain is automatically determined.

It has been found experimentally[3,4] that the ratio of the amounts of adenine to thymine, and the ratio of guanine to cytosine, are always very close to unity for deoxyribose nucleic acid.

It is probably impossible to build this structure with a ribose sugar in place of the deoxyribose, as the extra oxygen atom would make too close a van der Waals contact.

Fig. 179. No. 99. Watson and Crick. The first and last pages of the two-page, single-paper offprint, with Watson's signature on the second page.

The previously published X-ray data[5,6] on deoxyribose nucleic acid are insufficient for a rigorous test of our structure. So far as we can tell, it is roughly compatible with the experimental data, but it must be regarded as unproved until it has been checked against more exact results. Some of these are given in the following communications. We were not aware of the details of the results presented there when we devised our structure, which rests mainly though not entirely on published experimental data and stereochemical arguments.

It has not escaped our notice that the specific pairing we have postulated immediately suggests a possible copying mechanism for the genetic material.

Full details of the structure, including the conditions assumed in building it, together with a set of co-ordinates for the atoms, will be published elsewhere.

We are much indebted to Dr. Jerry Donohue for constant advice and criticism, especially on interatomic distances. We have also been stimulated by a knowledge of the general nature of the unpublished experimental results and ideas of Dr. M. H. F. Wilkins, Dr. R. E. Franklin and their co-workers at King's College, London. One of us (J. D. W.) has been aided by a fellowship from the National Foundation for Infantile Paralysis.

J. D. WATSON
F. H. C. CRICK

Medical Research Council Unit for the Study of the Molecular Structure of Biological Systems,
Cavendish Laboratory, Cambridge.
April 2.

[1] Pauling, L., and Corey, R. B., *Nature*, **171**, 346 (1953); *Proc. U.S. Nat. Acad. Sci.*, **39**, 84 (1953).

[2] Furberg, S., *Acta Chem. Scand.*, **6**, 634 (1952).

[3] Chargaff, E., for references see Zamenhof, S., Brawerman, G., and Chargaff, E., *Biochim. et Biophys. Acta*, **9**, 402 (1952).

[4] Wyatt, G. R., *J. Gen. Physiol.*, **36**, 201 (1952).

[5] Astbury, W. T., Symp. Soc. Exp. Biol. 1, Nucleic Acid, 66 (Camb. Univ. Press, 1947).

[6] Wilkins, M. H. F., and Randall, J. T., *Biochim. et Biophys. Acta*, **10**, 192 (1953).

Printed in Great Britain by Fisher, Knight & Co., Ltd., St. Albans.

molecular level that their paper may be considered the most significant single contribution to biology and medicine in the twentieth century.

In the early 1950s, several independent groups of researchers in both England and America were attempting to discover the structure of DNA, the extraordinarily complex molecule that had been identified in 1944 as the substance of the gene. At King's College in London, Maurice Wilkins, using X-ray diffraction, was able to demonstrate the overall helical structure of DNA, and Rosalind Franklin, his research associate, had succeeded in making X-ray diffraction photographs of DNA that clearly showed two helically arranged polynucleotide chains. Meanwhile Erwin Chargaff, at Columbia University in New York, had demonstrated that the amount of adenine in DNA equals the amount of thymine, and the amount of cytosine equals the amount of guanine. Using this information, James Watson and Francis Crick, both then affiliated with the Cavendish Laboratory at Cambridge University, began constructing cardboard and metal models of the molecule. By late February 1953 the two had arrived at a structure in which neither they nor their colleagues could find any flaw, and this structure was first announced in the present paper.

Watson and Crick's DNA model consists of two antiparallel (i.e., each running in a direction opposite to the other) helical strands of sequential deoxyribonucleotides, each deoxyribonucleotide consisting of a base (either adenine, thymine, cytosine, or guanine), a deoxyribose sugar, and a phosphate. The two strands are held together by hydrogen bonds between complementary bases in the two strands, forming a double helix. The bases on each strand can be arranged in any order, but since each base is complementary to only one other, the hydrogen bonds between the two strands are restricted to adenine-thymine and cytosine-guanine pairs. It was this restricted pairing in their model that enabled Watson and Crick to suggest how DNA might replicate itself: because the two strands of the DNA chromosome are complementary, each strand, upon cell division, can serve as the template for a complementary strand. Watson and Crick's model thus provides an explanation of how genetic material can be passed on to succeeding generations of cells.

When Watson and Crick's paper was submitted for publication in *Nature*, Sir Lawrence Bragg, the director of the Cavendish Laboratory at Cambridge, and Sir John Randall of King's College agreed that the paper should be published simultaneously with those of two other groups of researchers who had also prepared important papers on DNA: Maurice Wilkins, A. R. Stokes, and H. R. Wilson, authors of "Molecular Structure of Deoxypentose Nucleic Acids," and Rosalind Franklin and Raymond Gosling, who submitted the paper "Molecular Configuration in Sodium Thymonucleate." The three papers were published in *Nature* under the general title "The Molecular Structure of Nucleic Acids." Shortly afterwards, Watson and Crick published their paper "Genetical Implications of the Structure of Deoxyribonucleic Acid," in which they elaborated on their proposed DNA replication mechanism.[1] In 1962, Watson, Crick, and Wilkins shared the Nobel Prize in Physiology or Medicine.

JMN

Two offprints exist of Watson and Crick's paper: a single sheet containing the Watson and Crick article only, and a fourteen-page pamphlet containing the papers of all three research groups. The pamphlet pages are smaller in size than the single leaf, which has the same dimensions as the leaves of the journal, and the layout is different, the single-leaf offprint being printed in two columns like the journal, the pamphlet in single-column pages. The page breaks are different in each of the two offprints and the journal, as is the placement of the illustrations relative to the text. Despite these differences, all three versions appear to have been printed from the same setting of type, except that in the two offprints one paragraph of text has been reset to accommodate the placement of the diagram of the DNA molecule. This was embedded in the text of the journal article but stands at the head of a column, without flanking text, in each offprint. It has recently been stated that in 1953 *Nature* was set in Monotype and that plates made from this setting were used to print the journal, whereas the offprints were printed from the standing type.[2] The differences in imposition between the journal and the two offprints are consistent with this procedure.[3]

[ED.]

1. *Nature* 171 (1953): 964–67.
2. William Patrick Watson, *Catalogue Five: Science, Medicine and Natural History* (London, 1994), no. 145.
3. For an effort to establish the priority of the two offprints, see the Introduction.

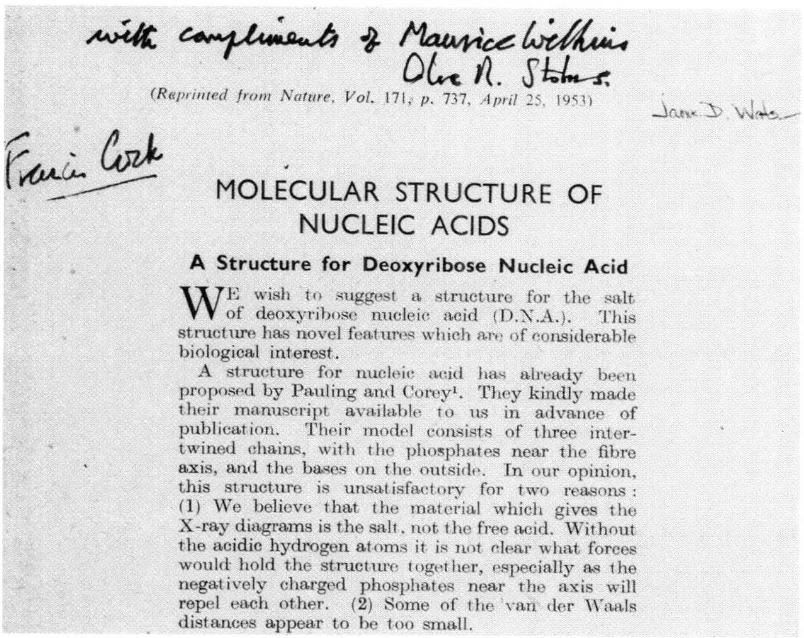
(Reprinted from Nature, Vol. 171, p. 737, April 25, 1953)

MOLECULAR STRUCTURE OF NUCLEIC ACIDS

A Structure for Deoxyribose Nucleic Acid

WE wish to suggest a structure for the salt of deoxyribose nucleic acid (D.N.A.). This structure has novel features which are of considerable biological interest.

A structure for nucleic acid has already been proposed by Pauling and Corey[1]. They kindly made their manuscript available to us in advance of publication. Their model consists of three intertwined chains, with the phosphates near the fibre axis, and the bases on the outside. In our opinion, this structure is unsatisfactory for two reasons: (1) We believe that the material which gives the X-ray diagrams is the salt, not the free acid. Without the acidic hydrogen atoms it is not clear what forces would hold the structure together, especially as the negatively charged phosphates near the axis will repel each other. (2) Some of the van der Waals distances appear to be too small.

Fig. 180. No. 99. Watson and Crick. A copy of the three-paper offprint signed by Crick, Watson, Wilkins, and Stokes.

1973, *British Journal of Radiology*, 46, 1016–1022

Computerized transverse axial scanning (tomography): Part I. Description of system

G. N. Hounsfield

Central Research Laboratories of EMI Limited, Hayes, Middlesex

(*Received February, 1973 and in revised form July, 1973*)

Abstract

This article describes a technique in which X-ray transmission readings are taken through the head at a multitude of angles: from these data, absorption values of the material contained within the head are calculated on a computer and presented as a series of pictures of slices of the cranium. The system is approximately 100 times more sensitive than conventional X-ray systems to such an extent that variations in soft tissues of nearly similar density can be displayed.

For many years past, X-ray techniques have been developed along the same lines, namely the recording on photographic film of the shadow of the object to be viewed. Recently, it has been realized that this is not the most efficient method of utilizing all the information that can be obtained from the X-ray beam. Oldendorf (1961) carried out experiments based on principles similar to those described here, but it was not then fully realized that very high efficiencies could be achieved and so, picture reconstruction techniques were not fully developed.

As the exposure of the patient to X rays must be restricted, there is an upper limit to the number of photons that may be passed through the body during the examination, and so to the amount of information that can be obtained. It is, therefore, of great importance that the method of examination ensures that all the information obtained is fully utilized and interpreted with maximum efficiency.

In the conventional film technique a large proportion of the available information is lost in attempting to portray all the information from a three-dimensional body on a two-dimensional photographic plate, the image superimposing all objects from front to rear. In order that any one internal structure may be seen, it must clearly stand out against the variations of the materials in front and behind it.

The technique to be described divides the head into a series of slices, each being irradiated via its edges; the radiation is confined to the slice and for this reason, unlike conventional X-ray techniques, the information derived from any object within the slice is unaffected by variations in the material on either side of the slice. Data are processed and displayed by digital computer methods.

A report on this work was presented at the April 1972 Annual Congress of the British Institute of Radiology (Ambrose and Hounsfield, 1973). A short account has also appeared in the *New Scientist* (*Technology Review*), 1972.

Principles of the Method

The aim of the system is to produce a series of images by a tomographic method as illustrated in Fig. 1. Each image shown at the bottom of the figure is derived from a particular slice.

In the actual equipment, the patient is scanned by a narrow beam of X rays. The X-ray tube, detectors, and collimators are fixed to a common frame, as shown in Fig. 2, those rays which pass through the head being detected by two collimated sensing devices (scintillation detectors) which always point towards the X-ray source. Both X-ray source and detectors scan across the patient's head linearly taking 160 readings of transmissions through the head as shown in scan 1 on the scanning sequence diagram (Fig. 3). At the end of the scan the scanning system is rotated 1 deg. and the process is repeated, as shown in scans 2 and 3. This continues for 180 deg. when 28,800 (180 × 160) readings of transmission will have been taken by each detector. These are stored in a disc file for processing by a mini computer. A picture is reconstructed from the data by the following method:

A separate detector measures the intensity of the X-ray source and the readings taken from this can be used to calculate absorption by the material along the X-ray beam path, where

$$\text{Absorption} = \log \frac{\text{Intensity of X rays at source}}{\text{Intensity of X rays at detector}}$$

If the body is divided into a series of small cubes each having a calculable value of absorption, then the sum of the absorption values of the cubes which are contained within the X-ray beam will equal the total absorption of the beam path. Each beam path, therefore, forms one of a series of 28,800 simultaneous equations, in which there are 6,400 variables and, providing that there are more equations than variables, then the values of each cube in the slice can be solved. In short there must be more X-ray readings than picture points.

Fig. 181. No. 100. Hounsfield. Opening page of the journal article.

100

SIR GODFREY NEWBOLD HOUNSFIELD
(b. 1919)

Computerized Transverse Axial Scanning (Tomography): Part I. Description of System.

In: *British Journal of Radiology* 46 (1973): 1016–22.

[journal number] Vol. 46, No. 552, December 1973: 58 leaves, pp. i–xxxii 1015–1088 [10]. Printed wrappers.

[article] pp. 1016–1022. Fig. 1–10: 1 line-block and 9 halftone illustrations in text.

GM 2700.4.

Calculating machines and computers have been used to compile and analyze medical statistics since the 1860s, but the first significant application of electronic computer technology in the practice of medicine did not occur until the invention of computed tomography (CT) in 1973. Computed tomography provided the first means for visualizing, in three dimensions, virtually all types of tissue within the body. The principle of CT evolved from the work of the Austrian mathematician Johann Radon, who demonstrated in 1917 that the image of a three-dimensional object could be constructed from an infinite number of two-dimensional projections of the object;[1] however, this concept was not applied to medicine until over forty years later, when Allen M. Cormack published a paper stating that changes in tissue density could be computed from X-ray data.[2] Cormack never constructed a practical machine based on his work, probably because the computers of his day were inadequate to handle such numerous and complex calculations, and his findings received little attention at the time. It remained for Godfrey Hounsfield of the British firm EMI, working entirely independently from Cormack, to produce the first practical CT scanner, the clinical prototype of which was installed in early 1972. For their contributions to CT technology, Hounsfield and Cormack were awarded the Nobel Prize in Physiology or Medicine in 1979. This was the first time that researchers trained not in the medical sciences but in mathematics and engineering received the Nobel Prize in Medicine.

Hounsfield's scanner proved to be an immediate success, and improvements were not long in coming. Hounsfield's machine was designed only for brain scanning, but machines were soon developed that could apply CT to the entire body, although anatomical motion remained a serious problem in first-generation scanners. Later scanners, taking advantage of the enormous improvements in computer technology over the next two decades, dramatically increased the speed of scanning and image reconstruction. For example, in 1972, acquisition of data from a single X-ray projection or "slice" took 4½ minutes, with an extra 1½ minutes required to construct the image on screen; by 1980, with continuing improvements in both hardware and software, the time required for these operations had been reduced to 9.8 seconds. As the development of computer hardware and software continued to advance at an ever more rapid pace, there were parallel advances in CT speed. Image quality also steadily improved, and the coarse 3-mm. pixel images of the early machines gave way to sophisticated high-definition images. Parallel development of other scanning modalities led to other computerized imaging systems such as Magnetic Resonance Imaging (MRI). Only twenty years after the invention of CT, computer technology of one sort or another is applied in most fields of medicine and in nearly all fields of medical research.

JMN

1. J. H. Radon, "Über die Bestimmung von Funktionen durch ihre Integralwerte längs gewisser Mannigfaltigkeiten," *Berichte über die Verhandlungen der königlich sächsischen Gesellschaft der Wissenschaften zu Leipzig, Mathematisch-physische Klasse* 69 (1917): 262–77.

2. Allen M. Cormack, "Representation of a Function by Its Line Integrals, with Some Radiological Applications," *Journal of Applied Physics* 34 (1963): 2722–27; 35 (1964): 2908–13.

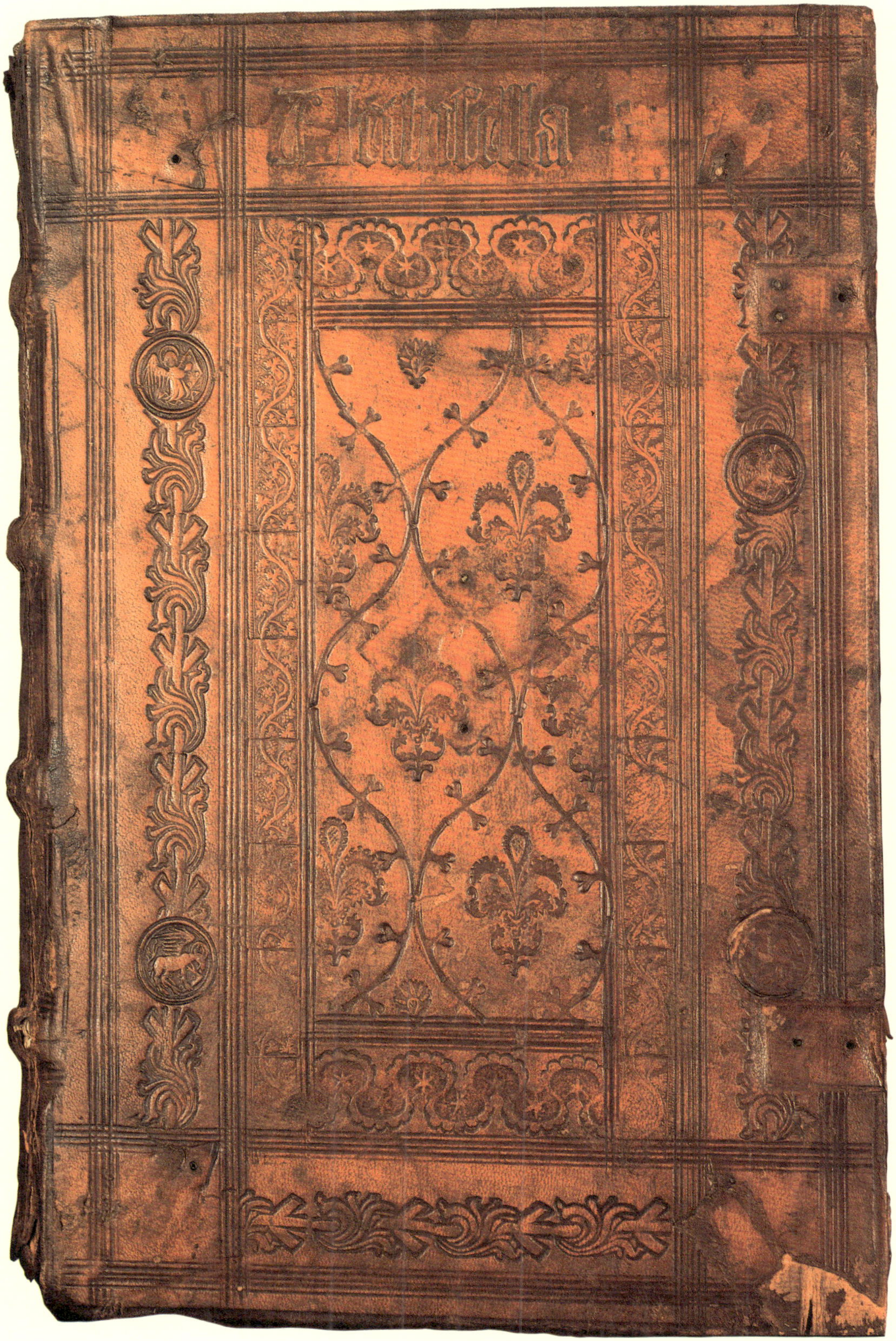

PLATE I. No. IC. Hippocrates. The *Articella* (1483), in a contemporary Nuremberg binding, a copy that once belonged to Hartmann Schedel, compiler of the *Nuremberg Chronicle*. This edition of the *Articella* contains the first printing of the Hippocratic Oath.

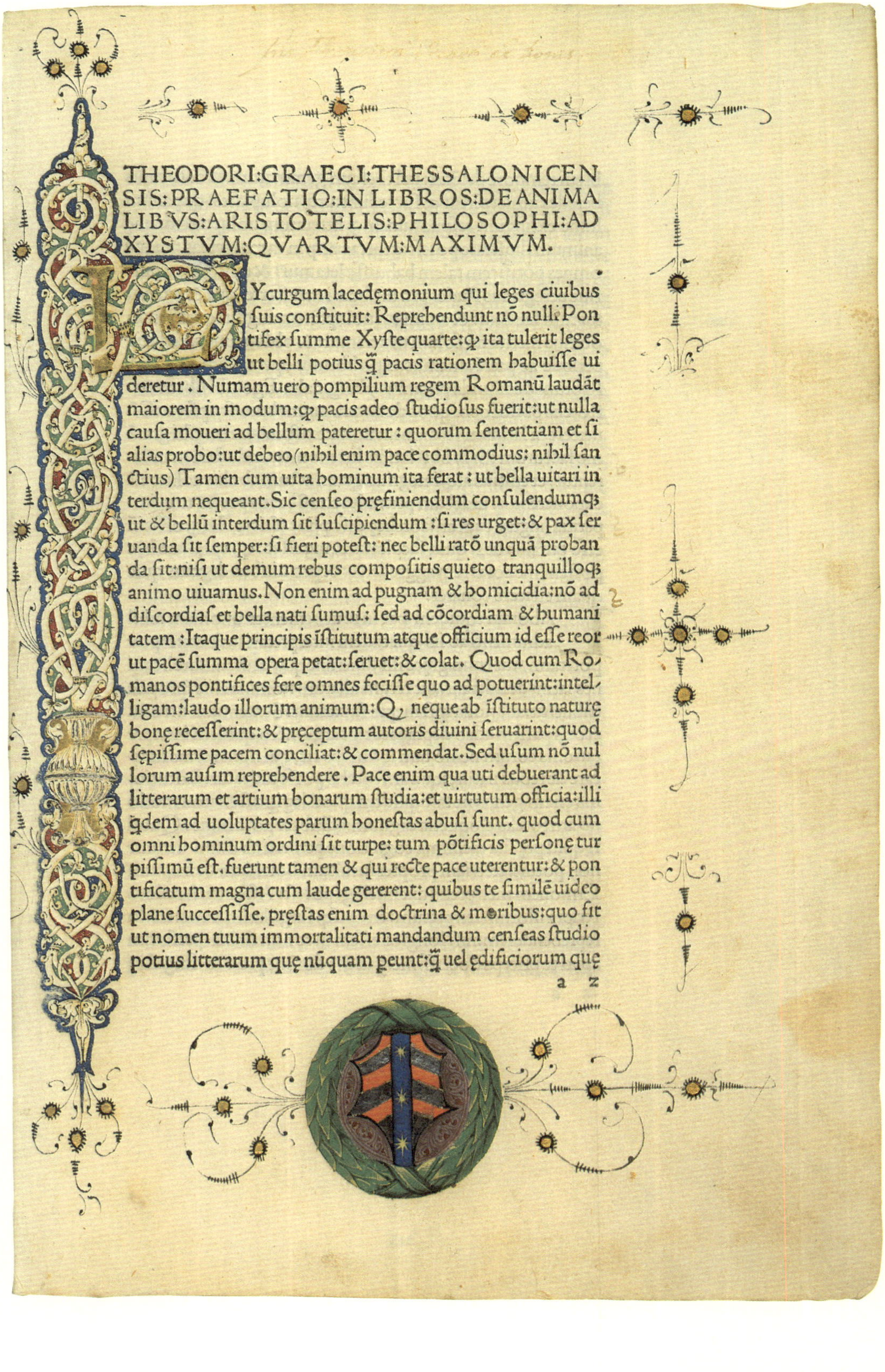
THEODORI:GRAECI:THESSALONICENSIS:PRAEFATIO:IN LIBROS:DE ANIMALIBVS:ARISTOTELIS:PHILOSOPHI:AD XYSTVM:QVARTVM:MAXIMVM.

LYcurgum lacedęmonium qui leges ciuibus
suis constituit: Reprehendunt nõ nulli. Pon
tifex summe Xyste quarte: q ita tulerit leges
ut belli potius q̃ pacis rationem habuisse ui
deretur. Numam uero pompilium regem Romanũ laudãt
maiorem in modum: q pacis adeo studiosus fuerit: ut nulla
causa moueri ad bellum pateretur: quorum sententiam et si
alias probo: ut debeo (nihil enim pace commodius: nihil san
ctius) Tamen cum uita hominum ita ferat: ut bella uitari in
terdum nequeant. Sic censeo prefiniendum consulendumq;
ut & bellũ interdum sit suscipiendum: si res urget: & pax ser
uanda sit semper: si fieri potest: nec belli ratõ unquã proban
da sit: nisi ut demum rebus compositis quieto tranquilloq;
animo uiuamus. Non enim ad pugnam & homicidia: nõ ad
discordias et bella nati sumus: sed ad cõcordiam & humani
tatem: Itaque principis ĩstitutum atque officium id esse reor
ut pacẽ summa opera petat: seruet: & colat. Quod cum Ro
manos pontifices fere omnes fecisse quo ad potuerint: intel
ligam: laudo illorum animum: Q, neque ab ĩstituto naturę
bonę recesserint: & pręceptum autoris diuini seruarint: quod
sępissime pacem conciliat: & commendat. Sed usum nõ nul
lorum ausim reprehendere. Pace enim qua uti debuerant ad
litterarum et artium bonarum studia: et uirtutum officia: illi
q̃dem ad uoluptates parum honestas abusi sunt. quod cum
omni hominum ordini sit turpe: tum põtificis personę tur
pissimũ est. fuerunt tamen & qui recte pace uterentur: & pon
tificatum magna cum laude gererent: quibus te similẽ uideo
plane successisse. prestas enim doctrina & moribus: quo fit
ut nomen tuum immortalitati mandandum censeas studio
potius litterarum quę nũquam peunt: q̃ uel ędificiorum quę

a 2

PLATE II. No. 2A. Aristotle. An illuminated leaf from a copy of the Latin *editio princeps* of *De animalibus* (1476).

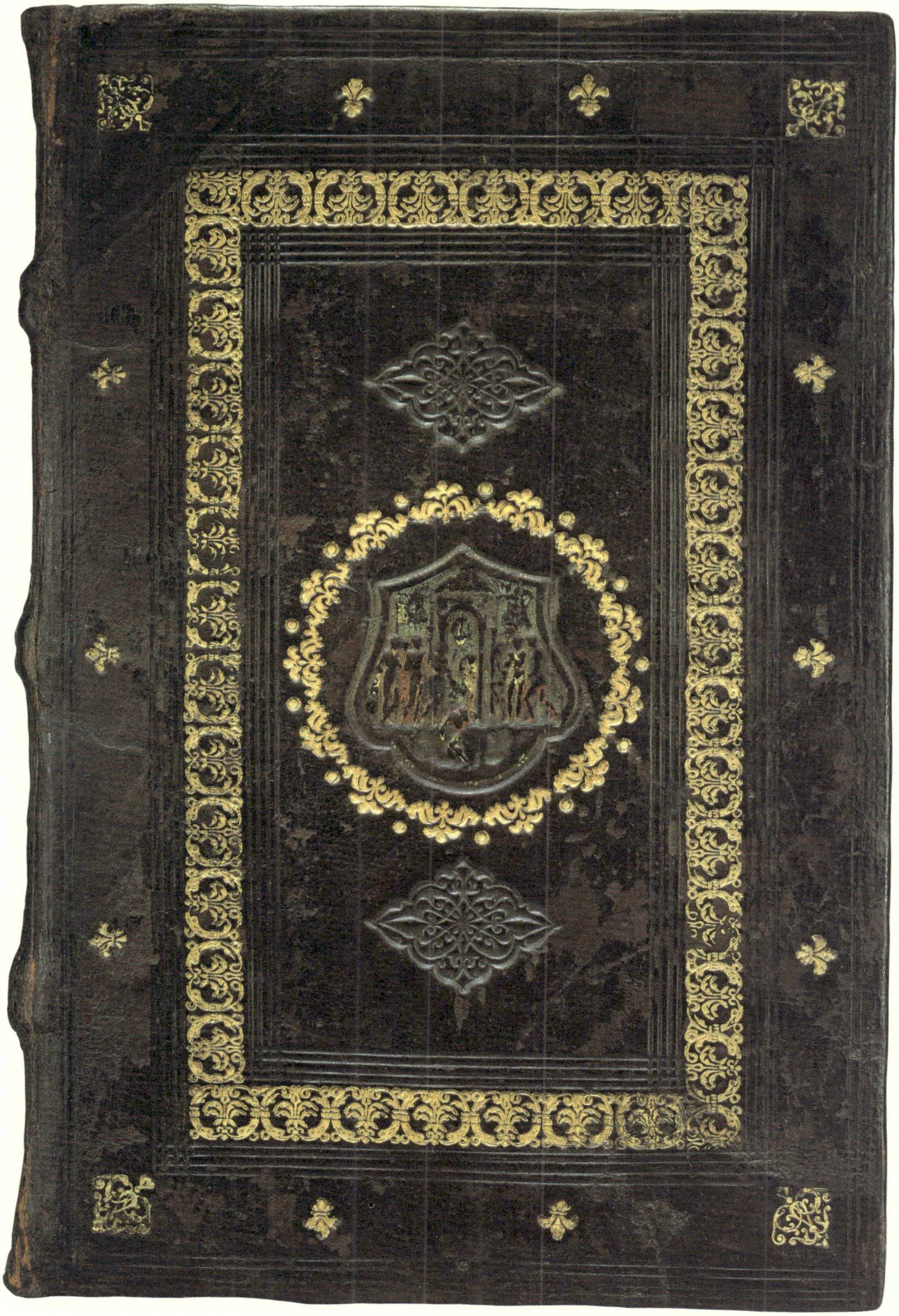

PLATE III. No. 2B. Aristotle. Volume II (1497) of the *Opera omnia* printed by Aldus Manutius. This copy was bound for Jean Grolier, ca. 1510–13, when he was resident in Milan as treasurer and receiver-general of the French in Lombardy.

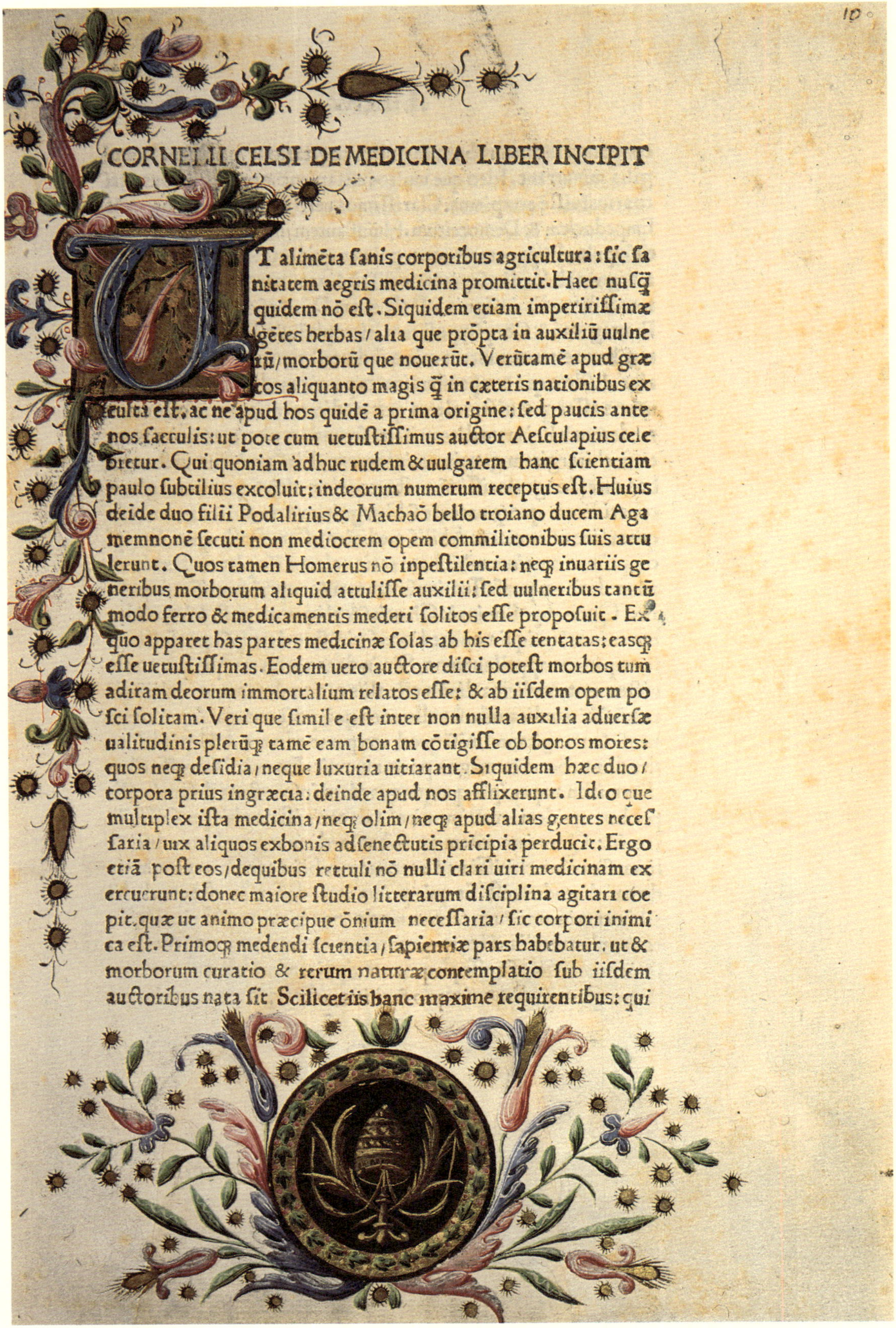

CORNELII CELSI DE MEDICINA LIBER INCIPIT

VT alimēta sanis corporibus agricultura: sic sa
nitatem aegris medicina promittit. Haec nusq̄
quidem nō est. Siquidem etiam imperitissimae
gētes herbas / alia que prōpta in auxiliū uulne
rū / morborū que nouerūt. Verūtamē apud grae
cos aliquanto magis q̄ in caeteris nationibus ex
culta est, ac ne apud hos quidē a prima origine: sed paucis ante
nos saeculis: ut pote cum uetustissimus auctor Aesculapius cele
bretur. Qui quoniam adhuc rudem & uulgarem hanc scientiam
paulo subtilius excoluit: indeorum numerum receptus est. Huius
deide duo filii Podalirius & Machaō bello troiano ducem Aga
memnonē secuti non mediocrem opem commilitonibus suis attu
lerunt. Quos tamen Homerus nō inpestilentia: neq̄ inuariis ge
neribus morborum aliquid attulisse auxilii: sed uulneribus tantū
modo ferro & medicamentis mederi solitos esse proposuit. Ex
quo apparet has partes medicinae solas ab his esse tentatas: easq̄
esse uetustissimas. Eodem uero auctore disci potest morbos tum
adiram deorum immortalium relatos esse: & ab iisdem opem po
sci solitam. Veri que simile est inter non nulla auxilia aduersae
ualitudinis plerūq̄ tamē eam bonam cōtigisse ob bonos mores:
quos neq̄ desidia / neque luxuria uitiarant. Siquidem haec duo /
corpora prius ingraecia: deinde apud nos afflixerunt. Ideo que
multiplex ista medicina / neq̄ olim / neq̄ apud alias gentes neces
saria / uix aliquos exbonis adsenectutis pricipia perducit. Ergo
etiā post eos / dequibus rettuli nō nulli clari uiri medicinam ex
ercuerunt: donec maiore studio litterarum disciplina agitari coe
pit. quae ut animo praecipue omnium necessaria / sic corpori inimi
ca est. Primoq̄ medendi scientia / sapientiae pars habebatur. ut &
morborum curatio & rerum naturae contemplatio sub iisdem
auctoribus nata sit Scilicet iis hanc maxime requirentibus: qui

PLATE IV. No. 4. Celsus. Illuminated leaf from a copy of the 1478 edition of *De medicina* at the College of Physicians of Philadephia. Osler described this volume as a "superb copy."

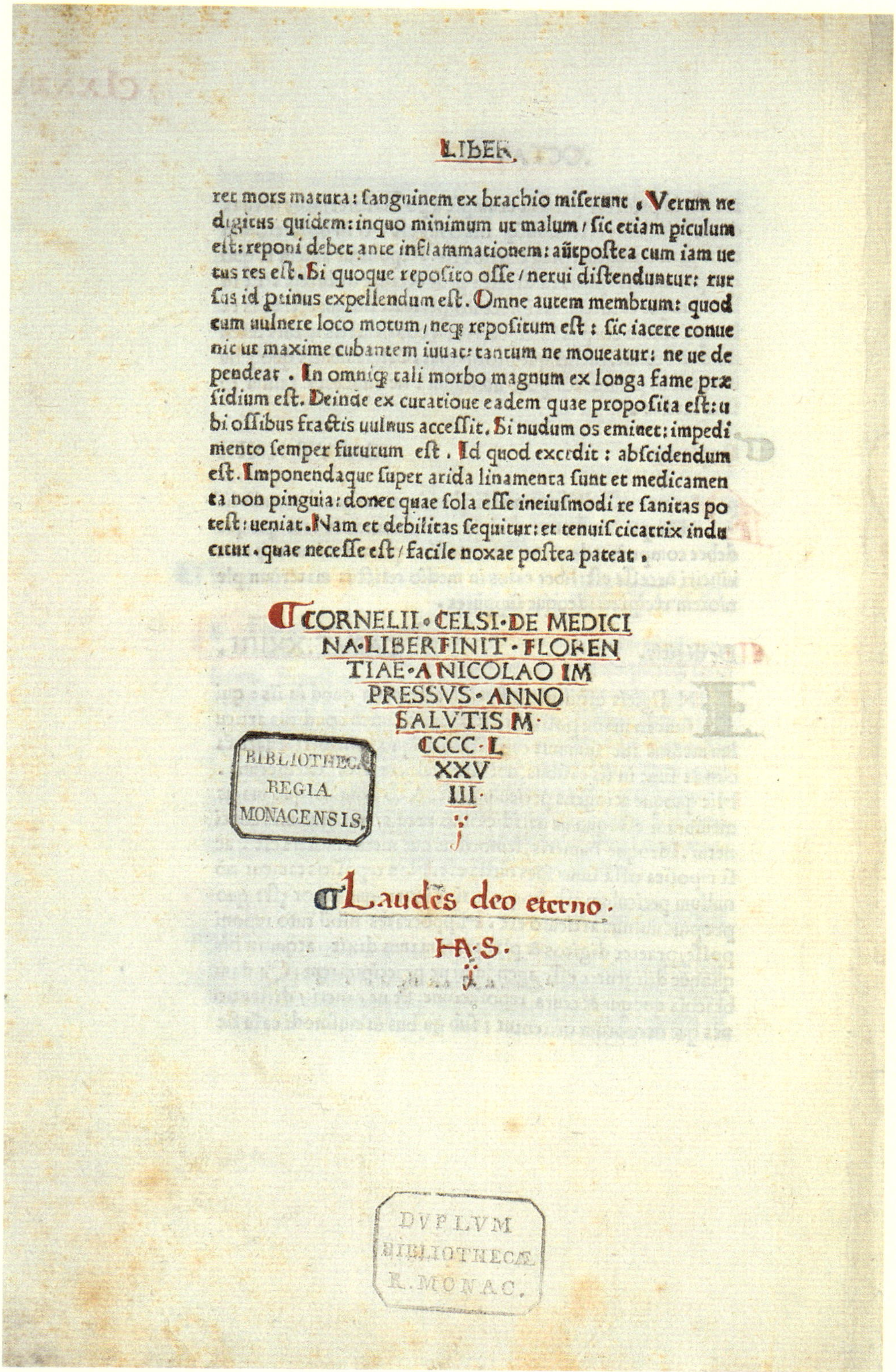

LIBER

ret mors matura: sanguinem ex brachio miserunt. Verum ne digitus quidem: inquo minimum ut malum / sic etiam piculum est: reponi debet ante inflammationem: aut postea cum iam ue tus res est. Si quoque reposito osse / nerui distenduntur: rur sus id ptinus expellendum est. Omne autem membrum: quod cum uulnere loco motum / neq3 repositum est: sic iacere conue nit ut maxime cubantem iuuat: tantum ne moueatur: ne ue de pendeat. In omniq3 tali morbo magnum ex longa fame præ sidium est. Deinde ex curatione eadem quae proposita est: u bi ossibus fractis uulnus accessit. Si nudum os eminet: impedi mento semper futurum est. Id quod excedit: abscidendum est. Imponendaque super arida linamenta sunt et medicamen ta non pinguia: donec quae sola esse ineiusmodi re sanitas po test: ueniat. Nam et debilitas sequitur: et tenuis cicatrix indu citur. quae necesse est / facile noxae postea pateat.

CORNELII · CELSI · DE MEDICI
NA · LIBER FINIT · FLOREN
TIAE · A NICOLAO IM
PRESSVS · ANNO
SALVTIS M ·
CCCC · L
XXV
III ·

Laudes deo eterno ·
H A S ·

PLATE V. No. 4. Celsus. Colophon page from a copy of the 1478 *De medicina* that belonged to Hartmann Schedel, compiler of the *Nuremberg Chronicle*. This copy was rubricated by Schedel himself, and the rubricator's inscription, signed with Schedel's initials, appears below the colophon.

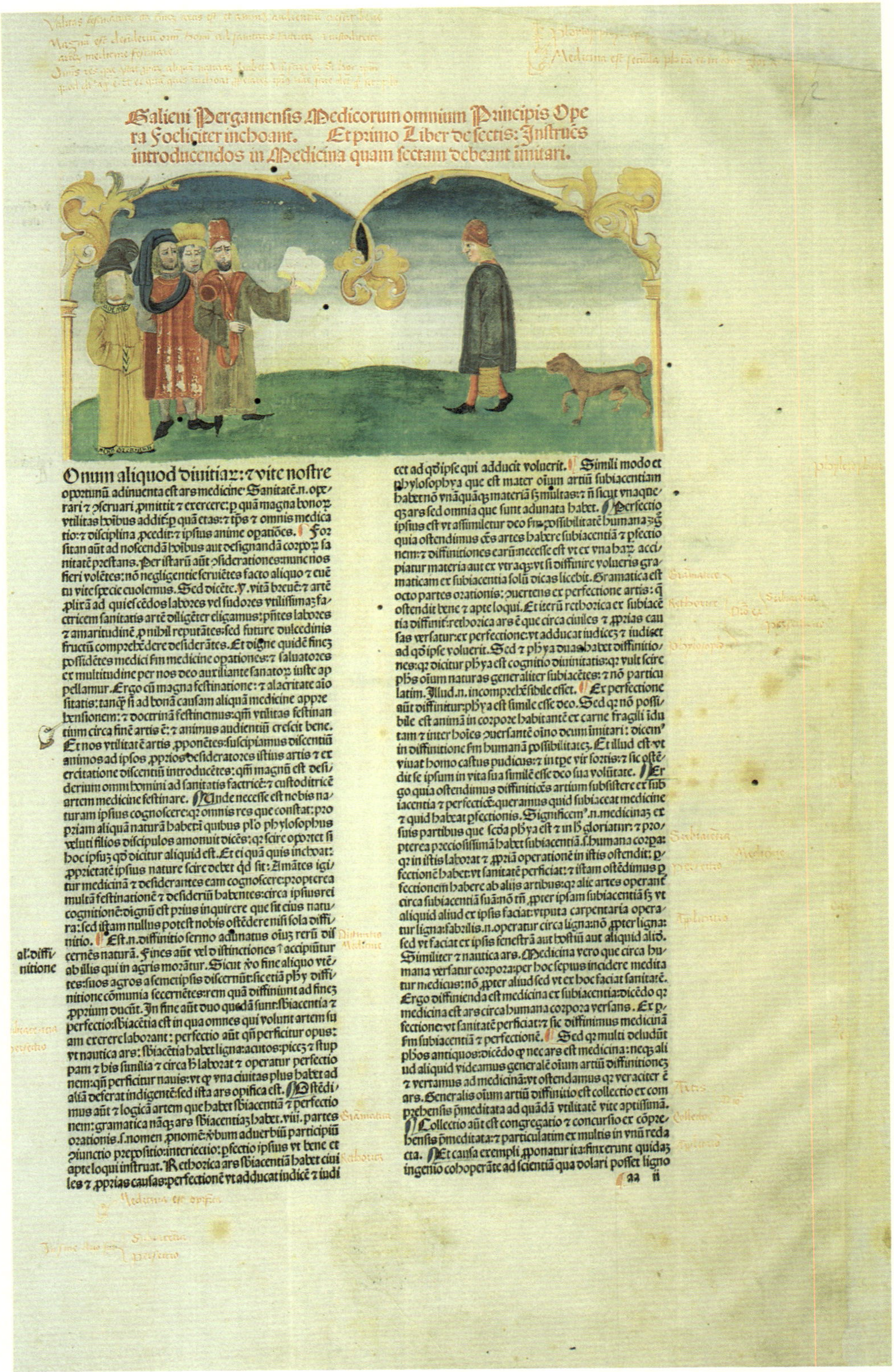
Galieni Pergamensis Medicorum omnium Principis Opera Foeliciter inchoant. Et primo Liber de sectis: Instruens introducendos in Medicina quam sectam debeant imitari.

Omnium aliquod diuitiarum: et vite nostre

PLATE VI. No. 5A. Galen. Illuminated leaf from a copy of the *editio princeps* (1490) of Galen's works in Latin.

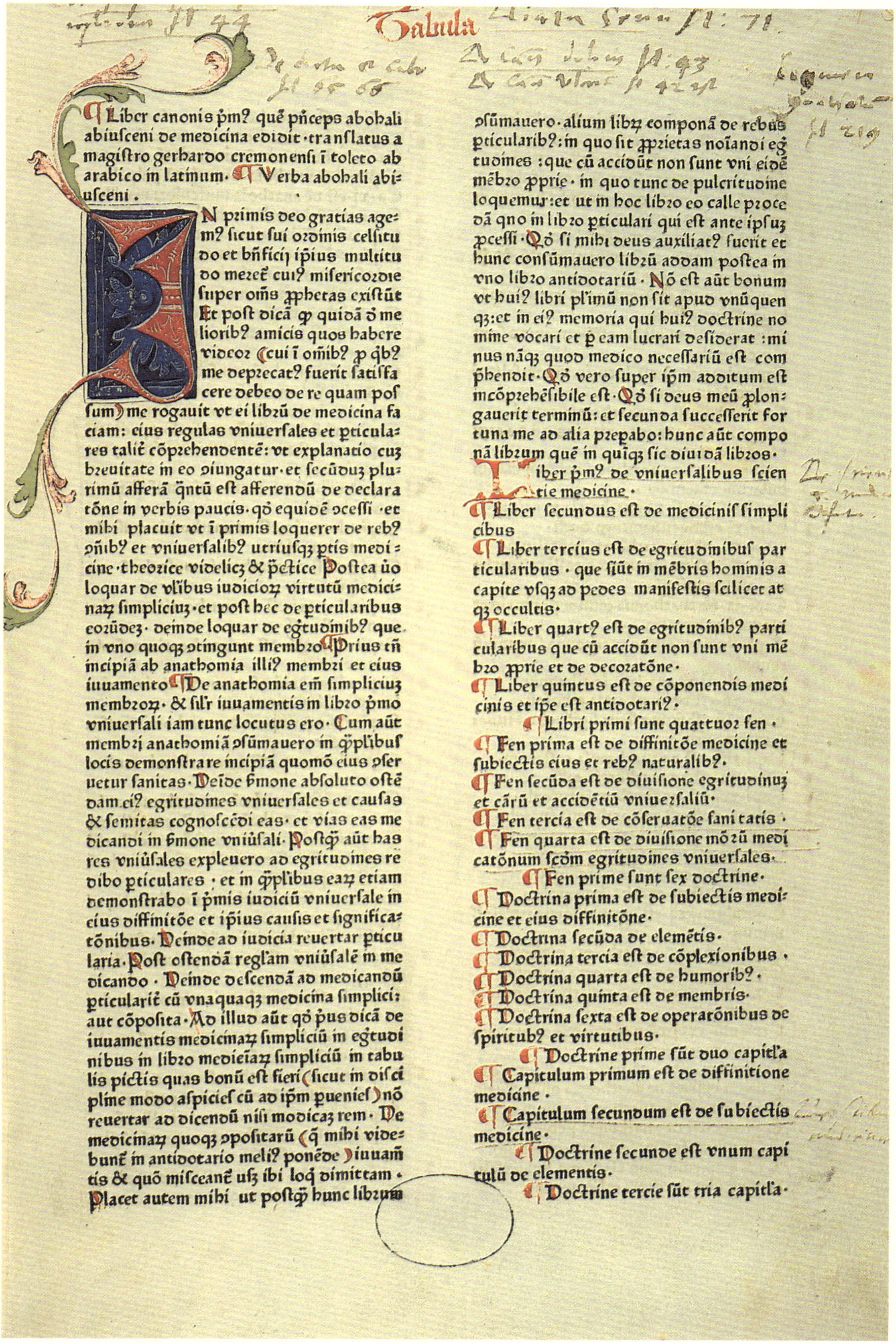

Tabula

¶ Liber canonis p̄m⁹ quē p̄nceps abobali abiusceni de medicina edidit · translatus a magistro gerbardo cremonensi ī toleto ab arabico in latinum. ¶ Verba abobali abiusceni.

In primis deo gratias agemus sicut sui ordinis celsitudo et beneficii ipsius multitudo merett cui⁹ misericordie super oms ꝓphetas existūt Et post dicā q quidā d̄ melioribus amicis quos habere videor (cui ī omib⁹ ꝓ qb⁹ me deprecat⁹ fuerit satisfacere debeo de re quam possum) me rogauit vt ei librū de medicina faciam: eius regulas vniuersales et p̄ticulares talie cōp̄hendentē: vt explanatio cuz breuitate in eo diungatur · et secūdū plurimū afferā qntū est afferendū de declaratōne in verbis paucis · qd equidē ocessi · et mihi placuit vt ī primis loquerer de reb⁹ cōib⁹ et vniuersalib⁹ vtriusqz p̄tis medicine · theorice videlicz & p̄ctice Postea uo loquar de vlibus iudicioꝝ virtutū medicinaꝝ simplicium · et post hec de p̄ticularibus eorūdez · deinde loquar de egtudinib⁹ que in vno quoqz otingunt membro · ¶ Prius tn̄ incipiā ab anathomia illi⁹ membri et eius iuuamento · ¶ De anathomia em̄ simpliciuz membroꝝ · & sil'r iuuamentis in libro p̄mo vniuersali iam tunc locutus ero · Cum aūt membri anathomiā ɔsūmauero in q̄plibus locis demonstrare incipiā quomō eius ɔseruetur sanitas · Deīde s̄mone absoluto ostēdam ei⁹ egritudines vniuersales et causas & semitas cognoscēdi eas · et vias eas medicandi in s̄mone vniūsali · Postq̄ aūt has res vniūsales expleuero ad egritudines redibo p̄ticulares · et in q̄plibus eaꝝ etiam demonstrabo ī p̄mis iudiciū vniuersale in eius diffinitōe et ipius causis et significatōnibus · Deinde ad iudicia reuertar p̄ticularia · Post ostendā reglam vniūsale in medicando · Deinde descendā ad medicandū p̄ticularit cū vnaquaqz medicina simplici aut cōposita · Ad illud aūt qd p̄us dicā de iuuamentis medicinaꝝ simpliciū in egtudinibus in libro medicinaꝝ simpliciū in tabulis pictis quas bonū est fieri (sicut in disciplīne modo aspicies cū ad ip̄m p̄uenies) nō reuertar ad dicendū nisi modicaz rem · De medicinaꝝ quoqz ɔpositarū (q̄ mihi videbunt in antidotario meli⁹ ponēde) iuuamtis & quō misceant ul̄ ibi loq dimittam · Placet autem mihi ut postq̄ hunc librum ɔsūmauero · alium libꝝ componā de rebus p̄ticularib⁹: in quo sit ɔprietas noīandi egtudines: que cū accidūt non sunt vni eidē mēbro ɔprie · in quo tunc de pulcritudine loquemur: et ut in hoc libro eo calle procedā quo in libro p̄ticulari qui est ante ipsuz p̄cessi · ¶ Qd si mihi deus auxiliat⁹ fuerit et hunc consūmauero librū addam postea in vno libro antidotariū · ¶ Nō est aūt bonum vt hui⁹ libri p'imū non sit apud vnūquenqz: et in ei⁹ memoria qui hui⁹ doctrine nomine vocari et p̄ eam lucrari desiderat: minus nāqz quod medico necessariū est comp̄hendit · ¶ Qd vero super ip̄m additum est incōp̄hēsibile est · ¶ Qd si deus meū ɔlongauerit terminū: et secunda successerit fortuna me ad alia p̄parabo: hunc aūt componā librum quē in quiqz sic diuidā libros ·

Liber p̄m⁹ de vniuersalibus sciencie medicine ·

¶ Liber secundus est de medicinis simplicibus

¶ Liber tercius est de egritudinibus particularibus · que siūt in mēbris hominis a capite vsqz ad pedes manifestis scilicet atqz occultis ·

¶ Liber quart⁹ est de egritudinib⁹ particularibus que cū accidūt non sunt vni mēbro ɔprie et de decoratōne ·

¶ Liber quintus est de cōponendis medicinis et ipe est antidotari⁹ ·

¶ Libri primi sunt quattuor fen ·

¶ Fen prima est de diffinitōe medicine et subiectis eius et reb⁹ naturalib⁹ ·

¶ Fen secūda est de diuisione egritudinuz et cārū et accidētiū vniuersaliū ·

¶ Fen tercia est de cōseruatōe sanitatis ·

¶ Fen quarta est de diuisione mōꝝ medicatōnum scdm̄ egritudines vniuersales ·

¶ Fen prime sunt sex doctrine ·

¶ Doctrina prima est de subiectis medicine et eius diffinitōne ·

¶ Doctrina secūda de elemētis ·

¶ Doctrina tercia est de cōplexionibus ·

¶ Doctrina quarta est de humorib⁹ ·

¶ Doctrina quinta est de membris ·

¶ Doctrina sexta est de operatōnibus de spiritib⁹ et virtutibus ·

¶ Doctrine prime sūt duo capitl'a

¶ Capitulum primum est de diffinitione medicine ·

¶ Capitulum secundum est de subiectis medicine ·

¶ Doctrine secunde est vnum capitulū de elementis ·

¶ Doctrine tercie sūt tria capitl'a ·

PLATE VII. No. 7B. Avicenna. Illuminated leaf from a copy of the undated Strassburg edition of Avicenna's works in Latin.

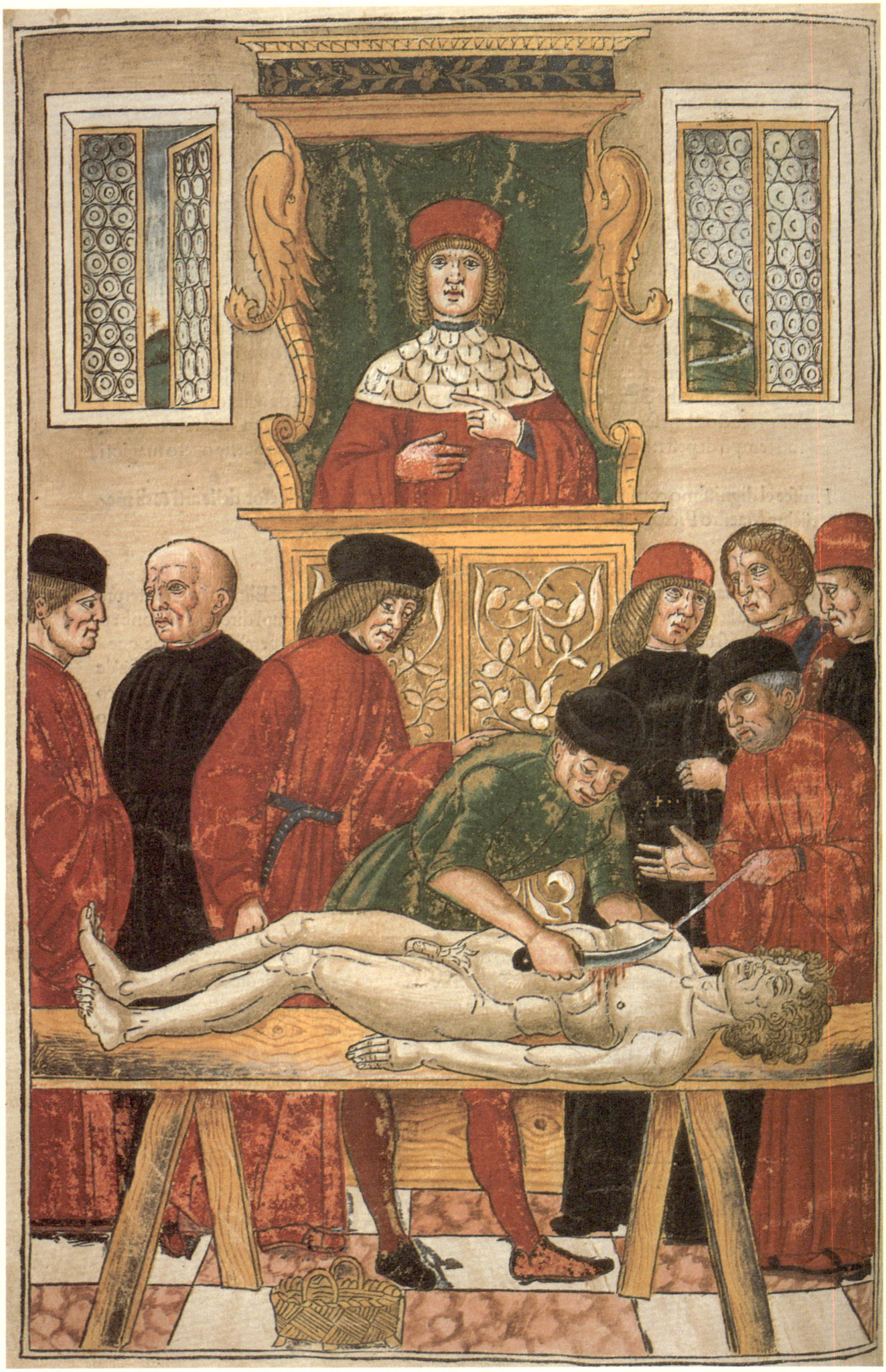

PLATE VIII. No. 10B. Johannes de Ketham. "Lesson in Dissection," from the Italian edition of 1493/94. In this copy the original woodcut was colored in red, green, and yellow, and this was further enhanced with hand-coloring. The red coloration of the professor's right hand and the prosecutor's left hand is evidence that the original coloring may have been applied by stencil.

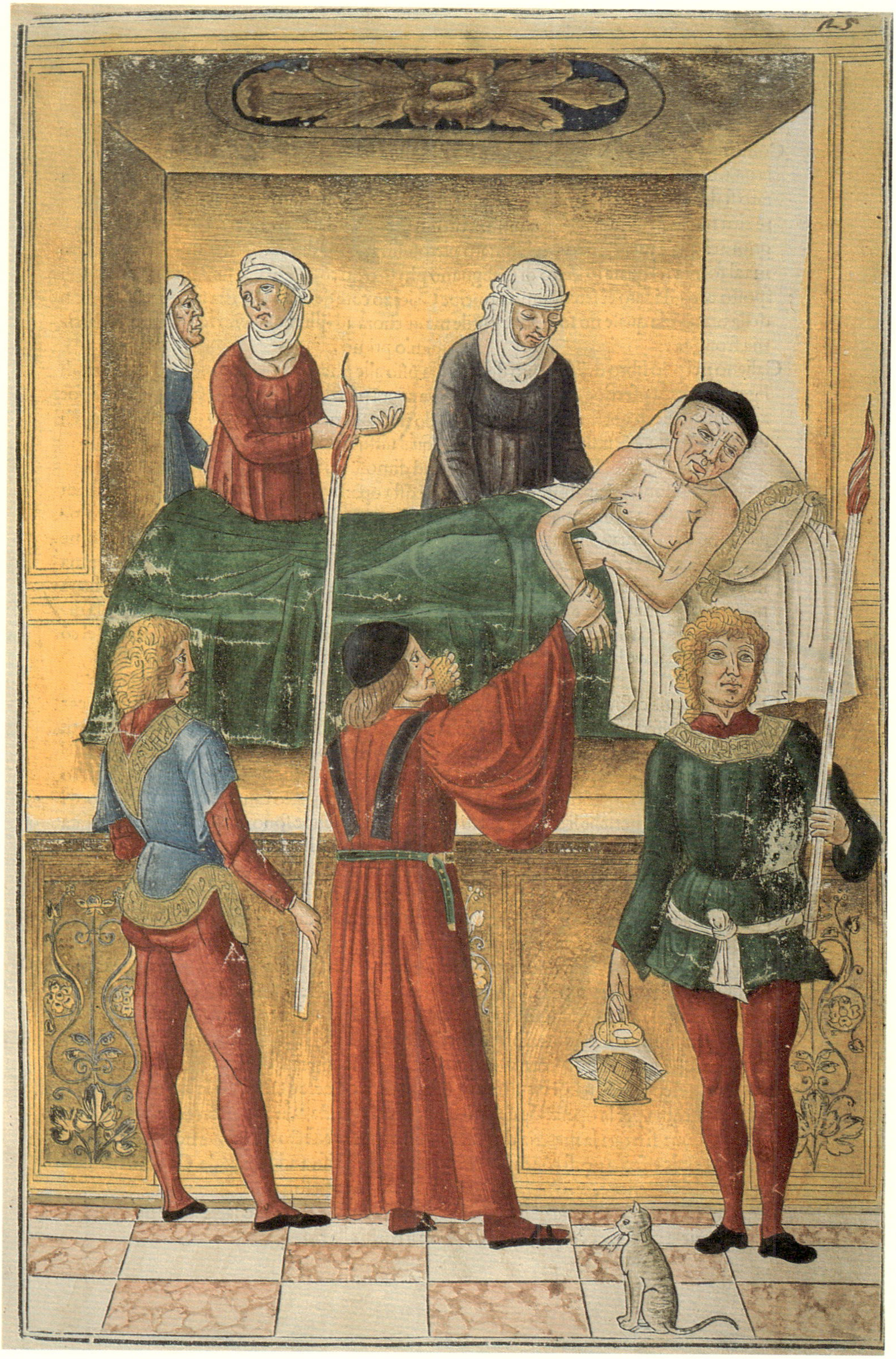

PLATE IX. No. 10B. Johannes de Ketham. "Doctor's visit to a plague patient," from the Italian edition of 1493/94. In this copy, the original woodcut has been colored by hand.

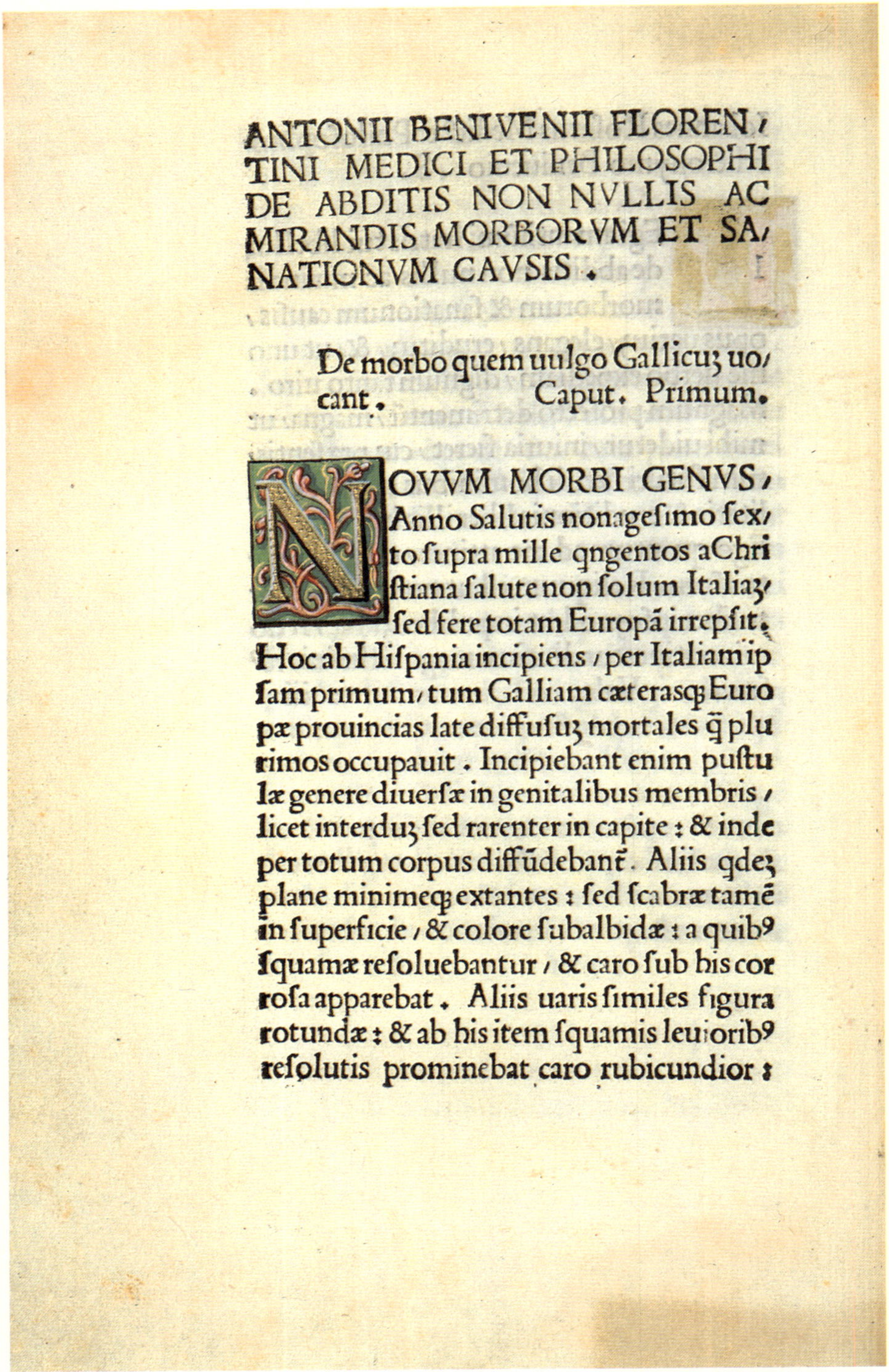
ANTONII BENIVENII FLOREN/
TINI MEDICI ET PHILOSOPHI
DE ABDITIS NON NVLLIS AC
MIRANDIS MORBORVM ET SA/
NATIONVM CAVSIS.

De morbo quem uulgo Gallicu; uo/
cant. Caput. Primum.

NOVVM MORBI GENVS/
Anno Salutis nonageſimo ſex/
to ſupra mille qngentos a Chri
ſtiana ſalute non ſolum Italia;/
ſed fere totam Europã irrepſit.
Hoc ab Hiſpania incipiens / per Italiam ip
ſam primum / tum Galliam cæterasq; Euro
pæ prouincias late diffuſu; mortales q̃ plu
rimos occupauit. Incipiebant enim puſtu
læ genere diuerſæ in genitalibus membris /
licet interdu; ſed rarenter in capite: & inde
per totum corpus diffũdebant̃. Aliis qde;
plane minimeq; extantes: ſed ſcabræ tamẽ
in ſuperficie / & colore ſubalbidæ: a quibꝰ
ſquamæ reſoluebantur / & caro ſub his cor
roſa apparebat. Aliis uaris ſimiles figura
rotundæ: & ab his item ſquamis leuioribꝰ
reſolutis prominebat caro rubicundior:

PLATE X. No. 12. Benivieni. Illuminated page from a copy of the first edition.

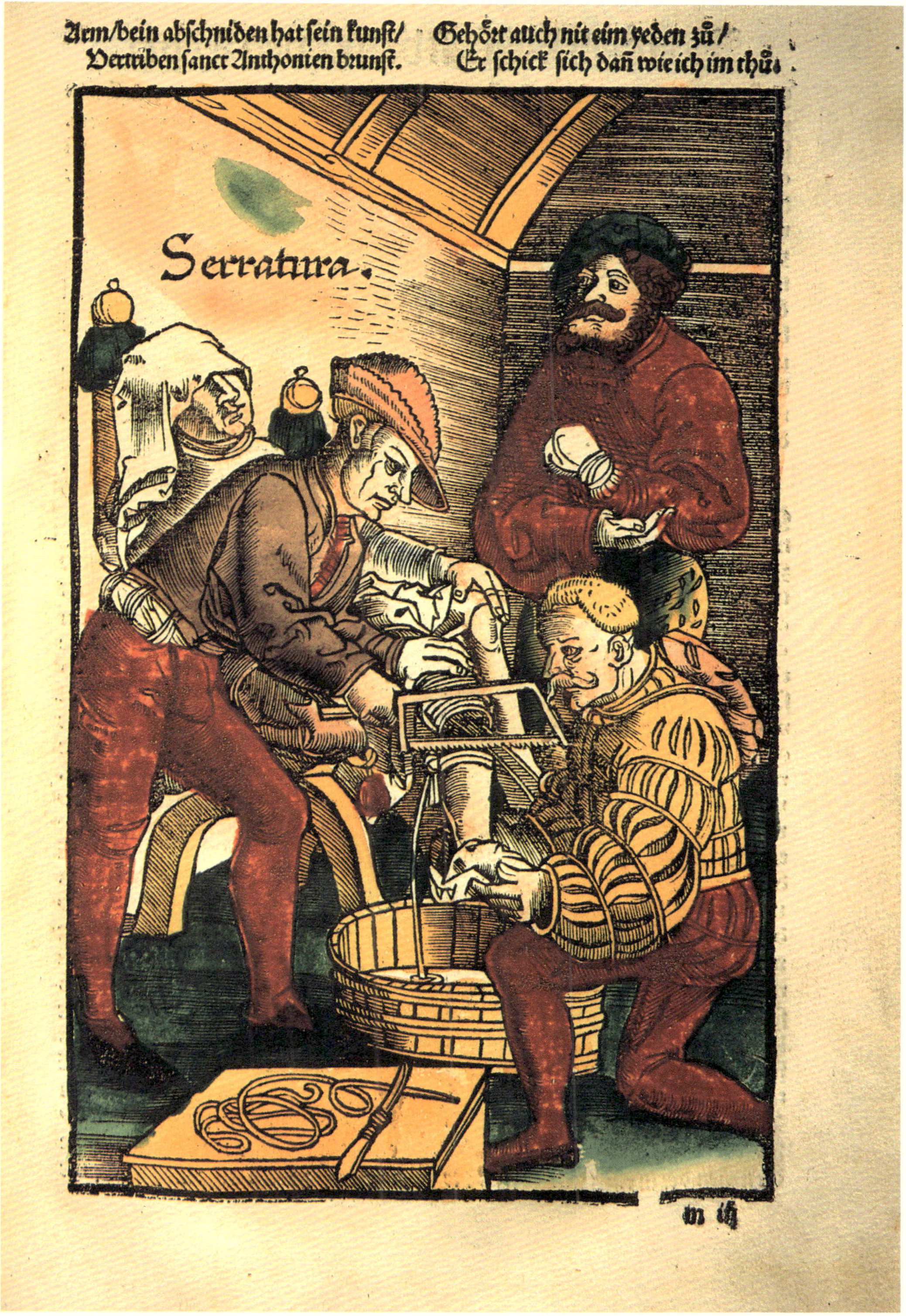
Arm/bein abschniden hat sein kunst/
Vertriben sanct Anthonien brunst.
Gehört auch nit eim yeden zů/
Er schick sich dañ wie ich im thů.
Serratura.

PLATE XI. No. 14. Gersdorff. Hand-colored woodcut of an amputation.

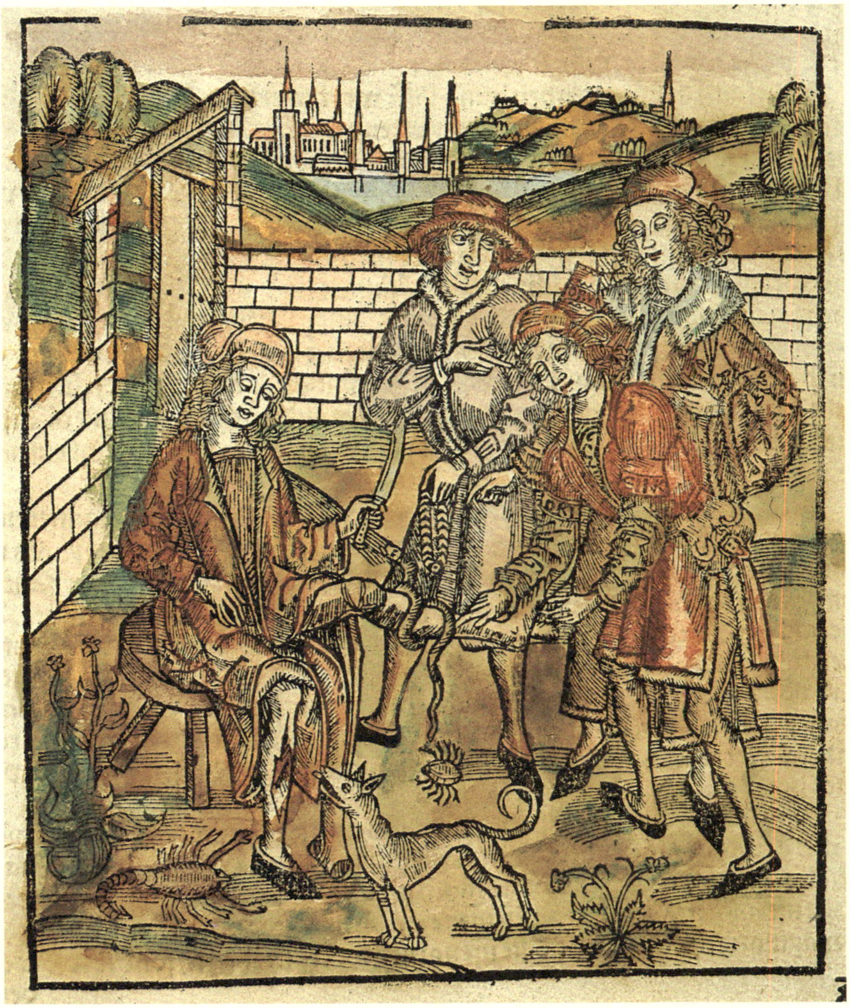

PLATE XII. No. 16. Paracelsus. Hand-colored woodcut.

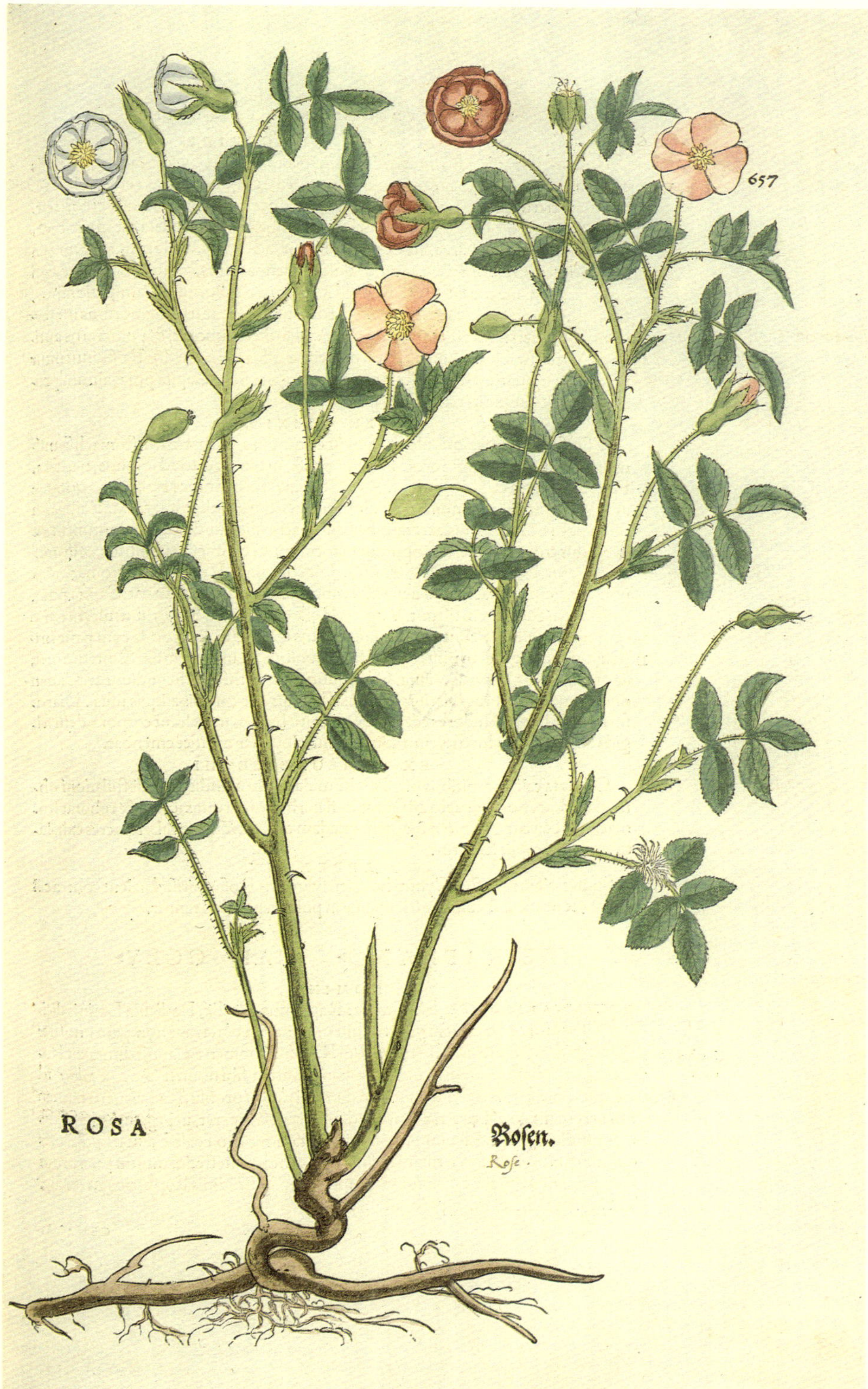

PLATE XIII. No. 17. Fuchs. Hand-colored woodcut of the genus *Rosa*, showing white, pink, and red flowers on the same plant. This copy is typical of those colored under the direction of the publisher Isingrin; these copies share features—such as the particular coloration and placement of the red, pink, and white blossoms in this illustration—that are not usually found in copies colored later by their owners.

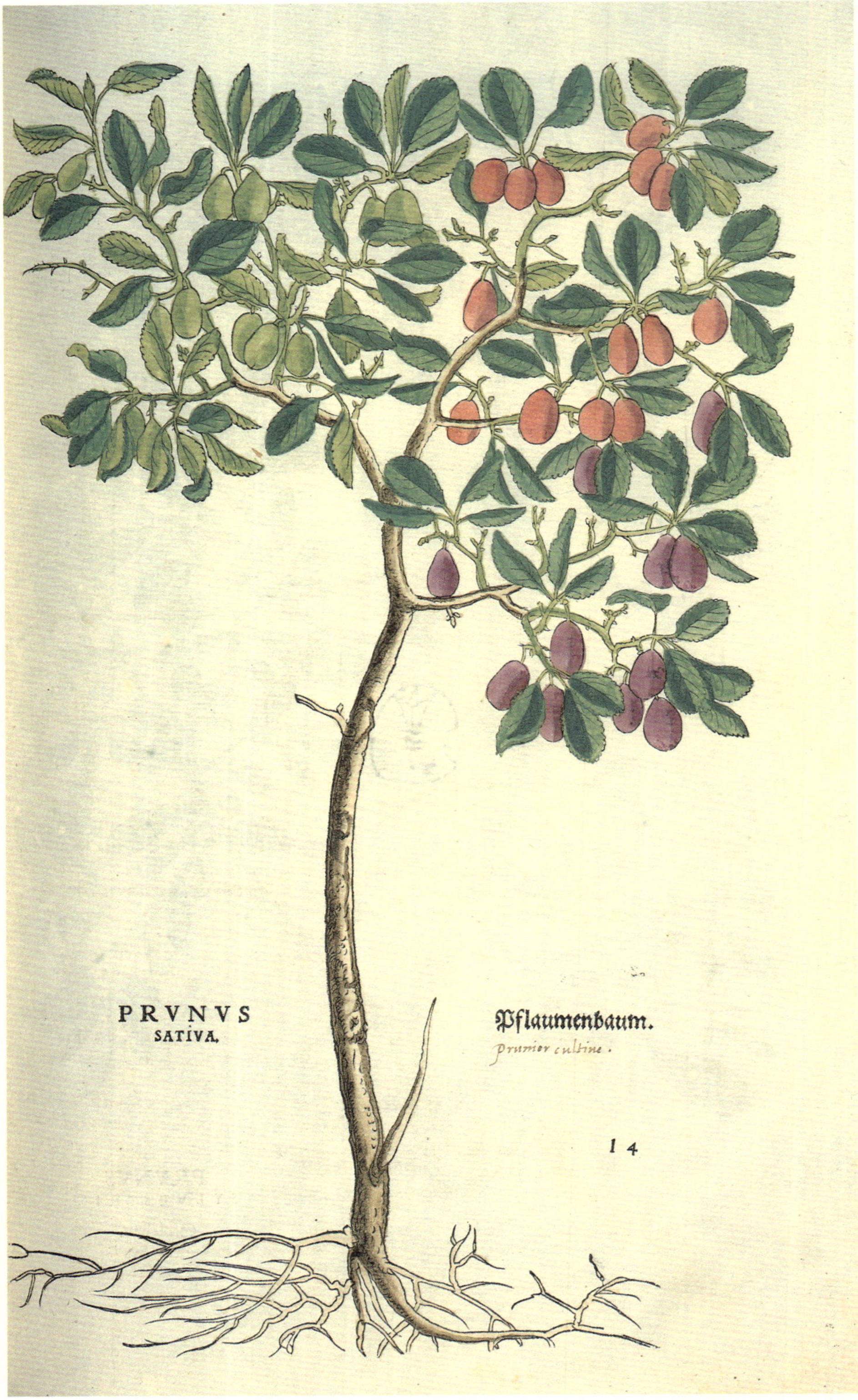

PLATE XIV. No. 17. Fuchs. Hand-colored woodcut of the genus *Prunus*, with green, red, and purple plums on the same tree. The coloring accords well with Fuchs's descriptions in the text, which indicates that Fuchs may have had some control over the coloring.

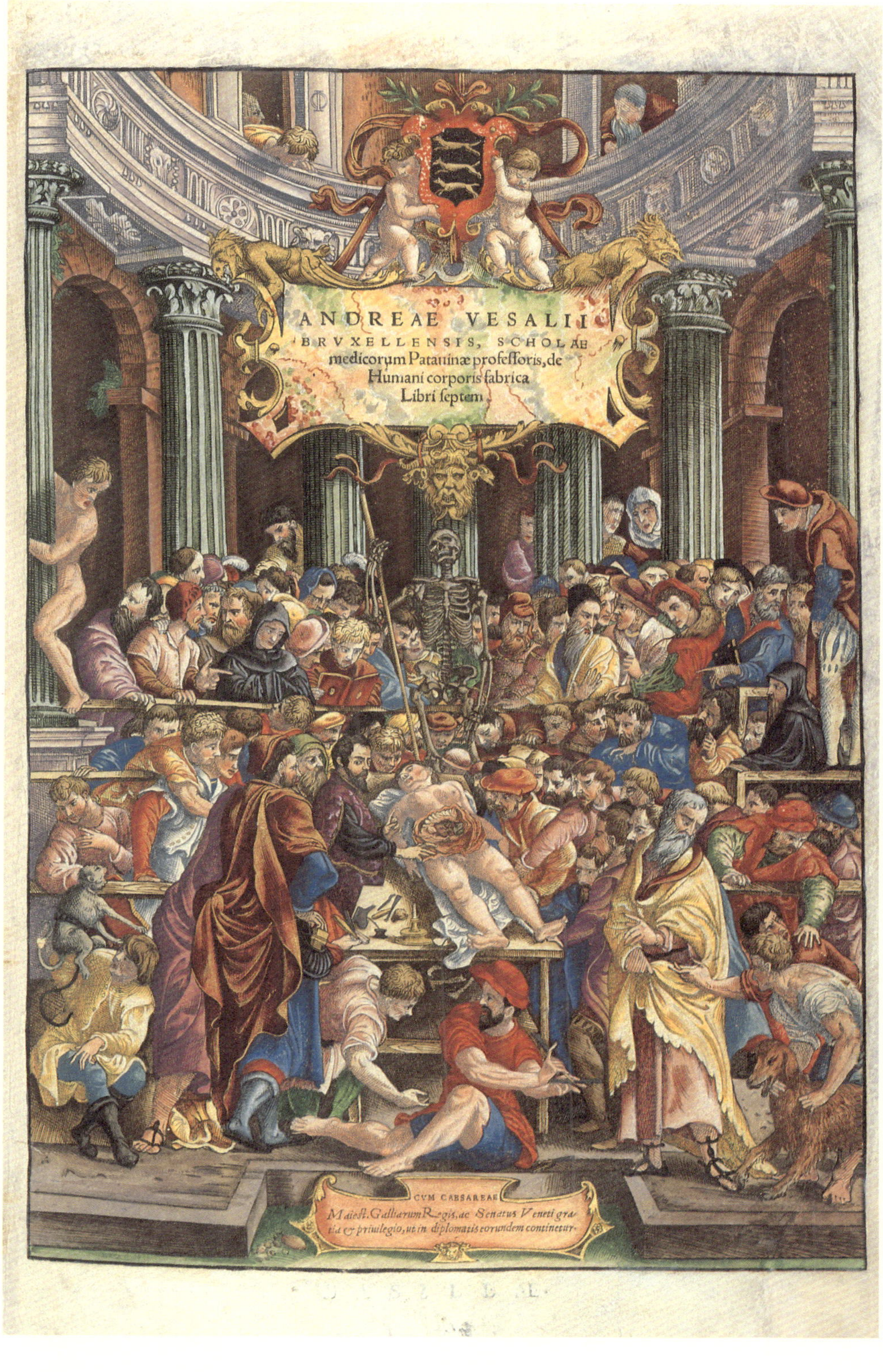

PLATE XV. No. 18A. Vesalius. Hand-illuminated title page from the dedication copy of *De humani corporis fabrica* (1543), presented to the Holy Roman Emperor Charles V.

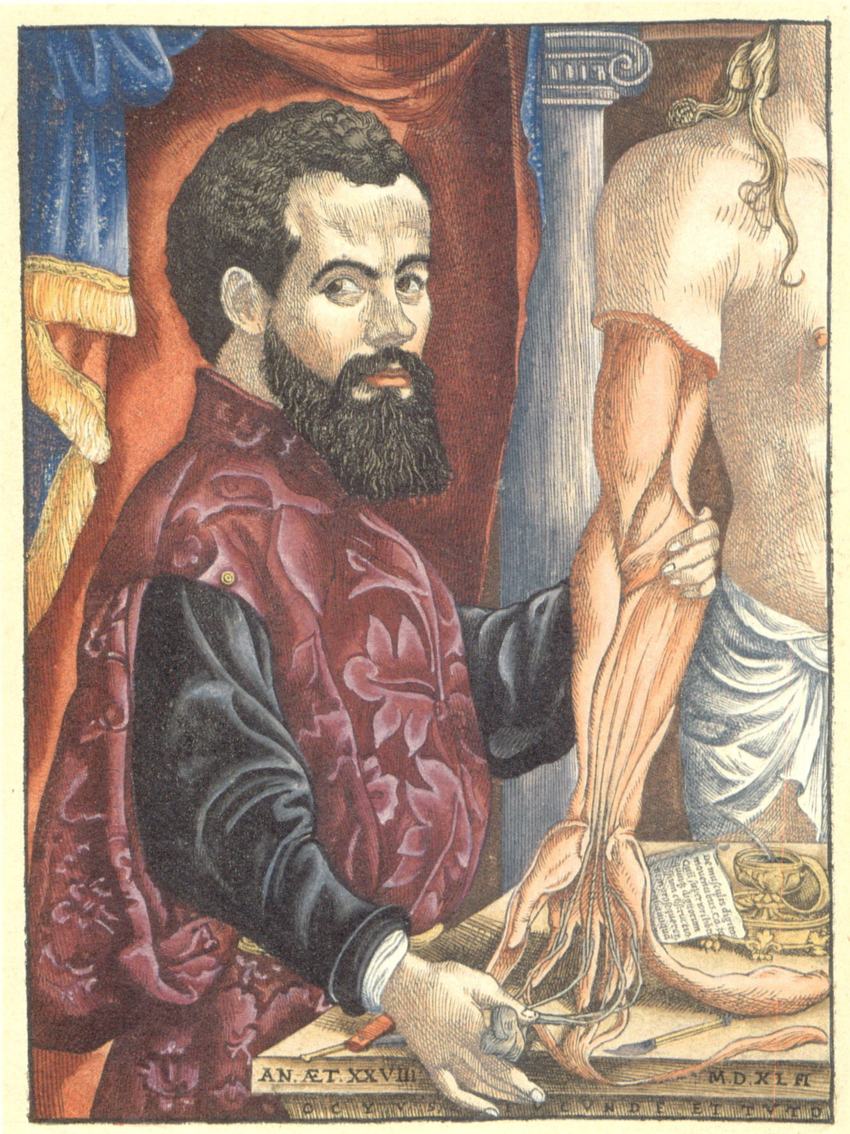

PLATE XVI. No. 18A. Vesalius. This hand-colored version of the portrait in *De humani corporis fabrica* is the only contemporary record of Vesalius's complexion and hair color.

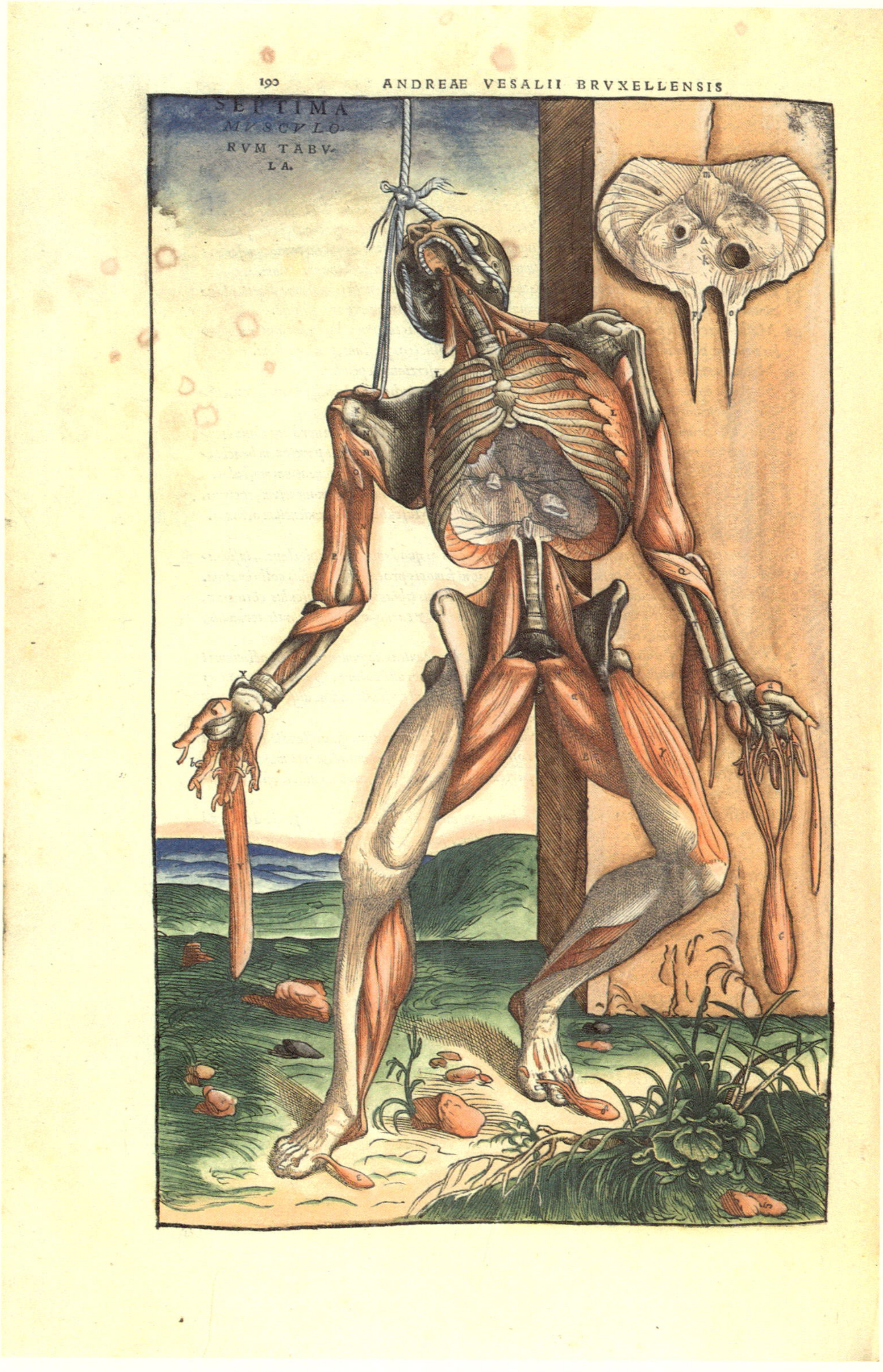

PLATE XVII. No. 18A. Vesalius. Hand-colored muscleman from *De humani corporis fabrica* (1543). The object hanging on the pillar to the right of the figure is the dissected diaphragm muscle.

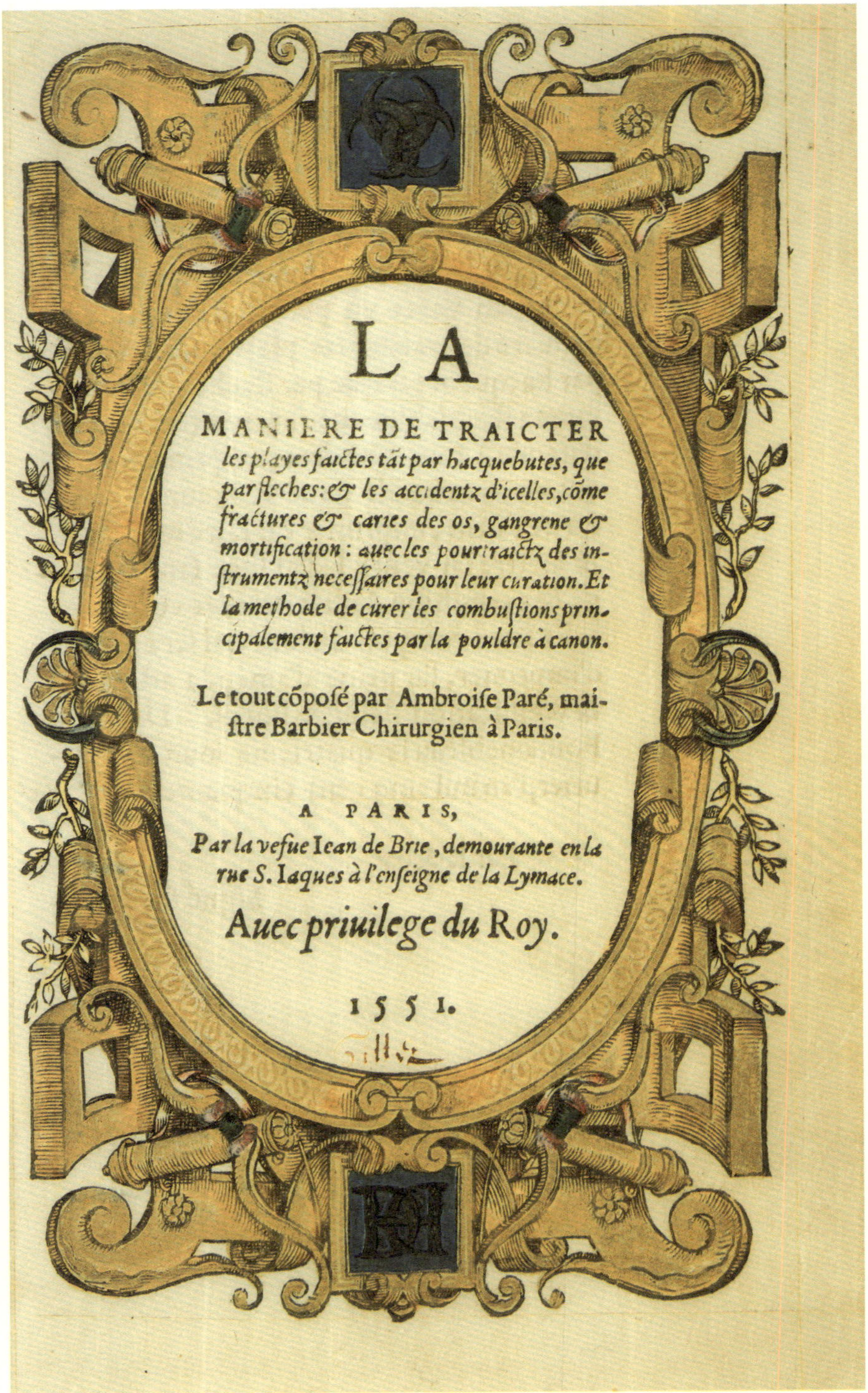

LA

MANIERE DE TRAICTER les playes faictes tãt par hacquebutes, que par fleches: & les accidentz d'icelles, cõme fractures & caries des os, gangrene & mortification: auec les pourtraictz des instrumentz necessaires pour leur curation. Et la methode de curer les combustions principalement faictes par la pouldre à canon.

Le tout cõposé par Ambroise Paré, maistre Barbier Chirurgien à Paris.

A PARIS,

Par la vefue Iean de Brie, demourante en la rue S. Iaques à l'enseigne de la Lymace.

Auec priuilege du Roy.

1551.

PLATE XVIII. No. 19B. Paré. Illuminated title page from the Yemeniz—Didot—Hoe—Bishop—Cushing copy of *La maniere de traicter les playes* (1551), one of three known copies printed on vellum.

PLATE XIX. No. 19B. Paré. Contemporary Grolieresque binding on the Yemeniz—Didot—Hoe—Bishop—Cushing copy of *La maniere de traicter les playes* (1551).

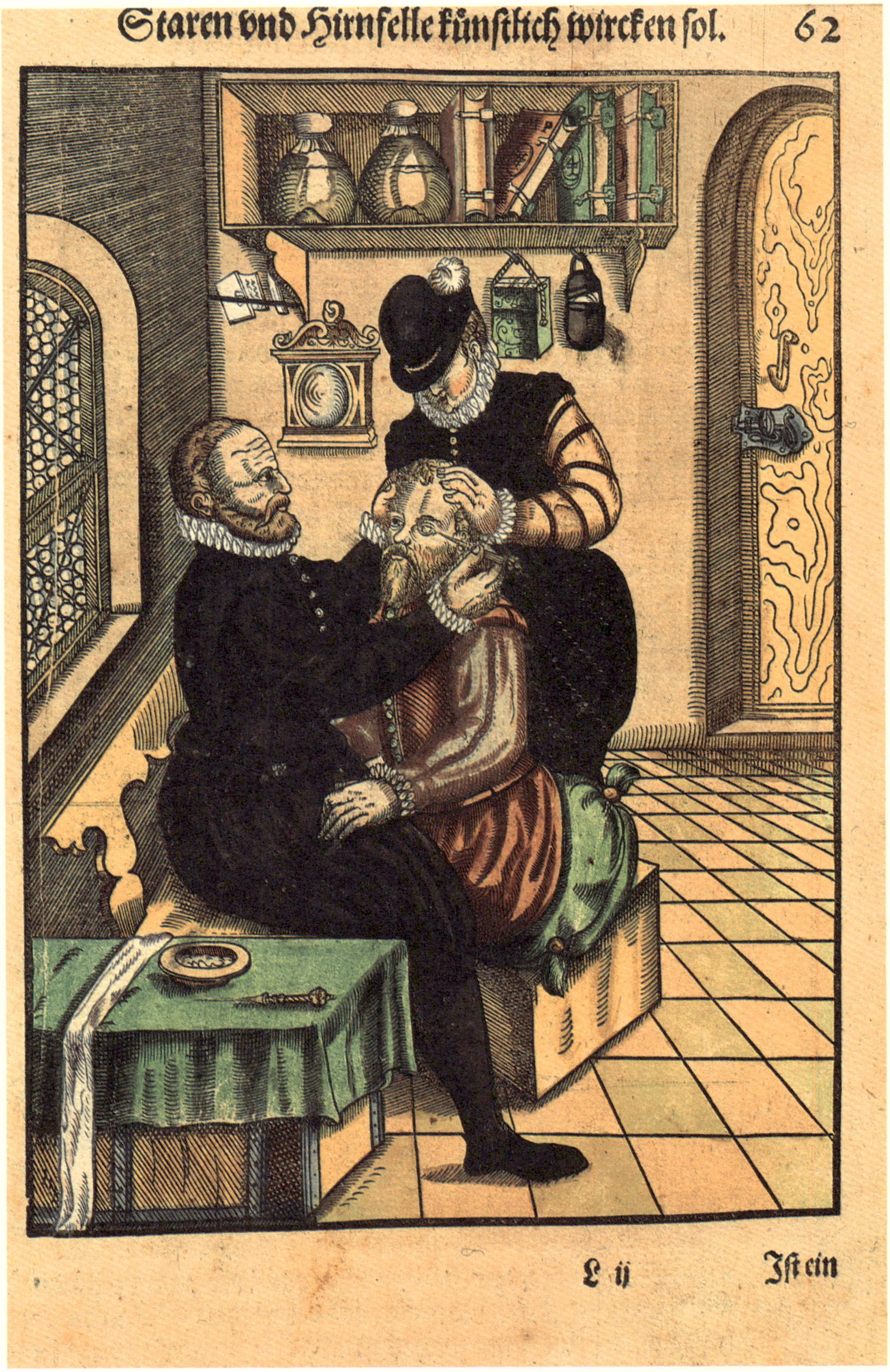
Staren vnd Hirnfelle künstlich wircken sol. 62

L ij Ist ein

PLATE XX. No. 22. Bartisch. Hand-colored woodcut of a cataract operation.

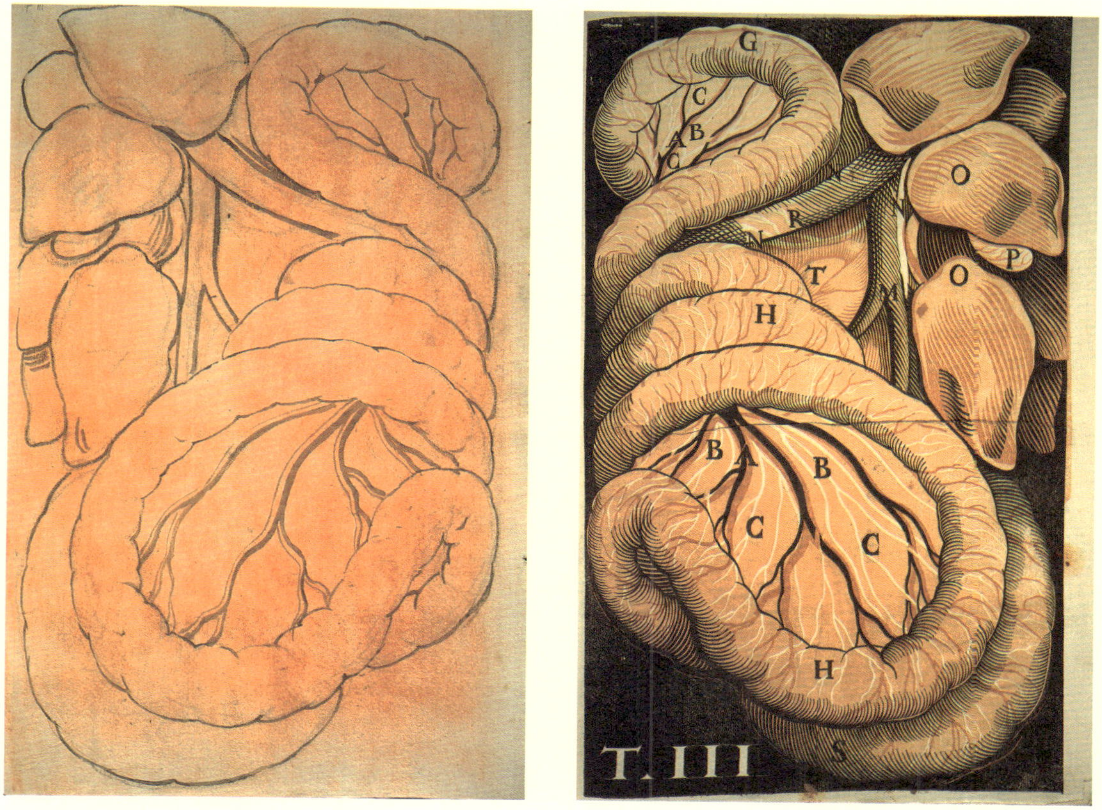

PLATE XXI. No. 26. Aselli. Artist's original drawing for Plate III, and a later proof of the plate, one of the first medical illustrations printed in colors.

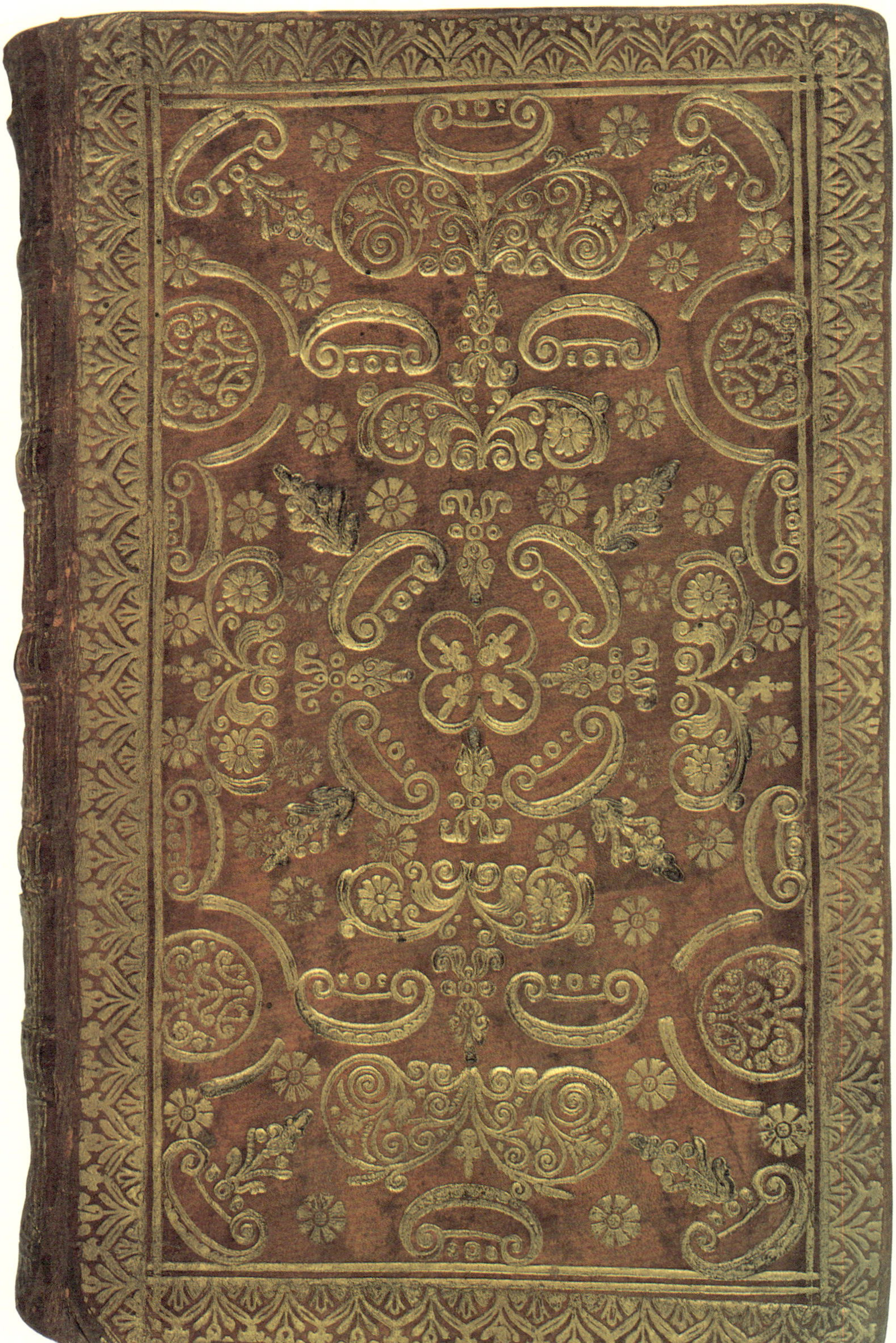

PLATE XXII. No. 39. Boerhaave. Richly gilt eighteenth-century Dutch binding on a copy of *Institutiones medicae.* Such elaborate and beautiful bindings are uncommon on medical books of this type, which were meant for use, not for show.

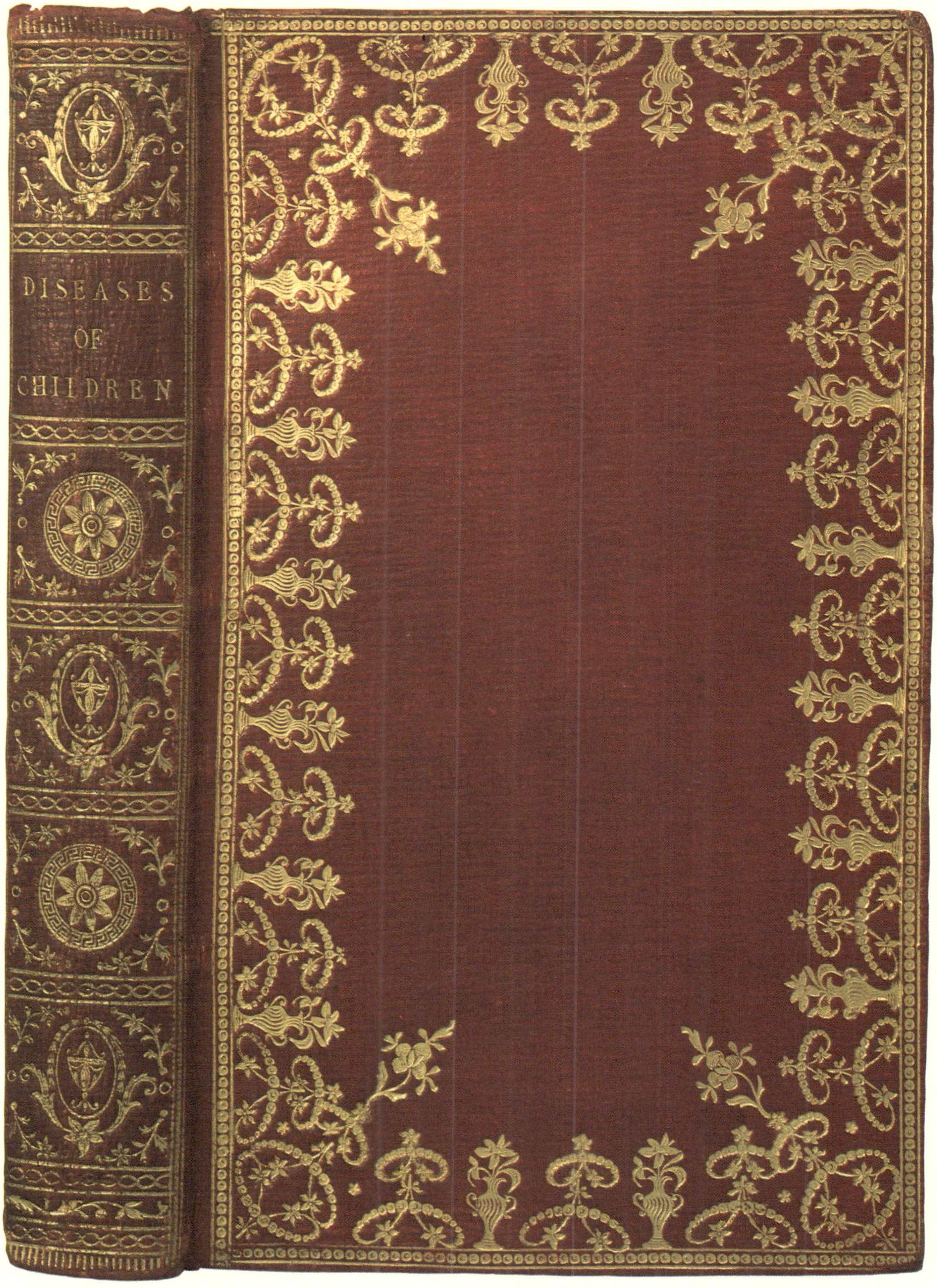

PLATE XXIII. No. 48. Underwood. Gilt morocco binding on the dedication copy of *A Treatise on the Diseases of Children*, presented to Queen Charlotte, consort of King George III of England.

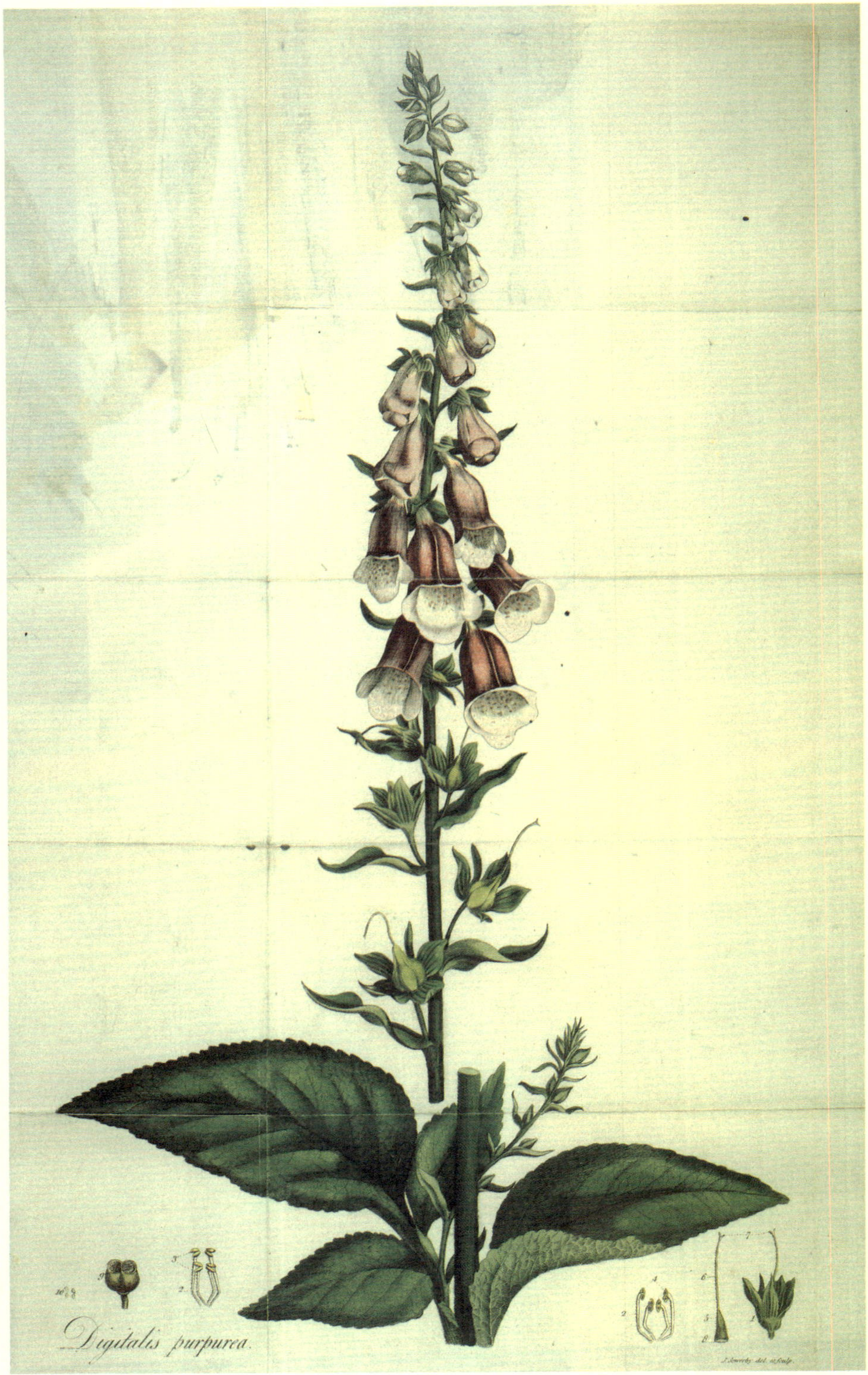

PLATE XXIV. No. 49. Withering. The hand-colored plate of the foxglove plant by James Sowerby.

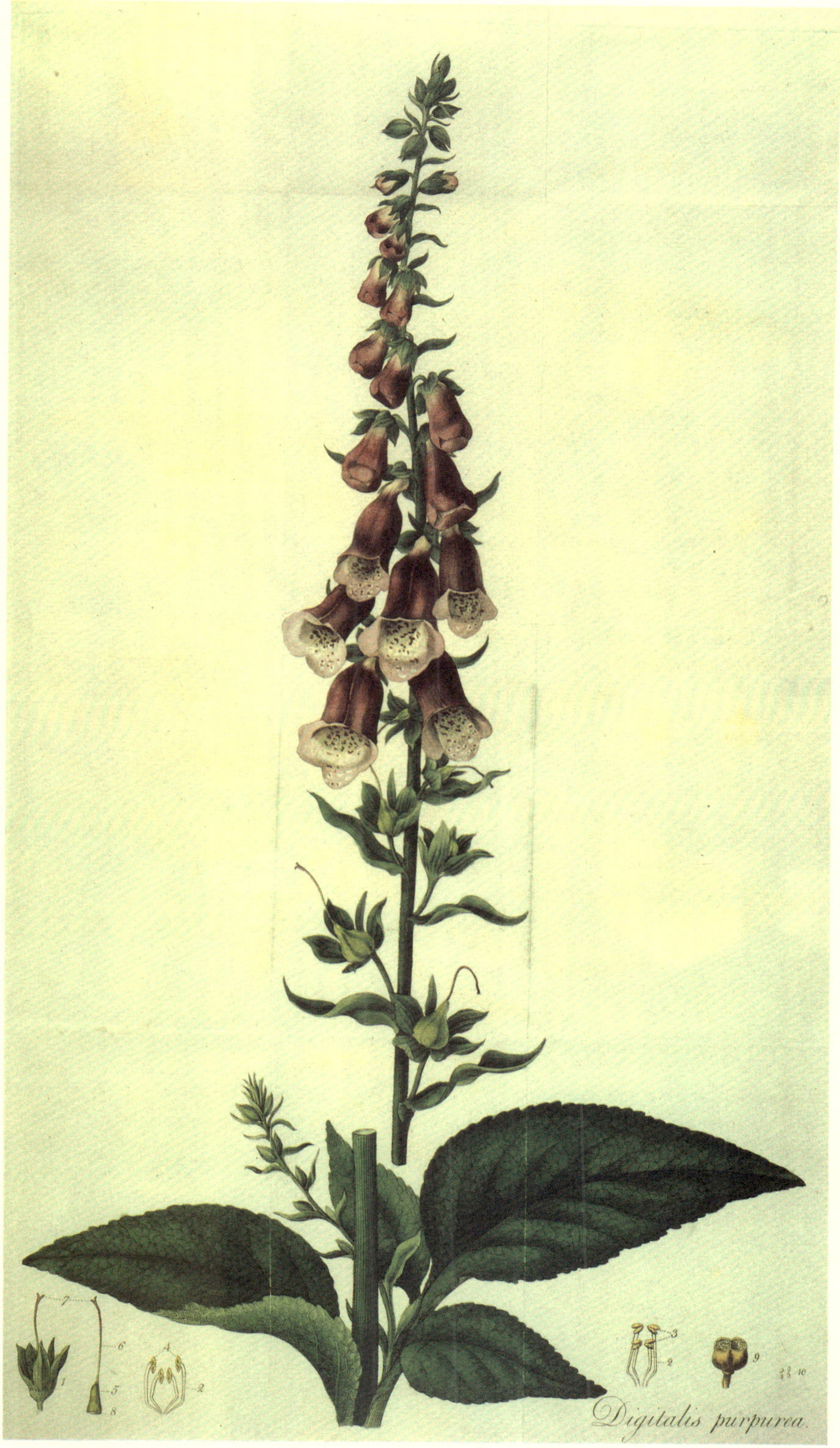

PLATE XXV. No. 49. Withering. The hand-colored plate of the foxglove plant from *Flora Londinensis.*

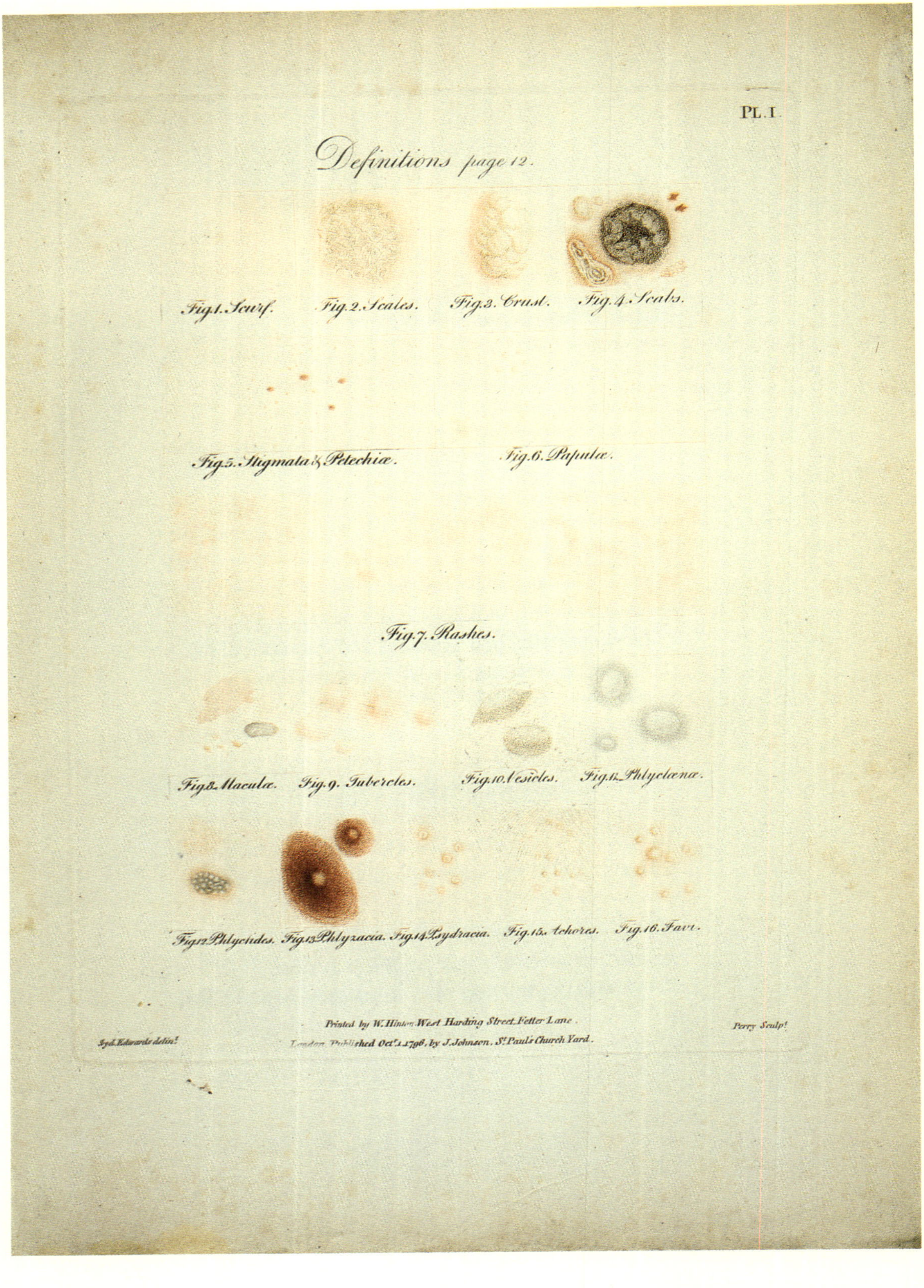

PLATE XXVI. No. 55. Willan. Plate I from *On Cutaneous Diseases*, illustrating Willan's classification of skin lesion types.

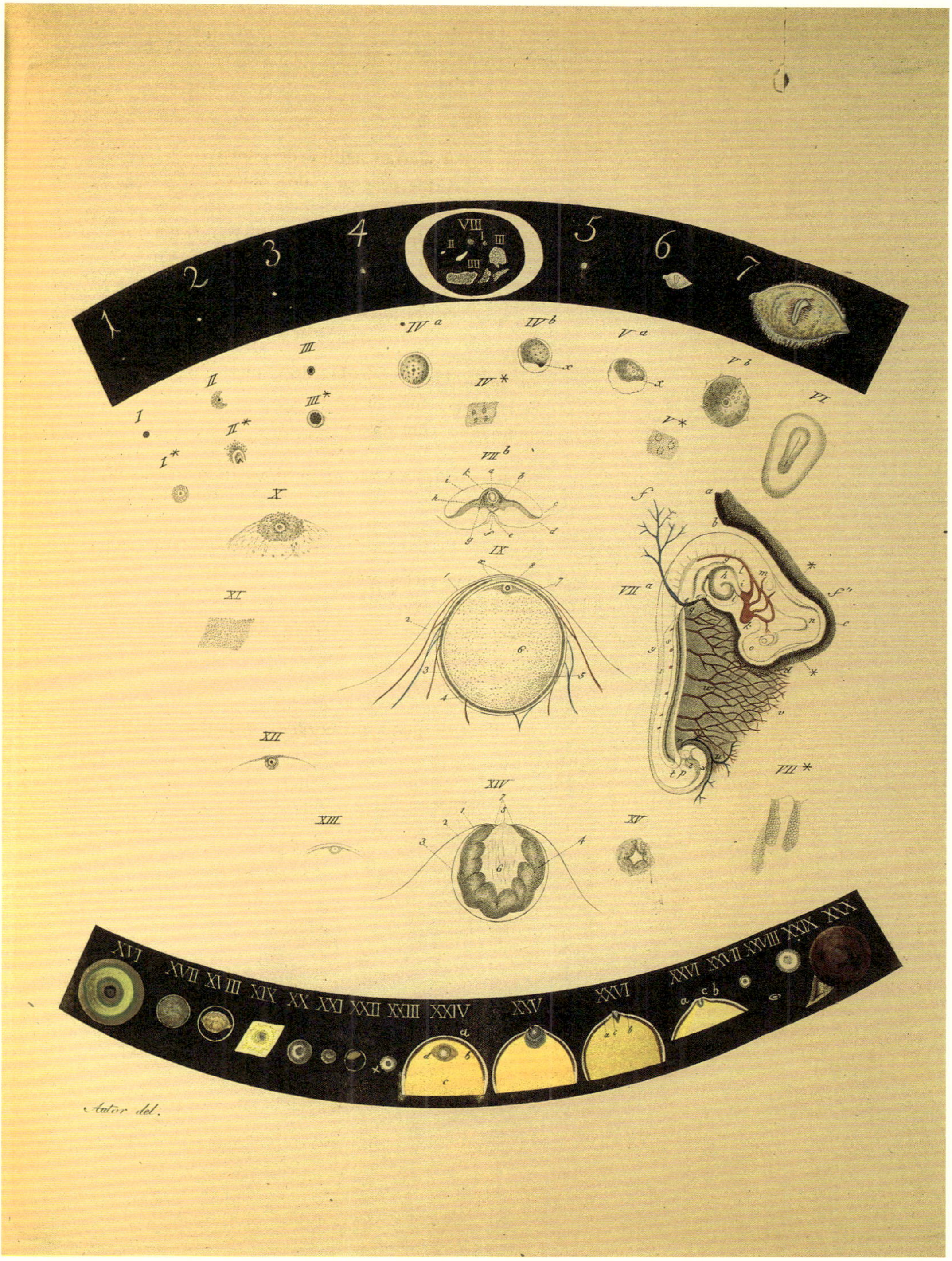

PLATE XXVII. No. 59. Baer. Plate showing the development of the mammalian ovum.

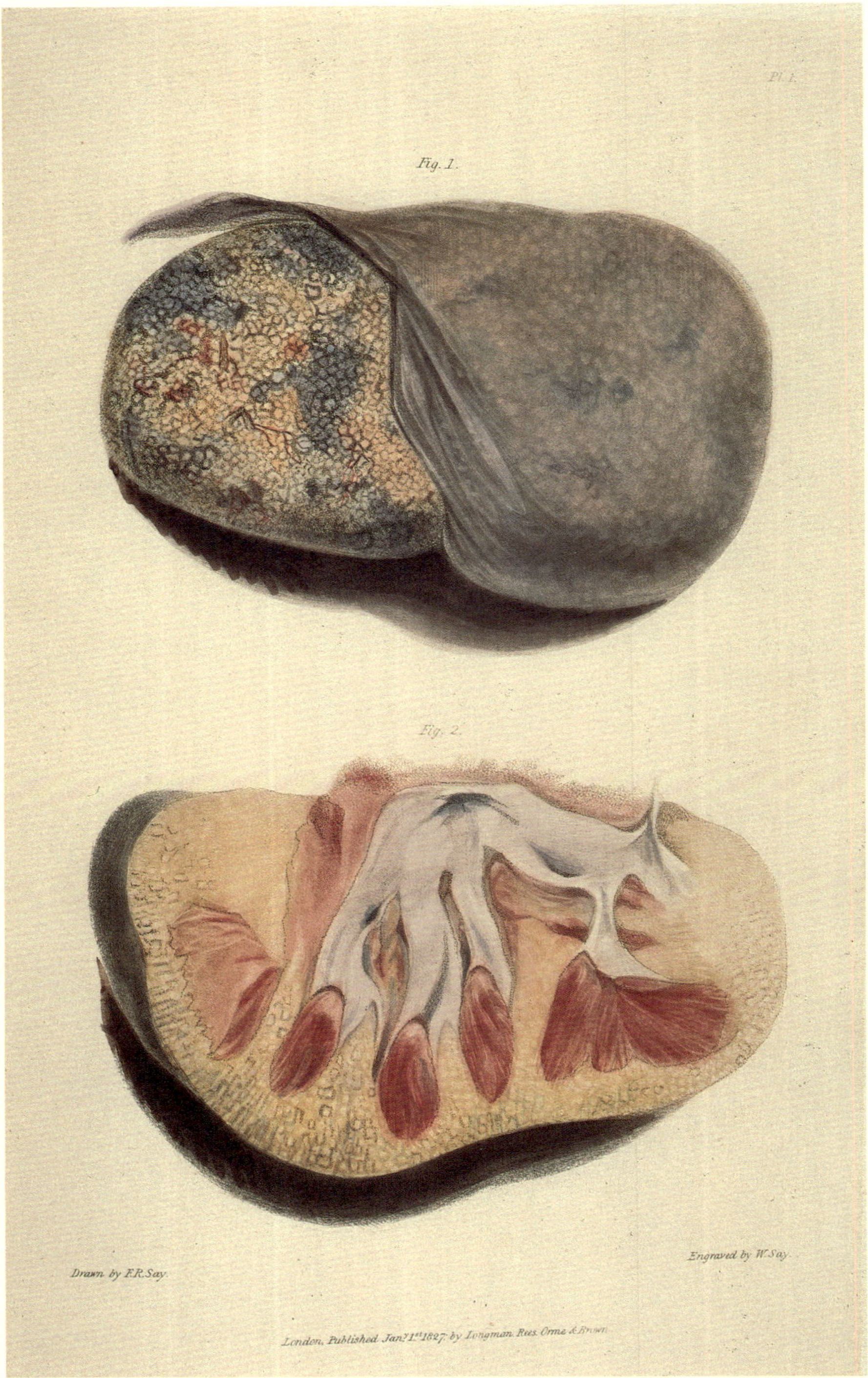

PLATE XXVIII. No. 60A. Bright. Plate I from the first volume of *Reports of Medical Cases* (1827).

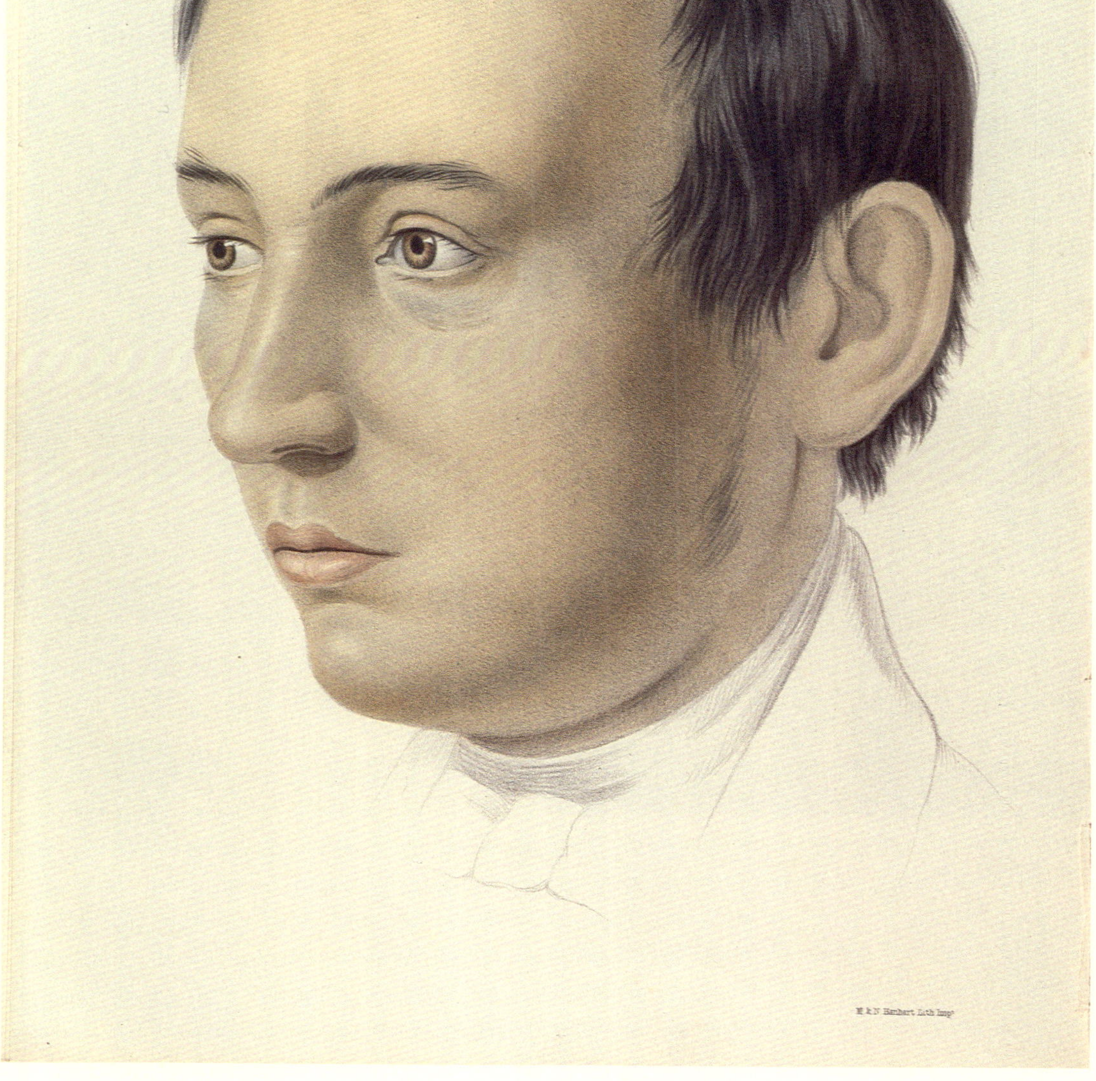

PLATE XXIX. No. 60C. Addison. Addison started his career as a dermatologist and thus gave careful attention to the bronze-colored pigmentation of the skin that is one of the chief symptoms of Addison's disease.

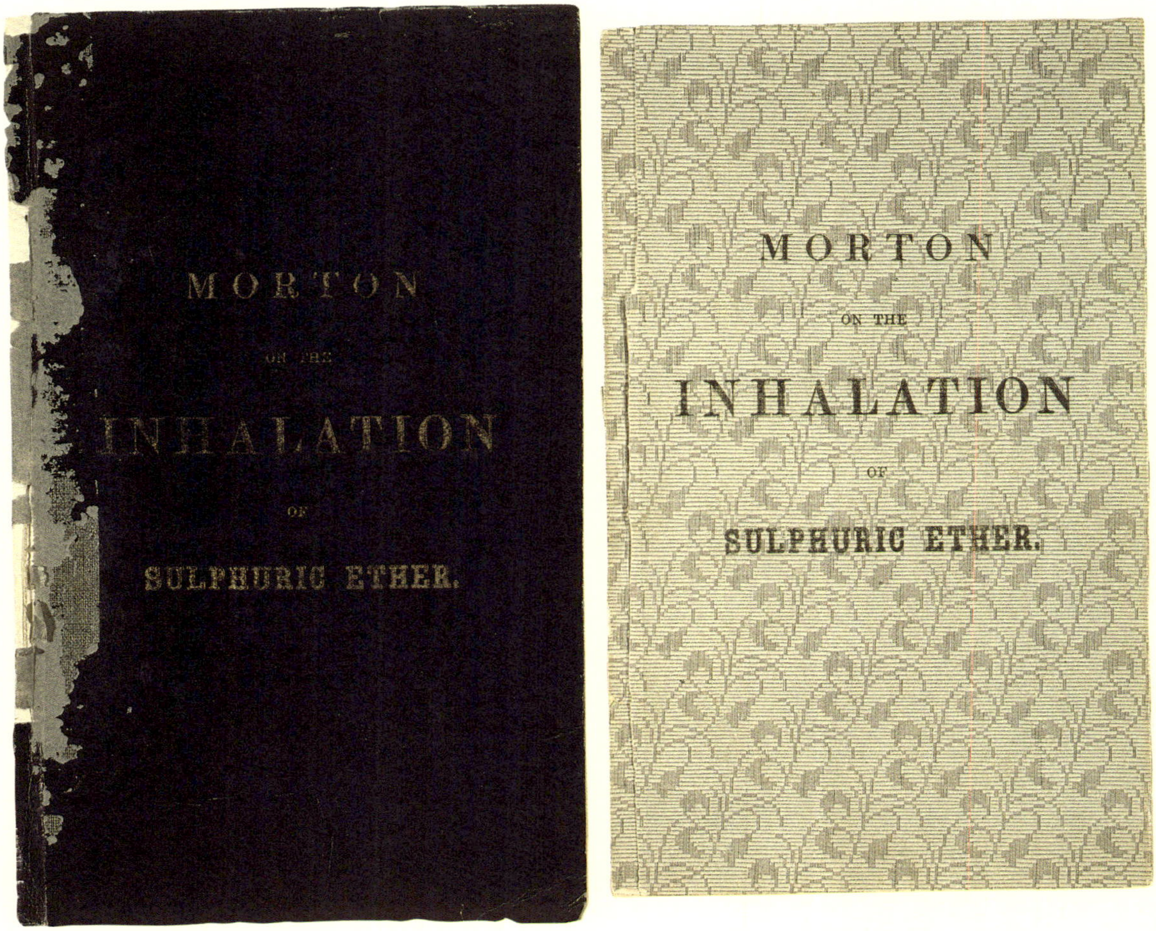

PLATE XXX. No. 64C. Morton. Two copies of *Remarks on the Proper Mode of Administering Sulphuric Ether by Inhalation*, in different colored wrappers.

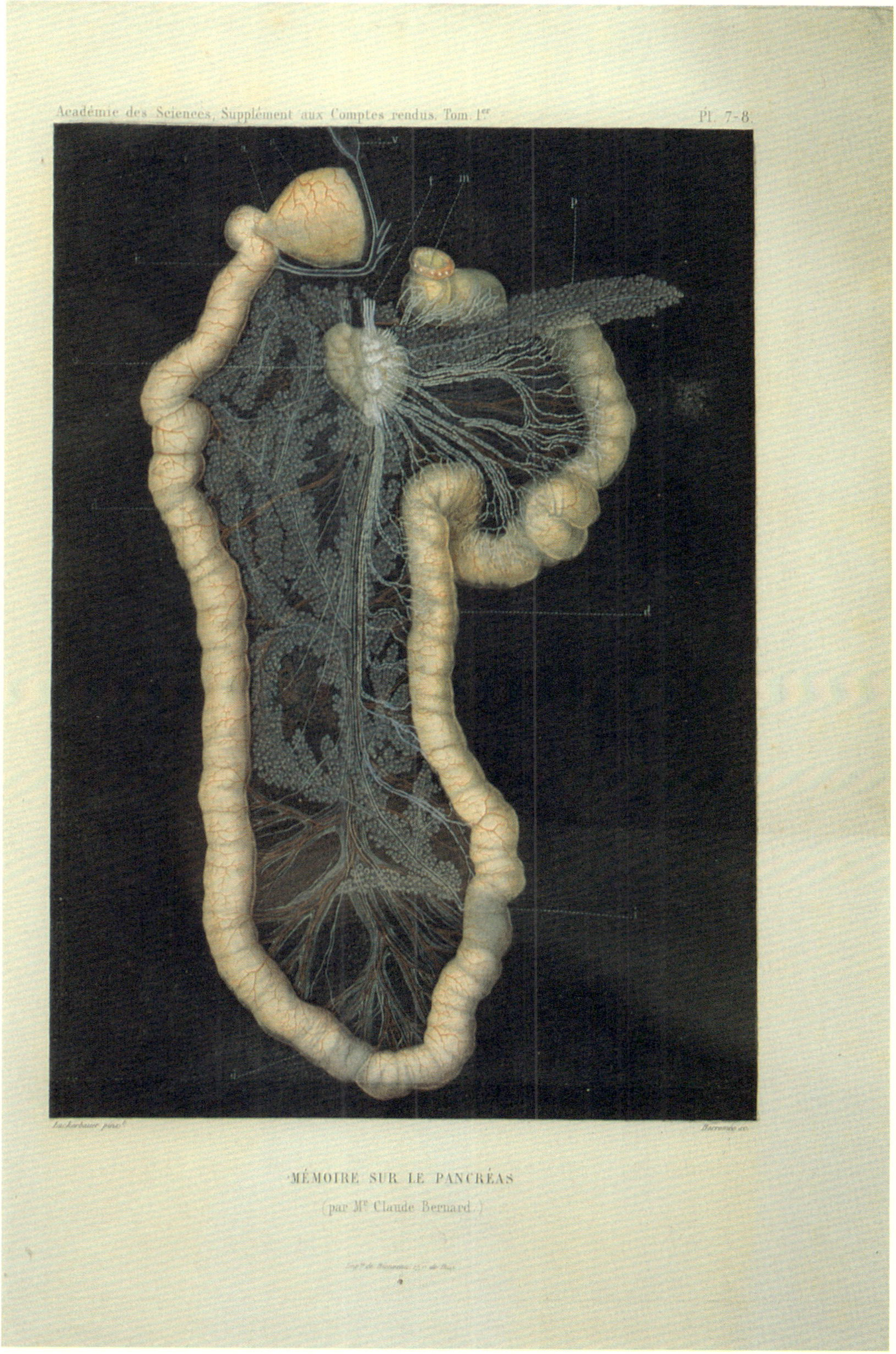

PLATE XXXI. No. 67B. Bernard. Hand-colored plate from *Mémoire sur le pancréas* (1856).

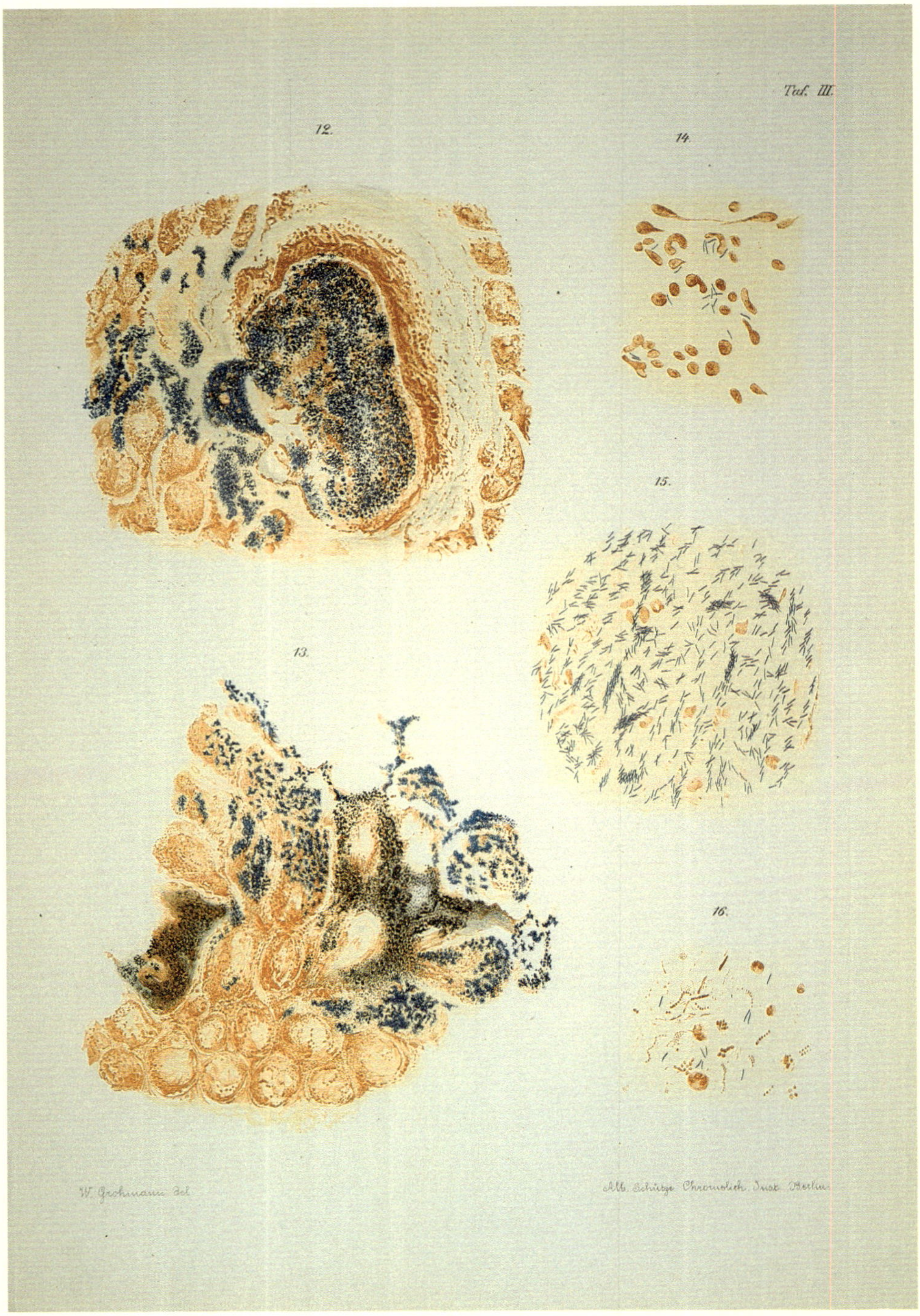

PLATE XXXII. No. 80. Koch. Illustrations of *Bacillus tuberculosis*, from "Die Aetiologie der Tuberkulose."

COPIES EXHIBITED

These copies were exhibited at the Grolier Club, 20 September–23 November 1994. Copy descriptions include, as applicable: catalogue number; citation (author, short title, abbreviated imprint); binding description; leaf size; additional copy description; provenance; comments; references; and lender.

1A Hippocrates. *Hippocratis Coi medicorum omnium longe principis, octoginta volumina.* Rome: F. M. Calvus, 1525.

Contemporary Italian blind-stamped morocco, rebacked in calf, remains of four tawed ties.
282 x 202 mm.
Gustavo Camillo Galletti (stamp)—Baron Horace de Landau (bookplate).

HASKELL F. NORMAN, M.D.

1B Hippocrates. *Omnia opera Hippocratis* [Greek]. Venice: Aldus, 1526.

Late eighteenth- or early nineteenth-century calf, panelled in gilt and blind.
307 x 210 mm.
Not rubricated; scattered early Greek marginalia.

HASKELL F. NORMAN, M.D.

1C Hippocrates. "Iusiurandum." In: *Articella.* Venice: H. Liechtenstein, 1483.

Fifteenth-century blind-stamped morocco over wooden boards, two clasps lacking (Kyriss shop 65: Nuremberg, Franz Staindorffer).
325 x 215 mm.
Rubricated with red and blue Lombard initials, the larger ones divided, with green and mauve pen-flourishing; contemporary marginalia.
Hartmann Schedel (inscription, front pastedown: *Liber doctoris Hartmanni Schedel de Nuremberga*) —Johann Jakob Fugger.

EUGENE S. FLAMM, M.D.

2A Aristotle. *De animalibus.* Venice: J. de Colonia and J. Manthen, 1476.

Seventeenth- or eighteenth-century vellum.
305 x 210 mm.
Illuminated white vine initial and half border on f. a2^r, an illuminated white vine initial opening each book, rubricated with chapter initials in red or blue roman capitals; contemporary marginalia.
William Bateman (bookplate)—William Morris (bookplate)—Richard Bennett (bookplate)—J. Pierpont Morgan (bookplate).

THE PIERPONT MORGAN LIBRARY, NEW YORK

2B Aristotle. *Opera* [Greek]. Venice: Aldus Manutius, 1495–98. 5 vols.

Volume 2 only: Brown morocco, gold- and blind-tooled, rebacked with original spine laid down, traces of four pairs of green silk ties, edges painted in a floral pattern of red and green. On each cover is a painted stamp based on a plaquette by the medallist IO.F.F. The upper cover shows Marcus Curtius riding into the chasm in the Roman forum, the lower, Horatius Cocles defending the Sublician bridge against Lars Porsenna. Made in Milan for Jean Grolier, ca. 1510–13.
311 x 205 mm.
Jean Grolier (inscription, f. K6^r: *Joannis Grolierij Lugdunensis et amicorum*; marginalia possibly in his hand).
Austin 28.1; Hobson 46b, 47b; Needham 41; Nixon 2.

THE PIERPONT MORGAN LIBRARY, NEW YORK

3A Dioscorides. *De materia medica.* Colle: J. de Medemblick, 1478.

Sixteenth-century blind-tooled mottled brown calf over wooden boards, rebacked, two brass clasps.
307 x 204 mm.
Johann Valentin Mammery (seventeenth-century inscription on former front pastedown, now lifted).

THE PIERPONT MORGAN LIBRARY, NEW YORK

3B Dioscorides. *De materia medica* [Greek]. Venice: Aldus Manutius, 1499.

Red morocco spine, red paper sides (French, ca. 1820).
303 x 208 mm.
Lacks the scholia on Nicander.
Scipio Carteromachus (i.e., Scipione Forteguerri, 1466–1515), whose *Oratio de laudibus literarum graecarum* was published by Aldus Manutius in 1504 (marginalia in his hand, according to a note by Renouard)—Petrus Andossillanus (ca. 1600) (inscription, title page: *Est Petri Andosillani*)—P. Le Cray (ca. 1650–1700) (inscription, title page: *Est nunc P. Le Cray*)—A.-A. Renouard (1765–1853), bibliographer of the Aldine press—Rudolph August Witthaus, M.D. (1846–1915), author of *General Medical Chemistry* (1881), *The Medical Student's*

Manual of Chemistry (1883), *Medical Jurisprudence* (1894–96), and other works on chemistry and toxicology (bookplate)—Emil Starkenstein (1884–1942), author of works on pharmacology, immunology, and medicine (bookplate).
Ahmanson-Murphy 26.

THE AHMANSON-MURPHY ALDINE COLLECTION, UCLA SPECIAL COLLECTIONS

4 Aulus Cornelius Celsus. *De medicina*. Florence: N. Laurentii, 1478.

COPY 1: Red morocco, gilt.
Illuminated coat of arms over obliterated stamp on f. A1r [bound first in this copy], illuminated initial and partial border (restored) on f. π2r; rubricated with red and blue Lombard initials.
275 x 197 mm.
Giorgio Antonio Vespucci, uncle of Amerigo Vespucci (signature above colophon: *Georgii Antonii Vespucii liber*)—Henry Huth (bookplate).

THE COLLEGE OF PHYSICIANS OF PHILADELPHIA

COPY 2: Modern morocco, blind-stamped in the style of the fifteenth-century, over wooden boards, two clasps; metal bosses, strap ends, and catchplates reused from a fifteenth-century binding.
287 x 214 mm.
Rubricated by Hartmann Schedel with red and blue Lombard initials, paragraph signs, underlines, capital strokes, and foliation (signed, f. hh4v: *Laudes deo eterno HA.S.*); verses in Schedel's hand on flyleaf.
Hartmann Schedel (ownership inscription from original pastedown remounted inside front cover: *Liber doctoris Hartmanni Schedel de Nuremberga*; rubrication in his hand, signed with his monogram)—Royal Library, Munich (bookplate, stamp, and duplicate stamp)—Charles H. Truax (sale catalogue, 1910)—Edward Clark Streeter (bookplate).
Ff. π2.5 and hh1.4 were for a period of time missing from this book. In the course of preparing One Hundred Books Famous in Medicine, Haskell F. Norman recognized three of these leaves (ff. π5, hh1, and hh4) at the Louise Darling Biomedical Library at UCLA, which acquired them with its Benjamin Collection in 1964. By courtesy of the Louise Darling Biomedical Library, these leaves have been returned to the New York Academy of Medicine and reunited with the book.
Benjamin 141; New York Academy of Medicine, *The Malloch Room Newsletter* (No. 9, Fall/Winter 1994), pp. 1–5.

THE NEW YORK ACADEMY OF MEDICINE

5A Galen. *Opera*. Venice: P. Pincius, 1490. 2 vols.

Contemporary blind-tooled pigskin over wooden boards, lacking three of four metal clasps (Kyriss shop 104: Leipzig).
415 x 283 mm. (vol. I); 425 x 280 mm. (vol. II).
Miniature on the opening text page of each volume, rubricated with red and blue Lombard or cadel initials and paragraph signs; copious fifteenth-century annotations.
Harvey Cushing (bookplate).

THE HARVEY CUSHING/JOHN HAY WHITNEY MEDICAL LIBRARY, HISTORICAL LIBRARY, YALE UNIVERSITY

5B Galen. *Opera* [Greek]. Venice: Aldus, 1525. 5 vols.

Brown calf, gilt.
417 x 273 mm.
Large-paper copy.
James Toovey (bookplates). According to a note in the book, it also belonged to Jacques de Thou, the Prince de Soubise, Cardinal Loménie de Brienne, and A.-A. Renouard.

THE PIERPONT MORGAN LIBRARY, NEW YORK

6 Rhazes. *Liber ad Almansorem*. Milan: L. Pachel and U. Scinzenzeler, 1481.

Modern binding of blind-stamped calf spine over bare wooden boards.
332 x 232 mm.
Not rubricated; occasional early marginalia.
Alouisius e Spingiola (seventeenth-century inscription, lower margin, f. z5r)—Jacobus Maximilianus I (bookplate).

HASKELL F. NORMAN, M.D.

7A Avicenna. *Canon medicinae*. Milan: Philippus de Lavagnia, 12 February 1473.

Not exhibited; no copies of this edition are recorded in North America.

7B Avicenna. *Canon medicinae*. [Strassburg: The R-Printer (Adolf Rusch), between 1475 and 1477].

Contemporary South-German or Austrian blind-tooled calf over wooden boards, two clasps.
345 x 245 mm.
Rubricated with large red and blue initial on f. 2r, red Lombard initials, headlines, paragraph signs, and capital strokes; contemporary marginalia, cropped by binder.

Deleted stamps.

THE BOSTON MEDICAL LIBRARY IN THE FRANCIS A. COUNTWAY LIBRARY OF MEDICINE

8A Guy de Chauliac. *Chirurgia* [French]. Lyons: [Nicolaus Philippi and Marcus Reinhart for] Barthélemy Buyer, 28 March 1478.

Not exhibited; the only known copy of this edition is in the Bibliothèque Nationale, Paris.

8B Guy de Chauliac. *Chirurgia* [Italian]. Venice: N. Girardengus, 1480.

Modern vellum spine, white cloth sides.
292 x 195 mm.
Partially rubricated by a late hand; early annotations on endleaves.

THE COLLEGE OF PHYSICIANS OF PHILADELPHIA

9 Paolo Bagellardo. *De infantium aegritudinibus et remediis.* [Padua]: B. de Valdezoccho and M. de Septem Arboribus, 1472.

Modern blind-ruled calf.
202 x 138 mm.
Rubricated with red Lombard initials.

HASKELL F. NORMAN, M.D.

10A Johannes de Ketham. *Fasciculus medicinae.* Venice: J. and G. de Gregoriis, 1491.

Contemporary German blind-tooled leather over wooden boards, metal bosses, lacking one of two clasps, formerly chained.
430 x 290 mm.
Five of the illustrations hand-colored; rubricated with red Lombard initials and paragraph signs. Bound with: Michael Savonarola, *Practica medicinae.* Venice: Andreas de Bonetis, 10 May 1486 [Goff S-297].
Harvey Cushing (bookplate).

THE HARVEY CUSHING/JOHN HAY WHITNEY MEDICAL LIBRARY, HISTORICAL LIBRARY, YALE UNIVERSITY

10B Johannes de Ketham. *Fascicolo di medicina.* Venice: J. and G. de Gregoriis, 1493/94.

Modern black blind-panelled leather over wooden boards, two clasps.
310 x 210 mm.
With the stencil-colored illustration, further enhanced by hand-coloring; the other illustrations hand-colored; illuminated with a coat of arms, and a colored roman initial on a gold ground; early marginalia, cropped by the binder. The first leaf supplied in facsimile.
Morosini family of Venice (coat of arms, f. a2^r)—Harvey Cushing (bookplate).

THE HARVEY CUSHING/JOHN HAY WHITNEY MEDICAL LIBRARY, HISTORICAL LIBRARY, YALE UNIVERSITY

11 Gabriele Zerbi. *Gerontocomia.* Rome: E. Silber, 1498.

Eighteenth-century German sheepskin, rebacked in modern calf with the original gilt spine laid down; gilt armorial centerpieces on front and back covers.
195 x 134 mm.
Lacks quire 18, the "Emendationes errorum."
Deleted stamp—Heinrich von Bünau (armorial binding).

THE BOSTON MEDICAL LIBRARY IN THE FRANCIS A. COUNTWAY LIBRARY OF MEDICINE

12 Antonio Benivieni. *De abditis nonnullis ac mirandis morborum et sanationum causis.* Florence: P. Giunta, 1507.

Eighteenth-century gilt sheep, gilt spine, marbled sides.
204 x 135 mm.
Illuminated chapter initials in two styles: in the first part of the book, colored initials on flat gold grounds, probably sixteenth-century Italian work; for the final chapters, later colored initials with gold or silver pen-flourishing.

HASKELL F. NORMAN, M.D.

13A Eucharius Rösslin. *Der swangern Frauwen vnd Hebammen Rosegarten.* Strassburg: M. Flach, 1513.

Sixteenth-century German blind-stamped calf over wooden boards, metal bosses, one metal clasp (the strap renewed).
180 x 135 mm.
Bound with seven additional works on the weather, medicine, herbs, and cookery; all were printed in Augsburg and range in date from 1494 to 1519. Tipped to the rear flyleaf is a note by William Osler, dated Oxford, January 1915, about other copies of Rösslin's work.
Various early inscriptions, some deleted.

THE COLLEGE OF PHYSICIANS OF PHILADELPHIA

13B Eucharius Rösslin. *Der swangern Frawen vnd Hebammen Roszgarten.* [Hagenau]: H. Gran, [ca. 1515].

Olive gilt-ruled morocco, by Roger de Coverly & Sons.
203 x 146 mm.
Harvey Cushing (bookplate).

THE HARVEY CUSHING/JOHN HAY WHITNEY MEDICAL LIBRARY, HISTORICAL LIBRARY, YALE UNIVERSITY

13C Eucharius Rösslin. *Der swangern Frawen vnd Hebammen Rosegarten.* [Cologne: A. von Aich, ca. 1518].

Contemporary blind-tooled calf spine over bare wooden boards, remains of one clasp.
198 x 140 mm.

THE REYNOLDS HISTORICAL LIBRARY, UNIVERSITY OF ALABAMA AT BIRMINGHAM

14 Hans von Gersdorff. *Feldtbuch der Wundtartzney.* Strassburg: J. Schott, 1517.

Contemporary blind-tooled pigskin spine, orange vellum sides, lacking four tawed ties.
243 x 175 mm.
Illustrations hand-colored. Lacks the plate of the viscera man; the skeleton bound in as a double plate.
Monasterij Weingartensis 1659 (inscription, title page)—Koniglicher Hand Bibliothek (armorial stamp, title page)—George William Norris, M.D. (bookplate).

THE COLLEGE OF PHYSICIANS OF PHILADELPHIA

15 Giacomo Berengario da Carpi. *Commentaria cum amplissimis additionibus super anatomia Mundini.* Bologna: H. de Benedictis, 1521.

Contemporary German blind-tooled calf over wooden boards, lacking two clasps.
207 x 150 mm.
Occasional early annotations.
Nicolaus Pol (c. 1470–1532), physician to the Holy Roman Emperor Maximilian I (inscription, front pastedown: *Nicolaus Pol Doctor 1494*; inscription, title page: *Pro D. Doctore Nicolao Poll*)—*Collegiate Ecclesie Intinensis [?] Anno 1632* (inscription, title page)—LeRoy Crummer (bookplate)—Herbert Evans (bookplate)—Lessing J. Rosenwald (bookplate).
Fisch, p. 153.

LESSING J. ROSENWALD COLLECTION, RARE BOOK AND SPECIAL COLLECTIONS DIVISION, LIBRARY OF CONGRESS

16 Paracelsus. *Der grossenn Wundartzney.* Augsburg: H. Steiner, 1536. 2 volumes bound together.

Sixteenth- or seventeenth-century green-stained vellum.
264 x 182 mm.
The woodcuts hand-colored.
Ad Bibliothecam Fratrum Minorum Conuentus Ratisbonae ad S. Saluatorem (seventeenth-century inscription, front pastedown)—*Anno 1729 Mensis Julij Johannis Georgij Andreae ex libris Dieterichs Operator et Chirurgus hujus Reviss. Monasterij Ordinarius* (inscription, second flyleaf)—Marcus L. Taft, M.D., gift from Edwin Smith, New York, 26 Jan. 1848 (inscriptions, second and third flyleaves)—Marcus P. Hatfield, Sept. 1870, from Mrs. M. L. Taft (inscription, second flyleaf)—Alfred E. M. Purdy, Feb. 1883 (inscription, second flyleaf)—Robert R. Terry, gift from Arthur H. Mann, Pittsburgh, 27 March 1964 (inscription, third flyleaf)—New York Academy of Medicine (deleted stamps).

THE LILLY LIBRARY, INDIANA UNIVERSITY, BLOOMINGTON

17 Leonhart Fuchs. *De historia stirpium commentarii insignes.* Basel: M. Isingrin, 1542.

Eighteenth-century mottled sheep, gilt spine.
365 x 240 mm.
Illustrations hand-colored under the publisher's supervision; contemporary annotations.
Ex libris Ludovici Folloppe pharmacopoei Calidobuensis 1710 (inscription partially over erasure, title page)—deleted stamp.

THE HOLDEN ARBORETUM, MENTOR, OHIO

18A Andreas Vesalius. *De humani corporis fabrica libri septem.* Basel: J. Oporinus, 1543.

Purple silk velvet, remains of eight blue silk ties.
420 x 277 mm.
Illustrations hand-colored and highlighted in gold by a contemporary artist highly skilled in miniature painting; no other completely colored copy like this one is known. The coloring of the portrait provides the only historical basis for our knowledge of Vesalius's complexion and hair color.
The dedication copy to the Holy Roman Emperor Charles V, presented to him on the eve of his 1543 military campaign in Gelders, as recorded in Vesalius's charter of ennoblement [see Charles O'Malley, *Andreas Vesalius of Brussels, 1514–1564*

(Berkeley, 1964), p. 189]—Jacques Mesnage, seigneur de Cagny (inscription, flyleaf: *Ce Livre a esté donné par l'empereur Charles le quint a Messire Jacques Mesnage chevalier seigneur et patron de Cagny Ambassadeur du Roy de France Francois premier aupres de sa personne*).

HASKELL F. NORMAN, M.D.

18B Andreas Vesalius. *De humani corporis fabrica librorum epitome.* Basel: J. Oporinus, 1543.

Modern calf, panelled in gilt and blind.
505 x 340 mm.

EUGENE S. FLAMM, M.D.

19A Ambroise Paré. *La methode de traicter les playes faictes par hacquebutes et aultres bastons à feu.* Paris: V. Gaulterot, 1545.

Contemporary limp vellum, remains of four tawed leather ties.
165 x 107 mm.

MATTHEW M. MALERICH, M.D.

19B Ambroise Paré. *La maniere de traicter les playes faictes tant par hacquebutes, que par fleches.* Paris: Widow of Jean de Brie, 1551.

Modern calf, with the sixteenth-century sides and spine laid down: the sides tooled in gilt in a Grolieresque pattern of interlaced scrolls and geometrical shapes outlined in gilt and darkened for contrast, the spine tooled in gilt with a gilt arabesque pattern.
164 x 103 mm.
One of three known copies printed on vellum (the others at the Musée Condé, Chantilly, and the Bodleian Library, Oxford). The woodcuts and floral woodcut initals have been illuminated in silver, gold, and colors.
Gillez (sixteenth-century inscription, title page) —Nicolas Yemeniz (bookplate)—Ambroise Firmin Didot (bookplate)—Robert Hoe (bookplate)—Cortlandt Field Bishop (bookplate)—Harvey Cushing (bookplate).

THE HARVEY CUSHING/JOHN HAY WHITNEY MEDICAL LIBRARY, HISTORICAL LIBRARY, YALE UNIVERSITY

20 Johann Weyer. *De praestigiis daemonum.* Basel: J. Oporinus, 1563.

Eighteenth-century sheep, gilt spine.
159 x 104 mm.
Sum Joannis Pauli He... Landishuti 1567 (inscription, title page)—*Ex libris Jo. Conradi Herwarth. C. Reg. Consiliarij Landishuti A. 1645* (inscription, title page)—stamp of a Hungarian library.

HASKELL F. NORMAN, M.D.

21 Bartolomeo Eustachi. *Opuscula anatomica.* Venice: V. Luchino, 1564.

Contemporary vellum.
200 x 140 mm.
Jo. Hier. Sbarallus (signature, title page)

HASKELL F. NORMAN, M.D.

22 Georg Bartisch. *Ophthalmodouleia. Das ist, Augendienst.* Dresden: M. Stöckel, 1583.

Eighteenth-century (?) leather spine, marbled sides; edges formerly gilt and gauffered.
305 x 190 mm.
All the illustrations and ornamental borders have been colored by a contemporary artist and highlighted in gold and silver.
Deleted signature (title page)—Hans Mehrer, 1583 (inscription, verso of title page)—Daniel Paulus Poetius 1678 (signature, title page)—Josiah Charles Trent, M.D. (bookplate).

DUKE UNIVERSITY MEDICAL CENTER LIBRARY, HISTORY OF MEDICINE COLLECTIONS

23 Gaspare Tagliacozzi. *De curtorum chirurgia per insitionem.* Venice: G. Bindoni, 1597.

Modern blind-paneled calf.
346 x 242 mm.
One of four recorded copies on large and thick paper (the others at the Bibliothèque Nationale, Paris; the University Library, Bologna; and the Jerome P. Webster Collection, Columbia University).
Illegible early signatures (flyleaf)—deleted library stamp—"Property of J. H. Hunt, M.D., 419 Hart Street, Brooklyn, L. I." (stamp, flyleaf).

HASKELL F. NORMAN, M.D.

24 Giulio Casserio. *De vocis auditusque organis historia anatomica.* Ferrara: V. Baldini, 1601.

Contemporary mottled calf, gilt spine.
391 x 260 mm.
Gabriel Naudé (1600–53), librarian to Cardinals Richelieu and Mazarin (signature, engraved title) —Jean-Baptiste Colbert (1619–83), minister of finance under King Louis XIV of France (abbreviated signature, verso of flyleaf).

THE REYNOLDS HISTORICAL LIBRARY, UNIVERSITY OF ALABAMA AT BIRMINGHAM

25 Santorio Santorio. *Ars . . . de statica medicina.* Venice: N. Polo, 1614.

Contemporary limp vellum, remains of four green silk ties.
130 x 70 mm.
Fletcher (signature, title page).

HASKELL F. NORMAN, M.D.

26 Gaspare Aselli. *De lactibus siue lacteis venis.* Milan: G. B. Bidelli, 1627.

Original boards.
231 x 177 mm.
Printed on special thick paper.
Nicolas-Claude Fabri de Peiresc (1580–1637), patron of science and the arts (cipher, title page)—Jean-Paul Marat (1744–93), French political journalist, scholar-physician, and revolutionary (signature inside front cover)—John F. Fulton (bookplate).

THE HARVEY CUSHING/JOHN HAY WHITNEY MEDICAL LIBRARY, HISTORICAL LIBRARY, YALE UNIVERSITY

ALSO: An original sketch for Plate III.
Ink, pencil, and chalk on paper.
410 x 280 mm.
Part of an archive of original drawings and printed proofs of Aselli's plates now in the Historical Collections of the College of Physicians of Philadelphia.

THE COLLEGE OF PHYSICIANS OF PHILADELPHIA

27A William Harvey. *Exercitatio anatomica de motu cordis et sanguinis in animalibus.* Frankfurt: W. Fitzer, 1628.

Red gilt-ruled morocco, by Pawson & Nicholson.
177 x 144 mm.
One of five known thick-paper copies, with the errata sheet from a thin-paper copy tipped in.
Cropped seventeenth-century inscription (title page)—Samuel Lewis, M.D. (bookplate).

THE COLLEGE OF PHYSICIANS OF PHILADELPHIA

27B Girolamo Fabrici. *De venarum ostiolis.* Padua: L. Pasquati, 1603.

Eighteenth-century blind-panelled calf, rebacked.
412 x 273 mm.
In: Girolamo Fabrici, *Opera physica anatomica* (Padua: Sumptibus Roberti Meglietti, 1625). Lacks the separate title page for *De venarum ostiolis.*
William Harvey's copy, with his annotations. Only a few books from Harvey's library are known to have survived the Great Fire of London (1666), in which most of his library was destroyed; other surviving titles include Falloppio's *Opera* (1584), Galen's *Opuscula varia* (1640), and Sylvius's *De febribus commentarius* (1555) [see Geoffrey Keynes, *The Life of William Harvey* (London, 1966), p. 178].

THE LILLY LIBRARY, INDIANA UNIVERSITY, BLOOMINGTON

28A Jean Pecquet. *Experimenta nova anatomica.* Paris: S. Cramoisy & G. Cramoisy, 1651.

Contemporary limp vellum, lacking four tawed leather ties.
190 x 144 mm.
Unknown recipient (author's presentation inscription, verso of flyleaf: *Dono datus ab Authore Kalendis Julii anno domini M.D.C.LX.*).

HASKELL F. NORMAN, M.D.

28B Thomas Bartholin. *Vasa lymphatica.* Copenhagen: G. Holst, 1653.

Modern blind-ruled calf.
198 x 150 mm.
Humboldt (signature, title page)—Cambridge [Mass.] Public Library, presented by Morrill Wyman, M.D. (bookplate).

THE BOSTON MEDICAL LIBRARY IN THE FRANCIS A. COUNTWAY LIBRARY OF MEDICINE

28C Olof Rudbeck. *Nova exercitatio anatomica.* Västerås: E. Lauinger, 1653.

Nineteenth-century Japan vellum spine and corners, marbled sides.
181 x 147 mm.

HASKELL F. NORMAN, M.D.

29 Francis Glisson. *Anatomia hepatis.* London: W. Dugard for O. Pullein, 1654.

Contemporary speckled calf, rebacked.
167 x 108 mm.
Arnold C. Klebs (stamp, rear flyleaf).

THE HARVEY CUSHING/JOHN HAY WHITNEY MEDICAL LIBRARY, HISTORICAL LIBRARY, YALE UNIVERSITY

30 Marcello Malpighi. *De pulmonibus observatio anatomica.* Bologna, 1661.

Modern marbled boards, rebacked.
153 x 110 mm.

THE JOHN CRERAR COLLECTION OF RARE BOOKS IN THE HISTORY OF SCIENCE AND MEDICINE, UNIVERSITY OF CHICAGO LIBRARY

31 René Descartes. *De homine.* Leiden: P. Leffen & F. Moyard, 1662.

Nineteenth-century vellum, gilt spine, rebacked with the original spine laid down.
190 x 150 mm.
Lyre-shaped symbol stamped in bronze ink (title page and last page)—Henry Gore Clough (signature, title page)—James Scott, M.D. (bookplates)—C. S. Sherrington (signature, title page: *C. S. Sherrington Caius Coll. Camb. 1888*)—William Osler (note in his hand, verso of flyleaf: "Given to me viii.16.14 by C. S. Sherrington"; preceded by a note in Sherrington's hand: "E libris Gulielmi Osler 1914").
W. W. Francis, the first Osler librarian, annotated the book as follows: "After Osler's death Sherrington got this book off the shelf, brought it to me with a twinkle in his eye, and told me he had LENT it to O. in 1914. About 1916 he found the book when O. was out, saw that O. had written 'Given to me ...', hadn't the heart to disillusion him, and so he (S.) added the 'E libris Gulielmi Osler 1914' acquiescing in the expropriation!" [Quoted by permission of the Osler Library, McGill University].

THE OSLER LIBRARY OF THE HISTORY OF MEDICINE, MCGILL UNIVERSITY, MONTREAL

32A Thomas Willis. *Cerebri anatome.* London: J. Flesher for J. Martyn and J. Allestry, 1664.

Contemporary calf, rebacked.
205 x 153 mm.
Quarto edition.
Charles Cockburn (bookplate).

HASKELL F. NORMAN, M.D.

32B Thomas Willis. *Cerebri anatome.* London: T. Roycroft for J. Martyn and J. Allestry, 1664.

Contemporary vellum.
155 x 97 mm.
Octavo edition.
Albrecht von Haller (1708–77), German physiologist, one of the founders of neurology (signatures dated 1726 and 1745, title page and flyleaf).

THE MOODY MEDICAL LIBRARY OF THE UNIVERSITY OF TEXAS MEDICAL BRANCH, GALVESTON

33 François Mauriceau. *Des maladies des femmes grosses et accouchées.* Paris: J. Henault [et al.], 1668.

Modern brown morocco spine and corners, marbled sides, by Bernard C. Middleton.
235 x 177 mm.
Alfred M. Hellman (bookplate).

LAWRENCE D. LONGO, M.D.

34 Richard Lower. *Tractatus de corde.* London: J. Redmayne for J. Allestry, 1669.

Contemporary blind-tooled calf, rebacked, with original spine laid down.
168 x 108 mm.
First issue, with the cancellandum A6.
Devon and Exeter Hospital Library (bookplate and inscription; sold as a duplicate, June 1860)—Norman Moore, M.D., St.B.H. 1884 (signature, title page)—John F. Fulton (his note regarding issues laid in).

THE HARVEY CUSHING/JOHN HAY WHITNEY MEDICAL LIBRARY, HISTORICAL LIBRARY, YALE UNIVERSITY

35 Thomas Sydenham. *Observationes medicae circa morborum acutorum historiam et curationem.* London: A. C[lark] for W. Kettilby, 1676.

Contemporary gilt-ruled calf, rebacked, with original gilt spine laid down.
177 x 112 mm.
College of Jesuits, Paris (inscription, title page: *Collegii Parisiensis Soc. Jes.*; IHS ciphers on spine)—Nicolas Fouquet (1615–80), finance minister to King Louis XIV of France in the early years of his reign (cipher in center panel of spine)—Joseph-Ignace Guillotin (1738–1814), inventor of the guillotine (signature dated 1764, flyleaf).

HASKELL F. NORMAN, M.D.

36 Guichard Joseph Duverney. *Traité de l'organe de l'ouie.* Paris: E. Michallet, 1683.

Contemporary calf, gilt spine.
165 x 87 mm.
Dr. Lannois (presentation inscription, flyleaf: *A mon ami le Dr. Lannois affectueuse hommage . . .*).

SPECIAL COLLECTIONS, THE LIBRARY AND CENTER FOR KNOWLEDGE MANAGEMENT, UNIVERSITY OF CALIFORNIA, SAN FRANCISCO

37 Antoni van Leeuwenhoek. *Ondervindingen en beschouwingen der onsigbare geschapene waarheden, waar in gehandeld werd vande eyerstok.* Leiden: D. van Gaesbeeck, 1684.

Modern vellum.
200 x 159 mm.

Bound with three other works published by Leeuwenhoek in 1684 [Norman 1301, 1305, 1306].

HASKELL F. NORMAN, M.D.

38 Bernardino Ramazzini. *De morbis artificum diatriba.* Modena: A. Capponi, 1700.

Eighteenth-century vellum.
174 x 112 mm.

SPECIAL COLLECTIONS, THE LIBRARY AND CENTER FOR KNOWLEDGE MANAGEMENT, UNIVERSITY OF CALIFORNIA, SAN FRANCISCO

39 Herman Boerhaave. *Institutiones medicae.* Leiden: J. vander Linden, 1708.

COPY 1: Eighteenth-century paneled calf, rebacked.
155 x 94 mm.
Interleaved and annotated with manuscript additions and anatomical drawings.
John Redman Coxe (1773–1864), American physician, possibly inherited from his grandfather John Redman (1722–1808), a medical student at the University of Leiden in 1747–48 (signature, front pastedown and title page).

ANONYMOUS LENDER

COPY 2: Mid-eighteenth-century Dutch morocco, richly gilt.
153 x 98 mm.
John F. Fulton (bookplate).

THE HARVEY CUSHING/JOHN HAY WHITNEY MEDICAL LIBRARY, HISTORICAL LIBRARY, YALE UNIVERSITY

40 Pierre Fauchard. *Le chirurgien dentiste, ou traité des dentes.* Paris. J. Mariette, 1728. 2 vols.

Contemporary sprinkled calf, gilt spines.
162 x 90 mm.
Dr. Charreau (signature, title page; stamps: *Charreau docteur medecin*)—Harvey Cushing (bookplate).

THE HARVEY CUSHING/JOHN HAY WHITNEY MEDICAL LIBRARY, HISTORICAL LIBRARY, YALE UNIVERSITY

41 Stephen Hales. *Statical Essays: Containing Haemastaticks.* London: For W. Innys, R. Manby, and R. Woodward, 1733.

Contemporary mottled calf, gilt-ruled, rebacked with original spine laid down.
193 x 120 mm.
Ron C. Belasque (signature, flyleaf)—Edward Neville da Costa Andrade (bookplate).

PAUL KLIGFIELD, M.D.

42 Nicolas Andry. *L'orthopédie ou l'art de prévenir et de corriger dans les enfans, les difformités du corps.* Paris: La veuve Alix; Lambert & Durand, 1741. 2 vols.

Contemporary gilt-blocked calf, gilt spines.
162 x 96 mm. (vol. I), 162 x 92 mm. (vol. II)
Bignon family of Anjou (armorial binding).

SPECIAL COLLECTIONS, THE LIBRARY AND CENTER FOR KNOWLEDGE MANAGEMENT, UNIVERSITY OF CALIFORNIA, SAN FRANCISCO

43A William Smellie. *A Treatise on the Theory and Practice of Midwifery.* London: For D. Wilson, 1752. *A Collection of Cases and Observations in Midwifery.* London: For D. Wilson and T. Durham, 1754. *A Collection of Preternatural Cases and Observations in Midwifery.* London: For D. Wilson and T. Durham, 1764. [3 vols.]

Contemporary sprinkled sheep, gilt-ruled.
200 x 119 mm.
American Antiquarian Society, Worcester (stamps, vols. [I] and [II])—Massachusetts Medical College Library/Harvard Medical School Library (bookplate, vol. [III]).

THE BOSTON MEDICAL LIBRARY IN THE FRANCIS A. COUNTWAY LIBRARY OF MEDICINE

43B William Smellie. *A Sett of Anatomical Tables, with Explanations, and an Abridgement of the Practice of Midwifery.* London, 1754.

Modern calf spine and corners, older marbled sides.
570 x 360 mm.

LAWRENCE D. LONGO, M.D.

44 James Lind. *A Treatise of the Scurvy.* Edinburgh: Sands, Murray and Cochran, for A. Millar, 1753.

Contemporary gilt-ruled calf.
201 x 128 mm.
Early signatures, deleted, one dated 1754 (title page and dedication page)—Samuel H. Rose (purchase inscription, partially deleted, title page) —William Wattles (signature, title page)—James F. Wattles (signature, front pastedown)—record of the birth of Solomon Gardner, 19 Nov. [18]29 (inscription, rear pastedown).

THE HARVEY CUSHING/JOHN HAY WHITNEY MEDICAL LIBRARY, HISTORICAL LIBRARY, YALE UNIVERSITY

45 Leopold Auenbrugger. *Inventum novum ex percussione thoracis humani.* Vienna: J. T. Trattner, 1761.

Blue wrappers.
220 x 150 mm.
First issue, without the errata list; untrimmed and partially unopened.
L. Jonker (stamp on remnant of old flyleaf)—William Osler (bookplate).

THE OSLER LIBRARY OF THE HISTORY OF MEDICINE, MCGILL UNIVERSITY, MONTREAL

46 Giovanni Battista Morgagni. *De sedibus, et causis morborum per anatomen indagatis.* Venice: Remondini, 1761. 2 vols.

Brown morocco, gilt-ruled, by Hyman Zucker.
378 x 237 mm.
John Morgan (1735–89), founder of the first medical school in the United States (now the School of Medicine, University of Pennsylvania) and one of the founders of the College of Physicians of Philadelphia (author's presentation inscriptions, title pages).
After receiving his medical degree from the University of Edinburgh in 1763, Morgan embarked on a grand tour of Europe, during which he had the pleasure of meeting the eighty-two-year-old Morgagni in Padua. Morgan presented a copy of his medical dissertation to Morgagni, who in turn gave the young Philadelphian a copy of the first edition of his famous *De sedibus*, inscribing both volumes of the work for Morgan. The inscription on the title page of Volume I reads: *Viro experientissimo et humanissimo D. Di. Joanni Morgan Auctor* (Gift of the author to the most skillful and accomplished Dr. John Morgan). The inscription on the title page of Volume II reads: *Viro de Re anatomico bene merito Do. Dr. Joanni Morgan Auctor* (Gift of the author to Dr. John Morgan, highly deserving in anatomy).

THE COLLEGE OF PHYSICIANS OF PHILADELPHIA

47 Franz Anton Mesmer. *Mémoire sur la découverte du magnétisme animal.* Geneva & Paris: Didot le jeune, 1779.

Contemporary mottled sheep, gilt spine.
161 x 103 mm.
Society of Harmony, the organization established by Mesmer and his followers to promote and disseminate his ideas (stamp and inscription, flyleaf: *Appartenant à la Société de l'harmonie de France, et faisant partie de Sa Bibliothèque*).

HASKELL F. NORMAN, M.D.

48 Michael Underwood. *A Treatise on the Diseases of Children.* London: For J. Mathews, 1784.

Red straight-grain morocco gilt, edges gilt.
156 x 96 mm.
The dedication copy, bound for Queen Charlotte (1744–1818), consort of King George III of England (note on flyleaf: "Bought at the sale of Queen Charlotte's books in June 1819")—Richard Southwell Bourke (1822–72), Lord Nass, from 1867 sixth Earl of Mayo (bookplate)—Lady Nass (inscription).

HASKELL F. NORMAN, M.D.

49 William Withering. *An Account of the Foxglove, and Some of Its Medical Uses.* Birmingham: M. Swinney for G.G.J. and J. Robinson, 1785.

COPY 1: Calf spine, marbled sides.
208 x 129 mm.
With the uncolored plate by James Sowerby.
Presentation copy to Mr. Freer, probably Mr. J. Freer, junior surgeon in Birmingham, who communicated to Withering a case reported in this work (inscription, title page: "Mr. Freer from the Author"; bookplate of John Freer, Surgeon)—Bath Medical Library (stamp, verso of title page).

THE LILLY LIBRARY, INDIANA UNIVERSITY, BLOOMINGTON

COPY 2: Nineteenth-century blue polished sheep spine, rebacked in blue morocco with the original spine laid down, blue pebble cloth sides.
217 x 134 mm.
With the hand-colored plate by James Sowerby.
Deleted purchase inscription, dated 1835 (half-title).

THE BOSTON MEDICAL LIBRARY IN THE FRANCIS A. COUNTWAY LIBRARY OF MEDICINE

COPY 3: Early nineteenth-century speckled sheep, gilt-ruled spine.
210 x 127 mm.
With the hand-colored plate from *Flora Londinensis.*
Gift of Hermann Ludwig Blumgart, M.D. (bookplate).

THE HARVARD MEDICAL LIBRARY IN THE FRANCIS A. COUNTWAY LIBRARY OF MEDICINE

50 Luigi Galvani. "De viribus electricitatis in motu musculari commentarius," *De Bononiensi Scientiarum et Artium Instituto atque Academia Commentarii* 7 (1791): 363–418.

OFFPRINT, FIRST ISSUE: Nineteenth-century vellum spine and corners, marbled sides.

284 x 210 mm.
Bound with two copies of the 1792 edition and several pamphlets on Galvani by Silvestro Gherardi.
Silvestro Gherardi (annotations in his hand)—John F. Fulton (bookplate).

THE HARVEY CUSHING/JOHN HAY WHITNEY MEDICAL LIBRARY, HISTORICAL LIBRARY, YALE UNIVERSITY

OFFPRINT, SECOND ISSUE: Pastepaper boards.
292 x 208 mm.
Harvey Cushing (bookplate; signature on flyleaf).

THE HARVEY CUSHING/JOHN HAY WHITNEY MEDICAL LIBRARY, HISTORICAL LIBRARY, YALE UNIVERSITY

51A Matthew Baillie. *The Morbid Anatomy of Some of the Most Important Parts of the Human Body.* London: For J. Johnson and G. Nicol, 1793.

Modern calf spine, marbled sides.
212 x 130 mm.
George C. Julius (bookplate)—Harvey Cushing (bookplate).

THE HARVEY CUSHING/JOHN HAY WHITNEY MEDICAL LIBRARY, HISTORICAL LIBRARY, YALE UNIVERSITY

51B Matthew Baillie. *A Series of Engravings, Accompanied with Explanations, Which are Intended to Illustrate the Morbid Anatomy of Some of the Most Important Parts of the Human Body.* London: W. Bulmer for J. Johnson and G. and W. Nicol, 1803.

Nineteenth-century red straight-grain morocco spine and corners, marbled sides.
322 x 245 mm.
The complete volume as published in 1803.
Thomas Edgar Fakenham Norf. (signature, title page)—Dr. Thor Jager (bookplate).

THE CLENDENING HISTORY OF MEDICINE LIBRARY, UNIVERSITY OF KANSAS MEDICAL CENTER

52 John Hunter. *A Treatise on the Blood, Inflammation, and Gun-Shot Wounds.* London: J. Richardson for G. Nicol, 1794.

Modern calf spine and corners, marbled sides.
260 x 196 mm.
Harvey Cushing (bookplate).

THE HARVEY CUSHING/JOHN HAY WHITNEY MEDICAL LIBRARY, HISTORICAL LIBRARY, YALE UNIVERSITY

53 Edward Jenner. *An Inquiry into the Causes and Effects of the Variolae Vaccinae.* London: For the author by S. Low, 1798.

Contemporary sheep.
265 x 215 mm.
Bound with: Edward Jenner, *Further Observations on the Variolae Vaccinae, or Cow Pox* (London, 1799).
John Clinch (author's presentation inscription, title page: "For the Rev. John Clinch his affectionate friend the author")—M. F. Gavin, M.D. (bookplate).
Jenner presented this copy to his boyhood friend, the Rev. John Clinch, who also studied with John Hunter before emigrating to Newfoundland in 1786 as a doctor-missionary. From 1800 on, Clinch was actively involved in the practice of vaccination, working for a time in Newfoundland with Jenner's nephew George Jenner, who reported some of Clinch's vaccination cases to the *Medical and Physical Journal* in 1801.

THE BOSTON MEDICAL LIBRARY IN THE FRANCIS A. COUNTWAY LIBRARY OF MEDICINE

54 Philippe Pinel. *Traité médico-philosophique sur l'aliénation mentale, ou la manie.* Paris: Richard, Caille et Ravier, An IX [1800–01].

Untrimmed in original purple wrappers.
212 x 135 mm.

HASKELL F. NORMAN, M.D.

55 Robert Willan. *On Cutaneous Diseases.* Vol. I. London: For J. Johnson, 1808.

Nineteenth-century sheep spine and corners, marbled sides.
272 x 217 mm.
The complete volume as published in 1808.
Louis Heermann (signature, title page).

THE HARVEY CUSHING/JOHN HAY WHITNEY MEDICAL LIBRARY, HISTORICAL LIBRARY, YALE UNIVERSITY

56 Dominique Jean Larrey. *Mémoires de chirurgie militaire.* Paris: J. Smith, 1812–17. 4 vols. *Relation médicale de campagnes et voyages.* Paris: J.-B. Ballière, 1841.

Nineteenth-century polished tan calf, spines gilt, arms stamped in blind on the covers within a gilt panel.
202 x 122 mm.
Second issue of Volumes I and II; Volume IV with the preliminary quire in 4 and no quire 31. The *Relation médicale* not exhibited.

Lord Charles Stuart, the British ambassador to France (cropped presentation inscription, half-title of vol. I: *A son excellence Lord Stuart ambassadeur de S.M.B . . . hommage de l'auteur . . . Larrey*).

THE LILLY LIBRARY, INDIANA UNIVERSITY, BLOOMINGTON

57 René Théophile Hyacinthe Laennec. *De l'auscultation médiate.* Paris: J.-A. Brosson & J.-S. Chaudé, 1819. 2 vols.

COPY 1: Untrimmed in original mauve printed wrappers.
215 x 135 mm.
With the original leaf a*2.

HASKELL F. NORMAN, M.D.

COPY 2: Red pebble-grain cloth spines, marbled sides. Vol. I rebacked with original spine laid down.
205 x 124 mm.
With the cancel leaf a*2.
Guillaume François Laennec, Laennec's uncle (author's presentation inscription, title page of vol. I: *Optimo patruo alteri patri . . . Laennec DM*).

THE HARVEY CUSHING/JOHN HAY WHITNEY MEDICAL LIBRARY, HISTORICAL LIBRARY, YALE UNIVERSITY

58 François Magendie. "Expériences sur les fonctions des racines des nerfs rachidiens," *Journal de physiologie expérimentale et pathologique* 2 (1822): 276–79.

Journal volume: Modern tan calf spine, marbled sides.
198 x 120 mm.

ARTHUR E. LYONS, M.D.

59 Karl Ernst von Baer. *De ovi mammalium et hominis genesi.* Leipzig: L. Voss, 1827.

Modern cloth spine, marbled sides, original cream printed wrappers bound in.
273 x 215 mm.

THE NEW YORK ACADEMY OF MEDICINE

60A Richard Bright. *Reports of Medical Cases.* London: Longman, 1827–31. 2 vols. in 3.

Original brown paper boards, rebacked in modern red morocco.
332 x 255 mm.
John Collins Warren (1778–1856), the first surgeon to perform an operation using surgical anesthesia (signature, front pastedown)—Warren family (bookplate).

THE HARVARD MEDICAL LIBRARY IN THE FRANCIS A. COUNTWAY LIBRARY OF MEDICINE

60B Thomas Hodgkin. "On Some Morbid Appearances of the Absorbent Glands and Spleen," *Medico-Chirurgical Transactions* 17 (1832): 68–114.

OFFPRINT: Nineteenth-century sheep spine and corners, marbled sides.
208 x 133 mm.
Bound with twenty-one other pamphlets on medical subjects.
A. Coleman, a graduate of the University of Pennsylvania Medical School (1832) who taught botany and medical jurisprudence at the Geneva (New York) Medical College from 1834 to 1836 (author's presentation inscription, title page: "From Dr. Thos. Hodgkin of London to A. Coleman 1833 May 4").

SUNY HEALTH SCIENCE CENTER LIBRARY AT SYRACUSE

60C Thomas Addison. *On the Constitutional and Local Effects of Disease of the Supra-Renal Capsules.* London: S. Highley, 1855.

Original green diagonal-weave embossed cloth stamped in gilt and blind, rebacked.
325 x 245 mm.
Francis Minot (bookplate)—James J. Minot (signature, flyleaf)—George R. Minot (1885–1950), who shared the Nobel Prize for Physiology or Medicine in 1934 for his part in the discovery of a cure for pernicious anemia, also called Addison's anemia (signature, flyleaf).

THE BOSTON MEDICAL LIBRARY IN THE FRANCIS A. COUNTWAY LIBRARY OF MEDICINE

61 William Beaumont. *Experiments and Observations on the Gastric Juice, and the Physiology of Digestion.* Plattsburgh: F. P. Allen, 1833.

Original full sheep, one of fifty copies so bound for presentation; rebacked in calf, with gilt-ruled spine.
218 x 134 mm.
William Dunlap, possibly the Canadian physician William Dunlop (1792–1848) (author's presentation inscription, title page: "To Wm. Dunlap Esqr. with the respects of the Author")—Samuel Smith Purple, M.D. (1822–1900), a founder of the New York Academy of Medicine and collector of early

American medical publications (signature dated 1845, flyleaf).

HASKELL F. NORMAN, M.D.

62 Theodor Schwann. *Mikroskopische Untersuchungen über die Uebereinstimmung in der Struktur und dem Wachsthum der Thiere und Pflanzen.* Berlin: Sander, 1839.

Nineteenth-century green paper boards.
200 x 123 mm.
Gilbert Breschet (1784–1845), French anatomist (author's presentation inscription, front pastedown: *Herrn Prof. Breschet empfiehlt sich hochachtungsvoll der Verfasser* [The author commends himself respectfully to Prof. Breschet])— August Weismann (1834–1914), formulator of the first modern cell-based theory of inheritance (note in Dobell's hand, front pastedown)—Clifford Dobell (1866–1949), biographer of Antoni van Leeuwenhoek (signature dated 1914, front pastedown).

THE LILLY LIBRARY, INDIANA UNIVERSITY, BLOOMINGTON

63 Edwin Chadwick. *Report . . . from the Poor Law Commissioners, on an Inquiry into the Sanitary Condition of the Labouring Population of Great Britain.* London: W. Clowes & Sons, 1842. *Local Reports on the Sanitary Condition of the Labouring Population of England.* London: W. Clowes & Sons, 1842. *Reports on the Sanitary Condition of the Labouring Population of Scotland.* London: W. Clowes & Sons, 1842. *A Supplementary Report on the Results of a Special Inquiry into the Practice of Interment in Towns.* London: W. Clowes & Sons, 1843. [4 vols.]

Original purple morocco-grain cloth.
214 x 133 mm.

HASKELL F. NORMAN, M.D.

64A Henry Jacob Bigelow. "Insensibility During Surgical Operations Produced by Inhalation," *Boston Medical and Surgical Journal* 35 (1846): 309–17, 379–82.

JOURNAL VOLUME: Individual numbers in original printed self wrappers, gathered and folded but unbound.
240 x 153 mm.

HASKELL F. NORMAN, M.D.

64B William T. G. Morton. *To Surgeons and Physicians.* [Boston], 1846. Advertising circular.

Unbound.
194 x 250 mm. (unfolded).
One of three known copies. Addressed to "Dr. Alfred Hitchcock, Ashby, Mass." and postmarked "Boston, Mass., Nov. 23."

THE HISTORICAL DIVISION, CLEVELAND MEDICAL LIBRARY ASSOCIATION

64C William T. G. Morton. *Remarks on the Proper Mode of Administering Sulphuric Ether by Inhalation.* Boston: Dutton and Wentworth, 1847.

COPY I: Original blue wrappers, title printed in gilt on the front wrapper.
Jonathan Mason Warren (1811–67) (author's presentation inscription, flyleaf: "J. Mason Warren, MD, Compliments of W.T.G. Morton")—Warren family (bookplate).
175 x 110 mm.

THE HARVARD MEDICAL LIBRARY IN THE FRANCIS A. COUNTWAY LIBRARY OF MEDICINE

COPY 2: Original floral patterned wrappers, title printed in black on the front wrapper.
167 x 104 mm.

THE BOSTON MEDICAL LIBRARY IN THE FRANCIS A. COUNTWAY LIBRARY OF MEDICINE

65 Hermann von Helmholtz. *Beschreibung eines Augen-Spiegels zur Untersuchung der Netzhaut im lebenden Auge.* Berlin: A. Förstner, 1851.

Original yellow printed wrappers.
228 x 140 mm.
Olga Helmholtz, wife of the author (author's presentation inscription, inside front wrapper: *Seiner Olga, zum Gedächtnisse daran, dass ihr Auge das erste war, dessen Hintergrund sich dem forschenden Auge entschleierte, der Verfasser* [To his Olga, in remembrance that her eye was the first to reveal its interior to the searching eye, the Author]).

HASKELL F. NORMAN, M.D.

66A J. Marion Sims. "On the Treatment of Vesico-Vaginal Fistula," *American Journal of the Medical Sciences,* N.S. 23 (1852): 59–82.

JOURNAL VOLUME: Contemporary sheep spine and corners, marbled sides.
214 x 134 mm.
Illegible signature (title page).

LAWRENCE D. LONGO, M.D.

66B J. Marion Sims. *Clinical Notes on Uterine Surgery.* New York: W. Wood & Co., 1866.

Publisher's gray-green pebble-grain cloth.
225 x 144 mm.
T. Sidney Scales, College of Physicians and Surgeons, New York 1867 (inscription, flyleaf).

LAWRENCE D. LONGO, M.D.

67A Claude Bernard. *Recherches sur une nouvelle fonction du foie.* Paris: L. Martinet, 1853.

THESIS PUBLICATION: Unopened in original blue printed wrappers.
276 x 220 mm.

THE HARVEY CUSHING/JOHN HAY WHITNEY MEDICAL LIBRARY, HISTORICAL LIBRARY, YALE UNIVERSITY

67B Claude Bernard. *Mémoire sur le pancréas.* Paris: J.-B. Ballière, 1856.

MONOGRAPH PUBLICATION: Unopened in original tan printed wrappers.
276 x 220 mm.

HASKELL F. NORMAN, M.D.

68 Henry Gray. *Anatomy, Descriptive and Surgical.* London: J. W. Parker & Son, 1858.

Original brown bead-grain cloth, blind-paneled, rebacked in modern calf.
257 x 158 mm.
Oliver Wendell Holmes (bookplate).
Holmes was professor of anatomy and physiology at Harvard Medical School at the time Gray's *Anatomy* was published. Holmes's bookplate illustrates the chambered nautilus, the subject of his most famous poem.

THE BOSTON MEDICAL LIBRARY IN THE FRANCIS A. COUNTWAY LIBRARY OF MEDICINE

69 Rudolf Virchow. *Die Cellularpathologie.* Berlin: A. Hirschwald, 1858.

COPY 1: Nineteenth-century red morocco-grain sheep spine and corners, marbled sides, the original buff printed wrappers bound in.
222 x 135 mm.
Smithsonian Institution (author's presentation inscription, front wrapper: "To the Smithsonian Institution, Washington, U.S. America, the author").

RARE BOOK AND SPECIAL COLLECTIONS DIVISION, LIBRARY OF CONGRESS

COPY 2: Original printed boards, black cloth spine.
223 x 138 mm.

HASKELL F. NORMAN, M.D.

70A Charles Darwin and Alfred Russel Wallace. "On the Tendency of Species to Form Varieties; and on the Perpetuation of Varieties and Species by Natural Means of Selection," *Journal of the Proceedings of the Linnean Society,* Zoology 3 (1859): 45–62.

OFFPRINT: Plain buff wrappers.
223 x 141 mm.
Inscribed in Darwin's hand on front wrapper: "CD & Wallace," and on back wrapper: "Wallace & Self."

THE HOUGHTON LIBRARY, HARVARD UNIVERSITY

70B Charles Darwin. *On the Origin of Species.* London: J. Murray, 1859.

Original green cloth (Freeman, variant B), with thirty-two pages of Murray's advertisements (third issue), dated June 1859, at the end.
200 x 125 mm.
Presentation copy to Charles Kingsley (1819–75), Anglican clergyman, naturalist, and author (inscription in the hand of a publisher's clerk on verso of flyleaf: "From the Author"; inscription on title page in Kingsley's hand: "Charles & Fanny Kingsley 1862 [corrected to 1860]"). Kingsley acknowledged receipt of the book in a letter to Darwin dated 18 November 1859 [*The Life and Letters of Charles Darwin,* ed. Francis Darwin, vol. 2 (London, 1887), p. 287].

JEREMY M. NORMAN

ALSO: The only extant proof copy of *On the Origin of Species,* showing the second through the fourth rounds of revision.
Unbound.
200 x 125 mm.

SPECIAL COLLECTIONS, LEHIGH UNIVERSITY LIBRARIES

ALSO: The title leaf from Darwin's autograph manuscript of *On the Origin of Species.*
202 x 125 mm.
The manuscript of *On the Origin of Species* was broken up, some of it being used for scratch paper in the Darwin family.

THE AMERICAN PHILOSOPHICAL SOCIETY

71 Florence Nightingale. *Notes on Nursing: What It Is, and What It Is Not.* London: Harrison & Sons, [1860].

Original charcoal bead-grain cloth on soft cardboard, with three blind rules framing cover, and plain yellow endpapers.
220 x 136 mm.

Miss Bevington (presentation printed in gilt, front cover: "Miss Bevington with Best Wishes from Florence Nightingale")—Rev. W. Chawner (presentation inscription from Nightingale's mother, flyleaf: "To the Rev'd W. Chawner with Mrs. Nightingale's kind regards").

The earliest state of binding, endpapers, and typesetting, without the translation notice (Skretkowicz, group 1).

THE LILLY LIBRARY, INDIANA UNIVERSITY, BLOOMINGTON

72A Ignaz Philipp Semmelweis. *Die Aetiologie, der Begriff und die Prophylaxis des Kindbettfiebers.* Pest, Vienna & Leipzig: C. A. Hartleben, 1861.

COPY 1: Black cloth spine, marbled sides.

224 x 145 mm.

Carl Siegmund Franz Credé (1819–92), professor of obstetrics at Leipzig (signature, title page and flyleaf)—illegible signatures (flyleaf).

Credé was known for initiating the prophylaxis of gonorrhea in the eyes of the newborn, i.e., *ophthalmia neonatorum*, by the instillation of silver nitrate, and for his method of expression of the placenta. Credé's review of Semmelweis's work, published in the *Monatsschrift für Geburtskunde und Frauenkrankheiten* in 1861, was on the whole favorable, although he noted that to disagree with Semmelweis did not necessarily imply that one was ignorant, or indeed murderous. Twenty-five years later, in his *Gesunde und kranke Wöchnerinnen*, Credé wholeheartedly endorsed Semmelweis's doctrine.

LAWRENCE D. LONGO, M.D.

COPY 2: Unopened in original pink printed wrappers.

236 x 150 mm.

DEPARTMENT OF SPECIAL COLLECTIONS, UNIVERSITY OF CHICAGO LIBRARY

72B Oliver Wendell Holmes. "The Contagiousness of Puerperal Fever," *New England Quarterly Journal of Medicine and Surgery* 1 (1843): 503–30.

OFFPRINT: Original buff printed wrappers.

235 x 140 mm.

Dr. Abel Lawrence Peirson (1794–1853) (author's presentation inscription, front wrapper: "Dr. Peirson With the Author's respects").

THE BOSTON MEDICAL LIBRARY IN THE FRANCIS A. COUNTWAY LIBRARY OF MEDICINE

72C Oliver Wendell Holmes. *Puerperal Fever as a Private Pestilence.* Boston: Ticknor and Fields, 1855.

Original pink printed wrappers.

240 x 150 mm.

Dr. Henry J. Bigelow (1818–80), author of the first description of the use of sulfuric ether as an anesthetic (author's presentation inscription, front wrapper: "Dr. H. J. Bigelow With the regards of O. W. Holmes").

THE BOSTON MEDICAL LIBRARY IN THE FRANCIS A. COUNTWAY LIBRARY OF MEDICINE

73A J. Henry Dunant. *Un souvenir de Solferino.* Geneva: J.-G. Fick, 1862.

Modern green morocco spine, green paper boards decorated with cut-out designs, original brown printed wrappers bound in.

258 x 169 mm.

Alfred-Auguste Cuvillier-Fleury (1802–87), French man of letters (author's presentation inscription, front wrapper: Monsieur Cuvillier-Fleury).

THE MOODY MEDICAL LIBARY OF THE UNIVERSITY OF TEXAS MEDICAL BRANCH, GALVESTON

73B John Pringle. *Observations on the Diseases of the Army, in Camp and Garrison.* London: For A. Millar, D. Wilson, and T. Payne, 1752.

Modern mottled calf.

202 x 122 mm.

With manuscript corrections throughout, presumably in Pringle's hand, in preparation for a new edition.

Walter C. Alvarez (pencilled signature, flyleaf).

DUKE UNIVERSITY MEDICAL CENTER LIBRARY, HISTORY OF MEDICINE COLLECTIONS

74 Gregor Mendel. "Versuche über Pflanzen-Hybriden," *Verhandlungen des naturforschenden Vereines Brünn* 4 (1865): 3–47.

OFFPRINT: Stapled, as issued.

223 x 144 mm.

Illegible signature and erased inscription, title page.

THE LILLY LIBRARY, INDIANA UNIVERSITY, BLOOMINGTON

75 Joseph Lister. "On a New Method of Treating Compound Fracture, Abscess, etc. With Observations on the Conditions of Suppu-

ration," *Lancet*, 1867, 1: 326–29, 357–59, 387–89, 507–9; 2: 95–96.

Modern gray paper boards.
273 x 190 mm.
The pages containing Lister's article, extracted from the *Lancet* and bound together.

THE HARVEY CUSHING/JOHN HAY WHITNEY MEDICAL LIBRARY, HISTORICAL LIBRARY, YALE UNIVERSITY

76 David Ferrier. *The Functions of the Brain.* London: Smith, Elder, & Co., 1876.

Publisher's green sand-grain cloth, panelled in black; rebacked in green cloth with original spine laid down.
200 x 140 mm.
Henry Pickering Bowditch (1840–1911), an American physiologist (author's presentation inscription, flyleaf: "H. P. Bowditch 1876 from the Author").

THE HARVARD MEDICAL LIBRARY IN THE FRANCIS A. COUNTWAY LIBRARY OF MEDICINE

77 Paul Bert. *La pression barométrique.* Paris: G. Masson, 1878.

Publisher's sand-grain maroon cloth, panelled in blind.
240 x 150 mm.
Illegible signature (flyleaf)—"Dr. E. Letersec, Médecin de la Marine, Brest" (stamp, flyleaf and title page).

HASKELL F. NORMAN, M.D.

78 Louis Pasteur. "Sur les maladies virulentes, et en particulier sur la maladie vulgairement appelée *choléra des poules*," *Bulletin de l'Académie de Médecine* 44, 2me série, 9 (1880): 121–34.

OFFPRINT: Original blue-green printed wrappers.
222 x 138 mm.

HASKELL F. NORMAN, M.D.

79 Alphonse Laveran. "Un nouveau parasite trouvé dans le sang de plusieurs malades atteints de fièvre palustre," *Bulletins et mémoires de la Société médicale des hôpitaux de Paris*, 2me série, Mémoires, 17 (1880): 158–64.

JOURNAL VOLUME: Modern black cloth.
244 x 151 mm.

DUKE UNIVERSITY MEDICAL CENTER LIBRARY, HISTORY OF MEDICINE COLLECTIONS

80 Robert Koch. "Die Aetiologie der Tuberkulose," *Mittheilungen aus dem kaiserlichen Gesundheitsamte* 2 (1884): 1–88.

JOURNAL VOLUME: Original gray-green printed boards, rebacked, original black cloth spine laid down.
305 x 217 mm.

JEREMY M. NORMAN

81 Emil Adolph von Behring and Shibasaburo Kitasato. "Ueber das Zustandekommen der Diphtherie-Immunität und der Tetanus-Immunität bei Thieren," *Deutsche medicinische Wochenschrift* 16 (1890): 1113–14.

JOURNAL VOLUME: Contemporary blue cloth spine, marbled paper sides.
313 x 237 mm.
Janus Foundation, San Francisco (bookplate).

JEREMY M. NORMAN

82 William Osler. *The Principles and Practice of Medicine.* New York: D. Appleton, 1892.

COPY 1: Rebound with brown morocco spine, brown cloth sides; the original brown morocco spine and brown pebble-grain cloth sides laid down.
235 x 150 mm.
First issue.
Grace Revere Gross (author's presentation inscription, flyleaf: "Grace Revere Gross from her friend Wm. Osler Feb 25, 1892, Phila.").
Osler inscribed this copy to Grace Revere Gross, the woman who would later become his wife. In his *Life of Osler*, Cushing records that Osler proposed to Mrs. Gross (who was the widow of a physician) by tossing the book in her lap with the words: "There, take the darn thing; now what are you going to do about the man?"—certainly one of the more bookish offers of marriage on record.

THE OSLER LIBRARY OF THE HISTORY OF MEDICINE, MCGILL UNIVERSITY, MONTREAL

COPY 2: Contemporary tan calf spines and corners, marbled sides, gilt spines, gilt edges. Bound in two volumes.
235 x 150 mm.
Second issue.
Osler's interleaved and annotated copy.

THE OSLER LIBRARY OF THE HISTORY OF MEDICINE, MCGILL UNIVERSITY, MONTREAL

83A Wilhelm Conrad Roentgen. "Eine neue Art von Strahlen. (Vorlaufige Mittheilung.)," *Sitzungsberichte der physikalisch-medicinischen Gesellschaft zu Würzburg*, 1895: 132–41.

OFFPRINT: Lacking the original printed wrappers. Bound with 83B in modern red cloth.
214 x 140 mm.
Unknown recipient (author's presentation inscription in English, first page: "With the Author's Compliments").

THE OSLER LIBRARY OF THE HISTORY OF MEDICINE, MCGILL UNIVERSITY, MONTREAL

83B Wilhelm Conrad Roentgen. "Eine neue Art von Strahlen. II. Mittheilung," *Sitzungsberichte der physikalisch-medicinischen Gesellschaft zu Würzburg*, 1896: 11–19.

OFFPRINT: Original orange printed wrappers. Bound with 83A in modern red cloth.
214 x 140 mm.
Unknown recipient (author's presentation inscription in English, front wrapper: "With respectful compliments").

THE OSLER LIBRARY OF THE HISTORY OF MEDICINE, MCGILL UNIVERSITY, MONTREAL

ALSO: Two original X-ray photographs made by Roentgen:
Photograph of a gun barrel, 170 x 122 mm.; on cardboard mount, 310 x 230 mm.
Photograph of Frau Roentgen's hand, 180 x 130 mm.; on cardboard mount, 230 x 160 mm.

THE HARVARD MEDICAL LIBRARY IN THE FRANCIS A. COUNTWAY LIBRARY OF MEDICINE

84A Henri Becquerel. "Sur les radiations émises par phosphorescence," *Comptes rendus hebdomadaires des séances de l'Académie des Sciences* 122 (1896): 420–21.

JOURNAL VOLUME: Black morocco spine, blind-panelled green cloth sides.
263 x 207 mm.

HASKELL F. NORMAN, M.D.

84B Marie Curie, Pierre Curie, and Gustave Bémont. "Sur une nouvelle substance fortement radioactive, contenue dans la pechblende," *Comptes rendus hebdomadaires des séances de l'Académie des Sciences* 127 (1898): 1215–17.

JOURNAL NUMBER: Original pink printed wrappers.
284 x 228 mm.

HASKELL F. NORMAN, M.D.

85 Ivan Petrovich Pavlov. *Lekstii o rabotie glavnikh pishtshevavritelnikh zhelyoz* [Lectures on the Work of the Principal Digestive Glands (Russian)]. St. Petersburg: I. N. Kushnereff, 1897.

Early twentieth-century light green cloth spine, marbled sides.
180 x 124 mm.

THE LILLY LIBRARY, INDIANA UNIVERSITY, BLOOMINGTON

86 Santiago Ramón y Cajal. *Textura del sistema nervioso del hombre y de los vertebrados.* Madrid: N. Moya, 1899–1904. 2 vols. in 3.

Green morocco spines, marbled sides, original wrappers for fascicles bound in.
246 x 157 mm.
Unknown recipient (author's presentation inscription, front wrappers and title pages: "Presented by the Author")—Royal Microscopical Society (stamp).

ARTHUR E. LYONS, M.D.

87 Sigmund Freud. *Die Traumdeutung.* Leipzig & Vienna: F. Deuticke, 1900.

Brown paper boards.
220 x 145 mm.
One of two author's copies received by Freud in October 1899.
Wilhelm Fliess (author's presentation inscription, title page: *Seinem theuern Wilhelm z. 24 Okt. 1899* [For his dear Wilhelm, 24 Oct. 1899]).

HASKELL F. NORMAN, M.D.

88A Karl Landsteiner. "Ueber Agglutinationserscheinungen normalen menschlichen Blutes," *Wiener klinische Wochenschrift* 14 (1901): 1132–34.

OFFPRINT: Unbound.
222 x 144 mm.
Harvey Cushing (presentation copy, signed "Karl Landsteiner" on a slip of paper attached to first page).

THE HARVEY CUSHING/JOHN HAY WHITNEY MEDICAL LIBRARY, HISTORICAL LIBRARY, YALE UNIVERSITY

88B Karl Landsteiner. "Zur Kenntnis der antifermentativen, lytischen und agglutinierenden Wirkungen des Blutserums und der Lymphe," *Centralblatt für Bakteriologie, Parasitenkunde und Infektionskrankheiten*, 1. Abt., 27 (1900): 357–62.

OFFPRINT: Original cream printed wrappers.
224 x 151 mm.
Harvey Cushing (presentation copy, signed "Karl Landsteiner" on front wrapper).

THE HARVEY CUSHING/JOHN HAY WHITNEY MEDICAL LIBRARY, HISTORICAL LIBRARY, YALE UNIVERSITY

ALSO: Letter from Karl Landsteiner to Harvey Cushing, 28 April 1937, presenting 88A, 88B, and other offprints.

THE HARVEY CUSHING/JOHN HAY WHITNEY MEDICAL LIBRARY, HISTORICAL LIBRARY, YALE UNIVERSITY

89 Willem Einthoven. "Galvanometrische registratie van het menschelijk electrocardiogram." In: *Herinneringsbundel Professor S. S. Rosenstein* (Leiden: E. Ijdo, 1902): 101–6.

Publisher's gray-green cloth, title printed in white on front cover.
264 x 171 mm.

PAUL KLIGFIELD, M.D.

90 Charles S. Sherrington. *The Integrative Action of the Nervous System.* New York: C. Scribner's Sons, 1906.

Publisher's dark green ribbed cloth.
222 x 146 mm.
Unknown recipient (author's presentation inscription, half title: "With kind regards C.S.S.").

ARTHUR E. LYONS, M.D.

91A Ross G. Harrison. "Observations on the Living Developing Nerve Fiber," *Proceedings of the Society for Experimental Biology and Medicine* 4 (1907): 140–43.

OFFPRINT: Unbound.
243 x 172 mm.
"Lafayette B. Mendel, Yale University, New Haven, Conn." (stamp).

THE HARVEY CUSHING/JOHN HAY WHITNEY MEDICAL LIBRARY, HISTORICAL LIBRARY, YALE UNIVERSITY

91B Ross G. Harrison. "The Outgrowth of the Nerve Fiber as a Mode of Protoplasmic Movement," *Journal of Experimental Zoology* 9 (1910): 787–846.

OFFPRINT: Modern morocco spine, pastepaper sides.
250 x 177 mm.

THE HARVEY CUSHING/JOHN HAY WHITNEY MEDICAL LIBRARY, HISTORICAL LIBRARY, YALE UNIVERSITY

92 Paul Ehrlich and Sahachiro Hata. *Die experimentelle Chemotherapie.* Berlin: J. Springer, 1910.

Contemporary blue cloth spine, marbled sides.
235 x 153 mm.
Hans Sachs (1877–1945), Ehrlich's pupil, co-worker, and bibliographer (author's presentation inscription, title page: *S. lieben Prof. H. Sachs freundschaftlich, P. Ehrlich* [To his dear Prof. H. Sachs, in friendship, P. Ehrlich]).

HASKELL F. NORMAN, M.D.

93 Harvey Williams Cushing. *The Pituitary Body and Its Disorders.* Philadelphia & London: J. B. Lippincott, 1912.

COPY 1: Red morocco.
243 x 160 mm.
First issue, with integral title leaf.
Cushing's working copy, interleaved and augmented with inserted notes, letters, and photographs.

THE HARVEY CUSHING/JOHN HAY WHITNEY MEDICAL LIBRARY, HISTORICAL LIBRARY, YALE UNIVERSITY

COPY 2: Publisher's red vertical-ribbed cloth.
243 x 159 mm.
Second issue, with cancel title leaf.

THE HARVEY CUSHING/JOHN HAY WHITNEY MEDICAL LIBRARY, HISTORICAL LIBRARY, YALE UNIVERSITY

94 Casimir Funk. *Die Vitamine.* Wiesbaden: J. F. Bergmann, 1914.

COPY 1: Original black patterned-sand-grain cloth over cardboard.
244 x 165 mm.
Unknown recipient (author's presentation inscription, half title: *Meinem lieben Richard von seinem Casimir* [For my dear Richard from his Casimir]).

HASKELL F. NORMAN, M.D.

COPY 2: Untrimmed in original blue printed wrappers.
258 x 173 mm.

HASKELL F. NORMAN, M.D.

95A F. G. Banting and C. H. Best. "The Internal Secretion of the Pancreas," *Journal of Laboratory and Clinical Medicine* 7 (1922): 251–66.

OFFPRINT: Bound with 95B and fourteen other pamphlets by Banting.
252 x 165 mm.
Harvey Cushing (book plate and signature, flyleaf of volume).

THE HARVEY CUSHING/JOHN HAY WHITNEY MEDICAL LIBRARY, HISTORICAL LIBRARY, YALE UNIVERSITY

95B F. G. Banting and C. H. Best. *The Internal Secretion of the Pancreas.* Read before the Academy of Medicine [Toronto], February 7th, 1922.

Bound with 95A and fourteen other pamphlets by Banting.
227 x 152 mm.
Harvey Cushing (author's presentation inscription, first page: "To Dr. Harvey Cushing Compliments F. G. Banting").

THE HARVEY CUSHING/JOHN HAY WHITNEY MEDICAL LIBRARY, HISTORICAL LIBRARY, YALE UNIVERSITY

96 Alexander Fleming. "On the Antibacterial Action of Cultures of a Penicillium, with Special Reference to Their Use in the Isolation of *B. Influenzae," British Journal of Experimental Pathology* 10 (1929): 226–36.

OFFPRINT: Original orange printed wrappers.
250 x 185 mm.
Medical Research Council Library (stamp on wrapper, signed "P. Dudley").

THE LILLY LIBRARY, INDIANA UNIVERSITY, BLOOMINGTON

97 Alfred Blalock and Helen B. Taussig. "The Surgical Treatment of Malformations of the Heart in Which There Is Pulmonary Stenosis or Pulmonary Atresia," *Journal of the American Medical Association* 128 (1945): 189–202.

OFFPRINT: Original blue printed wrappers.
216 x 136 mm.
W. Bruce Fye (author's presentation inscription, front wrapper: "To Dr. Bruce Fye from Helen B. Taussig").

W. BRUCE FYE, M.D.

98A J. F. Enders, T. H. Weller, and F. C. Robbins. "Cultivation of the Lansing Strain of Poliomyelitis Virus in Cultures of Various Human Embryonic Tissues," *Science* 109 (1949): 85–87.

OFFPRINT: Unbound.
266 x 198 mm.
Grolier Club (author's presentation inscription: "For the files of the Grolier Club, Thomas H. Weller, April 12, 1993").

98B Jonas E. Salk. "Studies in Human Subjects on Active Immunization Against Poliomyelitis. I. A Preliminary Report of Experiments in Progress," *Journal of the American Medical Association* 151 (1953): 1081–98.

OFFPRINT: Original light gray printed wrappers.
217 x 138 mm.
Signed by Salk on the front wrapper.

JONAS SALK, M.D.

99 James D. Watson and Francis H.C. Crick. "A Structure for Deoxyribose Nucleic Acid," *Nature* 171 (1953): 737–38.

JOURNAL NUMBER: Original printed wrappers.
254 x 176 mm.

JEREMY M. NORMAN

OFFPRINT (1-paper version): Unbound.
255 x 180 mm.
Signed on the last page by James D. Watson.

COLD SPRING HARBOR LABORATORY ARCHIVES

OFFPRINT (3-paper version): Stapled, as issued.
210 x 141 mm.
Signed on the first page by Maurice Wilkins, Alec Stokes, Francis Crick, and James D. Watson.

MATTHEW M. MALERICH, M.D.

100 G. N. Hounsfield. "Computerized Transverse Axial Scanning (Tomography): Part I. Description of System," *British Journal of Radiology* 46 (1973): 1016–22.

JOURNAL VOLUME: Modern blue cloth, original printed wrappers bound in.
260 x 190 mm.

THE NEW YORK ACADEMY OF MEDICINE

LENDERS TO THE EXHIBITION

The American Philosophical Society
Philadelphia, Pennsylvania

Clendening History of Medicine Library
University of Kansas Medical Center
Kansas City, Kansas

Cleveland Medical Library Association
Historical Division
Cleveland, Ohio

Cold Spring Harbor Laboratory Archives
Cold Spring Harbor, New York

The College of Physicians of Philadelphia
Philadelphia, Pennsylvania

Francis A. Countway Library of Medicine
Boston, Massachusetts

Duke University Medical Center Library
History of Medicine Collections
Durham, North Carolina

Eugene S. Flamm, M.D.
Philadelphia, Pennsylvania

W. Bruce Fye, M.D.
Marshfield, Wisconsin

The Holden Arboretum
Mentor, Ohio

The Houghton Library
Harvard University
Cambridge, Massachusetts

Paul Kligfield, M.D.
New York, New York

Lehigh University Libraries
Special Collections
Bethlehem, Pennsylvania

The Library of Congress
Rare Book and Special Collections Division
Washington, D.C.

The Lilly Library
Indiana University
Bloomington, Indiana

Lawrence D. Longo, M.D.
Loma Linda, California

Arthur E. Lyons, M.D.
San Francisco, California

Matthew M. Malerich, M.D.
Bakersfield, California

Moody Medical Library
Blocker History of Medicine Collections
University of Texas Medical Branch
Galveston, Texas

The New York Academy of Medicine
New York, New York

Haskell F. Norman, M.D.
Ross, California

Jeremy M. Norman
San Francisco, California

The Osler Library of the History of Medicine
McGill University
Montreal, Quebec, Canada

The Pierpont Morgan Library
New York, New York

Reynolds Historical Library
University of Alabama
Birmingham, Alabama

Verne L. Roberts, M.D.
Durham, North Carolina

Jonas E. Salk, M.D.
San Diego, California

State University of New York
Health Science Center Library
Syracuse, New York

University of California, Los Angeles
Department of Special Collections
Los Angeles, California

University of California, San Francisco
The Library and Center for Knowledge Management
Special Collections
San Francisco, California

University of Chicago Library
Department of Special Collections
Chicago, Illinois

James D. Watson, Ph.D.
Cold Spring Harbor, New York

Yale University
Harvey Cushing/John Hay Whitney Medical Library
New Haven, Connecticut

One anonymous lender

SUBSCRIBERS

Daniel M. Albert, M.D.
Elmer L. Andersen
John K. Ashton, M.D.
Kenneth Auchincloss
Gabriel Austin

George M. Barringer
Victor A. Basile
Wayne E. Batcheler
Terry Belanger
David E. Belch
Abel E. Berland
Peter C. Berry
W. Gordon Binns, Jr.
Lyman G. Bloomingdale
Fred J. Board
George M. Bowles
Wilson J.C. Braun, Jr.
Catherine Tyler Brody
Thomas Bryson

John C. Carson, M.D.
David Giles Carter
Daniel D. Chabris
Carlo Alberto Chiesa
Bernard Clavreuil
James B. Cummins, Jr.
Clifford Currie

William Drenttel
Barbara C.M. Dudley

Henry N. Ess, III

Joseph J. Felcone
Franklin Feldman
Eugene S. Flamm, M.D.
Robert Fleck
Helmut N. Friedlaender

Morris A. Gelfand
Jack Golden
Richard L. Golden, M.D.

Robin G. Halwas

Richard A. Harris
William H. Helfand
John E. Herzog
Jonathan A. Hill
Kenneth E. Hill
Anthony R.A. Hobson
Frederic K. Howard
Alfred H. Howell
K. Garth Huston, Jr.
Martin W. Hutner

Colta Ives

David Jacoby, M.D.
André Jammes

Paul Kligfield, M.D.
Peter Kraus

Richard M. Lan
A. Dean Larsen
Edmond L. Lincoln
Kenneth A. Lohf
Lawrence D. Longo, M.D.
Joyce H. Lowinson, M.D.
Arthur E. Lyons, M.D.

Bryan Maggs
Stephen C. Massey
Bruce McKittrick
Alexander Canaday McLeod
David J. Menke, M.D.
Davis W. Moore
Andrew B. Myers

Andrew T. Nadell, M.D.
Kenneth Nebenzahl
James W. Needham
Haskell F. Norman, M.D.
Jeremy M. Norman

James O'Halloran

John R. Payne
Michael A. Peich

Alton E. Peters

Richard C. Ramer
Kenneth D. Rapoport, M.D.
William S. Reese
Kenneth W. Rendell
W. S. Roberts
S. Wyman Rolph, III
Robert J. Ruben, M.D.
Robert Rulon-Miller, Jr.

Mary C. Schlosser
Fred Schreiber
Paul M. Schyve, M.D.
Thomas P. Sculco, M.D.
Spenser E. Sherman, M.D.
Carolyn L. Smith
Clinton I. Smullyan, Jr.
George E. Staehle, M.D.
Eliot Hungerford Stanley
Roderick D. Stinehour

Frank S. Streeter
Herman R. Sussman

G. Thomas Tanselle
Fl. Tulkens †
Decherd Turner
George H. Tweney

Gerald N. Wachs, M.D.
Alexander D. Wainwright
Ruth and Josiah Wedgwood
Allen B. Weisse, M.D.
Thomas Whitridge
Benson R. Wilcox, M.D.
Margaret W. Winkelman
Daniel Woodward
William P. Wreden †

Charles Zitner
Philippe Zoummeroff

INDEX OF AUTHORS

Numbers refer to catalogue entries.

PHOTO CREDITS

Ahmanson-Murphy Aldine Collection, UCLA Special Collections, Los Angeles: Figure 7.

American Philosophical Society, Philadelphia: Figure 129.

Cleveland Health Sciences Library, Historical Division: Figure 118.

Cold Spring Harbor Laboratory Archives: Figure 179 (Offprint from *Nature* 171 [1953]: 737–38. Reproduced by permission. Reprint courtesy of James D. Watson, Director, Cold Spring Harbor Laboratory).

College of Physicians of Philadelphia: Figures 8, 9, 13, 19, 46, 47, 85. Color plates IV, XI, XXI.

Francis A. Countway Library of Medicine, Boston: Figures 12, 17, 81, 90, 98, 109, 112, 119, 126, 135, 136, 153. Color plates VII, XXIV, XXV, XXX.

Duke University Medical Center Library, History of Medicine Collections: Figures 38, 139, 146. Color plate XX.

Eugene S. Flamm, M.D.: Figures 3, 4, 30, 31. Color plate I.

W. Bruce Fye, M.D., M.A.: Figure 175 (© 1945, American Medical Association. Offprint from *JAMA* 128 [1945]: 189–202. Reproduced by permission).

Grolier Club: Figure 176 (© American Association for the Advancement of Science. Offprint from *Science* 109 [1949]: 85–87. Reproduced by permission).

Holden Arboretum, Mentor, Ohio: Color plates XIII, XIV.

Houghton Library, Harvard University: Figure 130.

Paul Kligfield, M.D.: Figures 160, 161.

Lehigh University, Special Collections: Figure 128.

Library of Congress, Rare Book and Special Collections Division: Figures 26, 127.

Lilly Library, Indiana University: Figures 28, 48, 49, 89, 103, 114, 115, 132, 140, 156, 173 (Reproduced by permission of Blackwell Scientific Publications, Ltd.). Color plate XII.

Lawrence D. Longo, M.D.: Figures 121, 122, 134.

Arthur E. Lyons, M.D.: Figures, 157, 162, 163.

Matthew M. Malerich, M.D.: Figures 32, 33, 180 (Offprint from *Nature* 171 [1953]: 737–38. Reproduced by permission).

Moody Medical Library, Blocker History of Medicine Collections, University of Texas Medical Branch, Galveston: Figures 59, 138.

New York Academy of Medicine: Figures 108, 137, 181 (From the *British Journal of Radiology* 46 [1973]: 1016–22. Reproduced by permission). Color plates V, XXVII.

Haskell F. Norman, M.D.: Figures 5, 11, 18, 29, 50, 51, 53, 58, 62, 63, 64, 67, 68, 69, 70, 71, 74, 75, 77, 78, 79, 88, 94, 95, 96, 97, 99, 100, 102, 104, 107, 110, 116, 124, 131, 141, 142, 143, 145, 148, 152, 154, 155, 167, 169, 170. Color plate XXXI.

Jeremy Norman and Co., Inc.: Figures 1, 2, 14, 23, 24, 25, 27, 35, 36, 37, 39, 40, 42, 44, 60, 61, 65, 66, 76, 80, 82, 83, 84, 86, 87, 92, 101, 106, 113, 117, 120, 136, 144, 147, 158, 166, 174, 178 (From *Nature* 171 [1953]: 737–38. Reproduced by permission). Color plates X, XV (© 1991 by Jeremy Norman & Co., Inc.), XVI (© 1991 by Jeremy Norman & Co., Inc.), XVII (© 1991 by Jeremy Norman & Co., Inc.), XXIII, XXVI, XXVIII, XXIX, XXXII.

Osler Library, McGill University, Montreal: Figures 55, 56, 57, 149, 150, 151.

Pierpont Morgan Library, New York: Figures 6 (PML 23585), 10 (PML 1346+). Color plates II (PML 313; © The Pierpont Morgan Library, 1993), III (PML 19117; © The Pierpont Morgan Library, 1993).

Reynolds Library, University of Alabama at Birmingham: Figures 22, 41, 43.

Jonas E. Salk, M.D.: Figure 177 (© 1953, American Medical Association. Offprint from *JAMA* 151 [1953]: 1081–98. Reproduced by permission).

State University of New York at Syracuse, Health Science Center Library: Figure 111.

University of Chicago Library: Figures 54, 133.

Yale University, Harvey Cushing/John Hay Whitney Medical Library, New Haven: Figures 15, 16, 20, 21, 34, 45, 52, 91, 93, 105, 123, 159, 164, 165, 168, 171, 172. Color plates VI, VIII, IX, XVIII, XIX, XXII.

Fifteen hundred copies of this book
have been printed in Robert Slimbach's Adobe Garamond type
on Mohawk Superfine paper at The Stinehour Press.
Design by Jerry Kelly.